Toward a Healthy Lifestyle

TOWARD A HEALTHY LIFESTYLE

THROUGH ELEMENTARY HEALTH EDUCATION

WITH AN ATLAS OF INSTRUCTIONAL MATERIALS

JOHN J. BURT
UNIVERSITY OF MARYLAND

LINDA BROWER MEEKS
THE OHIO STATE UNIVERSITY

SHARON MITCHELL POTTEBAUM
THE OHIO DEPARTMENT OF HEALTH

WADSWORTH PUBLISHING COMPANY
BELMONT, CALIFORNIA

A DIVISION OF WADSWORTH, INC.

ISBN 0-534-00776-7

Health Editor: Marshall Aronson
Editorial/Production Services: Phoenix Publishing Services, San Francisco
Photographs: Elizabeth Crews
Cover Design: Robert Haydock

Printed in the United States of America
7   8   9   10—90   89   88   87   86

Library of Congress Cataloging in Publication Data

Burt, John J.
    Toward a healthy lifestyle through elementary health education.

    Bibliography: p.
    Includes index.
    1. Health education (Elementary)   I. Meeks, Linda Brower, joint author.   II. Pottebaum, Sharon Mitchell, joint author.   III. Title.
LB1587.A3B87   372.3'7   80-346
ISBN 0-534-00776-7

For our belief in the family's role in a healthy lifestyle
and individual responsibility for one's health,
we dedicate this book to:

ANN, EME, KEITH, and JOE

JOE, LOUISE, BOB, DOROTHY, RAY, PAM, BOB, TIMMY, and CAM

JIM, ELSIE, BETH, RALPH, LARRY, SANDY,
MARGARET, WILLIAM, BILLY, MEG, and KRISTEN

CONTENTS

vii

B TEACHING ABOUT SELF-ACTUALIZATION AND SELF-CONCEPT 54

CHAPTER 6
A FAMILY LIFE EDUCATION, INCLUDING DIVORCE, AGING, AND DEATH 65

B TEACHING ABOUT INTERPERSONAL RELATIONSHIPS AND FAMILY LIFE EDUCATION, INCLUDING DEATH AND DIVORCE 77

CHAPTER 7
A DRUGS, ALCOHOL, AND TOBACCO 101

B TEACHING ABOUT DRUGS, ALCOHOL, AND TOBACCO 116

PART III: **TOWARD A HEALTHY BODY**

CHAPTER 8
A THE HUMAN BODY 143

CONTENTS

CONTENTS

PREFACE

Toward a Healthy Lifestyle Through Elementary Health Education is a testimony of our belief in children, in their need to assume individual responsibility for their own health, and in the importance of the role that the family and school play in the process of a child's achieving a healthy lifestyle. We believe that children learn to make choices concerning their lifestyles starting at birth. Parents begin teaching this process by modeling a healthy behavior and by involving their children in the decision-making process. Teachers play a vital role in the elementary school by setting a healthy example and by continuing to teach about and put into action the decision-making process.

This textbook is designed with the needs of the elementary teacher in mind. We have provided a theoretical perspective for the teacher with a rationale for teaching health in the elementary school and a clear explanation of the lifestyle approach and the decision-making process. In addition to the theoretical base, a sequential curriculum including content, methods, materials, and evaluation techniques is provided. In order to use this curriculum most effectively, an A and B chapter format was utilized. The A chapters contain carefully outlined content material that gives the elementary teacher the health information background necessary to teach. The B chapters include lesson plans that employ varied and creative methods of instruction for the classroom, repeating material from the A chapters as needed. The activities in these lessons are designated by the symbols ○, □, ☆ (○ = primary, □ = intermediate, ☆ = upper) to help the teacher easily locate ideas for teaching at the appropriate grade level. These lessons have been field tested to give the teacher an added feeling of confidence. The Atlas provides exciting overlays, materials, and games that can easily be used in the classroom.

Toward a Healthy Lifestyle Through Elementary Health Education is a textbook designed for teachers by teachers with the future health of children in mind.

John Burt
Sharon Pottebaum
Linda Meeks

ACKNOWLEDGMENTS

The expertise and assistance received from our colleagues and good friends in completing this textbook demonstrate their dedication to a healthy lifestyle and to the well-being of elementary school-children.

We are grateful to the following teachers for examining and field testing many of the teaching activities:

Mary Alice Beetham, The Ohio State University

Floa Ripley, Upper Arlington School System

Rick Bond and Jack Hanlon, Grandview School System

Doris Utgard, Scioto Darby School District

Curriculum Team, Southwestern City School District

Dave Abbott, Maumee School District

We are grateful to the following persons whose expertise in the area of health behavior and lifestyle contributed to the quality of this textbook:

Nancy Reynolds, Dental Health
Phil Heit, School Health Services
Elaine Vitello, Environment
Dave Corbin, Environment and Consumer Health
David Schoedinger, Death Education
Charlene Montonaro, Nutrition
Pat Mann, Drugs

We would like to thank the following reviewers for their helpful comments: Richard Borstad, University of Minnesota; William T. Brennan, Indiana University; Lorraine G. Davis, University of Oregon; Thomas L. Dezelsky, Arizona State University; James Eddy, Pennsylvania State University; Karen King, University of North Carolina; David Phelps, Oregon State University; Michael W. Tichy, Portland State University; and Len Tritsch, Oregon State Department of Education.

We are grateful for the careful work of our typists who diligently worked on this tedious task: Mary Ann Mead; Chris Riddlebaugh; Dorothy Benke; Karen Miksch.

We are grateful to our editor, Roger Peterson, for his many contributions and suggestions that helped to make this textbook a reality.

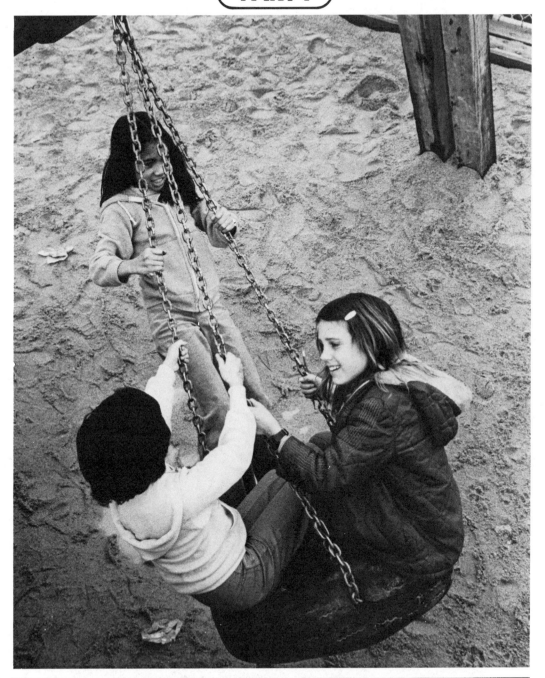

PART I

INTRODUCTION

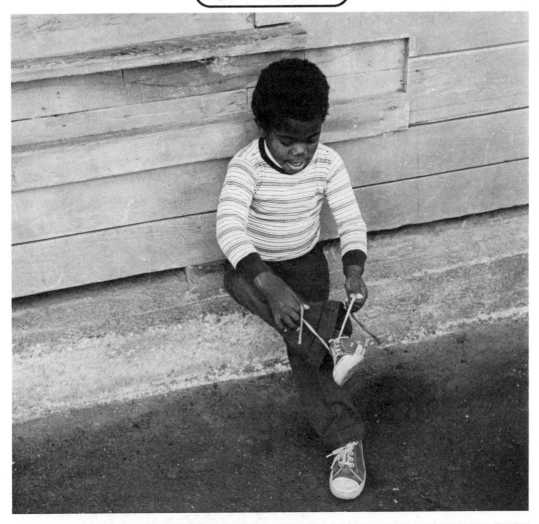

CHAPTER 1

HEALTH EDUCATION IN THE ELEMENTARY SCHOOL

Emily Burns was the kind of elementary school student that parents and teachers dream about but seldom have in their families or classrooms. She was beautiful, cooperative with her teachers, and helpful to her classmates. Emily was exemplary in the student role of "developing one's abilities," and she never received a grade lower than A. It appeared she was "just who the elementary curriculum was designed to benefit." One day when she was fourteen years old and in the eighth grade, Emily received a B. The next day she committed suicide.

In fourteen years of life and eight years of school, Emily never learned the difference between what you do and what you are. She never had a chance to make an A in "What It Means to Be Human." She never learned to accept fallibility and grow as a result of her mistakes. She never learned to be mortal and use that mortality to order her lifestyle. She never learned what it means to be susceptible to disease and use that fact to build health. In fact, Emily never understood very much about the human condition.

Most eighth graders in the United States don't commit suicide. But they do share Emily's ignorance of what it means to be human and healthy. Thus elementary schools are now beginning to focus attention on the relative importance of what you are and what you do. This focus has rendered it increasingly obvious that every elementary teacher must also be a health teacher. Indeed, any contemporary elementary school that does not give high priority to emotional development, self-concept, sexuality, physical health, environmental health, safety, and general happiness might properly be termed antiquated. In view of this, the authors present this book to future elementary teachers who might be interested in or committed to the claim that what a student learns or does not learn during elementary school is highly significant in future attempts to select a lifestyle that is fulfilling and healthy.

HEALTH EDUCATION: A NECESSARY PRIORITY IN TODAY'S ELEMENTARY SCHOOLS

The natural interest of elementary students and teachers in health matters has perpetuated at least a minimal concern

for health education throughout history. Recently, however, health education has again surged into the American limelight. The impetus for this change in status flows directly from the heart of several widespread human problems. Hence we shall begin our discussion with a consideration of seven trends that support health education as a necessary priority in our country:

1. Widespread dissatisfaction with poor quality lifestyles
2. A change in the nature of national health problems
3. A resurgence of humanism
4. The urgency of health problems of youth
5. A reexamination of the concept of mental health
6. A reevaluation of priorities in education
7. A move toward accountability in education

Widespread Dissatisfaction with Poor Quality Lifestyles

Throughout history a high percentage of the human population has felt oppressed by a poor quality lifestyle. Depending on their economic status, the discontented settled for bread and circuses, guzzled wine and felt badly that time was passing, or gave up on what they really wanted in favor of absorbing work or play. Today, the problem of poor quality lifestyle is as serious as it ever has been. Indeed, some suggest that it is our most serious contemporary human problem.

Many people are speaking out about dissatisfaction with their lifestyles, and considerable attention is being focused on the topic of human liberation. To date, however, our thinking about poor quality lifestyles remains ambiguous, and we hesitate to move into new territory.

On the other hand, we often feel trapped in our present lifestyles. There are times when we can't "find a way out," or just as things seem better, something beyond our apparent control comes along to mess up our lives again. We feel that we are the victims of a lifestyle trap, or that everything and everyone is against us. We feel that we are no longer in charge of our lives. It was these widespread feelings of "replacement" or "possession by outside factors" that prompted Rollo May to write (3), "The central core of modern man's neurosis is the undermining of his experience of himself as responsible."

Those individuals "possessed by" outside factors or those who feel their responsibility for their own lifestyles has been undermined constitute an increasing percentage of the total population. The dispossessed come from all economic, social, genetic, and educational levels. There appears to be no class immunity.

Much of our desperation over poor quality lifestyles seems to stem from the fact that we are not the masters of our fates. Recently, for example, a man named Raymond Southerland came to the National Institutes of Health with the following history. Ray was a community relations police officer making $15,000 a year. In the previous year he had been runner-up for policeman of the year for saving a girl whose car had flipped over into a canal. One might have guessed that Ray Southerland at age 37 had a satisfying lifestyle. But Ray had come to NIH to be studied. His son Jeffrey had lymphatic leukemia and died at age four;

his son Steve had his leg amputated to prevent the spread of bone cancer; his son Michael appeared to be cured of cancer; and now Ray had developed a brain tumor. Only a very insensitive poet-philosopher could say, "But remember Raymond Southerland, you are the master of your fate." Most of us know better. In fact, most of us understand all too well what Raymond Southerland meant when he said: "I don't fear dying. . . . I fear leaving the family. . . . I guess because I love them so much. . . . It is so hard to build a life. Things come along and you keep fighting them." Fortunately, most humans don't have it as tough as Ray Southerland. But all humans are connected to this problem. We try to plan a quality lifestyle and "things come along." There are times when like Stephen Southerland (one of the surviving boys), we all feel that we ought to write a book and entitle it: *Nowhere to Run.* The feeling that there is nowhere to run often gives people the notion that they are trapped in a lifestyle from which there is no escape, that is, they feel possessed by their lifestyle.

Widespread feelings that people are victims of poor quality lifestyle traps have resulted in a careful examination of current lifestyles. As a consequence of this examination, it is now generally appreciated that while humans cannot avoid death or disease, they do have the capacity to understand their condition and to create and enjoy *high level wellness.* In fact, they want it more than almost anything else! Hence, understanding what one is in both disease and high level wellness is a rapidly rising priority for our entire society. This is the purpose to which health education addresses itself.

A Change in the Nature of National Health Problems

Advances in science and medicine have resulted in significant changes in the nature of national health problems. These changes have been aptly traced by a recent President's Committee on Health Education:

Until fairly recent times, mankind's most threatening foes were famine and contagion. The first killed millions by starvation; the second by infection. Only since the middle of the 19th century has man been able to fight with reasonable success against those natural enemies. And even in the enlightened last century, the fight has been really successful only in the industrially advanced nations of the world.

While economic and agricultural progress have eradicated famine in most lands, public health physicians have played a major role in controlling infectious diseases by discovering the benefits of purifying water, disposing of sewage, keeping food clean and providing plumbing and sanitation.

Largely because of the reduction in infectious diseases, the average life expectancy of Americans has risen from 47 to 70 years since 1900, while the death rate has been more than cut in half.

Epidemics in the United States once featured such diseases as cholera and smallpox, tuberculosis and influenza, ill-defined fevers and gastro-intestinal disorders. Many children died of scarlet fever, diphtheria and other childhood diseases. Patients by the hundreds languished in hospitals for long periods, for medicine could neither cure the individual nor prevent the epidemics.

Today, communicable disease has almost disappeared from the list of the most common causes of death. In its place, physicians and health educators are faced with new antagonists: diseases caused not by famine or contagion, but by aging, by our sedentary way of life, by nutritional excesses and dietary fads, by urbanization, by changes in the physical environment and by a mobile population whose movements have reduced traditional ties to the community and have compromised the traditional personal acquaintance between patient and physician (4).

The new antagonists are conditions that are more susceptible to treatment with changes in lifestyle than to treatment with drugs. Hence health education becomes a high priority for those interested in national health problems. To be most effective, the evaluation of lifestyle alternatives should begin in elementary school.

A Resurgence of Humanism

The present age may be characterized as predominantly humanistic, for humanistic concepts and values seem to pervade all of contemporary life. Within this prevailing climate of humanism, an early concern of Plato and Aristotle has once again come into full bloom—the concept of self-actualization. Maslow defines self-actualizing people as those who:

are gratified in all their basic needs embracing affection, respect, and self-esteem. They have a feeling of belongingness and rootedness. They are satisfied in their love needs, because they have friends, feel loved and love-worthy. They have status, place in life, and respect from other people, and they have a reasonable feeling of worth and self-respect (1, p. 127).

Rendered popular by the research and writing of A. H. Maslow, the concept of self-actualization has had a profound effect on priorities in American education. For example, today's schools focus much of their attention on personal decision making.

In this atmosphere of humanism, concern with self-actualization, and personal decision making, health education occupies an important integrating role. That is, much of what is learned in elementary school and many of the decisions that are made are really secondary to a more important accomplishment: the selection and evaluation of a lifestyle that is healthy and promotes happiness. This latter process is a primary purpose of health education.

The Urgency of Health Problems of Youth

Although physical problems like tooth decay, malnutrition, and infectious diseases still plague the young, the most pressing problems of youth involve their emotional health, sexuality, safety, drug behavior, and overall happiness. In recent times, these latter problems have been attended by a sense of urgency, importance, and controversy. Hence health education has experienced greatly increased public awareness. In general, this increased awareness has been accompanied by increased support for health education in the schools. For example, the national PTA recently adopted the following resolution:

Whereas, the National PTA is vitally interested in the teaching of health in the public schools, and

Whereas, The school curriculum has been fragmented into separate programs in such areas as drug abuse, venereal disease, environmental health and family life education, and

Whereas, many local school districts have combined health and physical education programs, and

Whereas, there is a need for a comprehensive program of health instruction in our schools which will meet the total needs of all children and youth, therefore, be it

Resolved, that the National PTA lend its full and active support to the development of

an identifiable comprehensive school health education program.

The immediate health problems of youth have always provided impetus for health education in the elementary schools.

A Reexamination of the Concept of Mental Health

In the early 1960s, Dr. Thomas S. Szasz proposed a new concept of mental health stating:

It is customary to define psychiatry as a medical speciality concerned with the study, diagnosis and treatment of mental illness. This is a worthless and misleading definition. Mental illness is a myth. Psychiatrists are not concerned with mental illnesses and their treatments. In actual practice they deal with personal, social, and ethical problems in living (6).

Spurred on by sociologists and encouraged by humanist ethics, educators began to realize by the 1970s that in actual practice they also dealt with personal, social, and ethical problems in living—that they were, in fact, holding hands with psychiatry. Like psychiatrists, teachers also found themselves dealing with matters of sexuality, drug behavior, self-concept, and happiness. Within this new concept of mental health it is currently fashionable for psychiatrists and educators to work together to improve learning.

A Reevaluation of Priorities in Education

During the 1960s the educational community suddenly awakened to the fact that relevant subject matter, creative teaching, and interesting approaches were not the most important factors in effective learning. It also became obvious that teacher enthusiasm, although very important, was really a secondary factor. Even in the most carefully arranged teaching situations, it was the students' view of themselves that ultimately affected their ability to learn. A student with a history of success (success identity) and a high self-image was sometimes an effective learner and sometimes an ineffective learner. On the other hand, a student with a history of failure (failure identity) and a poor self-image consistently experienced learning blocks from the very beginning.

This finding made teachers aware of the extreme importance of good emotional health. Although the importance of the emotional life had been discussed at great length in their respective teacher training institutions, firsthand observation was startling to many teachers. Thus by the 1970s most elementary teachers were sensitive to the importance of a success identity for effective learning, and the importance of emotional health had become widely appreciated.

A Move Toward Accountability in Education

A recent emphasis on accountability in education is another trend that has contributed significantly to the contemporary importance of health education. During the late 1960s and early 1970s educators were called on to specify the goals of education to the public. Although this question initially evoked a flurry of statements about general goals, concepts, creative teaching, and multi-media, it soon became apparent that a basic shift in focus was necessary—from the teacher to the student and from the learning process to learning outcomes. Teachers were no longer so concerned with finding the "best" teaching method as with determining whether students were learning. As it became obvious that learning outcomes could only be measured in terms of student behavior, educators began to build their curricula around precise behavioral objectives whose outcomes could be measured.

In turn, behavioral objectives indirectly accentuated the importance of health education: that is, piecemeal behavioral objectives were often without unity and needed health education to bring them into focus. Statements identifying, describing, listing or demonstrating specific objectives all became more meaningful when they were fitted into the context of "selecting a lifestyle that is healthy and promotes happiness."

THE ELEMENTARY TEACHER AS A TEACHER OF HEALTH

Contemporary problems of living make it necessary for all elementary teachers also to be health teachers. In many ways, teachers already know much of the content of any health curriculum. They know what it is like to suffer with fever, chills, nasal congestion, headaches, toothaches, and stomachaches. They know what it is like to be angry, lonely, depressed, and unhappy. Living has made them aware of many time-tested rules of safety. They probably know more about where babies come from than about the source of atomic energy. However, possessing an abundance of health information does not automatically make a person a health educator. "Health education is an instrument in the hands of the user, and an intricate process in the experience of the learner. Its primary objective is to influence attitudes and health behavior of the learner"(2). This is best accomplished when (a) instruction fulfills a need and creates a readiness on the part of the learner; (b) the environment is both physically and emotionally conducive to learning; (c) opportunities are provided for the learner to practice what he is taught; and (d) the learning experience is pleasant.

The ultimate goal of a comprehensive school health program is to help every young person to achieve his [or her] full potential through becoming responsible for his [or her] personal health decisions and practices, through working with others to maintain a biological balance helpful to [humanity] and the environment, and through becoming a discriminating consumer of health information, health services, and health products (5, p. 16).

The school attempts to carry out this mission by providing health and safety education, health services, and a healthy environment. Whether we plan it or not, health education *will* occur. It will come from families, peers, religion, mass media, and the experiences of living. Much of this education will be negative and reinforce myths of previous generations. Therefore, we ask every elementary school teacher to give immediate and serious attention to the quantity and quality of their health teaching.

REFERENCES

1. A. H. Maslow, "The Good Life of the Self-Actualizing Person," *The Humanist 27* (1967).

2. William A. Mason, M.D., M.P.H., Medical Director of Atlanta Planned Parenthood Association.

3. Rollo May, *Love and Will* (New York: Norton, 1969).

4. The Report of the President's Committee on Health Education, 1973. Department of Health, Education, and Welfare, Health Services and Mental Health Administration.

5. Society of State Directors of Health, Physical Education, and Recreation, "A Statement of Basic Beliefs," *School Health Review* (March-April 1974): 16.

6. Thomas S. Szasz, *The Myth of Mental Illness* (New York: Dell, 1961).

CHAPTER 2

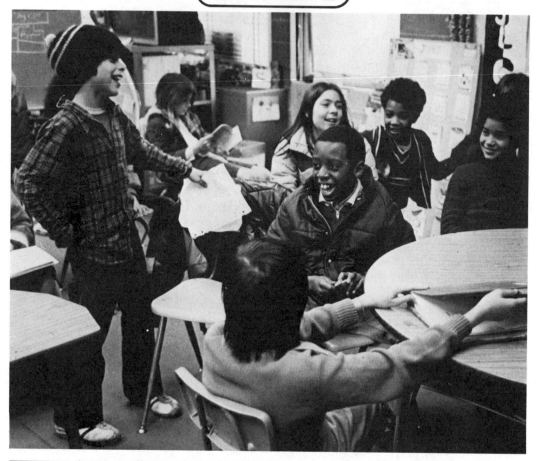

HEALTH EDUCATION: AN APPROACH TO LIFESTYLE ALTERNATIVES

History reveals that there has never been a commonly accepted definition of health. However, a recent study (2) of 292 health educators throughout the United States suggested that the three most common definitions were:

1. It is the quality of life involving dynamic interaction and interdependence among the individual's physical well-being, mental and emotional reactions, and the social complex in which the individual exists. (48 percent of those

studied selected this definition)

2. It is the ability of an individual to interact effectively, physically, psychologically, and socially with the environment in which that individual and society function. (25 percent selected this definition)

3. A state of complete physical, mental, and social well-being and not merely the absence of disease or infirmity. (17 percent selected this definition)

Likewise, there has been no specific agreement on the definition of health education. Nevertheless, the following working definition has evolved from the National Education Association and the American Medical Association:

Health education . . . may be defined as the process of providing learning experiences which favorably influence understanding, attitudes, and conduct in regard to individual and community health.

In view of the lack of any consensus about the nature of health and health education, it is not surprising that health education throughout the United States is organized in a variety of ways. These include organization by topics, concepts, body systems, and behavioral objectives. In addition, several states and many local units have developed their own approaches to organizing the health curriculum. This variety of approaches has received a mixed reaction from health education professionals. On the one hand, many experience a "sense of community" only when a kind of universal approach is the mode. On the other hand, many, including the authors, feel that progress is generally related to the number of viable alternatives. According to this view, a large number of alternatives affords individual teachers an opportunity to incorporate the most attractive aspects of different approaches into their personal styles of teaching.

The present text represents yet another approach to health education—a lifestyle approach. The authors hope that readers will review this approach as one of a number of alternatives and will incorporate any useful portion into their personal teaching styles. In keeping with this philosophy, the text is designed for use by teachers committed to any of several approaches to health education. That is, the health information and strategies for teaching that constitute the major part of this text are easily adapted to any method of organizing the health curriculum. On the other hand, those who find the lifestyle approach compatible with their own philosophy may use the text without any adaptations.

RATIONALE OF THE LIFESTYLE APPROACH

Dr. John Knowles, president of the Rockefeller Foundation, recently wrote: "People have been led to believe that national health insurance, more doctors, greater use of high-cost, hospital-based technologies will improve health. Unfortunately, none of them will. The next major advances in health will come from the assumption of individual responsibility for one's own health and a necessary change in lifestyle for the majority of people."

A fundamental assumption of the lifestyle approach to health education is that present and future health depends on assumption of individual responsibility and subsequent changes in lifestyle. It is important to emphasize that this is quite different from changes in lifestyle not preceded by assumption of responsibility. In the former, one evaluates the alternatives in lifestyle, selects one of the alternatives, and then stands responsible for that selection. In the latter, the selection of alternatives in lifestyle is generally motivated by external factors: rewards, punishments, or social pressures. This difference between internal and external motivations for changes in lifestyle is critically important to an understanding of the lifestyle approach to health education. Let's explore the dynamics of this difference.

Mark Twain once wrote: "Nothing so needs reforming as other people's habits." Unfortunately, most of the world views the health educator as a person likely to talk to them about reforming their habits (drinking, smoking, too much food, too many drugs, not enough exercise, or mistaken sexual behavior). Hence the health educator often gets a cold reception even from the elementary student. The lifestyle approach attempts to reverse this image. It retains the assumption that health education is primarily concerned with established and yet-to-be established patterns of living and thinking. But these habits are labeled alternatives in lifestyle. Subsequently, the purpose of health education moves from a focus on breaking bad habits to a new purpose: evaluation and intelligent selection of the alternatives in lifestyle.

In addition to its focus on internal motivation, the lifestyle approach also provides an organizational plan that attempts to avoid fractionization of health education into seemingly unrelated topics, unconnected body systems, or academic concepts. Rather, it views the scope of health education as including the total lifestyle. Thus the focus is not sex, drugs, nutrition, body systems, or the environment; more properly, it is lifestyle decisions. The lifestyle approach to health education involves three steps:

1. Identifying the alternatives in lifestyle
2. Evaluating these alternatives (or reevaluating in the case of old habits)
3. Intelligent selection of personal alternatives (or change in lifestyle in the case of old habits)

The lifestyle approach to health education provides a framework around which a highly meaningful curriculum can be developed. It is an approach that incorporates the warranted assumptions of history into arguments that speak for and against contemporary patterns of living and thinking. Further, the approach is instantly relevant; the student does not have to inquire, why is my lifestyle important to me? Even one's fellow students would consider that a strange question.

THE TAXONOMY OF LIFESTYLES

Lifestyle is a somewhat unwieldy concept from the elementary teacher's view, and effective study requires the establishment of a taxonomy of lifestyles. Hence our first step in planning a health education program for the elementary student will be the dissection of lifestyles into a number of component parts.

If one recorded all of one's activities for a week, they could probably be grouped in a number of well-defined categories. These categories, in turn, would represent individual components of one's total lifestyle. Using this method, the authors have identified twelve lifestyle components, and the resultant taxonomy is presented in Figure 2-1. The individual components are discussed here.

Coping Style

Starting very early in life, each individual develops a style of coping with a variety of life stresses. Some withdraw, while others make it a habit to face reality. Many escape with drugs, vacations, or even work, while a few threaten suicide. Some are easily upset, while others remain remarkably calm in the face of great stress. But whatever the pattern of response, each individual develops a coping style. This style, in turn, is part of the individual's total lifestyle.

The substructure of one's coping style develops before or during the elementary years. It is thus important for the elementary teacher to discuss such coping styles as not coming to school when a stressful day is anticipated, sleeping too much to escape life, placing unreasonable blame on either oneself or others, withdrawing from friends or life in general, or overreacting to minor stresses.

Relating Style

Each of us fights a personal battle, attempting to overcome our feelings of aloneness in the midst of a world of billions. In fact, history is a record of people's struggles with the "aloneness problem"—their attempts to gain recognition and appreciation, to belong, to be more than just chemical and physical processes, and to find themselves.

To overcome our aloneness, we develop a style of relating to others. The style might be heterosexual, homosexual, or purely psychic. It is characteristic of some to exploit or to be exploited. Others relate in a style that allows both parties in a relationship to flourish better than either could alone. But with or without careful study of the alternatives, each person develops a style of relating.

Elementary school is a very important time to discuss friendship. What is a friend? What should friends expect of each other? What should not be expected? What qualities do you look for in a friend? What causes friendships to end? These are all significant questions in the exploration of relating style.

Risk-taking Style

One of the prices of our existence is that we are mortal and subject to disease. To live is to be at risk. It is characteristic of some to be so deeply concerned about this that their total lifestyle is thwarted. The style of others suggests that they almost reject their mortality. Between these two extremes, most of mankind engages in trade-offs between present goals and long-range health risks—each developing an individual style.

Risk taking is a topic of high interest for elementary students, often evolving around the "I-dare-you" or chicken" model. Important discussion questions include: Why is risk taking exciting? What would life be like if you never took a risk? How do you know when a risk is worth taking? Why do we like to watch others take risks? What are healthy risks? Unhealthy risks?

Decision-making Style

People have the power to focus both the direction and intensity of consciousness, or to suspend thinking and let their minds drift passively. Hence to think is an act of choice. Some individuals select a decision-making style in which they only partially focus their consciousness, declining to struggle with any matter that does not come easily. Such individuals are fond of saying: "I have a block against X, or Y, or Z." Others are apostles of feeling and intuition rather than rationality. Yet others are characterized by predestinarianism—a style in which the directions to consciousness read: stand by to react to whatever cards life deals us. A

FIGURE 2-1 Taxonomy of lifestyles

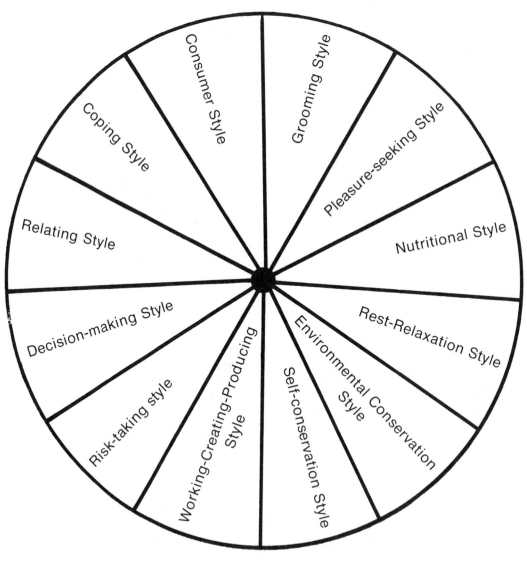

few display cognitive self-assertiveness, using, in the words of John Stuart Mill, "observation to see, reasoning and judgment to foresee, activity to gather materials for decision, discrimination to decide, and when he has decided firmness and self-control to hold to his deliberate decision" (1, p. 71). Whatever the style, there is no denying its relationship to mental health.

The following example may be valuable for discussion with elementary students. A man in Crown Point, Indiana, who was later found innocent by reason of insanity, called a number of women to say: "I am a doctor, and your husband has just collapsed at work from a scalp infection. Because you may also be infected, I want you to set your hair on fire immediately." Several women made a decision to do as they were told.

Elementary school is a very important time to discuss the questions: When should you do what you are told, and when should you make your own decisions? What opinions should you respect when making decisions? How does making a good decision make you feel? A bad decision?

Working-Creating-Producing Style

To have the fruits of one's working-creative-productive efforts accepted as worthwhile by one's self and others is probably a necessary condition for sanity. It is characteristic of some to be productive but not creative. Others are both creative and productive. Some are neither productive nor creative. Indeed, some might even be labeled destructive, but each has a style that may or may not promote happiness.

Self-conservation Style

Until recently humanity's major health problems were infectious diseases. Advances in science, however, have considerably reduced the risk of mortality from infection. In the modern world, degenerative diseases are of prime concern. Hence one thinks about conserving one's heart, arteries, pancreas, gall bladder, teeth, eyes, and so on.

For those who take self-conservation seriously, revision of several lifestyle components may be necessary. For others, self-dissipation may be the style. Whatever the choice, the alternatives are worthy of study.

Elementary students exhibit a great interest in the question: What can I do to increase the number of years that I will live? At present, one of the most important answers to this question is "avoid degeneration" or "avoid wearing out." Thus self-conservation commands interest. But what is self-conservation? Do you wear out from exercising or not exercising? From thinking too much or not thinking enough? Do you wear out from not eating the right foods or from eating too much? Do you wear out from working or not working? These are important questions for the elementary student.

Environmental Conservation Style

For hundreds of years we have taken land, water, and air for granted. That is, environmental conservation has not been a part of our previous lifestyles. Now the ravaged, polluted condition of the earth has almost overnight become one of the chief issues of our times. In view of this problem, a few people have modified their lifestyles willingly; others have been forced to accept changes. But many exhibit complete indifference.

With each passing year the number of alternatives in styles of environmental conservation are reduced, and unless each of us gives serious consideration to our personal patterns of conservation and dissipation, the lifestyles of all may be unfavorably modified in the near future.

Rest and Relaxation Style

Transcendental meditation, yoga, biofeedback, and sleeping pills are very much a part of the contemporary lifestyle. Tennis, golf, and swimming are the first choice of some. Others watch birds, listen to music, or smoke marijuana. For many, this component of lifestyle is so natural that a serious study of the alternatives seems to be a waste of time.

On the other hand, an effective style of rest and relaxation is a very difficult matter for some, even among young children. It now appears that we may have underestimated the significance of seriously studying the balanced life.

Nutritional Style

Food and fluid intake are essential to life, but for most people dining is more than just intake of nutrition. It includes such alternatives as what, when, where, and how much to eat. It is becoming increasingly clear that intelligent decisions about these alternatives are important to health.

Many people develop a nutritional style to gain or lose weight. Indeed, weight loss and weight gain may be an almost constant factor in one's total lifestyle. Again, the alternatives are many and

the implications for health are significant.

Pleasure-seeking Style

Despite its seeming simplicity, pleasure seeking is one of the most difficult of tasks. It is rendered difficult by lack of criteria to judge success. How does one know when one is being successful in pleasure seeking? People ask about their pleasures: Am I doing as well as I should? Would I accumulate more pleasure if I invested in another activity? Would my profits increase if I used another method?

Deciding between the alternative styles of pleasure seeking is not an easy business, but constant study and revision of one's pleasure-seeking style is an interesting and profitable undertaking.

Pleasure seeking is a complex topic for elementary students, but it cannot be neglected. Interesting questions include: Why is it sometimes pleasurable to eat and other times unpleasant? Why is it sometimes pleasurable to exercise and other times unpleasant? What makes something pleasurable? Why does a pleasurable activity become less fun when you do it too often? Why do different people find different things pleasurable? What does pleasure have to do with "planning your life"? What is the difference between short-range and long-range pleasure? What is healthy pleasure seeking? Unhealthy pleasure seeking?

Consumer Style

There are several aspects of the consumer style that relate to health and safety. These include the selection of physicians, hospitals, drugs, food, beverages, agents of transportation, recreational equipment, shoes, and clothing. Consumers may develop a style that includes careful evaluation of the potential health and safety risks of products and services, or they may ignore these risks. The alternatives in style are obviously significant.

Grooming Style

Differences in grooming style are perhaps more obvious than differences in other lifestyle components. Some of these differences have major implications for health; others are of little consequence.

Daily attention to skin, hair, teeth, mouth, gums, and general body cleanliness are part of the lifestyle of most people. Menstrual protection is a part of the female lifestyle. Evaluation of alternatives in grooming style appear to be especially significant for the elementary student.

REFERENCES

1. John Stuart Mill, *On Liberty* (New York: Liberal Arts Press, 1956).

2. Janet Shirreffs, "Investigating the Meaning of Health and the Scope and Nature of Health Education," *Health Education* (January-February 1978): 1–52.

FURTHER READINGS

Defining Health Education

Dolfman, Michael L., "Toward Operational Definitions of Health," *Journal of School Health* 44 (April 1974): 206–209.

Joint Committee on Health Education Terminology, "Definitions of Health Education," *School Health Review* (November-December 1973).

Joint Committee on Health Education Terminology, "New Definitions," *Journal of School Health* 44 (January 1974): 33–37.

Philosophy of Health Education

Association for the Advancement of Health Education, "Blueprint for Progress," *Health Education* (January-February 1975): 7–11.

Aubrey, Roger F., "Health Education: Neglected Child of the Schools," *Journal of School Health* 42 (May 1972): 285–289.

Burt, John, et al., "Philosophical Perspectives," *Health Education* (January-February 1975): 12–14.

Burt, John, "Rational Selection of Lifestyle Components," *School Health Review* (March-April 1974): 4–9.

Cooper, Theodore, "An Instrument of Prevention," *Public Health Reports* 91 (May-June 1976).

Douse, Mike, "Health Hints or Health Philosophy?" *Journal of School Health* 43 (March 1973): 195–197.

Galli, Nicholas, "Foundations of Health Education," *Journal of School Health* 46 (March 1976): 158–165.

Hoyman, Howard S., "New Frontiers in Health Education," *Journal of School Health* 43 (September 1973): 423–430.

Means, Richard K., "Can the Schools Teach Personal Responsibility for Health?" *Journal of School Health* 43 (March 1973): 171–175.

Nolte, Ann, "The Relevance of Abraham Maslow's Work to Health Education," *Health Education* (May-June 1976): 25–27.

Pottebaum, Sharon, "A Philosophy of Health Education from Children's Literature," *Health Education* (May-June 1977): 6–7.

Salk, Jonas, "What Do We Mean by Health?" *Journal of School Health* 42 (December 1972): 582–584.

CHAPTER 3

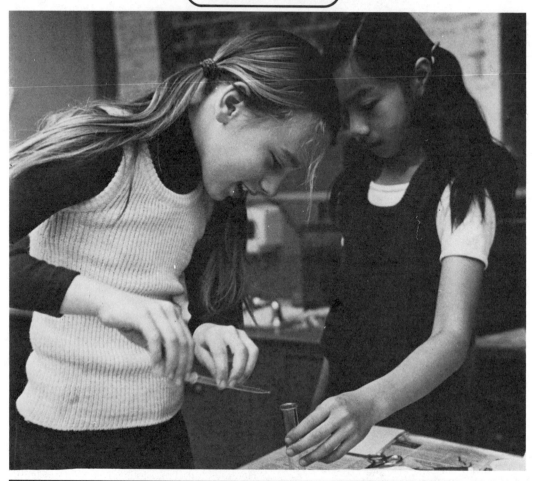

LIFESTYLE EDUCATION: PLANNING AND IMPLEMENTING THE HEALTH EDUCATION PROGRAM

"Planning without action is futile and action without planning is fatal" (5, p. v).

Each new year finds the teacher faced with the task of getting recharged and refueled for the task ahead. This usually involves a list of resolutions designed to improve one's general effectiveness as a teacher. Occasionally, it involves such critical questions as: What is the purpose of what I am doing? Is it really important? Does it make a difference? In the case of new teachers, questions include:

Will my methods work? Will I be able to control the class? Do I have enough planned to get through the day? But whether the teacher is experienced or a beginner, at least eight factors deserve careful consideration before the beginning of each teaching year:

1. Developing or Revising a Personal Philosophy of Teaching
2. Planning an Atmosphere Conducive to Learning
3. Planning the Health Education Curriculum
4. Constructing Behavioral Objectives
5. Organizing the Content
6. Selecting Learning Experiences
7. Using Available Media
8. Evaluation

DEVELOPING OR REVISING A PERSONAL PHILOSOPHY OF TEACHING

Developing a sound philosophy of teaching is the single most important thing that a teacher must do. A sound philosophy of teaching incorporates the teacher's general philosophy of life and insures that the teacher really believes in what he or she is doing.

The first step in integrating one's philosophy of life with one's philosophy of teaching is to resolve the question: Do the things that I believe in and the kind of person I am render me suitable for the profession of teaching? This is a very personal value judgment, and unfortunately there are no objective criteria by which to make it. There is, however, one psychological dynamic that in the experience of the authors seems to be characteristic of most good teachers:

1. I like and value myself.
2. This enables me to like and value the projects that are my life.

3. I have selected teaching as one of my major life projects, and I have confirmed the fact that I like and value teaching.
4. This authentic like and value that I associate with teaching enables me to exhibit enthusiasm for my work and zest for living.
5. My enthusiasm and zest are easily recognized by my students. Further, my students rank these characteristics very high on their list of what is important. In fact, they rank them so high that it is seldom possible to be judged a good teacher in the absence of this authentic enthusiasm and zest.

Teachers may find it valuable to relate their personal cases to this psychological dynamic as they attempt to integrate personal and teaching philosophies.

In addition to integrating one's personal philosophy of life into one's teaching, it is important to decide the question: What do I want for my students? The authors would like their students to be able to make intelligent decisions about the alternatives in their lifestyles. Others may have different objectives. The important thing is to understand clearly what one wants for the students.

Rather than attempting to channel students into a particular mold, the authors believe in helping the students "taste life" and providing experiences whereby the students can make more intelligent decisions about their personal lifestyles.

Kahlil Gibran has aptly described this approach to teaching:

No man can reveal to you ought but that which already lies half asleep in the dawning of your knowledge.
The teacher who works in the shadow of the temple among his followers, gives not of his wisdom but rather of his faith and lovingness.

If he is indeed wise, he does not bid you enter the house of his wisdom; but rather leads you to the threshold of your own mind (4, p. 56).

Leading people to the threshold of their own minds is another way of saying: "As a teacher, I would like my students to become authorities on their own lifestyles." This implies a helpful, rather than directing or controlling, posture toward one's students.

PLANNING AN ATMOSPHERE CONDUCIVE TO LEARNING

Having established the objective, the next step is to create an environment that is conducive to reaching it. In the lifestyle approach suggested by the authors, the task is to create an environment in which students can become authorities on their own lifestyles.

The importance of the learning environment is suggested by the following poem (11). The poem was given to a teacher by a high school senior shortly before the student committed suicide.

About School

He always wanted to say things. But
  no one understood.
He always wanted to explain things.
  But no one cared.
So he drew.

Sometimes he would just draw and it
  wasn't anything. He wanted to carve
  it in stone or write it in the sky.
He would lie out on the grass and look
  up in the sky and it would be only

him and the sky and the things
  inside that needed saying.

And it was after that, that he drew the
  picture. It was a beautiful picture.
  He kept it under the pillow and
  would let no one see it.
And he would look at it every night
  and think about it. And when it was
  dark, and his eyes were closed, he
  could still see it.
And it was all of him. And he loved it.

When he started school he brought it
  with him. Not to show anyone, but
  just to have with him like a friend.

It was funny about school.
He sat in a square, brown desk like all
  the other square, brown desks and
  he thought it should be red.
And his room was a square, brown
  room. Like all the other rooms. And
  it was tight and close. And stiff.

He hated to hold the pencil and the
  chalk with his arm stiff and his feet
  flat on the floor, stiff, with the
  teacher watching and watching.
And then he had to write numbers.
  And they weren't anything. They
  were worse than the letters that
  could be something if you put them
  together.
And the numbers were tight and
  square and he hated the whole
  thing.

The teacher came and spoke to him.
  She told him to wear a tie like all
  the other boys. He said he didn't
  like them and she said it didn't
  matter.

After that they drew. And he drew all

yellow and it was the way he felt
about morning. And it was
beautiful.
The teacher came and smiled at him.
"What's this?" she said. "Why don't
you draw something like Ken's
drawing? Isn't that beautiful?"
It was all questions.

After that his mother bought him a tie
and he always drew airplanes and
rocket ships like everyone else. And
he threw the old picture away.
And when he lay out alone looking at
the sky, it was big and blue and all
of everything, but *he* wasn't
anymore.

He was square inside and brown, and
his hands were stiff and he was like
anyone else. And the thing inside
him that needed saying didn't need
saying anymore.

It had stopped pushing. It was
crushed. Stiff.
Like everything else.

The school environment described in
this poem is the antithesis of the security
and warmth that students need to be
themselves and to become authorities on
their own lifestyles. Unless students have
opportunities to be themselves and take
risks on new behavior, they are blocked
from actualizing their individuality. It is
essential to establish an atmosphere of
trust and respect for individual differences. Such a classroom atmosphere is
highly related to personal risk taking. It
takes trust to risk. It takes trust to share
one's creativity with a group. It takes
trust to express and test beliefs in a
classroom. In the absence of trust, very
little self-disclosure can take place.

Hence, students cannot come to "own"
their behavior and direct their lives, and
they become frustrated.

PLANNING THE HEALTH EDUCATION CURRICULUM

The health educator can select from a
variety of approaches to curriculum design. Although each approach differs in
its orientation, each includes a framework for organizing health instruction to
meet the needs of the learner, to convey
subject matter in a meaningful way, and
to evaluate the effects of instruction.

The School Health Curriculum Project

One significant approach to the preventive aspects of health-related problems
was undertaken in 1969 by the National
Clearinghouse for Smoking and Health, a
division of the Center for Disease Control
of the Federal Department of Health, Education and Welfare. The project was The
School Health Curriculum (SHCP), also
known as the "Berkeley Model" (7, p.
2).* The goals of this model follow those
of many health curricula: imparting
knowledge, developing healthy attitudes,
and changing one's behavior. The curriculum initially focused on four body
systems: fourth grade—digestive, fifth
grade—respiratory, sixth grade—circulatory, and seventh grade—nervous. Recently completed units for grades K–3
stress Happiness Is Being Healthy (K),

*Works of Olsen, Redican, Stone, and David were
also consulted for this discussion of the Berkeley
Model.

Super Me (first grade), Sights and Sounds (second grade) and The Body . . . Its Framework and Movement (third grade).

The tasks used for accomplishing the Model's objectives are exemplified by the multilevel, multimedia, and multimethod approaches employed. Books, filmstrips, pamphlets, transparencies, cassette tapes, anatomical models, and slides are a few of the materials being used in the different grade levels. By implementing a multiplicity of teaching methods, such as lectures, role-playing, panel discussions, games, plays, skits, and independent study, the SHCP provides students with numerous learning activities.

Competency-based Approach

A competency-based approach to curriculum design specifies minimum performance levels for students to complete at the various grade levels. An excellent example of a competency-based curriculum is the newly developed WOW Health Education Curriculum Guide (16). This guide specifies performance levels expected at primary, intermediate, junior high, and senior high school levels. The competencies are reached through exploring attitudes, beliefs, and values; combining these with knowledge; and using the combination effectively in the decision-making process. The four content areas selected for the design of this approach are mental health, physical health, safety, and community health. There are directions and suggestions for effectively covering the competencies included in each of the four areas. These directions and suggestions were field-tested by teachers in Washington, Oregon, and Wisconsin as the guide was developed, thus making it very practical.

Unit Approach

The unit approach to curriculum design breaks health into several units or areas. The teacher decides on the amount of time to be allotted to each unit. Often the same amount of time is spent on each unit, and areas are grouped together to become units with approximately equal value to the curriculum. This traditional approach to health education has remained popular for several reasons. Teachers who feel obliged to cover as much as they can often use the unit approach because it organizes the school year into blocks of time linked to curriculum units. Teachers organizing their curriculum around a textbook selected for their classroom often plan units to correspond to the scope and sequence of the text. Student teachers and beginning teachers often use the unit approach to make use of units developed during their professional preparation. Units can also be organized around teacher strengths and weaknesses. Some teachers plan to use their best units during the busiest times of the year, such as the beginning of the year, the end of the year, and before holidays. Thus, the unit approach allows for teacher control and provides a framework for covering as many topics as possible during an allotted time period.

Conceptual Approach

The conceptual approach to curriculum design stresses key concepts as "basic central ideas, an understanding of which opens the door to an entire field of knowledge. The concepts serve as the major organizing elements of the curriculum" (6, p. 15).

The School Health Education Study,

1961–1965, has been the backbone for many conceptual models in health education. This study, often referred to as SHES, uses three key concepts—growing and developing, interacting, and decision-making—as the unifying threads of the curriculum. Ten specific concepts serve as the major organizing elements reflecting the scope of health education in the curriculum.

The strength of the School Health Education Study is that it provides a conceptual framework for the ever-changing knowledge rather than relying on an informational base soon to become outdated.

The State of New York has also developed a comprehensive course of study featuring the conceptual approach. The program is known as the New York State Health Strands Program (15). There are five different "health strands": physical health, sociological health problems, mental health, environmental and community health, and education for survival. Teaching guides focus on the subjects to be emphasized in each of the health strands. The guides employ a "cookbook" approach, consisting as they do of detailed lesson plans that (a) outline content, (b) state fundamental concepts, (c) suggest teaching aids and learning activities, and (d) include supplementary information for the teacher.

Another example of the conceptual approach is the Framework for Health Instruction in California Public Schools (3). The curriculum is organized into ten content areas: consumer health; mental-emotional health; drug use and abuse; family health; oral health, vision, and hearing; nutrition; exercise, rest, and posture; disease and disorders; environmental health hazards; and community health resources.

Concepts are developed for each of the ten content areas at the primary, intermediate, junior high, and senior high school levels. The framework includes a unique approach to interrelating the concepts in the ten content areas. It is organized by a Roman numeral numbering system that is consistent in each of the content areas. Thus, a teacher wanting to find out how a particular concept is covered in more than one content area merely looks for the same Roman numeral.

The Theme Approach

The theme approach to curriculum design takes a central idea or philosophy to give perspective to the development of health instruction. Howard Hoyman, professor emeritus at the University of Illinois, discussed several different themes in his article "New Frontiers in Health Education"(8). Some of the themes that Hoyman developed are: human life cycle approach; personality-lifestyle approach, human potentialities approach; ethical approach; ecological approach; preventive-constructive approach; and community experience approach.

As the elementary teacher examines the varied approaches to health instruction and curriculum, something becomes evident. The approaches are not mutually exclusive; most curricula carefully combine the assets of several different approaches.

CONSTRUCTING BEHAVIORAL OBJECTIVES

After the health education curriculum has been chosen, it is necessary to establish goals. Long-range goals describe the desired outcome to be expected at the completion of the curriculum. If these outcomes are stated specifically, they clarify the intent of classroom instruction and specify the desired behavior that students will demonstrate after each lesson or experience. The statements are called "behavioral objectives."

A behavioral objective is a statement of what a learner is to be like when he has successfully completed a learning experience. How are objectives written that describe the desired behavior of the learner? First, identify the terminal behavior by name; specify the kind of behavior that will be accepted as evidence that the learner has achieved the objective. Second, try to define the desired behavior further by describing the important conditions under which the behavior will be expected to occur. Third, specify the criteria of acceptable performance by describing how well the learner must perform to be considered acceptable (10, p. 3).

Consider the following objective: the student will be able to identify in writing the correct food group for at least 90 out of 100 foods appearing on a grocery list. The terminal behavior is identified by name (identify in writing the food groups). The conditions are described (foods appearing on a grocery list). The criteria of acceptable performance are specified (90 out of 100). Thus, the three steps in constructing behavioral objectives have been included.

A description of what students will be like when they have completed a learning experience can be a change that occurs in their thinking, feelings, or actions. Thus, behavioral objectives that describe outcomes desired can be classified in three domains: cognitive, affective, and psychomotor.

The objectives in the *cognitive domain* emphasize intellectual learning and problem-solving tasks. These objectives are divided into six classifications:

1. Knowledge objectives require students to reproduce or recall something that they have experienced previously in the same or similar form.
2. Comprehension objectives require students to reproduce or recall something previously experienced in a new form.
3. Application objectives require students to use previously experienced procedures or knowledge in new situations.
4. Analysis objectives require students to break down into its component elements something which they have not broken down previously.
5. Synthesis objectives require students to put something together which they have not put together previously.
6. Evaluation objectives require students to render judgments regarding something for which they have not rendered judgments previously (9, pp. 93–94).

"The *affective domain* contains behaviors and objectives which have some emotional overtone. It encompasses likes and dislikes, attitudes, values, and beliefs" (9, p. 56). The following classifications of objectives are in the affective domain:

1. Receiving objectives require students to recognize and receive certain phenomena and stimuli.
2. Responding objectives require students to demonstrate a wide variety of reactions to stimuli.
3. Valuing objectives require students to display a behavior with sufficient consistency.
4. Organization objectives require students to organize values into a system, determine the interrelationship among them, and establish dominant and pervasive ones.

5. Characterization by a value or value complex objectives require students to act consistently in accordance with the values they have internalized at this level.

The objectives in the *psychomotor domain* emphasize some muscular or motor skill, some manipulation of materials and objects, or some act that requires neuromuscular coordination level (2, p. 98–165). The following four classifications are psychomotor:

1. Gross bodily movement objectives require students to move entire limbs.
2. Finely coordinated movements require students to coordinate movements of the extremities usually with the eye and ear.
3. Nonverbal communication objectives require students to convey a message to a receiver without the use of words.
4. Speech objectives require students to communicate through speech such as public speaking (9, pp. 68–74).

In each of the approaches to curriculum discussed, special emphasis should be placed on describing all three domains of behaviors as desirable outcomes.

ORGANIZING THE CONTENT

Behavioral objectives are an extension of the overall goal or purpose of the curriculum. When these objectives are clearly stated they operate as a thread that ties the curriculum together. The long-range goals and behavioral objectives provide a sound basis for: (a) organizing the content, (b) selecting the best learning experiences, (c) using media to the best advantage, and (d) evaluating the results. Thus, content becomes an extension of behavioral objectives.

Several suggestions may help the teacher to deal with content.

1. Ask what content is needed to perform the desirable outcomes (behavioral objectives).
2. Research the content thoroughly. It is generally advisable to be "overprepared." Students respect the teacher who is well read and current in the subject being taught.
3. Develop a system or organizing pattern for the information collected. Some teachers keep file boxes of index cards on various topics, adding cards when new information becomes available. Other teachers collect materials and organize notebooks by topic areas. When a particular behavioral objective is to be covered, the teacher consults the notebook and writes lectures or organized thoughts around these bits of knowledge.

SELECTING THE BEST LEARNING EXPERIENCES

Learning activities facilitate the completion of the behavioral objectives by helping students examine their knowledge, attitudes, and values. The learning activities should be creative and varied and should deal with content or background information, as well as clarifying values. In addition to the learning that accompanies structured activities, the students learn from the example set by the teacher.

How do we provide a variety of relevant teaching methods? One very helpful technique is to determine the behavioral objectives to be achieved, then review Table 3-1. This chart was developed by Dr. Glen Gilbert, Portland State University, for use with preservice and inservice teachers. Each method is rated according to the likelihood of that particular method's accomplishing the various types of objectives. Most frequently (MF) indicates that the method is usually used in this manner. Occasionally (O) indicates that it is sometimes used in this way and has the potential to be used in this manner. It is suggested that the teacher keep clearly in mind the objectives to be achieved by a class or course, then review the list, checking the methods that might achieve stated objectives. Following such an appraisal, the teacher should consider how each checked method might be implemented and then make a decision based on feasibility and likelihood of successful accomplishment of objectives. Following these guidelines should encourage innovation and discourage selection based only on ease of use.

Values Clarification

The role of the teacher in facilitating the learner's completion of the behavioral objectives is quite complex. In addition to imparting knowledge in a meaningful way, the teacher needs to provide a laboratory where students can examine the impact of their values and attitudes on their health behavior. To fill this need, many teachers have turned to the use of values clarification.

The focus is on how people come to hold certain beliefs and establish certain behavior patterns (14, p. 19). Valuing, according to Raths (13), is composed of several subprocesses:

PRIZING one's beliefs and behavior.
1. Prizing and cherishing
2. Publicly affirming, when appropriate
CHOOSING
3. Choosing from alternatives
4. Choosing after consideration of consequences
5. Choosing freely

ACTING on one's beliefs
6. Acting
7. Acting with a pattern, consistency, and repetition.

These seven subprocesses are to be applied to the student's current health beliefs and behavior patterns and to those that are emerging. When we talk about values clarification as a method, we are referring to strategies that provide the student an opportunity to use this seven step process. The following guidelines will help the teacher use this method effectively in the health education curriculum:

1. Provide appropriate skills. Cover the decision-making process and the seven subprocesses before using any values clarification strategies.

2. Be accountable. Identify objectives that report, explain, or justify the use of this strategy. Remember that a "fun" activity should also have a purpose.

3. Precede the valuing activity with appropriate knowledge. What information do the students need to make informed decisions?

4. Use the values clarification approach correctly. The role of the teacher is to use clarifying responses in the discussion of the strategy. A "clarifying response encourages someone to look at his life and his ideas and to think about them." A few examples of the clarifying responses developed by Simon (13):

—Where would that idea lead?

—What do we have to assume for things to work out that way?

—Is that a personal preference or do you think most people should believe that?

5. Evaluate the objectives. Simon says that students should "see the probable consequences of a choice and find out if they are willing to accept the consequences which may follow." Has the stu-

TABLE 3-1 SUMMARY OF TEACHING METHODS AND STRATEGIES ACCORDING TO LIKELIHOOD OF MEETING OBJECTIVES IN COGNITIVE, AFFECTIVE AND PSYCHOMOTOR DOMAINS

	Cognitive Knowledge	Affective Attitude	Psychomotor Action
1. Music	MF	O	O
2. Cartoons	MF	MF	
3. Brainstorming and buzz sessions	MF	O	O
4. Stories with fill-in-the blanks	MF	O	
5. Interviews	MF	O	MF
6. Pantomimes	MF	O	MF
7. Self-appraisal	O	MF	O
8. Panel discussions	MF	O	
9. Visitations to agencies	O	O	MF
10. Field trips	O	O	MF
11. Bulletin boards, displays, flannel boards	MF	O	
12. Transparencies	MF	O	
13. Review bees	MF		
14. Values clarification	O	MF	O
15. Mystery puzzles	MF		
16. Word-o-games	MF		
17. Anagrams	MF		
18. Crossword puzzles	MF		
19. Games	MF	O	O
20. Simulated situations or critical incidents	MF	MF	MF
21. Problem solutions*		MF	
22. Mock radio and T.V.	MF	MF	O
23. Personal health improvement projects	O	MF	MF
24. Movie, slide, or video tapes (student produced)	MF	O	MF
25. Debates	MF	O	O
26. Skits	MF	O	MF
27. Plays	MF	O	MF
28. Role playing	O	MF	MF
29. Self-tests	MF		
30. Surveys	O	MF	MF
31. Oral reports (individual or group)	MF	O	O
32. Guest speakers	MF	MF	
33. Computer assisted instruction	MF		
34. Programmed learning	MF		
35. Experiments	MF	O	MF
36. Demonstrations	MF	O	MF
37. Mobiles	MF		
38. Charts, transparencies or graphs	MF		
39. Models	MF		
40. Slides	MF	MF	O
41. Video tapes	MF	O	O
42. Auditory tapes or records	MF	O	O
43. Films and film strips	MF	O	O

*Refers to a specific technique called problem solution.

MF = Most Frequently; O = Occasionally. If blank, it is very rarely or never used in this way.

Glen Gilbert, "Toward a Variety of Teaching Methods in Health Education," *Health Education* (September/ October, 1978).

dent examined the consequences of different health behaviors in arriving at his decision?

There are many values clarification strategies that can be adapted to different lessons.

The Role of the Teacher

The teacher should provide an example or model of a person who is continually evaluating and selecting alternatives in health behavior. The alternative that the teacher selects is not the emphasis; the emphasis is the teacher's commitment to the process. The model the teacher exemplifies is important in gaining the respect of students. The importance of deeds matching words is expressed in the following poem:

I

I'd rather see a sermon
   Than hear one any day;
I'd rather one should walk with me
   Than merely show the way.
The eye's a better pupil,
   And more willing than the ear;
Fine counsel is confusing,
   But example's always clear.

II

I soon can learn to do it,
   If you'll let me see it done;
I can see your hands in action,
   But your tongue too fast may run.
And the lectures you deliver
   May be very fine and true,
But I'd rather get my lesson
   By observing what you do.
For I may misunderstand you
   And the high advice you give,
But there's no misunderstanding
   How you act and how you live!

Anonymous

USING AVAILABLE MEDIA

Effective teaching is the result of carefully selected objectives communicated to the student through a creative combination of methods and media. The vast and growing world of media has a significant effect on the curriculum. Media can assist in all phases of instruction:

Teachers can *introduce* new material with newspaper articles, curious objects, colorful pictures, provocative films, field trips, or speakers from the community. It is important to choose resources that will stimulate enthusiasm and suggest directions for study.

During the *developmental* phase of study, students will locate, examine, assess, and use or reject information in many different forms. Appropriate learning experiences may involve independent study, discussion and decision-making activities, films and slides, recordings, pictures, biological specimens, a torso with removable organs, and work with a microscope. Students should be encouraged to write for free or inexpensive materials and explore in individual ways.

Questions are raised and previous research and study activities are shared during the *organizational* phase of instruction. Students can prepare written reports illustrated with tables or graphs, develop slide presentations, design bulletin boards and displays, create models and original transparencies, or construct mobiles.

Instruction may be *summarized* through class-prepared displays, dramatizations, or presentations. These projects may be shared with other classes or parents. Films are also used to summarize health topics.

The use of media is often overlooked when it comes time for *evaluation*. A teacher might construct a buzz board so students can quiz themselves independently or display various medical instruments, teeth, etc., for the students to identify. Teachers should ask students to appraise the media they used and whether they think a different method would have been better.

When reviewing media for possible purchase, it is necessary to remember that while it may save planning and production time, it will also be more expensive and less adapted to local needs, since media are generally produced to satisfy needs in all parts of the country. The teacher should consider the instructional purposes. Is the content accurate, significant, and up-to-date? Is the item worth its price? Could another less expensive item produce the same results? Is the message appropriate to the age and background of the students? Has the item been field-tested?

EVALUATING THE RESULTS

Evaluation measures the performance of both the teacher and the student.

Student Performance

The evaluation of student performance by the teacher is the testing of the behavioral objectives. Within each objective there is a clear description of the behavior the student will perform, the conditions under which the behavior will be performed, and the criterion of acceptable performance. In constructing the behavior objectives, care should be taken to provide various means of evaluating the learner. Evaluation should be a learning experience as well as a means of holding students accountable. A variety of evaluative techniques are described in the following objectives:

Objective Test. After the unit on heart disease, the student will be able to answer 90 out of 100 multiple choice questions.

Position Paper. After the unit on smoking, the student will write a 150- to 200-word position paper on smoking that includes at least five well-documented statements to defend the position taken.

Bulletin Board. After the unit on grooming, the students will be divided into groups of four to make a bulletin board depicting four healthy grooming habits. Each student in the group will describe one habit depicted on the bulletin board.

Skits. After the unit on consumer health, the students will be divided into groups of five to develop a skit identifying three aspects of quackery.

"I Learned" Statements. After the lesson on epilepsy, the student will be able to complete at least ten "I learned" statements.

Art Project. After the lesson on safety, the student will draw a picture of a playground illustrating five aspects of safety. He or she will number these five aspects and describe them to the class.

Checklist. After the lesson on friendship, students will make a list of twenty traits of a good friend. They will ($\sqrt{}$) the traits they possess. They will write two or three sentences describing how they will work to attain the traits they do not yet possess.

Continuum. After the lesson on exercise, the students will place themselves on the following continuum. They will write a short paper about whether they are proud of their behavior.

Never	Daily
Ned or Nellie	Donna or Dan

Mobile. After the lesson on dental health, the student will make a mobile out of five foods that are good for snacking.

Oral Report. The student will select one food group for an oral report. In the report, the student will identify the function of the food group and mention ten foods belonging to that group.

Students are aided in the lifelong attempt to evaluate their behavior by a teacher who takes evaluation seriously. The teacher's example profoundly influences the students. If the teacher is not clear, how will students learn to evaluate themselves effectively? Examine the following comments written to students:

1. Excellent report!
2. This is not acceptable.
3. Confusing.

This kind of feedback is not very helpful to students carefully examining their behavior. Very little learning, if any, takes place. These comments should direct the student to (a) repeat desirable behavior or (b) reevaluate and change undesirable behavior. The comments could be stated differently:

1. I thought your report was excellent, because you included more than five types of quackery and your descriptions were so lifelike.
2. I would like you to draw another safety poster. Although your poster is attractive, I cannot clearly identify the safety slogan you are describing.
3. I have read your descriptions of menstruation, and I am not certain that you understand the cycle. I would like to go over this paper with you to avoid confusion.

Careful evaluation takes time but its impact cannot be overlooked. If students are expected to evaluate and select alternatives to unhealthy behavior when they leave the classroom, they must learn to evaluate themselves and others. The teacher can give students opportunities to assist in the evaluation of bulletin boards, skits, films, and so on. The teacher should also assist the students in self-evaluation and construction of individualized objectives. Here are some examples of a student's personal goals:

1. At the end of the month, I will be able to do twenty-five sit-ups each day. (Record weekly progress)
2. I am going to arrange my desk neatly and examine it daily. I want to have at least four neatness checks this week. (Record daily progress)
3. I am going to make an effort to listen carefully. I'll use the following scale to evaluate myself each day for a week.

Need to Improve	*Was OK*	*Was Pleased*
Monday ____	____	____
Tuesday ____	____	____

This approach to evaluation places emphasis on developing a plan for changing habits that the student finds undesirable and repeating desirable behaviors.

Teacher Performance

Teacher performance can be evaluated by the students or by the teacher himself. Examples of student evaluation of the teacher might be:

Open Ended

My health teacher was _____
The lesson on smoking _____
My favorite health issue _____
Next year I would _____

Value Continuum

My health teacher was:

Never prepared	Always prepared

Boring	Interesting

Detached	Personal

Unhealthy	Healthy

During health I learned:

about (heart disease)

Very little	A great deal

about (drugs)

Very little	A great deal

Value Ranking

Rank the following units from most learned to least learned using (1) first:

_____ Grooming
_____ Dental health
_____ Safety and first aid
_____ Nutrition
_____ Consumer health

Rank the following classroom activities. Use (1) for your favorite.

_____ Puppet shows
_____ Lecture
_____ Movies
_____ Oral reports
_____ Guest speakers

Likert Scales

Place a check in the column that best describes your feeling.

	Strongly Agree	Agree	Disagree	Strongly Disagree
1. The teacher knew many facts about health.				
2. The teacher demonstrated good health behavior.				
3. Health class was difficult for me.				

Feedback from students is helpful in planning future health lessons. In addition, teachers concerned with growth and improvement conduct frequent self-evaluations and record the results in the form of future directions and goals. For example:

1. I was displeased with my unit on safety. I want to develop a new set of objectives and more creative learning experiences for next fall.
2. My skills in group processes are lagging. I will see if the university has a summer workshop I can take.
3. The self-actualization lesson was a real high! I'll use the movie again.
4. This year I'd like to read at least one current medical report a week.

Evaluation is essential to teaching. Many teachers place this at the bottom of their priority list and yet beginning rather than ending with evaluation helps to insure a good program.

Hugh Prather has said, "When I see I am doing it wrong, there is a part of me that wants to keep on doing it the same way anyway and even starts looking for reasons to justify the continuation"(12). The beginning of the school year is an exciting opportunity to change those things that can be improved and to repeat those things that were successful.

INTRODUCTION

REFERENCES

1. Benjamin S. Bloom, et al., *Taxonomy of Educational Objectives—The Classification of Educational Goals, Handbook I: Cognitive Domain* (New York: McKay, 1956).

2. ———. *Taxonomy of Educational Objectives—The Classification of Education Goals, Handbook II: Affective Domain* (New York: McKay, 1956).

3. *Framework for Health Instruction in California Public Schools* (Sacramento: California State Department of Education, 1970).

4. Reprinted from *The Prophet*, by Kahil Gibran, with permission of the publisher, Alfred A. Knopf, Inc. Copyright 1923 by Kahil Gibran; renewal copyright 1951 by Administrators C.T.A. of Kahil Gibran Estate, and Mary G. Gibran.

5. Mary E. Hawthorne and J. Warren Perry, *Community Colleges and Primary Health Care: SAHE Report* (Washington, D.C.: American Association of Community and Junior Colleges, 1974).

6. *Health Education: A Conceptual Approach to Curriculum Design* (St. Paul, Minn.: 3M Education Press, 1967).

7. Phil Heit, "The Berkeley Model," *Health Education* 8:1 (January-February 1977).

8. Howard S. Hoyman, "New Frontiers in Health Education," *The Journal of School Health* 43:7 (September 1973).

9. Robert J. Kibler, Larry L. Barker and David T. Miles, *Behavioral Objectives and Instruction* (Boston: Allyn and Bacon, 1971), p. 93.

10. Robert Mager, *Preparing Instructional Objectives* (Belmont, Calif.: Fearon, 1962).

11. R. Mukerjii, "About School," *Colloquy*, January 1970.

12. Hugh Prather, *Notes to Myself* (Moab, Utah: Real People, 1970).

13. Louis Raths, Merrell Harmin, and Sidney Simon, *Values and Teaching* (Columbus, Ohio: Merrill, 1966).

14. Sidney B. Simon, Leland W. Howe and Howard Kirschenbaum, *Values Clarification* (New York: Hart, 1972).

15. *Suggested Outlines for the Development of Courses of Study in Health Education for Junior and Senior High Schools* (Albany, N.Y.: New York State Department of Education, 1970).

16. *WOW Health Education Curriculum Guide* (Washington State Department of Public Instruction, Olympia; Wisconsin State Department of Public Instruction, Madison; Oregon State Department of Education, Salem, 1975).

CHAPTER 4

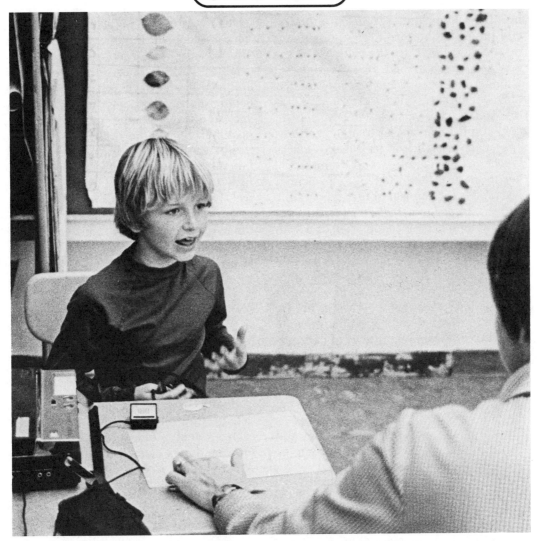

SCHOOL HEALTH SERVICES

"School, after all, is the one institution in our society that is inflicted on everybody, and what happens in school makes a difference—for good or ill" (5, p. 13).

The promotion and maintainence of schoolchildren's health is one of the major objectives of education. School health services represent one aspect of the total school program to meet the physical and emotional necessities of the developing child. School health services can be defined as the part of the school health program that appraises, protects, and promotes the health of students and of the personnel in the school. These services are provided by a variety of health professionals including physicians, nurses, dentists, counselors, social workers, and teachers as well as a variety of community agencies and organizations. The school health service "team" works together to (1) appraise and evaluate the health status of all students and school personnel; (2) counsel students, parents, and school personnel when necessary; (3) refer students and school personnel to appropriate health care services when a health status problem exists; (4) help to arrange a total school health program that enhances the health status of students and school personnel; (5) assist in the prevention and control of communicable diseases; (6) examine the school environment to assure that it provides sanitary conditions, safe facilities, and a conducive learning atmosphere; (7) provide procedures for dealing with emergency care for injury and illness of students or school personnel; and (8) examine the curriculum to be certain that it promotes the health status of students.

This definition of health services has implications for education that often go unrecognized by school personnel. Carl E. Willgoose states that health services help children become better informed of their assets and liabilities, which in turn helps develop lasting attitudes toward health providers (7). Through school health services, the student may learn to value both professional health services and the practice of having one's state of health evaluated regularly.

The classroom teacher is only one of many persons who play a role in the delivery of health services. Physicians, nurses, psychologists, health counselors, guidance counselors, administrators, and custodians are all significant to the health development of the elementary school child.

Those with the most important role in a child's health development are parents or guardians. They have the primary responsibility for maintaining the proper health care of their children. School health services are meant to encourage parents in developing behavior that will lead to physical, emotional, and social well-being for their children.

Through an ongoing collaborative relationship between parent and school, the health status of the child may be maintained at an optimum level. The school should inform parents of the emotional and physical development of their children. In cases where parental neglect, such as child abuse, is suspected, the school has the responsibility to intervene.

HEALTH APPRAISAL

Health appraisal is the term used for determining the total health status of each student. This appraisal is critical, for a student's classroom performance is directly related to his or her physical, mental, and emotional health status.

Health status is appraised by a variety of persons through observation, examination, and evaluation. The most important persons in health appraisal are the parents, the teacher, and the student's physician. The parent and teacher spend the most amount of time with the student and are able to make detailed observations. The physician has access to the student's medical examination and can provide an accurate health history. In addition to parent and teacher observation and the medical examination and health history of the physician, health appraisal includes screening tests, hearing tests, a dental examination, and a social and psychological evaluation. Each of these aspects will be discussed in more detail.

Teacher Observations

Next to parents, teachers have more contact hours with the elementary school child than any other adult. This places teachers in a special position to observe deviations from the norm. In this role, the teacher can suspect, detect abnormalities, and refer. The teacher should not diagnose or treat, except in emergency situations.

A child's nonverbal behavior, such as mannerisms, skin color, eyes, posture, and gait, or verbal behavior, such as complaints, voice tones, and frequency of verbal interactions with peers, both provide important clues to the child's overall health. If a teacher suspects a potential problem, the school nurse or the child's parents should be contacted. Both parents and teacher should refrain from making a diagnosis, since the limited backgrounds of each may not provide a correct judgment. They should consult a physician when in doubt.

Before teachers attempt to make decisions about student health problems, they must have the ability to differentiate between healthy and unhealthy conditions and behaviors. Table 4-1 lists conditions and behavior that may aid in the recognition of physical and emotional conditions requiring special attention.

Health History

Another method of appraising the health status of students is to determine "where they were," "where they are now," and "where they are going," in terms of physical and mental development. Knowledge of the student's health history can help the teacher deal with these concerns.

The student's cumulative health record provides information on such items as results of screening tests, teacher observations, physician's reports, dentist's reports, psychologist's findings, immunizations, medical conditions, scores on physical performance tests, and physical growth curves. This record follows the student from kindergarten through high school and should be kept up-to-date.

For the health record to be effective, several criteria must be met:

1. Data should be objective rather than subjective.

2. The record should be reviewed by the student's teacher at the beginning of each year.

3. The teacher's and school nurse's comments should be understandable to all teachers.

In some cases, students have a different teacher for each subject. In these circumstances how can each teacher have an understanding of the health status of all the students? The school nurse can examine the cumulative health records of each student, note any conditions that need teacher consideration, and send a note to each of the child's teachers.

Screening Tests

Screening tests, which may be performed by teachers, nurses, technicians, parent volunteers, or other trained personnel, uncover student health problems not detected by observation of pupil behavior. Although screening tests are commonly used for measuring growth and determining visual and hearing acuity, they are of value only in leading to remedial care (2, p. 13). The proper use of screening procedures will help secure a better understanding of how a student can achieve greater physical effectiveness and lead a healthier life.

TABLE 4-1 CONDITIONS REQUIRING SPECIAL ATTENTION

	Appearance	Behavior	Complaints
General Condition	Fever Very thin or overweight Extreme changes in weight Tired expressions, i.e., yawns, rubs eyes Very pale or flushed Rashes Nausea Poor posture	Lethargic Irritable toward peers Gets into accidents Not interested in school activities Eats too little or too much Uncoordinated	Wants to be excused from activities Wants to go home or to the nurse's office Stomachaches Headaches Dizziness Wants to lie down Numerous visits to the bathroom
Eyes	Crossed or turned out Repeated styes Watery Red Crusted eyelids	Holds books too close to eyes Squints or frowns Favors one eye Rubs eyes Excessive blinking Tilts head	Frequent headaches Dizzy spells Wants to sit near front of room Nausea Complains of not seeing clearly
Ears	Discharge from ear Cotton in ear Excessive wax in canal	Can't hear discussions or answers Picking in ear Tilts or turns head to one side Fails to answer questions correctly Monotone or poor voice pitch Speech problems Leans forward when someone speaks Shows no interest in what the teacher says	Asks for things to be repeated Complains of earaches or ringing noises Asks teacher to talk louder
Skin and Scalp	Rashes or sores Acne and blackheads Nits on hair Bald spots Hives Rough areas	Scratching Keeps certain areas covered	Itches Pain on touch
Nose, Throat, and Mouth	Irregular teeth Excessive tartar on teeth Cracks at corner of mouth Bad breath Persistent mouth breathing Bleeding gums Nasal discharge Stuffy nose	Coughing Wheezing Shortness of breath Does not smile Picks teeth	Toothache Sore throat Difficulty breathing

Vision Screening

According to the National Society for the Prevention of Blindness, one out of every four schoolchildren has an eye condition that requires attention by a health professional (6). School health personnel, rather than health professionals, are responsible for vision screening, because the objective of an eye exam is referral, not diagnosis.

The Snellen test for distant vision is the most commonly accepted of all vision screening tests and should be administered every two or three years in elementary school. Two types of Snellen charts may be used—the standard chart and the E chart (Figure 4-1).

The advantages of the Snellen test include: (a) it does not depend on reading speed; and (b) it is simple to administer. The disadvantages of this test are that students may memorize the chart or try to cheat by "peeking" through the side of the card covering one eye.

Other deficiencies of the eye should be considered aside from those revealed by the Snellen test. Before graduation from the primary grades, children should be tested for color blindness. Since almost 80 percent of children are born with hyperopia (far-sightedness), some schools consider this a worthy subject for screening (3). Opinions differ, however, and the decision to employ multiple eye screening tests is a local decision that should be based on recommendations from school administrators, nurses, teachers, physicians, and others who might examine the referred child.

Hearing Screening

Hearing tests should be given annually to elementary schoolchildren by health specialists rather than classroom teachers. About 85 percent of hearing problems will be evident by the third grade (4).

The sweep test and the threshold test are the most common tests used. In the sweep test, various sound frequencies are scanned. Children failing to hear two or more tones should be retested at another time. If the child fails again, the threshold test should be made. In this test, volumes are decreased in order to measure the lowest volume a child can hear. The threshold test is considered the best test of hearing acuity.

Medical Examinations

There are two types of medical examinations. The *periodic* medical examination is used to appraise the health of apparently normal and healthy schoolchildren. The *referral* examination requires a physician to check reported deviations from normal health (2, p. 14).

All children entering school for the first time should have a medical examination. They should be reexamined in the fourth or fifth grade and whenever deemed appropriate by school personnel.

Examination by a family physician is recommended, because (a) a more thorough appraisal may be conducted; (b) he or she may be familiar with the family and the child's health history; and (c) follow-up can be immediate. In cases where a child cannot be examined by a family physician, perhaps due to lack of money or willingness by the parents to arrange for an appointment, an examination by the school physician is the next best choice.

The school should provide the child with a standard form to be completed by the physician. This form should be placed in the child's cumulative record. However, the teacher or school nurse

FIGURE 4-1 Snellen Chart (Courtesy of National Society for the Prevention of Blindness)

LETTER CHART FOR 20 FEET
Snellen Scale

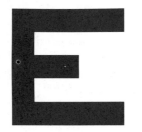

E   200 ft.

H N   100 ft.

D F N   70 ft.

P T X Z   50 ft.

U Z D T F   40 ft.

D F N P T H   30 ft.

P H U N T D Z   20 ft.

N P X T Z F H   15 ft.

should note any significant remarks made by the physician.

A thorough physical examination will:

1. Identify for the child the importance of being examined periodically

2. Provide children and their parents with information about the physical condition of the child

3. Detect obvious and subtle defects

4. Serve as a basis for the scheduling of future examinations and health counseling.

Unless deviations from the norm are followed up, physical examinations will be of no value.

Dental Examinations

About 95 to 99 percent of elementary schoolchildren suffer from dental problems. Yet half of all children in the country under the age of fifteen have never been to a dentist. Students of elementary school age should visit a dentist at least once a year, because this age group has the highest incidence of cavities. The child's dentist will determine if more frequent visits are necessary. As in the medical examination, the dentist should complete a standard form, which is then filed in the student's cumulative health record folder.

Some schools provide dental inspections as a supplement to the school health program. Though not used as a substitute for a dental examination by one's personal dentist, the dental inspection permits a dental hygienist to detect problems by using a mirror and explorer. New teaching aids allow children to conduct their own inspection under the guidance of the school nurse or dental hygienist.

Teachers, in addition to emphasizing prevention through brushing, should also stress the importance of flossing daily.

The procedures to be followed in dental screening should be determined locally by the school, health professionals, and community groups.

Social and Psychological Evaluation

Many physical problems are an outgrowth of emotional problems. A child's health may be affected by his ability to get along with the peer group, his teachers, or his parents.

The teacher can detect evidence of social and emotional problems by observing the student during play, when classroom formalities are not followed. When the teacher observes social or emotional deviations from the norm, she or he should consult appropriate personnel. School psychologists, social workers, and guidance counselors should work cooperatively with other community health personnel to offer children the best services possible.

Psychological examination of referred children should be conducted and results interpreted to classroom teachers by appropriate professionals. The results should be filed in the student's cumulative health record.

Among the reasons for psychological referral may be a lack of interest in schoolwork, withdrawal from other children, discipline problems, difficulty in playing with others, rapid deterioration in schoolwork, restlessness, aggressiveness toward others, apathy, and crying for no apparent reason.

Parents should be contacted before referral. A more effective program will evolve if parental cooperation is sought and received.

HEALTH COUNSELING AND FOLLOW-UP

As an important part of school health services, health counseling seeks to identify and follow up health problems by:

1. Providing students information about their health status as revealed by the health appraisal
2. Interpreting to parents the significance of their child's health condition
3. Encouraging and motivating parents to obtain needed care for their children
4. Encouraging and motivating children to be responsible for their own health
5. Promoting the health education of students and parents
6. Developing educational programs that can be adapted to meet the needs and abilities of exceptional children (1, pp. 111–112).

Revealing problems in a health appraisal is of little value unless counseling and follow-up procedures are implemented. Although follow-up is primarily a school responsibility, it often involves contact with community agencies and almost always with parents. Among those in the school who are integral parts in the counseling and follow-up programs are the teacher, health counselor, and school nurse.

Teacher

Elementary school teachers have the following counseling responsibilities:

1. They know and abide by ethical standards, such as those formulated by

the American Personnel and Guidance Association.

2. They know their limitations in the helping relationship and how to refer cases for additional help.

3. They counsel students who want guidance. "Forcing" help on a student who does not want it may produce negative results.

4. They provide the student non-judgmental and specific feedback.

Health Counselor

A school health counselor should have a strong background in counseling techniques as well as in health education. The health counselor should be responsible for planning contact with parents, discussing health problems with student and parents, monitoring follow-up procedures and student health progress, and working with school and community personnel. In many cases the health counselor is the school nurse.

School Nurse

A school nurse should possess all the attributes of a health counselor. Medical background and awareness of community health services enable the school nurse to work with parents, teachers, and children toward the child's achievement of high level wellness.

Some Things to Consider About Follow-Up

Direct verbal contact, either in person or by telephone, should be made with the parents, since mail may not reach them. Mail can get lost, be "intercepted," or go unacknowledged.

Parents must understand what the teacher or health counselor is telling them. Language barriers, lack of education, even hearing loss may cause misunderstandings. Teachers and health counselors should be "askable."

Follow-up should be confirmed either by a note or phone call from the source to which the child was referred. If no follow-up takes place, the teacher or health counselor should determine the reason why and take appropriate measures. These measures may take the form of acquiring free care or court-ordered medical care for the child.

Responsibilities of School Personnel

Parents who fail to take care of their children can be found guilty of child neglect. From 9:00 to 3:00 (in most schools), the teacher serves in *loco parentis* ("in the place of parents"). Therefore, failure on behalf of the teacher is also considered an act of negligence. School personnel should have access to written procedures specifying their responsibilities during an emergency and how parents are to be informed and counseled.

Providing Immediate Care

Since all teachers at one time or another will be required to administer first aid to an injured or ill child, they should know the appropriate actions to take. If they have not received training in college, the school nurse should conduct in-service workshops.

The teacher's responsibility is to administer *immediate* and *temporary* care to a student. In no case should the teacher diagnose an illness or injury. Medication should be administered only under the direction of a physician.

At least one teacher well versed in first aid procedures should be in the school building whenever students are involved in activities, whether during or after school hours.

All first aid procedures, as well as the events leading to the procedures, should be entered in the child's cumulative health record.

First aid supplies should be easily accessible to every teacher.

Before the first class meeting with students, school administrators should distribute to each faculty member detailed procedures for emergency care.

Informing Parents

Parents need to be notified of their child's accident or sudden illness. In a reassuring and calm manner, the school should notify the parents of the nature of the injury and the first aid precautions taken.

All students should have an Emergency Contact Card on file in the school. This card should contain the following information: 1. phone number of where the parent may be reached; 2. phone number of a secondary contact; 3. name and telephone number of family physician; and 4. a parent's authorization to send the child to a hospital.

Counseling Parents

An individual from the school who contacts the parent may guide that parent toward a responsible decision about the care of the child. The parent should be informed of the situation that led to the contact, the treatment facilities available, and possible alternatives if the child is not treated.

PREVENTION AND CONTROL OF COMMUNICABLE DISEASE

Before immunization vaccines were discovered, childhood diseases took a terrific toll of life and health. Today one hears little about the child who is condemned by polio to life in a wheelchair or the mentally retarded child who was a bright baby before suffering brain damage from measles. Yet these tragedies are still happening. Why? One reason is that many children never get immunized until they start school, although they are more apt to get childhood diseases before age six. Some children get one or two doses when they should have four or five doses for full protection, so they are just as likely to get the disease as the child who has had no immunizations at all. Many state health departments have adopted a number of recommendations made by the American Academy of Pediatrics to promote uniformity in the delivery of basic childhood immunizations, but differences still remain. Therefore teachers and health counselors should consult their own state health departments regarding the diseases to be immunized against and the types of communicable diseases that must be reported.

A child's parents should maintain an immunization record that can be entered on the cumulative health record when the child begins school.

Teacher's Role in Communicable Disease Prevention

The classroom teacher should refer children suspected of having communicable diseases to the school nurse. Rather than stressing perfect attendance, since this encourages children with communicable diseases to attend school, teachers should praise children for not coming to school when they have a communicable disease. The teacher should be aware of readmission and exclusion policies concerning communicable diseases and should incorporate instruction on communicable disease control and prevention in the curriculum.

REFERENCES

1. Joint Committee on Health Problems in Education, *School Health Services* (Chicago: AMA 1964).

2. Joint Committee on Health Problems in Education of the National Education Association and the American Medical Association, *Health Appraisal of School Children,* 4th ed. (Chicago: AMA, 1969).

3. Joint Study Committee of the American School Health Association and the National Society for the Prevention of Blindness, *Teaching About Vision* (New York: The Association, 1972).

4. Alma Nemir and Warren E. Schaller, *The School Health Program* (Philadelphia: Saunders, 1975).

5. Neil Postman and Charles Weingartner, *Teaching as a Subversive Activity* (New York: Dell, 1969).

6. *Vision Screening in the Schools* (New York: Society for the Prevention of Blindness, 1975).

7. Carl E. Willgoose, *Health Education in the Elementary School* (Philadelphia: Saunders, 1974).

PART II

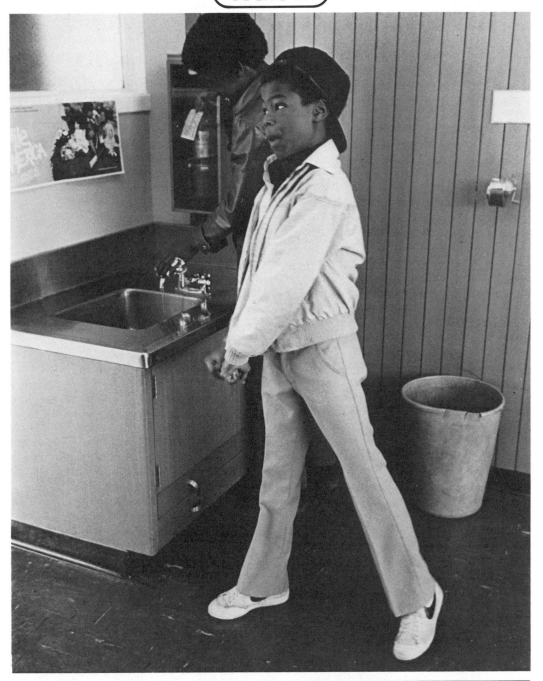

TOWARD A HEALTHY MIND

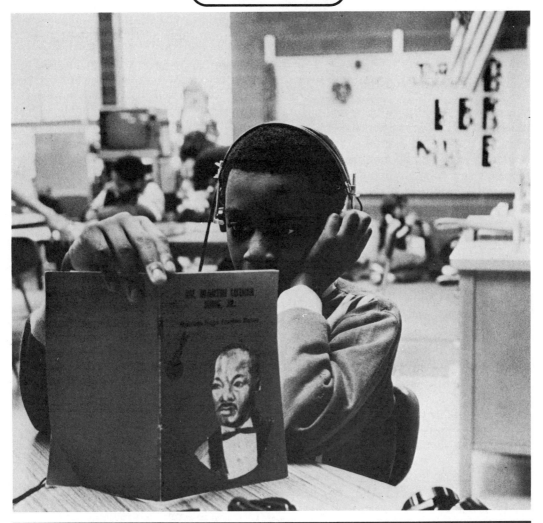

CHAPTER 5

PART A: SELF-ACTUALIZATION AND SELF-CONCEPT

In the total realm of health, few questions are as important as the question What do I think of what I am and what I am becoming? For the elementary student, this question is especially urgent and difficult and must be given serious consideration at every grade level. To this end, the authors have evolved eleven concepts that have been helpful to students in their struggles with what they are and what they are becoming. These concepts are introduced and discussed at an adult level in this chapter, and suggestions for incorporating them in the elementary curriculum are found in Chapter 5B.

GOOD SELF-CONCEPT

How would you like to be a one-person judge and jury at your own trial? In many ways, that is what happens when one renders a verdict on one's self-concept, for one's self concept always stems from a personal judgment about the self. Although this appears obvious, any effective understanding of self-concept must begin with a clear view of who is judging what.

For students, the idea of self-concept can be effectively communicated by explaining that self-concept is the grade given to one's self in a course entitled "Competence to Live."

Grade A might be represented by the judgment: I like myself and what I am becoming; I am competent to take care of myself, and I have a hand in my future. Grade F might be represented by the judgment: there is little hope for me; I am incompetent, and I have no hand in my future.

It is important for elementary-aged students to be aware of who assigns the grades for self-concept and to understand the difference between a healthy self-concept (grade A) and a poor self-concept (grade F). The acquisition of such knowledge at an early age is necessary, because it is easier to develop a healthy self-concept than to correct a poor one.

DEVELOPING A HEALTHY SELF-KNOWLEDGE

Many attitudes related to self-concept require attention at an early age. Among these, one of the most important is a heal-thy attitude toward self-knowledge. For example, Abraham H. Maslow writes:

From our point of view, Freud's greatest discovery is that the great cause of much psychological illness is the fear of knowledge of oneself—of one's emotions, impulses, memories, capacities, potentialities, of one's destiny. . . .

In general this kind of fear is defensive, in the sense that it is a protection of our self-esteem, of our love and respect for ourselves. We tend to be afraid of any knowledge that could cause us to despise ourselves or to make us feel inferior, weak, worthless, evil, shameful. We protect ourselves and our ideal image of ourselves by repression and similar defenses, which are essentially techniques by which we avoid becoming conscious of unpleasant or dangerous truths (4).

An early pattern of thinking must be established in which the temptation to hide things from oneself is resisted. This includes both negative and positive aspects of one's life. Perhaps the tendency is greater to hide from ourselves the negative aspects, those things that threaten self-esteem, self-love, and self-respect. We too often focus on our weaknesses and problems, overlooking our personal strengths and resources. A healthy attitude toward self-knowledge is to welcome to consciousness knowledge of both our strengths and weaknesses.

COPING WITH PROBLEMS OF LIFE

The way that we feel about ourselves is largely determined by how well we think we handle the cards that we are dealt in life. When we cope successfully, we like ourselves, while failure to handle our problems creates self-doubt.

Each of us starts to develop a self-concept very early in life, at a time when there are almost no standards by which to judge success. Thus, positive reinforcement of young children's behavior by parents and teachers is imperative. Obviously, the elementary school years are a significant time for establishing standards by which to judge success in living.

The authors believe that the greatest tragedy in education is the fact that discussion of the human condition, or what it means to be human, is reserved for graduate school rather than initiated in the elementary school. In the past, elementary schools have focused very little on the human condition. Rather, most of the emphasis has been on "what you do" or "what you are getting ready to do" or, perhaps, "what you should not do." Thus, success in elementary school has been judged primarily by whether a student achieves or fails to achieve certain grade-level standards.

Unfortunately, the preoccupation with "what you do" instead of with "what you are" could not occur at a worse time in the development of the individual. For it is at the elementary school level that students could profit most from understanding the human condition (i.e., understanding what they are and how they are similar and different from other humans). The discussion need not be a profound philosophical one, but it should include the communication of a few basic concepts that can be reexamined at all grade levels.

These basic concepts regarding human nature stem from the fact that "to be a human, one must symbolically agree" to be fallible, ignorant of much, susceptible to disease, mortal, capable of bad will, and possessed by a drive toward pleasure. All human beings share these characteristics, and with the possible exception of the last, they are generally considered liabilities. Each is a mark of what the French call *la condition humaine* —the human predicament. At first glance the traits seem relatively simple, perhaps not even especially important; but an understanding and appreciation of the human predicament in large part determines the grades that students assign themselves on self-concept.

Suppose we have a student who constantly makes mistakes in one aspect of life or another. The grade that this student would assign himself or herself on self-concept is primarily dependent upon the recognition of human fallibility. Students who clearly understand this idea are able to make mistakes and still like themselves. Students who do not understand the nature of human fallibility not only may come to hate themselves because they make mistakes but also may progress into adulthood without ever having developed healthy attitudes toward their fallibility.

Elementary schools should teach students to discover their limits rather than to deny them. This concept also applies to susceptibility to disease. Too many people are either reckless about their health or hypochondriacal. They reason either that they can take some preventive action that will guarantee good health or that there is no point in worrying about it. They say, for example, "There is no point in giving up smoking so long as there are all these other diseases that can strike me."

Unfortunately, very few people are willing to accept co-responsibility for their health. People's being co-responsible in this case means that they fully realize that there are factors beyond their control that affect their health status at the same time that they maintain the attitude that there are also many steps that they can take to positively affect their health. It is important to realize that one can never be more than a co-contributor to one's health and that there can never be any guarantee of health. We would all like to have a signed guarantee, but this would deny a factor of the human condition, namely that we are all susceptible to disease.

The elementary student soon confirms the fact that all people are susceptible to disease and can begin to develop a more general attitude toward all human limits. The following attitudes, for example, contribute significantly to self-concept:

1. The fact that I am susceptible to disease is no reason to give up on trying to be healthy.

2. The fact that I am fallible is no justification for giving up on reason.

3. The fact that I am capable of bad will toward others is no reason to give up on being a loving person.

4. The fact that I am ignorant of much is no reason to give up on learning.

5. The fact that I am mortal is no reason to give up on life.

6. The fact that I am pleasure-seeking is no reason to give up on self-control.

These attitudes allow us a role in our future. Although we cannot predict or determine the future, we can influence the course of events in our favor. Our individual efforts to change the direction of things make us co-creators of the future along with fate, evolution, cosmic happenings, and other living and nonliving factors. We are one of the partners. To give up the partnership, to sell out to fate, to reject individual responsibility for the future, is one of the most significant marks of an unhealthy child or adult. A pediatric psychiatrist told one of the authors that all of his patients had given up the co-creator role and that he could make no progress in therapy until the patients started to take a hand in the future. Although the co-creator role is difficult to sustain, it is indispensable to mental health.

UNDERSTANDING GENETIC DIFFERENCES

In addition to knowing the characteristics we all share as humans, it is necessary to understand that we are different and why we are different. Race, color, sex, height, body form, and a variety of abilities are all products of our genetic backgrounds. They are givens that we must learn to accept and work with. It is thus important that children learn to relate their self-concepts to what they do with their genetic potential rather than to what they inherited. No matter how inferior or superior our genetic backgrounds, in reality we are each proud or ashamed of what we do with what we have. The old saying, "Of those who are given much, in turn, much is expected," distorts the relationship of genetic background to self-concept. In truth, we expect much of ourselves no matter what our genetic backgrounds. The important thing is to be able to determine our limits realistically and to build a good self-concept within those limits.

This is a difficult task for both the elementary teacher and the student. The evidence is clear that students achieve more when more is expected of them. The evidence is equally clear that repeated failure tends to detract from learning. Hence, the task of teacher and student is one: to discover limits and to build self-concept within those limits.

This means that to be most effective, the teacher and student must respect each other and work together in an atmosphere in which both parties are aware of the following.

1. People inherit different abilities in different degrees, and all abilities are important. One person may think fast; another, run fast; and yet another, both think and run fast. The fast thinker may earn a million dollars in business or the fast runner may earn a million as a professional athlete. The third person may use either of those talents or both to earn a living. The important thing is for the students to discover and actualize the talents that they do have. A person who does not have athletic ability obviously cannot be a professional athlete. Blind or physically handicapped people cannot do certain things either, but there are other things that they might do very well. We must each discover our limits and stand responsible within those limits.

2. Many people participate in self-deception regarding their genetic differences. They claim to have no potential in certain areas and announce their lack of potential to the world. They say, for example, "I can't do math." This self-deception may reflect a lack of interest in math or an unwillingness to think deeply. Either way, a mathematical talent may be prevented from actualizing. Self-deception often keeps us from discovering our real limits.

MAKING DECISIONS

Upon awakening each day, one is stuck with the question: upon what, for how long, and with what intensity shall I focus my consciousness? The way that one goes about answering this question and the relative confidence that one places in various faculties (e.g., thinking, feeling, imitating, reasoning, or judging) in attempting to answer it constitutes one's decision-making style.

Human beings exhibit a variety of styles in decision making. Moreover, the same individual may employ more than one style. Some of the more common styles include: (a) mental take-it-easy-ism, (b) apostle of feeling and intuition, (c) predestinarianism, (d) cognitive self-assertiveness, and (e) replaced pilot.

Mental Take-it-easy-ism

People have the power to regulate the directions and actions of their own consciousness: to think is an act of choice. In reality, people are free at any moment to suspend their thinking and to let their minds drift. They may only partially focus their consciousness, declining to struggle with any matter that does not come easily. Many persons are not willing to exert the mental effort necessary to make their own decisions. Consequently, they select a decision-making style that is not very demanding and surrender to the pull of lethargic passivity. Mental take-it-easy-ism as a decision-making style ignores Kant's challenge: ". . . *sapere aude!* Have the courage to avail yourself of your own understanding."

Apostle of Feeling and Intuition

A decision-making style in which the individual seeks the wonders of the emotions and rejects rational regulation is a style that requires little planning, a style in which one simply follows feeling and intuition. We have labeled this style "apostle of feeling and intuition." In this style, one allows one's consciousness to move in the direction of the greatest pull rather than intentionally focusing it.

Predestinarianism

Predestinarianism is a decision-making style in which the individual feels that the events of life are predetermined. Those who adopt this style escape responsibility for their own successes or failures. Their lives are primarily matters of good or bad fortune, neither of which is deserved. They reject the role of co-creator of the future. Instead, the directions to their consciousness read simply: stand by. The lifestyles of those characterized by predestinarianism consist mainly of a series of adjustments to whatever cards life deals to them.

Cognitive Self-Assertiveness

Cognitive self-assertiveness is a decision-making style in which individuals proudly accept the role of co-creator. Realizing that people are not the masters of their own destiny, they nevertheless assert themselves and take charge of as much of the future as possible. They develop and constantly reevaluate their life plans.

Replaced Pilot

In sharp contrast to the style of cognitive self-assertiveness, an increasing number of people display a style in which they appear to have been replaced as pilots. Such individuals claim that they have been "taken over." Substitute pilots include anger, rage, eros, the divine, and the diabolical, to mention but a few.

At one time or another, everyone employs all the described decision-making styles. One must, however, learn to be aware of the style being used and must understand the consequences of heavy reliance on any style that denies one's role as co-creator and that may result in the destruction of one's self-concept.

SETTING GOALS

Goal-directed behavior produces feelings of worth and significance because it confirms our roles as co-creators of the future. Ivan Pavlov, winner of the 1904 Nobel Prize in physiology and medicine, has aptly described the significance of setting goals:

Purpose has a tremendous biological importance; it is the basic form of the vital energy of everyone. Only the life of those is full and strong who strive all their lives toward an always realizable but never realized goal or go with enthusiasm from one goal to another. . . . By the same token life ceases to be attractive as soon as the goal disappears. Do we not read quite often in the notes left by the suicides that they terminate life because it has no purpose or goal? It is true the goal of human life is boundless and inexhaustible. The tragedy of suicide consists precisely in that in most cases merely momentary impediment, or as we physiologists say a "breaking" of the goal-reflex occurs, and only in rare instances is this impediment a lasting one (5).

Elementary school is an important time to examine the process of setting goals and standards. It is a time when the process itself can easily be separated from a long list of rapidly changing goals and standards. It is a time when one can more easily accept advice about unrealistic goals or standards. It is a time when one's goals are usually shared without serious reservation. Most of all, it is an ideal time to discuss the relationship between goals and standards and one's self-esteem.

THE DIFFERENCE BETWEEN SELF-LOVE AND SELFISHNESS

Contemporary theology, philosophy, and popular thought are pervaded by the notions that self-love and selfishness are synonymous and that both are wrong. In contrast, many psychiatrists suggest that the belief in these notions constitutes our biggest hang-up.

Erich Fromm explains the problem (2):*

The selfish person is interested only in himself, wants everything for himself, feels no pleasure in giving, but only in taking. The world outside is looked at only from the standpoint of what he can get out of it; he lacks interest in the needs of others, and respect for their dignity and integrity. . . . Does not this prove that concern for others and concern for oneself are unavoidable alternatives? This would be so if selfishness and self-love were identical. But that assumption is the very fallacy which has led to so many mistaken conclusions concerning our problem. Selfishness and self-love, far from being identical, are actually opposites. The selfish person does not love himself too much but too little: in fact he hates himself. This lack of fondness and care for himself, which is only one expression of his lack of productiveness, leaves him empty and frustrated. He is necessarily unhappy and anxiously concerned to snatch from life the satisfactions which he blocks himself from attaining. He seems to care too much for himself but actually he only makes an unsuccessful attempt to cover up and compensate for his failure to care for his real self. . . . It is true that selfish persons are incapable of loving others, but they are not capable of loving themselves either.

Most elementary students develop an early understanding of the concept of

*From *Man for Himself* by Erich Fromm. Copyright 1947, © 1975 by Erich Fromm. Reprinted by permission of Holt, Rinehart, and Winston, Publishers.

selfishness. Seldom, however, are they introduced to the meaning of self-love.

The challenge of the future thus becomes: how can I as an elementary teacher foster self-love among students who, like myself, are fallible, ignorant of much, susceptible to disease, mortal, capable of bad will, and possessed by a drive toward pleasure? How can we love such liabilities? We can begin meeting the challenge by separating self-love from selfishness.

ACHIEVING A POSITIVE SELF-CONCEPT

A positive self-concept is generally referred to as self-esteem. Self-esteem is based on both self-respect and self-confidence. Nathaniel Branden has described the interrelationship of these concepts (1).

Man needs self-respect because he has to act to achieve values—and in order to act, he needs to value the beneficiary of his action. In order to seek values, man must consider himself worthy of enjoying them. In order to fight for his happiness, he must consider himself worthy of happiness.

The two aspects of self-esteem—self-confidence and self-respect—can be isolated conceptually, but they are inseparable in man's psychology. Man makes himself worthy of living by making himself competent to live: by dedicating his mind to the task of discovering what is true and what is right, and by governing his actions accordingly. If a man defaults on the responsibility of thought and reason, thus undercutting his sense of worthiness, he does so by evasion, he commits treason to his own (correct or mistaken) judgment, and thus will not retain his sense of competence.

Because one of the characteristics of the human condition is fallibility, people will always be able to label many of their past decisions as incorrect, logically unsound, or mistaken in some way. The ratio of sound to unsound decisions will, in turn, have a major influence upon self-confidence.

It is especially important for the elementary student to understand the difference between self-confidence and self-respect. If our behavior violates what we have decided to be right, we should properly place the blame on lack of willpower, leaving self-confidence intact.

Self-respect, however, is not directly related to the soundness or unsoundness of the decisions made but is more a function of bringing one's behavior in accord with what one has deliberately decided, whether the decision be sound or unsound. We maintain our self-respect by doing what we consider to be right. If what we considered to be right later turns out to be wrong, we should properly place the blame on mistaken judgment, leaving our self-respect intact.

BECOMING AN AUTHORITY ON ONE'S OWN LIFESTYLE

Young people may be guided in some good path and kept out of harm's way without becoming authorities on their own lifestyles. Such guidance, however, regardless of how well intended, is not in the best interest of students. It is the student who becomes an authority on his or her own lifestyle who enhances the probability of achieving self-esteem.

Students who learn to observe carefully, to think and reason about what they observe, and to make wise decisions based upon their observations and who, further, develop the self-control to hold to their decisions have reason to be proud of themselves and are justified in being self-confident and self-respecting.

To be considered worthwhile by one's

self and by others, one must behave originally, avoiding apelike imitation. To conform to custom merely renders one customary rather than individually worthy. In today's society, the young are attempting to render themselves uncustomary. These attempts at individuality are more than simple rejections of older lifestyles. In fact, becoming an authority on one's own lifestyle is a necessary condition for the development of mental health.

It is essential to mental health that individuals realize early in life that they stand responsible within the context of the human predicament for their own successes or failures in the selection of lifestyles that are actualizing and promote health and happiness. Although attempts to place the blame elsewhere (on a regular basis) are unhealthy, freedom and individual responsibility are not easily accepted. Have you stopped recently to consider how far we have moved from individual responsibility? If something goes wrong in our lives today, we have developed patterns of response whereby we immediately shift the blame to our parents, our genetic heritage, poor education, bad teachers, impulses, childhood traumas, gods, or bad luck.

Indeed, we have even reached a stage at which we are unwilling to accept responsibility in recreational aspects of our lifestyles. For example, how many times have you heard of a "poorly disciplined tree" running across the golf course and maliciously and unfairly attacking the ball of an innocent and highly skilled golfer? Or, how many times have you seen a tennis player miss a shot only to look down and verbally or otherwise express encouragement to his or her racquet?

In all aspects of our lives we have learned to be highly efficient blame-shifters. Rollo May was probably right when he noted in his book *Love and Will* that "the central core of modern man's neurosis is the undermining of his experience of himself as responsible."

RESPECTING INDIVIDUAL DIFFERENCES

Many words and a great number of books have been written on the topic of individuality. Yet many of our decisions and much of our behavior today requires only the faculty of apelike imitation. William Glasser has blamed the schools for a major portion of the repression of individuality. He writes (3):*

Education does not emphasize thinking and is so memory-oriented because almost all schools and colleges are dominated by the certainty principle. According to the certainty principle, there is a right and a wrong answer to every question; the function of education is then to ensure that each student knows the right answers to a series of questions that educators have decided are important. . . .

The unusual child who questions the certainty principle by saying that there may not be just one right answer, or any right answer, to a given educational question gets short shrift in the average classroom. Unless this unusual child has an unusual teacher, he will soon learn that although his thinking may receive brief recognition, in the end, regardless of how thoughtful his discussion may be, the payoff is the right answer. . . .

Taught formally from kindergarten about the value of our democratic way of life, children learn from experience that the major premise of a democratic society—that the people involved in any endeavor help determine its rules—does not apply to them. We wonder why there is so much confusion in our society over what democracy is. Could this confusion stem from the lack of experience in democracy in school?

*From *Schools Without Failure* by William Glasser. © 1969 by Harper & Row, Inc. Reprinted by permission.

In contrast to accepting the certainty principle, every elementary student ought to be encouraged to develop the attitude, "What I think and feel and what others think and feel is important even when we are wrong." Not only is this attitude important to the self-actualization process, but it is also an essential step in becoming truly educated.

SELF-ACTUALIZING

The following list of characteristics of the self-actualized individual was assembled from a variety of sources but primarily from the work of Abraham H. Maslow (4, p. 60). The traits are stated in the form of behavioral objectives, the attainment of which would render any elementary school truly outstanding. The self-actualizing person:*

has gratified the need for self-esteem, love, and identity and is no longer blocked by deficiencies in these areas.

is not in conflict with herself or himself.

is in harmony with the world; has overcome his or her separateness, yet experiences his or her uniqueness; has personal identity; and does not feel like an object.

is using his or her capacities to the fullest extent, does not feel that he or she is being wasted, and appears to operate effortlessly even when working to full capacity.

is her or his own pilot and is not dependent, driven, or passive.

has confidence in the ability to overcome problems.

is spontaneous, expressive, candid, natural.

*Taken from *Toward a Psychology of Being* by Abraham H. Maslow. © 1968 by Litton Educational Publishing Co. Reprinted by permission of D. Van Nostrand Company.

is creative.

has resolved the apparent conflict between selfishness and self-love.

exhibits zest for living.

has the ability to transcend ego and be objective.

has transcended the problem of becoming and is more concerned with being.

accepts herself or himself and avoids affectation.

tends to be problem-centered and enjoys the challenge of problems.

is characterized by an appreciation and richness of emotional reaction.

has a high frequency of satisfying experiences.

values truth, honesty, and simplicity.

exhibits little fear of the unknown, the new experience, or the strange and, in fact, is interested in them.

tends to laugh with rather than at others.

gives people or objects total attention.

accepts his or her sexuality. The individual likes being a male or female.

is not sexually promiscuous but enjoys sex more than those who are driven to indiscriminate sex.

accepts and enjoys responsibility.

avoids exploiting others and respects others as human beings.

accepts and appreciates physiological needs and does not consider physical or intellectual appetites evil.

would be described as rational, sensitive, responsible, interesting, authentic, loving, and appreciative.

There is no self-concept, however good, that cannot be seriously damaged by failure to understand any of the eleven concepts presented in this chapter. Communicating these concepts in elementary school will demand a high level of energy and creativity on the part of teachers and is not a job for one whose style is mental take-it-easy-ism.

REFERENCES

1. Nathaniel Branden, *The Psychology of Self-Esteem* (Los Angeles: Nash, 1969).

2. Erich Fromm, *Man for Himself* (Greenwich, Conn.: Fawcett, 1947).

3. William Glasser, *Schools Without Failure* (New York: Harper & Row, 1969).

4. Abraham H. Maslow, *Toward a Psychology of Being* (New York: Van Nostrand Reinhold, 1968).

5. I. Pavlov, *The Goal Reflex*. In "Concerning Suicide in Soviet Russia" (J. Choron). *Bulletin of Suicidology* (December 1968).

PART B: TEACHING ABOUT SELF-ACTUALIZATION AND SELF-CONCEPT

"One of the findings of the current research into Human Potentialities has been that the average, healthy, well-functioning person has a very limited awareness of his personality strengths and resources but has a much clearer idea of his weakness and problem areas. On the other hand, it has been found that the process of taking inventory of one's strengths and personality assets is experienced as strengthening, brings gains in self-confidence, and improves self-image" (4, p. 143).

Healthy, self-actualized children continually take stock of themselves yet accept their own being. They need to examine the behavior of others, evaluate how others affect them, and accept others. Children have the greatest chance of happiness and self-actualization if the elementary school curriculum acknowledges the following needs:

1. Students need to examine their strengths and weaknesses.

2. Students need to accept the feelings they experience at different times and to learn to channel their feelings into appropriate behavior.

3. Students need to recognize their uniqueness and to learn to accept themselves.

4. Students need to examine how they relate to others (e.g., are they cooperative? competitive?).

5. Students need to examine how others influence their behavior and decisions.

6. Students need to set their own standards.

7. Students need to recognize what it is to be functioning less than fully.

The following lessons on self-actualization and self-concept incorporate these student needs. The teacher can use the lessons or films from the "Inside/Out" (1) and "Self-Incorporated" (6) series.

Appropriate grade levels are suggested for each teaching strategy and appear as ○, □, ☆ in the left-hand column:

  ○ = most suited for the primary grades;
  □ = most suited for the intermediate grades;
  ☆ = most suited for the upper elementary grades.

"Inside/Out" is a unique series of thirty 15-minute color programs designed to help eight- to ten-year-olds achieve and maintain a sense of well-being. It uses a feelings approach to health education, recognizing that the way people live, the kinds of decisions they make, and how they feel are as important to their well-being as heredity, environment, and the medical care they receive. "Self-Incorporated" is a series of fifteen programs with a teacher's guide, designed to stimulate classroom discussion of the critical issues and problems of early adolescence. Its objective is to instill in eleven- to thirteen-year-olds a desire to learn skills for coping with these issues and problems.*

UNIT I: SETTING YOUR STANDARDS

According to the popular psychologist Murray Banks, "It is important to learn how to live with yourself, for unless you learn to live with yourself, no one else will ever want to live with you." How do you learn to live with yourself? The authors would like to suggest that you learn to live with yourself most compatibly if you like yourself. To like yourself, you need to have self-respect and you need to have control over your life.

The authors believe that this concept is critical to health education. People who like themselves, value what they are doing, and select their own lifestyles have the greatest opportunities for self-actualization. We have included the lesson Setting Your Standards to help students begin the regular examination of the direction in which they want their lives to head. The authors have equated

*Both series are available from National Instructional Television, Box A, Bloomington, IN 47401.

the directions with different kinds of pilots. The critical questions are Who pilots your life? and Are you proud of your pilot?

OBJECTIVES

1. Through lecture and discussion, the student will be able to describe five lifestyle standards, or ways by which people direct their lives: as lazy pilots, glider pilots, lucky pilots, or by piloting themselves or having copilot takeover.

2. Through role play, the students will be able to identify at least two difficulties that they might experience if they adopt one of the five lifestyle standards.

3. By recording and evaluating ten activities, the students will describe how being each of the five different pilots relates to their self-esteem and feelings of worth.

4. The students will express at least four characteristics they value in their flight through life.

MATERIALS

1. Pictures that illustrate the five different types of pilots: lazy pilot—elementary-aged child floating on a raft; glider pilot—mountain landscape, surgeon operating; lucky pilot—fortune teller, plane just above a mountain top; self-pilot—tall bridge under construction, single pilot in a small plane: copilot takeover—someone who is drunk.

2. Model airplanes (optional).

Methods

○ □ ☆

Discussion

The purpose of this lesson is to help students better understand the relationship between how they use their minds and what they think of themselves. The students are asked to think of themselves as pilots. They can pilot their lives as lazy pilots, glider pilots, or lucky pilots. They can pilot themselves or experience copilot takeover. Read through the lesson and look for or make pictures to use with the different examples.

Who Is My Pilot?

1. Show a picture of an elementary-aged child floating on a raft and ask the students to describe what goes on in their minds while viewing it. The reactions might serve as examples of passive daydreaming. Examples of other passive activities might be examined and a list made for this category. After completing the list, the category should be given a name such as "lazy pilot." Ask the students to describe a lifestyle that is piloted by someone who is lazy.

2. Show a picture of a mountain landscape and ask what, if anything, the scene makes them feel like doing. The category could be extended by discussion of the question: what are some things that people do simply because they feel like doing them? Show a picture of a surgeon performing an operation and ask the class to discuss the following questions. Why do most doctors think that it is not a good idea to operate on family members? What do you think about it? Are there times when feelings interfere with your decisions? How do you handle those situations? After discussing behavior in which people follow their feelings, derive a name for this category such as "glider pilot." Ask the students to describe a lifestyle that is piloted by someone who is a glider.

3. Show a picture of a fortune teller. You might have the class discuss the following questions. Suppose you could

look into the future and know exactly what is going to happen to you. How many would want to know: why or why not? If you knew, how do you think it would affect the way you think? Many people believe that people are in control of their own futures. What do you think? Following discussion of this category, a name might be derived through the use of a picture of a plane just missing a mountain top. A suggested name might be "lucky pilot." Have the students describe a lifestyle that is piloted by someone who is lucky.

4. Show a picture of a tall bridge being built and ask some of the following questions. How do engineers use their minds to build bridges? Should they build them according to the way they feel each day? What might happen if an engineer had a lazy mind? Who is responsible if the bridge falls down? What kinds of activities require you to think and reason? Is it important to think and reason about your life plans? In deriving a name for this category, show a picture of a single pilot in a small plane. A suggested name might be "piloting yourself." Have the students describe a lifestyle in which one is self-piloted.

5. Show a picture of a drunk person. Appropriate discussion questions may include the following. Is this person in control of himself or herself? Should he or she be allowed to drive? What would you do if you saw this person get into a car and start to drive? Can you name some other ways in which people lose control of themselves? Did you ever know people who said that the devil was controlling them? Find a picture to demonstrate the devil as copilot. A suggested name might be "copilot takeover." Ask the students to describe a lifestyle that is piloted by someone other than the pilot.

Problem Solving

The purpose of the problem-solving activity is to have the students become acquainted with the difficulties associated with adopting a lifestyle in which one makes decisions and sets standards for oneself.

○ ☐ ☆

1. Create a problem (appropriate grade level) that requires a solution.
2. Have the students attempt a solution to the problem while role playing lazy pilot, glider pilot, lucky pilot, piloting yourself, and copilot takeover.
3. Discuss the difficulties each pilot has.
4. Model airplanes can be labeled and kept in the room for a while as reminders of various lifestyles.

Evaluation

LIFESTYLE CONTENT

☐ ☆

Have the students make a list of ten activities in which they have participated during the past week and indicate by letters whether it made them feel (a) happy, (b) brave, (c) self-loving, (d) important, (e) worthwhile, (f) useful, (g) significant, or (h) needed.

☐ ☆

Finally, have the students complete the following incomplete sentences:

When I am a lazy pilot, I feel _____ .
When I am a glider pilot, I feel _____ .
When I am a lucky pilot, I feel _____ .
When I pilot myself, I feel _____ .
When I have copilot takeover, I feel

_____ .

LIFESTYLE VALUE

○ □

Have the students either make their own airplanes by folding construction paper or each bring a model airplane from home. Ask the students to describe what they would like to be like in their flight through life by placing appropriate words on the two wings, the tail, and the nose of the airplanes.

UNIT II: FOLLOW YOUR FEELINGS

Almost all the pleasures and pains of life are deeply involved with our emotions and feelings. Thus, health and happiness cannot be separated from people's struggle to examine their feelings. In developing healthy, happy lifestyles, how do we learn to recognize, confront, and accept our feelings? Several suggestions are given in the lesson Follow Your Feelings.

OBJECTIVES

1. Through pantomimes and skits, the student will describe what it is like to concentrate while under the influence of one of the following feelings: fear, anger, hate, sorrow, love, excitement, loneliness, jealousy.

2. The student will express his or her feelings through an art activity and will later describe those feelings.

3. The student will describe the frequency of experiencing emotions after completing an emotion diary.

4. The student will be able to describe eight different emotions when participating in the emotion barometer activity.

5. Through the use of a happy-face ac-tivity and completion of statements, the student will express her or his feelings.

MATERIALS

1. Cardboard for the spin wheel.
2. Happy faces.

Methods

□ ☆

Have the students write examples of how each of the following emotions might cause a person to make a wrong decision: fear, anger, hate, love, sorrow, loneliness, excitement, jealousy.

○ □ ☆

Discuss with the class some of the following points and questions: why is it that the same experience may produce different feelings in different people? Why do you think that some people are more easily upset than others? What do people mean when they say "Control your feelings"? Is it better to control your feelings or to follow your feelings? What kinds of problems occur when you follow your feelings? What kinds of problems occur when you completely control your feelings? Think of five things that you value in life. What feelings can you identify as being related to these things? Give some examples of how changing what you value might change how you feel. Do you tend to like or dislike people who can control their feelings? How does following your emotions make you feel about yourself?

□ ☆

Ask students to pantomime a person following various feelings and have the class try to identify the feeling.

Other students can pantomime a student attempting to concentrate (study, read, paint) while under the influence of various feelings. Again, the class might attempt to identify the feeling. Following the pantomimes, discuss the concept of following feelings.

□ ☆

Have each student keep an emotion diary for one week. In their diary they should record the emotions they felt, what brought on each emotion, how long the emotion lasted, whether the emotion was good or bad for them, and what they did about it.

Evaluation

LIFESTYLE CONTENT

Construct an emotion barometer out of cardboard (or wood) with a spin wheel, as shown in the accompanying diagram.

○ □

Each student can have a chance to spin the barometer. When it lands on an emo-

tion, the student must describe what the emotion is like and present a situation in which she or he has experienced that emotion.

LIFESTYLE VALUE

○ □ ☆

Give each student ten happy faces and ask each one to write a few words on one of the faces to describe himself or herself when happy. Have the students turn the faces over and each draw a picture of what his or her face is like today. The faces can be shared with the class.

○ □

Ask the students to complete the following incomplete statements:

When I am happy _____ .
When I am sad _____ .
Today I am _____ .

The happy-face activity can be repeated ten different times, saving all the faces in a booklet. Ask the students to examine all ten faces and consider the questions How do our feelings change? Why aren't all the faces alike?

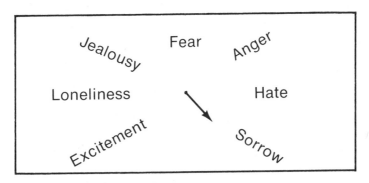

UNIT III: I'VE GOT TO BE ME

Why am I afraid to be me? Why am I afraid to tell you who I am? "I am afraid to tell you who I am, because, if I tell you who I am, you may not like who I am, and it's all I have" (5, p. 12).

The lesson I've Got To Be Me is designed to help young people identify who they are and share who they are proudly with their classmates. The acceptance of oneself is necessary in creating a lifestyle that is free of psychosomatic illnesses and in attaining self-actualization.

OBJECTIVES

1. Through the collage-advertisement activity, the students will identify things that they like about themselves.

2. After the mirror activity the students will be able to complete "I learned" statements about their self-images.

3. During What's in My Cup, the students will write down ten words each to describe themselves and will explain how they feel about each description.

4. Through making the Who Are You? bulletin board, the student will describe his or her uniqueness and learn to appreciate the uniqueness of others.

5. The student will express feelings about herself or himself by completing the winner-loser continuum.

MATERIALS

1. Magazines, glue, scissors, posterboard.
2. Large mirror.
3. Paper cup for each student.
4. Ink pad, student photographs.

Methods

○ □ ☆

Collage Advertisement

Have the students bring to class several magazines, glue, and scissors. Give each student a sheet of posterboard and ask the students to make posters to advertise themselves. After the students have completed their poster-collages, place them around the room and have the class guess what poster belongs to whom. Each student can explain his or her poster and can answer questions that other students might have. This activity helps students to know each other better and helps you as a teacher to identify positive reinforcements in your pupils.

○ □ ☆

Mirror

The mirror activity is aimed at examining the student's self-image. Obtain a full-length mirror. Have the students study themselves individually in the mirror for two to three minutes and write papers about what they see. The following starter questions are suggested,* but many more can be developed. Have you recently looked at yourself in a mirror? What did you see? Did you like what you saw? What changes would you make in your appearance? What do you like best and least about yourself? What bugs you the most about the way you behave? What could influence you the most to change? Who would you most like to pattern yourself after? In what way? Why?

○ □ ☆

Brown Bag

Have each student bring an important personal belonging in a paper bag.

*From a Columbus, Ohio, Youth Outreach Rap Session, January 1973.

("Fragile" might be written on bags with breakables.) The teacher should disclose one item at a time and ask the class to give possible reasons why someone might value the item. After each item is discussed, have the students claim their items and explain why they cherish them.

○ □

What's in My Cup?

Give each student a paper cup. Have the students each write on separate pieces of paper ten words to describe themselves and put the papers in their cups. Taking turns, each student can draw a word from her or his cup and describe how she or he feels about the description.

○ □

Who Are You?

Individuality can be emphasized by preparing a bulletin board display of photographs or drawings of students in the class, with names written underneath the pictures. Thumb prints on small pieces of paper can be attached next to the names.

□ ☆

Discussion Questions

Discuss the following questions with the students: what do you think is meant by the expression "Be yourself"? Have you ever noticed that some people completely change their behavior depending on who they are with? Why do you think they do this? Many people pretend that they are different from what they really are for short periods of time. Have you ever pretended this way? How did you feel while pretending? What are some factors that prevent young people from being what they want to be? List five of your favorite activities, then five of your least favorite activities. What are the major differences between these two groups? Do your favorite activities allow you to be more yourself than your least favorite ones? Do you think it is easier to be yourself when you are young or when you are older? Why?

Evaluation

LIFESTYLE CONTENT

□ ☆

Have each student write a paper called "How I Feel About Myself" or "What I Would Like to Be Like."

LIFESTYLE VALUE

□ ☆

Winner-Loser Continuum Have the students privately rate themselves along the following continua (5) after they ask themselves what they have accomplished and what their relationships are with others. One end of the continuum represents a person who is a loser, and the other, a person who is a winner.

How do you feel about yourself?
LOSER ＿＿＿＿＿＿＿＿＿＿WINNER
How do you feel about what you have accomplished in your life?
LOSER ＿＿＿＿＿＿＿＿＿＿WINNER
How do you feel about your relationships with others?
LOSER ＿＿＿＿＿＿＿＿＿＿WINNER

If the students are not satisfied with where they have placed themselves, ask them what they would like to change.

UNIT IV: COOPERATION AND COMPETITIVENESS

The elementary school affords the opportunity for building many skills and competencies. We see students discover many new words and meanings, examine numbers and configurations, dabble with paint, and sing new tunes. The things we learn to do build the foundation for a lifetime, yet life would be rather lonely with just these skills and few satisfying interpersonal relationships.

In the lesson Cooperation and Competitiveness, students examine one social skill—the ability to work with a group for the common good of all. The students will be able to see their reactions on a competitive-cooperative scale and will be able to evaluate whether they like what they see.

OBJECTIVES

1. After playing the Road Game, the student will be able to give three characteristics of cooperation.

2. After playing the Road Game, the student will be able to give three characteristics of competitiveness.

3. The students will describe whether they are cooperative or competitive in three situations and will say whether their behavior is what they would like it to be.

MATERIALS

1. Four large (approximately 2 × 2 feet) paper squares made of distinct colors, arranged as in the accompanying diagram.

Blue	Red
Yellow	Green

2. Four jars of tempera paint of the same four colors.

3. Four brushes, 1/2 to 1 inch wide.

4. Four dowel rods, each about 3 feet long.

5. One roll of masking tape.

6. Newspaper.

The masking tape is used to tape the paper squares together as shown in the diagram and is also used to tape the brush handles to the dowel rods so the students can paint while standing. The newspaper is placed under the colored paper to prevent spilling paint on the floor.

Methods

□ ☆

Divide the class into four equal groups and assign one colored square on the map to each group as its property. Each group is assigned a role to play, but these roles are to be kept secret from the other three groups.

Roles for the Road Game

Group 1—Members of group 1 are competitive and pushy and don't mind giving other people a shove to get them out of their way. They have had a hard life and need a lot of things. However, sometimes they have to be careful not to make people angry, because they find it is useful to be liked. Nevertheless, they'll do almost anything to get where they want to go.

Group 2—Members of group 2 are reasonable and try to respect the rights of others. They have found that often the best way to get what they want is to arrange things so that others get what they want. That seems to make them more willing to make concessions. Group 2 members feel that they get farther if they cooperate or swap, but they see the importance of persevering. They don't usually walk over other people but occasionally find it necessary.

Group 3—Members of group 3 are determined to accept their fate. They are primarily interested in thinking and dreaming, but as a group they know that survival can sometimes depend on concentrated activity. They worry about this need to go out into the world, because it conflicts with their ideas of being good and quiet and peaceful. They will have to be more inventive than other groups in order to get their goal by good and pure means. Like all people who try not to push others around, they can sometimes be pushed too far by others.

Group 4—Members of group 4 want to explore the whole world. They are very curious about things. They want to cover more ground than anyone else, but they don't always like to do things the way other people do. They don't always believe that the best road between two places is a straight line—they might miss something along the way. It's more fun to find out about things. They would like to do something great for the whole world, but, after all, they have to take care of themselves first.

Road Game Rules

After assigning the roles, the teacher reads the rules of the Road Game (2).

1. The object of the game is to build roads to the outside edge of the game squares. You build roads by painting lines on the game squares in the color of paint of your group's property. The group with the most roads at the end of the game is the winner.

2. You can build roads on your own property, but they will not count as roads at the end of the game.

3. Each road must begin at a point on your own property and arrive at the outside edge of the game squares on some other group's property in order to count.

4. You are permitted to speak freely within your own group but are to address other groups only through your leader.

5. You must receive permission from a group before you can enter its property to build a road. This must be obtained *each time* you build a road.

6. You must receive permission *each time* you wish to cross another *group's road* even in your own property.

7. Permission is obtained through a group's leader. This leader, however, must have unanimous approval from the group before giving permission. If one member of a group does not wish to give permission, the leader may not give it.

8. There will be a time limit for the game, but you will not know what it is. The game can end at any time.

9. The leaders do not paint roads.

The game then begins without intervention by the teacher. The game should be limited to ten to fifteen minutes. After the game is ended, the teacher declares one group the winner by counting the number of roads. The groups are given a chance to appeal the teacher's decision based on the various interpretations of the game's rules.

Discussion Questions

Discuss the following questions with the game participants: how could everyone have cooperated rather than competed for territory? How did you pick your leader? Did you vote? Did the leader just happen? Why? Why did you get so excited? It was only a game! Did you stick to the personality that you were assigned? Was it difficult? What happened to the way you behaved? (Students often drop the

63

personality but like to discuss why.) Can you guess what personality the other groups were assigned?

Evaluation

LIFESTYLE CONTENT

☐ ☆

Have each student write "Cooperation" on one side of a sheet of paper and "Competitiveness" on the other. As the students share their papers with their group, they can say three things about cooperation and three things about competitiveness.

LIFESTYLE VALUE

☐ ☆

Ask the students to consider the following:

1. The Road Game
2. What I Am Usually Like
3. What I Would Like to Be Like

Which statement would characterize their behavior in each of the above situations?

1. I cooperate with others and compete when necessary. When I compete, I treat others fairly.

2. I cooperate with others and do not compete even when necessary. I allow others to influence me to cooperate at my expense.

3. I compete with others and cooperate when necessary. I cooperate when it is to my advantage.

4. I compete with others and do not cooperate. I see cooperation as hurting my chances of making myself first or best.

Do students think they should be the same in each situation?

REFERENCES

1. *Inside/Out: A Guide for Teachers* 1973.

2. Thomas E. Linehan and Barbara Ellis Long, *The Road Game* (New York: Herder and Herder, 1970). Used by permission of the publisher, The Seabury Press, Inc.

3. James Muriel and Dorothy Jongeward, *Born to Win* (Reading, Mass.: Addison-Wesley, 1971).

4. Herbert A. Otto, *Human Potentialities* (St. Louis: Warren H. Green, 1968).

5. John S. J. Powell, *Why Am I Afraid To Tell You Who I Am?* (Niles, Ill.: Argus Communications, 1969).

6. *Self-Incorporated*, 1975.

CHAPTER 6

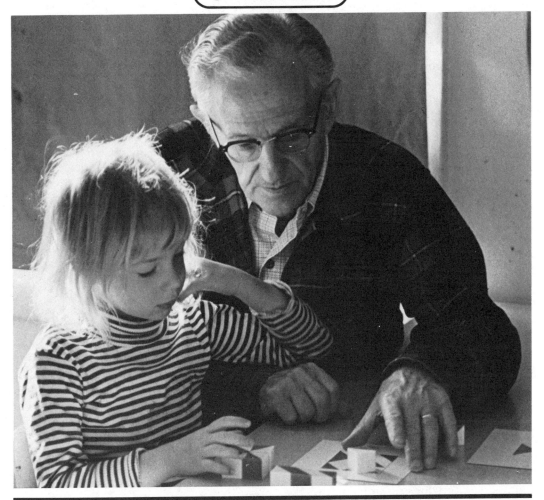

PART A: FAMILY LIFE EDUCATION INCLUDING DIVORCE, AGING, AND DEATH

This chapter is designed to provide the factual information required to teach about interpersonal relationships and family life in the elementary school. A major portion of the chapter, however, is devoted to sex education because of the large body of factual information required. Other parts of family life education (e.g., divorce and death) receive less emphasis, but in Chapter 6B these topics are treated in more detail. This arrangement stems from the fact that the latter topics require more creative teaching skills and less factual information.

SEX EDUCATION IN THE ELEMENTARY SCHOOLS

If strangers to our world observed the interactions of adults and children, they might deduce the following as a categorical imperative among adult human beings:

The existence of human sexuality is a classified secret that shall not be revealed to children, and if the secret should be accidentally uncovered, it is essential that it always be relegated to the realm of the negative.

This perspective of childhood as an "age of innocence" or of children living in a nonsexual society has resulted in child-rearing practices that have generally excluded sex education in the home and rendered it very difficult in the school setting.

It is very important that the elementary teacher recognize the basic opposition to sex education in the schools. On the one hand, society suggests that sexuality does not exist in the world of the child; while, on the other hand, sex education suggests not only that sexuality exists but also that it is good when used responsibly. Thus, a major conflict exists.

Chapter 6B includes suggestions for gaining support for sex education in the elementary school and methods and materials to implement the program. The present chapter is limited to the factual material that provides the foundation for elementary sex education.

MALE GROWTH AND DEVELOPMENT

About the seventh or eighth week of prenatal life, a special group of cells known as *testes* develop in male infants. Initially, the testes develop inside the body. Then during the eighth or ninth month of fetal life they slowly descend through a tunnel-like passageway to the outside of the body.

At birth, the male usually has two testes located outside the body and in the scrotum. In rare cases in which the testes do not normally descend, medical assistance may be required to locate them in the scrotum. Descent of the testes is important to male reproduction, because the temperature inside the body is too high for the testes to function normally. Thus, sperm cannot be produced at body temperature. Outside the body, however, the saclike structure (scrotum) that contains the testes is a few degrees below normal body temperature. In this environment sperm are readily produced.

The scrotum has two mechanisms for regulating the temperature of the testes. First, it has many sweat glands and sweats freely in a warm environment. Secondly, the scrotum contains muscles that contract and relax to raise or lower the testes. These muscles relax to lower the testes away from the body on a warm day. Conversely, they contract to raise the testes closer to the body, and thus increase their temperature, on a cold day.

The testes begin their function of producing male sex hormones and sperm when a boy is approximately ten years of age. At first, they produce only testosterone, a very powerful hormonal substance, which is released into the blood and proceeds to circulate to all parts of the body. This hormone causes the following extensive changes in the male body:

1. Growth and enlargement of the entire male reproductive system.

2. Development of longer vocal cords resulting in a deeper voice.

3. Development of pubic, facial, and other body hair.

4. Growth of muscles.

5. Development of sex drive.

6. Closure of the growing ends of long bones.

7. Development, in later life, of baldness, if there is a genetic potential for this condition.

In addition to hormonal production, the testes begin to produce sperm when a boy is approximately twelve or thirteen years of age, thus making him physiologically capable of reproduction.

Search for Sexual Identity

As the male continues to grow and develop, he becomes more and more psychologically involved with his sexual identity. In the past each male was left to work out the problems of sexual identity on his own or with others of the same age, but the problems were seldom discussed with adults. This situation has improved somewhat in recent years, and perhaps the time is not too far off when every male child will have a chance to discuss such topics as erection, ejaculation, masturbation, nocturnal emission, sex drive, sexual orientation, and concerns about the size and shape of the reproductive system, with a knowledgeable and understanding person. Female children should also have access to this information about male sexuality.

The following basic facts regarding male sexuality should be communicated to all elementary students:

1. The male reproductive role consists of producing sperm and assisting them to reach the female egg. This role involves two biological reactions known as (a) *erection* and (b) *ejaculation*.

a. Male erection may result from either psychological or physical stimuli. These stimuli cause blood to flow in and fill small compartments in the penis (erectile tissue). When these compartments are filled, the male penis becomes erect, and enables the male to deposit sperm safely inside the female body.

b. Ejaculation is the release of sperm by the male. The ejaculated material is called semen and contains sperm and substances to protect and nourish sperm during their trip to fertilize an egg.

2. Masturbation is a harmless and pleasurable act participated in by most males as a part of their normal sexual lifestyle. At one time in history, masturbation was thought to be a cause of mental illness, poor vision, and poor sexual adjustment; however, these beliefs have no scientific basis.

3. Nocturnal emission is a normal release of sperm or ejaculation during sleep that is experienced by approximately 90 percent of all males at least once and usually more often. It is almost always accompanied by dreams, but the dreamer often awakens in the process. Nocturnal orgasm is an entirely normal but involuntary mechanism that does not indicate any abnormality in mental, physical, or moral health.

4. Sex drive is one of several motivations that prompt males into pleasure-seeking behavior. The drive is partly hormonal and partly psychological and may move the male toward any of several sexual outlets, including exploiting others in an attempt to satisfy the drive. One of the major problems of sexuality stems from the fact that the sex drive is very high at a time when humans are least prepared for a sexual relationship, the teenage years. However, the feelings are normal and healthy.

5. Males may exhibit a sexual orientation in which they are attracted to females, other males, or both. Males who

feel sexually attracted toward females are known as *heterosexuals*. Males who feel sexually attracted toward other males are known as *homosexuals*. In general, less than 10 percent of all males are homosexual, but the fact that they represent a minority does not mean that they are physically or psychologically abnormal.

At the present time, the cause of homosexuality is unknown. Further, an attraction toward persons of the same sex is involuntary. Thus, making fun of homosexuals is a very unkind practice. Given different parents and a different childhood experience, any of us might have developed a different sexual orientation.

6. There is a considerable variety in the size and shape of the male reproductive system, but these differences are not significant in male sexual functioning.

Many male children worry excessively about the size of their penis. This situation is often further complicated by unkind and uninformed comments from peers.

For these reasons, all males should be informed at an early age that the size of the penis makes no difference in any aspect of the male sexual role, especially in sex and reproduction. It is tragic that so many males suffer unnecessarily because they never were afforded an opportunity to acquire this information.

FEMALE GROWTH AND DEVELOPMENT

About the tenth or eleventh week of prenatal life, a special group of cells known as *ovaries* develop in female infants. Two in number, the ovaries develop and remain inside the body.

The ovary resembles an almond in shape and is about 1½ inches long and 1 inch wide. The ovaries produce ova and hormones.

Between the ages of eleven and fourteen the ovaries stimulate development of the secondary sex characteristics in the female by releasing estrogen into the blood. This hormone circulates to many different groups of cells resulting in:

1. Enlargement of the breasts
2. Broadening of the pelvis
3. Development of soft, smooth skin
4. Deposition of fat in buttocks and thighs
5. Development of pubic and axillary hair
6. Closure of the growing ends of long bones

The Menstrual Cycle

In addition to hormonal production, the ovaries now begin to produce eggs. These eggs are produced from small sac- or podlike structures, known as *primary follicles*, that are contained in the ovaries at birth.

Beginning at puberty, a number of these primary follicles start to grow and develop at the beginning of each menstrual cycle. Ordinarily, one of these reaches full maturity midway through the cycle. This fully mature follicle is known as the *Graafian follicle*. All the other follicles degenerate. Thus, the ovary rejects several immature follicles each cycle.

The Graafian follicle contains the female egg, which is released near the middle of the cycle. This release is known as *ovulation*. The newly released egg is very fragile and requires special protection. In addition, it must be fertilized during the first twelve to twenty-four hours after it is released in order to develop into a baby.

Usually, the egg that is released from the ovary enters a long tube immediately adjacent to the ovary. These two tubes, one for each ovary, are known as the *right* and *left Fallopian tubes.*

After ovulation, the egg enters one end of the Fallopian tube and the sperm moves up the other end. The egg and sperm meet in the Fallopian tube and fertilization takes place.

A fertilized egg requires a safe place to grow and develop. Nature has provided such a location inside the female body. It is known as the *uterus.* Once an egg has been fertilized it moves down the Fallopian tube and into the uterus, where it implants itself in the lining and continues to grow. This process is known as *pregnancy.*

Approximately nine months after fertilization a fully developed baby emerges from the uterus and is delivered through a canal-like passageway known as the *vagina.*

Each month the uterus prepares itself to receive a fertilized egg. These preparations include development of a specialized lining for the inside of the uterus. This lining includes a rich blood supply and special secreting glands.

There is a highly sophisticated communication system between the ovaries and the uterus. At the beginning of each cycle, the ovaries signal the uterus to prepare its special lining. It accomplishes this through a chemical signal that travels from the ovaries through the blood to the uterus. The chemical messenger is known as *estrogen.* This substance is produced by the follicles that start to grow in the ovaries at the beginning of each cycle. Thus, the first phase of each menstrual cycle is known as the *estrogen phase.* This is a time of rapid growth in the lining of the uterus.

To receive the fertilized egg, one additional preparation is necessary: the lining of the uterus must secrete enough nutritious fluid to sustain the fertilized egg until it can implant itself. Thus, the second phase of the normal menstrual cycle is known as the *secreting phase.*

This phase is initiated by the release of a second hormonal substance from the ovary. Known as *progesterone,* this hormone is produced by the same structure that released the egg at the time of ovulation. Before ovulation this structure is known as the *Graafian follicle.* When it releases its egg, the remaining podlike structure continues to grow within the ovary. Known as the *corpus luteum,* this structure finally secretes progesterone.

Working together, estrogen and progesterone support the preparations for pregnancy that occur during the second phase of the menstrual cycle. Due to the addition of progesterone, this phase of the cycle is also known as the *progesterone phase.*

In the final phase of the menstrual cycle, there are two options. If the egg is fertilized, the work accomplished during the first two preparatory phases continues and supports pregnancy. If conception does not occur, the growth and development that occurred in the uterus during the early part of the cycle undergoes a self-destructive process.

In the absence of fertilization, the ovary stops secreting estrogen and progesterone. This results in a shutdown of the blood supply to the lining of the uterus. In turn, the lining of the uterus dies, and, together with a small quantity of blood, it is released as the menstrual flow. Accordingly, this phase is termed *menstruation.*

During menstruation, the female places an absorbent material inside or at the entrance of the vagina to collect the menstrual flow.

The uterus begins to develop a new lining, and bleeding stops about five days after the onset of menstruation. This is the end of the three-phase female cycle.

Search for Sexual Identity

As the female child continues to grow and develop physically, she, like the male, initiates a search for sexual identity. This search may be facilitated by a clear understanding of the following basic facts regarding female sexuality.

1. The female reproductive role consists of producing an egg, accommodating that egg during fertilization and implantation, supporting the fetus during pregnancy, and delivering a new individual.

During sexual intercourse sperm are deposited near the female's cervix, where they enter and travel through the uterus and enter the Fallopian tubes. The ultimate fertilization of an egg occurs in the upper portion of the Fallopian tube.

The moment at which an egg is fertilized by a sperm is termed *conception*. At this time all hereditary characteristics are established, including the sex of the unborn child.

It is always the sperm that determines whether the fetus is to be male or female. If a male-producing sperm fertilizes the egg, the new baby will be a boy. A girl results when the egg is fertilized by a female-producing sperm.

Fertilization usually occurs in the Fallopian tube. After conception, the fertilized egg takes three or four days to travel down to the uterus. Once inside the uterus, it spends an additional two to five days locating a proper place to implant itself. Just as a seed must be planted in good soil if it is to grow, a human egg must be planted if it is to produce a new individual. The only difference is that a human fertilized egg has no one to plant it; thus, it must plant itself. It is thought that the human egg digs a little tunnel for itself (possibly by releasing a chemical) and thereby attaches itself to the lining of the uterus.

The connection between mother and baby (somewhat like the roots of a plant) is known as the *placenta*. During pregnancy, the placenta supplies nutrition to the fetus and removes waste material. As the fetus grows and develops, the uterus enlarges to accommodate the size of the growing baby, which may reach seven to nine pounds. After approximately nine months, the lower end of the uterus opens and the baby is delivered through the vagina.

2. Masturbation is a harmless and pleasurable act participated in by most females as a part of their normal sexual lifestyle. Masturbation does not produce any acute or long-range health maladies in the female.

3. The female does not experience an ejaculation during sexual intercourse as does the male. Sexual orgasm in the female consists of a series of rapid muscular contractions that are very pleasurable, but there is no emission of fluids as in ejaculation. Sexual orgasm may occur as a consequence of sexual intercourse, masturbation, psychological stimulation, or dreaming. In each case, the final response is the same.

4. Sex drive exists in the female and is both hormonal and psychological in origin. At one time in history it was thought that the male had a far greater sexual drive than the female and that the female was mainly a passive partner. However,

recent research suggests that in the absence of strong social conditioning against the expression of sexual feelings, the female also exhibits a strong sexual drive.

5. Females may exhibit a sexual orientation in which they are attracted to males, other females, or both. Females who have an affectional preference for males are heterosexuals. Females who have an affectional preference for other females are homosexuals.

In general, female homosexuality is more widely accepted than male homosexuality. Nevertheless, the female homosexual is often the object of deeply hurting remarks, and it is very important that everyone realize that given other parents and a different early background, any of us might have developed a different sexual orientation.

6. There is considerable variety in the size and shape of the female breast, but these differences are not significant in female sexual functioning. The size of breasts is genetically and hormonally determined and little can be done to alter their size except through surgery. Silicone injections are not generally recommended.

CONTRACEPTION

A common mistake in sex education is the introduction of too much information at too early an age. On the other hand, it is important for elementary level students to understand certain basics without going into any real depth. One such topic is contraception.

The topic probably requires only the following factual information.

1. Conception is the fertilization of an egg. Contraception is the prevention of fertilization and is a concept that should be introduced in elementary school.

2. Today, pregnancy is avoided by couples not wishing to have children through a wide range of contraceptive techniques. These include:

   a. taking pills to avoid production of eggs,

   b. use of a variety of methods to prevent the egg and sperm from coming together,

   c. surgery to block off the roads that sperm or eggs must travel.

3. People who want to limit the number of children they have or who do not want to have children must select and learn to use some form of contraception. This is the responsibility of both the male and female.

DIVORCE: A SPECIAL CONSIDERATION

Why Teach About Divorce?

With the number of divorces that are currently taking place in our country, children will invariably be exposed to divorce in one form or another. Many will have parents who are divorced; others may have brothers or sisters who are divorced; and still others may have friends with divorced parents. No matter how children come into contact with divorce, they will need to deal with it both emotionally and cognitively. Educating about divorce will help children deal with current problems and situations as well as future encounters with divorce.

Discussion Topics

One of the major topics to be covered in class is "What is divorce?" Once the teacher makes it clear to the students what divorce is, a number of other subjects should be addressed. Some of these subjects are:

1. How many people are getting divorced.

2. Why people divorce.

3. Emotional reactions a child might have to divorce.

4. What a child can do to help the situation.

5. Where people go to get help with their family problems.

6. How parents might act during divorce.

How Many People Are Getting Divorced It may be easier for children to adjust to divorce if they understand that divorce is not uncommon and is probably affecting many friends (10). The teacher can make this point by presenting some basic statistics concerning divorce or perhaps by just asking the children how many of them know someone who is divorced.

Why People Divorce This is a major question for children. It is best to explain to children that people divorce for many different reasons, but basically, they just are not able to get along with one another well and are no longer happy together. The teacher should point out that everyone makes mistakes, and adults are no exception. Divorce is an attempt to correct a mistake (6). It is important for children to realize that divorce is not the fault of children. Many children feel guilty when divorce happens, thinking that in some way they have contributed to their parents' unhappiness (10). The teacher should stress that divorce is a problem between parents and is not caused by the children.

Emotional Reactions A Child Might Have To Divorce Some children may be willing to comment on their reactions to their parents' divorce or perhaps how friends

acted when their parents divorced. Children should realize that it is normal to feel great sadness and that crying is also normal and should even be encouraged if the child feels like crying. At the first news of the divorce, children are usually surprised, even though they might have known that parents were unhappy together. Later the child may feel frightened or angry at the parents for getting a divorce. Many times, children are told to "be brave" when it would be better for them to show their feelings. Besides some of the reactions mentioned previously, other feelings might occur. Often children feel nervous or tense; they may worry a great deal and feel confused. Fear of being abandoned is also common (10). These reactions and others should be brought out by the teacher and children in class so that the children realize typical reactions to divorce.

What a Child Can Do to Help Mention should be made of problems that people cannot handle on their own. Often the family situation is very confused or family members are having difficulty dealing with their own emotions or communicating well. Professional people can be a help to families in times of crises such as divorces (10). The teacher should mention psychiatrists, psychologists, marriage counselors, and family counselors, so that the children will know the type of help that is available. In addition, the teacher could specify that local agencies offer counseling services.

How Parents Might Act During Divorce A relevant topic for the classroom discussion is how parents often react to divorce and how they might act toward their children during this difficult time. The teacher can point out that children need to be very understanding of parents' feelings and actions, because parents are often preoccupied with their problems.

Some children have to face more difficult problems than a divorce in which both parents are concerned about the children. It may be carefully explained that some parents have so many problems of their own that they are simply not ready to be parents and thus act in ways that hurt their children very much. Examples of this are parents who abuse their children (10). The main focus of the talk about this sensitive topic could be on the child's feelings about being abused, but the discussion could also relate to understanding that the parent who has been unkind or harsh has a problem and needs help (10). If it becomes obvious that an absent parent simply does not care for his or her family and will not share responsibility for the family, it is best for the children to try to accept that fact and turn to other persons who will care for them (1, pp. 66–68).

Additional topics that the teacher may wish to address are visitation by a divorced parent and dealing with new family combinations that might occur as a result of the divorce or as a result of a parent's remarrying.

AGING: A SPECIAL CONSIDERATION

There appears to be a definite need in elementary school for education about the elderly and the aging process. The current generation has less contact with the elderly than previous generations due to the breakdown of the extended family. On the whole, the current generation is generally uneducated about aging (4, pp. 37–38). Martha John has listed a number of specific reasons for learning about the elderly:

a. It seems important for children to learn that warm, sensitive relationships can span generations.

b. Children need to see old age as a part of the total life cycle.

c. Learning about aging can help students face this [phenomenon] more realistically.

d. It seems important, also, for children to learn about the contributions the older age group makes to our society.

e. Studying about the elderly can give the student a more positive picture of the total life span that will hopefully be available to him or her.

f. The elderly frequently demonstrate values and ideals that have survived the tests of time (9, pp. 524–27).

Attitudes and Knowledge of Children About Aging and the Elderly

In order to be able to teach about aging, it is important for the teacher to understand what children know about aging and how they view the elderly, as well as how they view their own aging process. The results of a study conducted by Jantz and others (8, pp. 518–23) are relevant here. Children six and older did understand who "older people" were in our society. Children below the fourth grade, however, were not accurate in identifying an older person's age. Younger children tended to confuse age with size, for instance, believing that larger people were older and that people of the same size were the same age. Younger children did not realize that aging is continuous and relates to birth dates. Concepts of age became more accurate as the child grew older. Children's attitudes toward the elderly tended to be mixed, consisting of positive feelings of affect and negative feelings about the physical aspects of age. Most of the children did not perceive being old as positive.

When questioned about their activities with elderly persons, children in the Jantz study revealed that they had very few contacts with the elderly outside their own families. Additionally, passive activities were associated with the elderly while active involvements were associated with younger persons. Finally, most children did not perceive as positive their own aging process or the aging process in general.

Discussion Topics

Aging can be more effectively taught by teachers who have examined their own feelings about aging and are able to accept their own aging process. In addition, it is important to look at the ways in which the school influences attitudes toward aging by surveying educational materials to be certain that they do not show the elderly as a stereotyped group (12, pp. 70–73).

A number of topics concerning the elderly are relevant to the elementary school child (13, pp. 13–16). From kindergarten through grade three, the class might consider just what is *old* and what it means to be old. An examination of how it feels to be lonely is relevant to children, followed by a discussion of loneliness as related to the elderly. Elementary children are generally interested in how to help an older person. Such points as how to call for help in an emergency and an emphasis on making the home safe for the elderly by keeping toys out of the way are important to emphasize with younger children. In addition, children will benefit from a discussion of discrimination against the elderly in jobs and in the attitudes of the public. Young children can be informed of the numerous services (such as foster grandparent programs, senior student aides, and volunteer work) that are performed by the elderly. Finally, the teacher may focus on communication with grandparents or other older persons who have hearing or vision problems.

In grades four through six, the problems and concerns of aging may be dealt with in more detail. Health problems that affect communication, sensitivity, and mobility are a concern of the elderly and may be discussed with older children. This age level is capable of understanding about special diets for diabetes, low cholesterol, hypoglycemia (low blood glucose), obesity, and low sodium. Some general statistics about the elderly, such as the number nationwide and locally, may also be introduced. Many children have grandparents living in their homes. The contributions of the grandparents to the home should be outlined, as well as their social, spiritual, and financial needs. The children will also benefit from a discussion of how to show that they care about older persons. Emergency care may be elaborated on more with the older children than with the younger children. Fatigue and physical changes in the bones, muscles, hair, and digestion may be examined, as well as disorders affecting the vision, hearing, smell, taste, balance, touch, and speech. Other relevant topics for older children include preventive health measures, lifetime physical fitness, transportation services for the elderly, and available economic services (social security, medicaid, and medicare basics).

Goals of Education About Aging

Some basic goals for the teacher in teaching children about aging have been enumerated by Jantz and his coworkers (8, pp. 518–23). These goals are as follows:

a. to provide accurate information. about the elderly so that children will form positive realistic concepts and attitudes toward older people.

b. to enable children to assess their perceptions of the aging process and how aging will affect them.

c. to expose children to an unbiased look at the attributes, behaviors, and characteristics of the elderly in a wide variety of roles.

DEATH: A SPECIAL CONSIDERATION

The subject of death is important to the proper development and education of elementary schoolchildren. There are a number of reasons for discussing death with children. Some might argue that children are too young to understand about death; however, children do have some conception of death at least as early as age two. Children have definite ideas about death, which affect their emotional, psychological, and intellectual development. In addition, a child's own death or the death of a loved one is always a possibility. Furthermore, the death of a loved one should not be a child's first experience with having to discuss death (2).

Many elementary school teachers have a tendency to avoid the topic of death in the classroom, because they cannot fully comprehend the meaning of death themselves or simply because they have their own personal fears and anxieties about the subject. However, most elementary school teachers are capable of becoming competent in teaching about death. Bensley listed the following qualities necessary for a teacher in teaching about death:

a. The teacher must have come to terms with his or her own feelings, and to have admitted not only its existence, but to its full status in the dynamics of his total personality functioning.

b. The teacher needs to know about death and death education in order to teach it.

c. The teacher of death education needs to be able to use the language of death easily and naturally, especially in the presence of the young.

d. The teacher needs to be familiar with the sequence of developmental events throughout life, and to have a sympathetic understanding of common problems associated with them.

e. The teacher needs acute awareness of the enormous social changes that are in progress and their implications for changes in our patterns of death-related attitudes, practices, laws and institutions (2, p. 4).

How Children View Death

Maria Nagy reports that from three to five, children may see death as a type of departure or sleep and deny death as a final process (11). Between five and nine, it is thought that children may accept the idea of death, but not necessarily the fact that death is inevitable. Not until nine or ten is death recognized as an inevitable part of life that applies to all living organisms, including children themselves.

Nagy's results are helpful in obtaining an overall picture of how children view death, but this outline may overlook the influences of the child's experiences, life concerns, and self-concept. Myra Bluebond-Langner asserts that all views of death (death as separation, the result of intervention by a supernatural being, an irreversible biological process) are present at all stages of a child's development, but that the particular view the child displays at a specific time reflects his/her psychological and intellectual experiences at that time (3).

There is a great deal of debate concerning what concepts of death can be understood at a given age. This is probably due to the fact that children differ to a great extent in behavior, development, and environment (5, pp. 27–29). The most important point for the teacher to remember is that each child should be considered as an individual, each with his or her own view of death.

Topics for Discussion

Death-related places and events that are familiar to the children can be used by the teacher to introduce relevant concepts. The death of a pet, the life cycle of plants, a news report of a plane crash, a bomb scare, funerals, and cemeteries are all examples of places and events that can be used to initiate discussion of death (5, pp. 27–29).

Discussion topics could include questions that are often in the minds of children (7).

a. What is death?
b. What makes people die?
c. What happens when people die; where do they go?

Talk might also focus on the children's opinions about appropriate behavior at the time of death. For instance:

a. Should one cry?
b. Should one be buried or cremated?
c. What would you want for yourself or a loved one?
d. How do people feel and act when a loved one dies?

Talking to Children About Death

The manner in which the teacher relays information about death to the children is just as important as the information itself. If the teacher is not relaxed and at ease in discussing death, it may contribute to the development of fears and anxieties in the children (7).

There are a number of positive points that should be communicated, as well as some things that the teacher should not say. The child does not need a lot of details, but should always be told the truth. It is not good to tell stories and fairy tales about death. In the factual explanation of death, it should be made clear that with death life stops, that a dead person (or pet) will not return, and that the body will be buried or cremated. Every attempt should be made to establish an atmosphere in the classroom in which the children will feel free to express themselves (7).

Children often believe that by wishing someone dead, they may have caused the death of that person (3). By focusing on this point, the teacher can correct this mistaken idea.

Grollman (7) has outlined some explanations of death that are considered unhealthy and should be avoided by the teacher:

1. The dead person has gone on a long journey (the child might expect the person to return)

2. God took the loved one away because he wants the good in heaven (child might be afraid that all who were good would die)

3. The person died due to sickness (child might equate all sickness with death)

4. To die is to sleep (child might be afraid to sleep).

REFERENCES

1. Louise B. Ames, "Children and Divorce: What the Teacher Can Do," *Instructor* 79 (August/September 1969).

2. Loren B. Bensley, *Death Education as*

a *Learning Experience* (Washington, D.C.: ERIC Clearing House on Teacher Education, November 1975).

3. Myra Bluebond-Langner, "Meanings of Death to Children," *New Meanings of Death*, Herman Feifel, ed. (New York: McGraw-Hill, 1977).

4. Kenneth A. Briggs, "Aging: A Need for Sensitivity," *Health Education* (September/October 1977).

5. Marianne G. Everett, "Helping Parents Teach About Death," *Health Education* 7 (July/August 1976).

6. Earl A. Grollman, ed., *Explaining Divorce to Children* (Boston: Beacon, 1969).

7. Earl A. Grollman, *Explaining Death to Children* (Boston: Beacon, 1967).

8. Richard K. Jantz, et al., "Children's Attitudes Toward the Elderly," *Social Education* 41 (October, 1977).

9. Martha T. John, "Teaching Children About Older Family Members," *Social Education* (October 1977).

10. Eda LeShan, *What's Going to Happen to Me?* (New York: Four Winds, 1978).

11. Maria H. Nagy, "The Child's View of Death," *The Meaning of Death*, Herman Fiefel, ed. (New York: McGraw-Hill, 1959).

12. Kathy Serock, et al., "As Children See Old Folks," *Today's Education* 66 (March-April 1977).

13. James Terhune, "About Aging and Death," *Health Education* (November/December 1977).

PART B: TEACHING ABOUT INTERPERSONAL RELATIONSHIPS AND FAMILY LIFE EDUCATION INCLUDING DEATH AND DIVORCE

Family life education is education for love.

"Love," says Erich Fromm, "is the only satisfactory answer to the problem of human existence. Yet, most of us are unable to develop our capacities for love on the only level that really counts—a love that is compounded of maturity, self-knowledge, and courage. Learning to love, like other arts, demands practice and concentration. Even more than any other art, it demands genuine insight and understanding (3, p. 3).

Dr. Fromm mentions four skills needed to enhance love:

1. Labor: being willing to work and give of oneself for person(s) one loves.

2. Responsibility: evaluating the consequences of one's behavior as it relates to others and being prepared to help when needed.

3. Respect: refraining from exploiting others.

4. Understanding: trying to place oneself in the shoes of another.

Thus, family life education is education for and about love, and its main goal is to enrich one's life through meaningful interpersonal relationships.

It also helps children to understand breakdowns in communication, problems in living, and divorce. The term family life education is an accurate description for this kind of education. Why? Because the family is the best single source for the giving and receiving of love. The family survives on love, grows on love, and perpetuates itself through love.

This last phrase, "perpetuates itself," explains the *life* in family life education, which brings in another aspect of loving—the creation of new life. The life aspect of family life education includes information on the life cycle, sexuality, reproductive processes, and death. Children need information and understanding of this aspect of family life education in order to understand themselves and others.

Thus, family life education in the elementary school includes two broad aspects:

1. Education for and about love and close interpersonal relationships, breakdowns in relationships, and divorce.
2. Education about the life cycle including birth, growth, reproduction, aging, and death.

Children's future lifestyle has the greatest potential to be happy and self-actualizing if the family life education teaching plan considers the following needs of elementary schoolchildren:

1. Students need to be self-loving and have a feeling of worth (see Chapter 5B).
2. Students need to accept their bodies and to recognize individual differences in growth and maturation.
3. Students need to know where they come from, how life begins, and when life ends.
4. Students need to assume responsibilities within the family unit and develop respect for family members.
5. Students need to learn to form good friendships and to value the traits found in good friends.
6. Students need to appreciate the differences between boys and girls and yet not form stereotypes in role expectations.
7. Students need to recognize the function that marriage fills in our society.
8. Students need to examine breakdowns in communication and to examine divorce as a possible solution.

UNIT I: MY FAMILY

The family has the greatest impact on a child's life before and during elementary school. From the family, the child learns to relate to others, develops a concept of love, and forms an impression of what male and female roles are supposed to be.

A lesson on the family assists the teacher in helping children select a healthy lifestyle in two ways. First, it affords an opportunity for children to communicate information about their family to the teacher. The teacher will gain valuable information that may help in relating to the children throughout the year.

Second, the lesson on family helps children see that all families are not just like theirs. Through sharing activities, students will see that families have different lifestyles. Although many years will pass before the students will form their own families, the early appreciation of

Appropriate grade levels are suggested for each teaching strategy and appear as ○, □, ☆, in the left-hand column:

  ○ = most suited for the primary grades;
  □ = most suited for the intermediate grades;
  ☆ = most suited for the upper elementary grades.

family differences may help students more easily accept and adjust to differences in later years.

OBJECTIVES

1. After making a family album, students will describe what each person in their family does through "I learned" statements.
2. Students will describe different roles of parents.
3. Students will describe ways that they can help their family.
4. Students will make a poster or collage of a new family member that illustrates why new babies need so much attention.
5. Students will express their desire for compatible family relationships through role play.
6. Students will examine the household responsibilities of each family member by making a checklist to discuss with their family.
7. Students will examine ten things they love to do with their family.

MATERIALS

1. Leather or cardboard, yarn, manila filler paper.
2. Poster paper.
3. The book or record *Free to Be You and Me.*

Methods

○ □

For this unit, the students will make a family album (2).

Have the students design the cover on their cardboard or leather and title the album *Our Family.* Then they will punch holes in the cover and filler paper and bind the book with yarn. Each insert or manila sheet in the album can be a lesson. Many ideas about the roles of family members, the work and fun of the family, and family relationships can be discussed.

Each time that there is an insert to the album, offer an alternative activity. For example, if the topic is "Father," you might also use "My Favorite Man." This will be helpful to students who do not have a father. Other alternatives can be used for different inserts.

Below are some suggested inserts for the albums and questions to use for discussion.

Father at Work What do you like best about your father? Why does your father work? What kind of work does your father do? How can you help your father? What kind of work does your father do at home?

Mother at Work What do you like best about your mother? Does your mother work? What kind of work does your mother do? What kind of work does your mother do at home? How can you help your mother?

My Parents After the students have drawn the insert about father and mother, discuss the role of parents in the family. This would be a good time to read the poem "Parents Are People" from the book, *Free to Be You and Me* (9, p. 48), or play the *Free to Be You and Me* record.

My Brother and I Do you have a brother? Is your brother bigger or smaller than you? What kinds of things does your brother like to do? What have you learned from your big brother? Have you ever helped your little brother learn to do new things? What do you like best about your brother?

My Sister and I Do you have a sister? Is your sister bigger or smaller than you? What kinds of things does your sister like to do? What have you learned from your big sister? Have you ever helped your little sister do new things? What do you like best about your sister?

A New Family Member For the discussion of a new family member, bring a baby doll to class. Other materials necessary: diapers, safety pins, powder, wash cloth, towel, small tub, soap, baby bottle. As you discuss helping mother with the baby, you can show the children how to change the diapers. Emphasis should be placed on helping the new family member: Do any of you have a baby in your family? Is the baby a boy or a girl? What "special" things do mothers and fathers have to do for babies? Do mothers and fathers sometimes have to spend a lot of time with the baby? Why? What things do you like to do for the baby? Why does a baby need older brothers and sisters?

Our Family Works Together Arrange to have two empty bulletin boards, one for the boys and one for the girls. Have the boys look through magazines, cutting out picture examples of the work that they, their brothers, and fathers do around the house. They can also bring things from home. Have the girls look through magazines, cutting out picture examples of the work that they, their sisters, and mothers do around the house. They can also bring things from home. Do the bulletin boards look about the same?

Have the students draw a picture for the family album of the family working together with the title *Being Helpful*.

Sharing Have the students draw a pic-

ture of their family sharing something special, good or bad, together.

Housework After the students have drawn the inserts about sharing, working together, and being helpful, discuss housework. Read the poem called "Housework," from the book and record, *Free to Be You and Me* (9, pp. 54–59).

Ask the students whether there are any other pictures they want to color to include in their album. After they have added their own ideas, have them take their albums home to discuss with their family.

UNIT II: MY FRIENDS

The ability to relate to others in a fulfilling satisfactory manner is essential to the self-actualizing, healthy personality. This ability is often recognized when people mature. With maturation, people can evaluate the strengths and weaknesses in their relating style. These strengths and weaknesses are the product of many years of socialization.

In the young child, the ability to relate and the socialization process is often noticed first by the teacher. The elementary school is one of the first grounds for testing these abilities. A caring teacher who realizes the importance of the relating and socialization process to the development of a healthy lifestyle will do two things in the classroom. First, the teacher will observe the students, noting their strengths and weaknesses. These observations can be discussed with the child's parents. Second, the teacher will provide opportunities for strengthening the student's relating style in the classroom. The structuring of these activities helps both student and teacher to make an evaluation. As the students see themselves improving in "friendship making," they will gain self-confidence, which will strengthen their egos. The following lesson affords relating opportunities and opportunities for evaluation.

OBJECTIVES

1. The student will draw a picture and describe "A friend is. . . ."
2. After the puppet show, the student will describe what it is like to move, what it is like to leave a close friend, and what it is like to make a new friend.
3. Through the use of a friendship tree, the student will have the opportunity to make new friends.
4. After the puppet show, the student will be able to answer five multiple choice questions about friendship.
5. After the lesson, students will select from a list four things that make a good friend and will rank them in order of importance.

MATERIALS

1. Cardboard box, two sock puppets.
2. *Sesame Street* album with song "Somebody Come and Play."
3. Posterboard and wire pipe cleaners.

Method

○ □ ☆

As an introduction to a friendship, have each student draw a picture and describe "A friend is. . . ."

○ □

Puppet Show*

Make two puppets out of socks and a stage out of a cardboard box. The follow-

*This lesson was taught by Greg Smith and Willie Warren. If the teacher desires to discuss prejudice, make one puppet out of a white sock and another from a black sock.

ing friendship skit can be performed in three scenes. After each scene, there is a chance for class discussion. The show is simple and can be done by the students themselves.

Scene I Boy puppet is alone thinking about leaving his friends and moving into a new neighborhood. Puppet expresses great fear of the change in his routine daily activities. The idea of making new friends worries him. He begins to think of a close friend he has and how much he will miss him.

Scene II Boy puppet in his new neighborhood meets his first neighbor. She offers her friendship first and suggests a game. He rejects playing her game and calls it "sissy." He finally suggests a game of his own.

Scene III Boy puppet playing by himself. Girl puppet wants to join in the activity. In the process of trying to be part of the activity she disturbs the boy. He becomes very angry at the girl puppet and ignores her. The girl puppet leaves with a very sad face. The boy puppet says he is sorry. They decide to be friends and play.

○

Song

Play the record "Somebody Come and Play" from *Sesame Street*.*

○ □

Friendship Tree

Have each student make a friendship tree out of heavy poster paper and pipe cleaners. To make the tree, students will draw a large tree with several branches on sturdy poster paper, then use the pipe

*Peter Pan Records, a division of Peter Pan Industries, Newark, New Jersey 07105.

cleaners to make hooks on the branches, by pulling the pipe cleaners through the posterboard, securing them to the back with masking tape, and making small hooks in the front. Students will then make cardboard circles about two inches in diameter, and put a hole in each circle large enough to hang the circle on the pipe cleaner hook. Students should put their name or initials on several of the circles. During "friendship time" give the students a topic to learn about in pairs. Each student must learn something about the other student as they talk. When "friendship time" is over, let the students exchange a circle that has their name or initials on it and put the circle on their friendship tree.

Evaluation

LIFESTYLE CONTENT

○ □

Quiz: Circle the answer you think is best after having listened to the puppet show.

1. If I moved away from my friend,
    a. I could find a new friend.
    b. I could never have a friend again.
    c. I would never want any more friends.
2. To be my friend, you
    a. must be a boy.
    b. must be a girl.
    c. can be a boy or a girl.
3. If someone new moved into my neighborhood,
    a. I would wait for him or her to come to my house.
    b. I would make "fun" of him or her.
    c. I would go over to his or her house and make friends.
4. When I have a toy,
    a. I am willing to share it with others.

    b. I will always play with it by myself.
    c. I will hide it if someone comes near.
5. When I do something unfair to my friend,
    a. I pretend it did not happen.
    b. I will say that I am sorry.
    c. I don't know what to do.

○ □

Thought question: Ask each student what this saying by Robert Louis Stevenson means: "A friend is a present you give yourself."

LIFESTYLE VALUE

○ □

After reading the following ten traits, ask the students to choose the four items they think are the most important when making friends and rank them in order, number one being the most important.

What Makes A Good Friend For Me?

1. Always shares toys with me.
2. Always lets me have my way.
3. Will spend the night with me.
4. Isn't afraid of anything or anyone.
5. Always helps me when I'm in trouble.
6. Will always pick me first if captain on a team.
7. Will visit me when I am sick.
8. Will wait for me when I am late for school.
9. Will always let me sit by the window in a car or bus.
10. Will say nice things about my new clothes.

UNIT III: MY BEGINNING

Elementary children are normally curious about all the things around them, including themselves. They are fascinated by

82

the human body, its many parts, and their functions. They attempt to make sense out of things. This is one of the wonders and thrills of being an elementary teacher—watching children discover and grow.

A natural question from a young, curious child is, "Where did I come from?" Most psychologists and educators of sexuality and family living agree that the normal, naturally curious child will ask this question by the age of six or seven. They feel that children who have not asked their parents or an admired adult this question have thought about it and decided that it is not an appropriate question. In other words, children's "sixth" sense tells them that their parents or admired adults do not want to answer the question.

Perhaps adults do not want to hear the question, "Where did I come from?" because it requires a straightforward answer. It means talking about the difference between Daddy and Mommy and about how the sperm gets in Mommy. Many teachers fear such a discussion. To these teachers, sex education is frightening. "If I answer those questions, what will the child do?"

The teacher who has these fears might be comforted by a statement from Dr. Milton I. Levine, a physician and professor of clinical pediatrics at Cornell University Medical College in New York City:

There is no evidence whatsoever that sex education is harmful, that it excites curiosity or stimulates sex urges and desires. On the contrary, there is ample evidence that it aids children in gaining a wholesome attitude toward sex and an understanding of the normal sex attitudes, roles, and relationships.

A wholesome attitude toward sex is necessary if a child is to develop a healthy, self-actualizing lifestyle. When a significant adult is open and honest in answering children's questions, the children develop trust and feel that they can be honest about the questions to which they need answers.

The following lesson answers one of the first questions a child has regarding sexuality, "Where do babies come from?" The lesson is developed as a booklet to be read by the children at their own rate of mastery. The authors have granted permission for this booklet to be xeroxed. This will enable the children to take their booklets home after the lesson to have a sharing session with their parents.

OBJECTIVES

The student will be able to explain:

1. How conception takes place.
2. How the baby grows inside the mother.
3. Heredity and how we acquire traits.

MATERIALS

1. The booklet *Where Babies Come From.**
2. Felt board tic-tac-toe.

Method

☐

Students vary immensely in their ability to grasp and retain new concepts. This often presents the teacher with a problem in introducing a new unit. From the story "Where Babies Come From" the students learn at their own speed that:

1. The human body is made up of many parts called cells.
2. The cell is governed by DNA.
3. Half of the DNA in each cell comes from the mother and half from the father.

*Originally appeared in *Education for Sexuality: Concepts and Programs for Teaching* (Philadelphia: Saunders, 1975). The authors (John J. Burt, Jr., and Linda Brower Meeks) have granted permission to teachers to duplicate the booklet for their children.

4. All of the body's cells developed because of orders sent out by the DNA boss in the very first cell.

5. Half of the first cell comes from the mother and half of the first cell comes from the father.

6. Therefore, it takes both a mother and a father to have a baby.

7. To have a baby, the father puts his penis inside the mother's vagina so that the sperm that carry his half of the DNA can get into the mother's body to look for the egg.

8. Unless a man and a woman really love each other, they certainly will not be able to love and take care of children and that is why you should have a strong lasting relationship before you try to have children of your own.

Evaluation

LIFESTYLE CONTENT

☐

Make a tic-tac-toe felt board. Divide the students into two teams, an X team and an O team. The teams alternate to answer the following questions. Each time a team answers a question correctly, the team gets a turn on the tic-tac-toe board. The first team to make a tic-tac-toe is the winner.

Questions

1. The human body is made up of many tiny units called _____ .

2. What are the cells that allow you to move called?

3. How does a cell know how fast to grow or what job to do?

4. What is DNA?

5. What is the half of the DNA boss that comes from the mother called?

6. What is the half of the DNA boss that comes from the father called?

7. Where do the sperm and egg come together to form the first DNA boss?

8. How does the father's sperm get inside the mother?

9. After the sperm and egg come together, how long before a new baby is born?

10. Where in the mother's body does the baby develop?

11. Why are some babies born boys and some born girls?

12. How does the new baby get out of the mother?

13. When should people have babies?

14. Why are human babies more fortunate than fish babies?

LIFESTYLE VALUE

Select several cartoons from Sam Levenson's book, *Sex and the Single Child* (5) to discuss. Ask the students to describe how the cartoon character probably feels. Ask "What do you know that the cartoon child does not?"

Where Babies Come From

John Burt, Ed. D.
Linda Brower Meeks, M.S.

The human body is made up of many small parts called cells. The cells are like the bricks

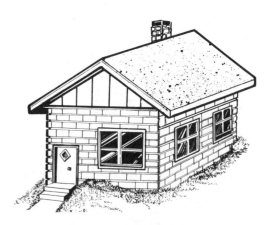

in a house: it takes many bricks to make a house and it takes many cells to make a boy or girl.

Some of your cells make it possible for you to move; these are called muscle cells. Other cells produce tears to wash your eyes. Some cells help you to fight disease and to get well when you are sick. The cells that allow you to think are called brain cells. The food that you eat is taken to your muscles through tunnels that have walls made of cells. Thus, cells make up all parts of your body.

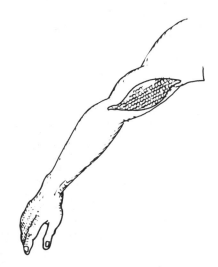

A car, like a person, is made of many parts. It has tires, an engine, windows, seats and other parts. But a car needs a driver to make it go. The driver decides how fast it will go and in what direction it will move.

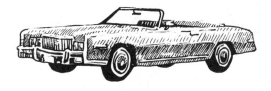

A train also has many parts but it needs an engineer to make it go. The engineer determines how fast and in what direction the train will move.

Each of the cells in your body has its own driver or engineer. His name is Mr. DNA. He

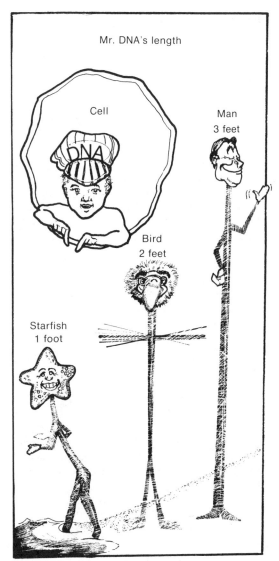

is not a real man, just a long string of chemicals. But scientists refer to him as the boss of the cell and we shall call him Mr. DNA.

Mr. DNA is a very bossy boss because he tells the rest of the cell just what to do and what not to do. But he is a good and wise boss that was passed on to you by your parents. Half of Mr. DNA in each of your cells came from your mother and half came from your father. And the DNA in the cells of your mother and father came from your grand-mothers and grandfathers. So you see, Mr. DNA has been around for a long time and has a great deal of wisdom. His wisdom or knowledge fills up 41 books that are kept right inside the cell.

Most books are written by putting the letters of the alphabet together in different ways to make words. But, Mr. DNA has a very short alphabet, made of only four letters. These letters are A, T, C, and G. Thus, Mr. DNA's books are hard to read. Some of the words look like this: TA CG AT CG. Scientists haven't learned to read Mr. DNA's code yet, but they do know that the four letters in his alphabet stand for four chemicals. It is a very hard code to understand.

When scientists first saw Mr. DNA's books they looked like tiny colored bodies. For lack of a better name, they were called colored bodies. But that was a long time ago and the scientists of that day used the Greek language. So Mr. DNA's books were called chromosomes (kro' mo sohms), the Greek word for colored bodies. Today, we know that they are like very tiny books that contain the knowledge that Mr. DNA needs to run his cell.

Mr. DNA is really a curled up string of chemicals. If he were taken out of the cell and uncurled, he would be about three feet long. Mr. DNA, in a cell of starfish, is about one foot long, and in the cell of a bird he is about two feet long.

There are many DNA bosses in your body: one in every single cell. They know when your body needs to grow and when it should stop growing. They know when to make new cells and when to replace old worn out ones. And when new cells are made, the old Mr. DNA makes a new Mr. DNA for the new cell.

When you are born, your body is already made up of many cells, each with its own DNA boss. But all of these cells developed because of orders sent out by the DNA boss in your very first cell.

Where do you think this first cell came from? Half of it came from your mother and half of it from your father. You see it takes both a mother and a father to have a baby.

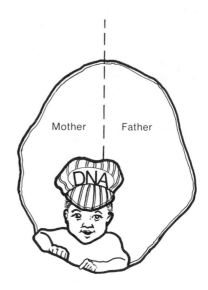

Mother   Father

A mother has a place in her body where this first cell can grow and develop. This place is about the size of a pear and is called the uterus (yoo' tuh rus). And as this first cell grows into many cells, the uterus gets bigger and bigger until it can hold a full size baby.

The mother's uterus is just below her navel (children sometimes call this the belly but-

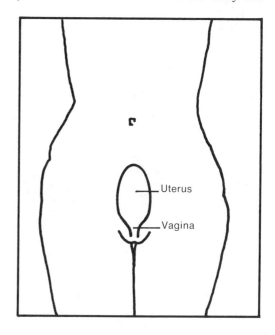

Uterus

Vagina

ton). It is shaped like a bottle except that the bottle is turned upside down so that it opens like a tunnel between the mother's legs. When you were born, you came out through this tunnel which is called the vagina (vuh jy' nuh).

The uterus then is the place where the first cell starts to grow and develop. And we know that half of the first cell comes from the mother and half from the father. But how do the two halves get together in the uterus?

Fortunately, the uterus has three tunnels leading into it. The tunnel that goes down to open between the mother's legs we already know as the vagina. And at the top of the uterus there are two more tunnels that connect with two egg factories. These factories are called ovaries (ova' ries). Each month an

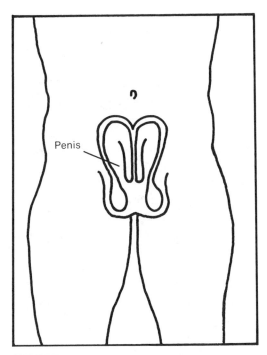

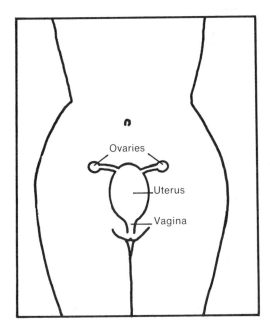

egg leaves the factory and goes down one of the tunnels toward the uterus. But eggs are only one-half of a DNA boss. They must combine with another half from the father before a new baby can start to grow.

The father also has a factory to make his half of the first DNA boss. This factory is found in a small sack just behind his penis

(pee' nis). When the mother and father decide to have a baby, the father puts his penis in the mother's vagina tunnel so that his half of Mr. DNA can get inside the mother's body. In just a few minutes, the father's DNA halves are swimming up the vagina to the uterus. These halves from the father are called sperm.

The sperm swim through the uterus and up to the tubes that lead to the egg factories. If an egg that has recently left the egg factory happens to meet one of the father's sperm, the two halves of the DNA boss zip themselves together and you have the first complete DNA boss. He now takes control and makes all future decisions about growth and development. He decides how tall you will be, what color your eyes will be and even what size shoes you will wear. All of this information is contained in Mr. DNA's library books or chromosomes.

Perhaps you have wondered why some babies are born girls and some boys. As you might expect, the answer is in Mr. DNA's 46 books. First, we should point out that 23 books come from the father and 23 books come from the mother. Thus, when the two halves of Mr. DNA are zipped together, he has a full new library of 46 books, or as scientists would say, 46 chromosomes. But not all new libraries are the same: some contain the knowledge needed to form a boy and others contain the knowledge needed to form a girl.

The 23 books or chromosomes that come from the mother never contain the information needed to form a boy. But some sperm carry a book of information about boys and some carry a book of information about girls.

If a sperm with one of these books about boys is zipped together with the egg, a new baby boy will be born. If a sperm with a book of girl information combines with the egg, the baby will be a girl. Thus, it is the type of book carried by the sperm that determines whether the baby will be a boy or girl.

After the sperm and egg combine in the tunnel between the uterus and the egg factory, the new cell starts to grow and to move down the tunnel to the uterus. It plants itself in the side of the uterus and starts to grow rapidly. After about nine months, it is a full grown baby. When the baby is ready to be born, the mother feels a slight pain and goes to the hospital. There the doctor helps the baby to come out of the tunnel between the mother's legs.

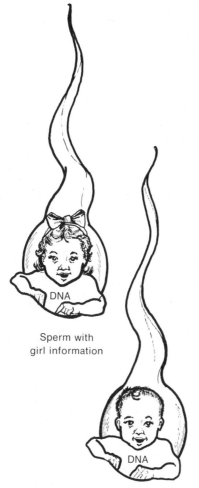

Sperm with
girl information

Sperm with
boy information

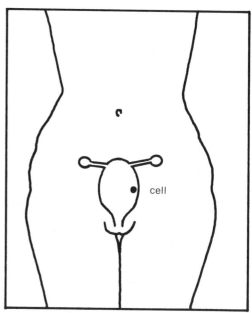

New cell will grow
into full grown baby
in about 9 months.

One day you may want to become a mother or a father, so you should know when and how to have babies.

First, you should know that girls don't produce eggs and boys don't produce sperm until about the time that they become teenagers. So young children couldn't become mothers or fathers even if they wanted to.

When you grow up, you may find a boy or girl that you like very much. Then you decide to get married. When you get married, you promise to love and take care of each other. This is very important because unless a man and woman really love and take care of each other, they certainly will not be able to love and take care of children. That is why you should have a strong and lasting relationship before you try to have children of your own.

P.S. You may also be interested to know how fish have babies since the mother and father fish never fall in love or get married. The mother just releases her eggs into the water, and the father releases his sperm into the water. The two halves of the DNA boss zip themselves together and form the first cell of a fish. Unfortunately, there is no uterus to protect the first fish cell so many of them don't get to grow up. Humans are lucky that they develop in their mother's uterus where they are protected. Humans are also lucky that they have a mother and father who love each other and who love and care for their babies. If mothers and fathers didn't love each other enough to plan to take care of their children, babies wouldn't be much better off than fish. Poor fish.*

UNIT IV: DIVORCE

Although parents like to shelter their children, it is not easy to shelter a child in a world where many things are happening around him. Since one out of three marriages now end in divorce, more than six million children are experiencing the trauma that surrounds a divorce.

Children may feel "afraid of the future, guilty for [their] own (usually imaginary) role in causing the divorce, hurt at the rejection [they] feel from the parent who

*Reprinted with permission. John Burt and Linda Brower Meeks, *Education for Sexuality: Concepts and Programs for Teaching*. Philadelphia: W. B. Saunders Co., 1975.

does not remain with [them], and angry at both parents for making a shambles of [their] world" (6, p. 523). Children may become depressed, hostile, disruptive, irritable, lonely, sad, accident-prone, or even suicidal; they may suffer from fatigue, insomnia, skin disorders, lack of appetite, or inability to concentrate; and they often lose interest in schoolwork and social life, partly because of shame and embarrassment (8, pp. 588–95).

The most important factor in children's adjustment to their parents' divorce is the way that the parents handle the children's anxieties and questions. Learning to express feelings and discuss anxieties, as well as having questions answered, is important if a child is to be healthy and self-actualized.

The following lesson on divorce provides a story for children to ask questions about. By being involved in the story, the child will express feelings, doubts, and fears. Some children will identify with the story. Other children will be exposed to a part of family life that is happening around them.

OBJECTIVES

1. After the story about Anne, students will draw a picture and explain some aspect of divorce.

2. Students will complete open-ended statements to express their feelings about divorce.

MATERIALS

1. Felt board, cutouts described in activity.

Methods

○ □

A Story About Anne may be simply read or illustrated by using a felt board and cutouts of a girl with a red baseball cap, a mother, a father, and two houses.

A Story About Anne

Anne was lying in her bed. She had had a really fun day. She was seven years old and just learning to play baseball.

Tonight Daddy had played catch with Anne. It was lots of fun. Anne smiled and laughed. She liked her daddy. Daddy had fun too.

Anne wished things were happy all the time. She wished very hard that Mommy and Daddy would smile all the time.

She could hear her mommy and daddy shouting as she lay in bed. She wondered what was wrong. Oh, how she wished that they would not shout! It made Anne feel very bad. Sometimes it made her tummy hurt.

At last Anne fell asleep.

When Anne woke up she stretched and yawned. She looked outside her window. Wouldn't it be fun to play baseball on such a nice day?

She hurried down to the kitchen for her breakfast. She wore a red baseball cap that Daddy had given her.

Mommy and Daddy were sitting at the kitchen table. Mommy drank a cup of coffee. Daddy read the newspaper. It was very quiet. Anne thought it was too quiet. Mommy and Daddy gave each other a funny look.

"Anne, Mommy and I want to talk to you," said Daddy. "You are very special to both of us. We have a problem to share with you."

Anne gulped. She felt very funny inside.

"You see, Anne, Mommy and I have a very hard time talking when we are to-gether. We fight with each other many, many times."

"When mommies and daddies argue all the time and don't have much fun, it may be better for them not to live to-gether. Mommy and I think that this would be best for us."

"We think it would be best if we lived in two different houses. You will live here with Mommy."

"But I don't like that much at all!" cried Anne. "I want to live with both of you. Why can't we be together?"

Mommy answered. It was hard for her to talk. She and Daddy knew that Anne was confused.

"It won't be easy for all of us to be apart, Anne, but it will be better than being together. Both Daddy and I love you. Daddy will take you to his house on weekends. He will play baseball with you."

Anne thought she was to blame. "If I am a good girl, will you stay Daddy?"

"Anne, it is not your fault that Mommy and Daddy have problems. You are a good little girl. We think it will be better for us all."

Anne was very quiet. She didn't feel much like breakfast. She ran out to play.

Maybe she was just dreaming. Maybe everything would be better. Maybe Daddy would be at home tonight. Maybe Daddy would not leave. Anne wished and hoped.

That night was lonely for Anne. Daddy was gone. Mommy held Anne close and told her that when parents live apart and are happier, they get a divorce.

A divorce means that a mommy and daddy never live together again. They do not belong to each other anymore.

Anne went to her bedroom to sleep. She was very sad. She felt lonely. Mommy told her that with time she would not feel so bad. It was hard for Anne to understand.

Questions

1. Why was Anne sad?
2. What is a divorce?
3. Why did Anne's parents get divorced?
4. Do you think Anne thought that the divorce was her fault?
5. How did Anne try to get her daddy to stay?
6. Will Anne still see her daddy?
7. Does Anne's mommy love her? Does her daddy love her?
8. Will it be easier for Anne when she gets more used to her daddy being gone?
9. Is Anne afraid? Angry? Hurt?
10. What questions do you think Anne has?
11. How did you feel about this story?
12. What do you know about divorce?
13. How do you feel about divorce?

Evaluation

LIFESTYLE CONTENT

○

Have each student draw a picture of some part of the story and explain the picture.

LIFESTYLE VALUE

□

Have each student complete the following open-ended statements:

1. Anne's mommy _____ .
2. Anne and her daddy _____ .
3. Divorce is _____ .
4. Anne felt _____ .
5. If I were Anne, I would _____ .

An alternative activity would be to show the film "Breakup" from the "Inside/Out" series, and follow the film with role playing and discussion.

UNIT V: THE AGING PROCESS*

In every culture there is an age structure. Within the age structure there are typical patterns of behavior related to the life cycle. The authors believe that the elementary school child can best understand these life stages by learning about them as they relate to the family.

The following lesson on the aging process is designed to introduce elementary schoolchildren to aging by studying the "Smith Family." By studying this family unit, the students learn the seven stages of the aging process and identify personal goals for their own lifeline.

OBJECTIVES

1. On completion of the story, "The Smith Family," the student will be able to identify by listing the seven stages of the aging process.
2. The student will be able to draw his or her lifeline and identify at least one personal goal for each stage.
3. On completion of the story, "The Smith Family," the student will cut out at least one illustration of the seven life stages, mount them on construction paper, and identify each illustration with the appropriate life stages of the aging process.

MATERIALS

1. A copy of the story "The Smith Family" (either a copy for each student or one copy for the teacher to read).

*This lesson was prepared with the help of Jerry Wright, Ph.D. candidate at The Ohio State University.

2. One worksheet per student for listing the seven life stages of the aging process.

3. Magazines, construction paper, rubber cement, marking pens, and scissors.

Methods

A STORY ABOUT THE SEVEN LIFE STAGES

Give each student a copy of "The Smith Family" to read, or read the story to the class.

The Smith Family

A human being belongs to the group of animals called Homo sapiens. We are all Homo sapiens: You, your mother and father, your brother and sisters, your grandparents, even the boys and girls who sit behind or across from you in school, and all of your friends.

But do you notice any differences in the appearance of your mother, your grandmother, father, grandfather, your brother, or perhaps your baby sister? Some are very small, while others are very big. What are some of the things they do? Do they work, play, or study? Do they sometimes do things together or alone and tell you that you are not old enough to join the activity?

Each of the members of your family are at different stages in their life. And at each stage, each individual sees himself or herself differently, develops differing attitudes and values, and sets different goals for the future. Let us observe a family much like yours and mine and see how each person is different. They are the Smith family.

Little Jimmy is the youngest member of the Smith family. Jimmy is twenty-one months old and, having learned to walk, is continuously broadening and exploring his new surroundings. Each new thing he sees, he must touch and identify with his own vocabulary. When little Jimmy is not exploring, he is taking a nap or crying for attention. Jimmy is in the stage of life known as infancy, the period from birth to age two.

Jimmy has an older sister, Amy, who is five, and an older brother, Tim, who is nine. Amy is a very busy little girl. She goes to kindergarten in the mornings, where she meets friends, plays, draws, and learns to read. In the afternoon she goes to her piano lesson, and in the evening she helps her mother and watches television. Tim likes to watch television too. But he and Amy fight over what shows to watch. Tim doesn't seem to like girls. They are all taller than he is and tease him a lot. He doesn't care much for school with the exception of recess. At recess he and his friends play baseball. Tim also plays on a little league team after school and on weekends. Both Amy and Tim need their rest and are usually in bed by 8 o'clock in the evening. This stage of life that Amy and Tim are experiencing is called childhood. Childhood is the period from three through eleven.

Amy and Tim have an older brother and sister, Bob, who is sixteen, and Susan, who is thirteen. Bob is in high school. He is very athletic and plays on the varsity football team. Bob recently got his driver's license and is always asking his mom and dad to let him borrow the car. He hopes to get a job this summer and save enough money to buy a car of his own. Bob is popular at school. He is class president, goes out on dates, and gets to stay up until ten during the week and eleven on the weekends.

At thirteen, Susan is slender and taller than the boys her age. Two years ago she was a tomboy, playing ball with Bob, climbing trees, and running with the wind. Now Susan is more serious. She is conscious of her appearance, wearing the right clothes, saying just the right things. Susan is also very popular. She enjoys school; is a top student; plays soccer; and belongs to Girl Scouts, the Honor Society, and the school band. Susan doesn't get to go out on dates, but she is allowed to stay up until eleven o'clock. Bob and Susan are in the life stage called adolescence. The adolescent stage of life spans the ages of twelve to eighteen.

Jimmy, Amy, Tim, Susan, and Bob have an older sister named Jane. Jane is twenty-two years old, and is away at college. She lives in a dormitory on the university campus and has a roommate. They sometimes have conflicts and arguments over study habits, playing the stereo too loud, and who should use the shower first. But they are able to work these problems out by talking. Jane has to study hard and make top grades, since she plans to enter medical school to become a doctor. However, Jane doesn't study all the time. On weekends she spends some time with her steady boyfriend or goes out with her friends. Jane also thinks about her future. She wants to finish school, set up a practice to help others, and perhaps get married and raise a family. Jane is in the stage of life known as young adulthood. The young adult stage spans the ages of nineteen to twenty-nine.

The parents of the Smith children are Mr. and Mrs. Smith, Jack and Nora. Jack works as an electrician for a construction firm. Mr. Smith has a lot of responsibility on his job. He works hard. His responsibility for work carries over to his family. With a wife and six children, Mr. Smith is very conscientious about community, national, and world problems. He tries to keep up on current affairs. There are many bills to pay. The children need food and clothing, and Jane's college tuition is very expensive. Bob also wants to go to college in a couple of years and that will be another expense to plan ahead for. After working hard during the week, Mr. Smith takes time to relax on the weekend. On Saturday morning he plays golf with friends and enjoys a ball game in the afternoon. Some Saturdays and Sundays he works around the house making minor repairs or building something in his workshop.

Nora Smith has made the readjustment to being a housewife and mother since little Jimmy was born. Mrs. Smith is a schoolteacher, but decided to take a couple of years off while Jimmy is small. She plans to return to teaching in the fall. Mrs. Smith has a lot of responsibility taking care of a big family. She goes shopping, prepares the meals, and cleans the house. She is active in the community, participating in fund drives and belonging to several clubs. In addition to their many responsibilities, Mr. and Mrs. Smith value the time that they spend together and with the entire family. Mr. and Mrs. Smith are in the stage of life called adulthood. The adulthood stage spans the ages thirty through forty-nine.

Mr. Smith's parents, Elmer and Julia, live across town. Elmer and Julia are known as Grandfather and Grandmother to the Smith children. Elmer recently retired from the railroad. Elmer's retirement pension and Julia's social security provide an average income. To supplement this income, Elmer has set up a woodworking shop in his basement. He builds a variety of items, such as doll furniture, candle holders, toy windmills, and clocks.

Julia Smith is also busy. She belongs to a women's club and occasionally knits and sews for supplemental income. Baking cookies is Grandma Smith's favorite pastime. She always has plenty of homemade cookies for the grandchildren when they visit. Elmer and Julie are both active in the church and enjoy taking short trips together. Elmer and Julia are in the stage of life known as middle age, the years fifty through sixty-nine.

Elmer Smith's mother, Ester, lives in a retirement home. Ester is Jack Smith's grandmother. She is the Smith children's great-grandmother. The whole Smith family goes to visit her often. Ester looks forward to their visits. Last year Ester's husband, Bill, died and she misses him very much. She has made many new friends at the retirement home and participates in a variety of daily activities. There are group trips to places of interest and transportation is provided weekly to a local shopping mall. Ester is in the stage of life called elderly, age seventy until death.

Each member of the Smith family has a particular lifestyle. All have things that are important to them, goals for the future, and present responsibilities. As each passes into another stage of life, goals and responsibilities change. New goals are set and responsibilities are seen differently. Not everyone will identify the same goals for each of life's stages, nor will each of us have exactly the same responsibilities. However, each of us will experience all seven stages: infancy, childhood, adolescence, young adulthood, adulthood, middle age, elderly.

Evaluation

LIFESTYLE CONTENT

☆

Each student will complete the following unfinished sentences.

1. Little Jimmy is in the _____ stage of life within the aging process.

2. Jimmy's older sister Amy is in the _____ life stage of the aging process.

3. Mrs. Nora Smith is in the life stage known as _____ .

4. Ages three through eleven are considered to be the _____ life stage of the aging process.

5. Elmer and Julia Smith are in the life stage known as _____ .

6. List four things that might be characteristic of Bob and Susan in the adolescence life stage:_____
_____   _____
_____ .

7. Persons between the ages of nineteen and twenty-nine are in the stage of life known as _____ .

8. The adolescence life stage includes ages _____ through _____.

9. Persons aged seventy to death are considered to be in the life stage known as _____ .

10. Mr. Jack Smith is in the life stage known as adulthood, ages _____ through _____.

LIFESTYLE CONTENT

☆

Each student will bring to class three or more old magazines containing pictures of family life. The student will select a picture to illustrate each of the seven life stages depicted in the Smith family story. Each picture will be mounted on construction paper and placed in order.

LIFESTYLE VALUE

☆

The students will draw a horizontal line across their paper and place a dot at each end of the line. Over the left dot, they will write in their birth date. The dot to the right represents death. Then they will place a dot on the line between their birth and death dates that represents their present life stage and indicate each of the seven life stages by placing them along the line. Under each life stage, they will indicate at least one goal they would like to achieve. (See Figure 6B-1).

Divide the students into groups of four or five and have them discuss their lifelines. One person in each group will share some of the ideas with the entire class. The following questions will be helpful in stimulating discussion:

1. What age do you consider elderly?

2. What are some of the things you consider to be characteristic of individuals in each of the seven life stages of the aging process?

3. How do you suppose you viewed older persons when you were in the infancy stage? In the childhood stage?

4. What are your goals at each of the stages of the aging process?

5. Consider how much time do you really have for a life of meaning?

UNIT VI: DEATH*

"Confronting death brings us face to face with ourselves. We cannot but search for the meaning of life when we try to understand death" (10, p. 3). An elementary curriculum focusing on the selection of healthy lifestyle components must include death education. This lesson was included to assist the teacher in this task.

The lesson focuses on a story and a question and answer session that deals with the four developmental phases a child experiences during grief. The four phases are: (a) announcement: telling the death, in an experimental sense including affective, abreactive recall of details and feelings along with the perception that this death represented a significant loss; (b) acknowledgement: dealing with the irreversibility of the loss, not just immediate fact, and the realization that it is always going to be this way; (c) mourn-

*This lesson was written in consultation with David Schoedinger, Funeral Director, Schoedinger Funeral Home, Columbus, Ohio.

FIGURE 6B-1 Lifeline Activity

0–2 Infancy Goals	3–11 Child-hood Goals	12–18 Adoles-cence Goals	19–29 Young Adult-hood Goals	30–49 Adult-hood Goals	50–69 Middle Age Goals	70 Elderly Goals

* *   *

Birth   Present   Death
Date   Age   Date

ing: expressing directly and dealing with feelings of anger, guilt, and vulnerability and working through personal implications relative to the child's life space (that is, developmental state, family situation) and dealing with annihilation fantasies that the loved one's "abandonment" evokes; and (d) renewal: incorporating the deceased, exploring the environment for appropriate replacement objects to meet one's needs, perceiving and planning for the future without the deceased, recognizing that although a loved one is dead, the child is alive and has inner resources as well as environmental resources that can facilitate survival and growth (4, p. 396).

Often teachers would rather not deal with a discussion of death in the classroom. This is due partly to their own feelings of denial and repression and may reflect the way that death was handled in their homes as they were growing up. Denial and repression of emotion are incompatible with the emergence of a healthy, self-actualizing personality. Thus, students should have the benefits of discussing the emotions surrounding all of life's phases from birth to death. It is our responsibility to assist children in this process.

OBJECTIVES

1. By drawing and explaining a picture, the students will express what is meant by "living."

2. After the story "New Clothes for Old," the students will explain what it means to be dead.

3. By visiting a funeral home and cemetery, the students will answer: What happens when someone dies? What arrangements does the family make? What happens to the body?

4. When the lesson is complete, the students will complete an objective examination on feelings and facts about death.

5. The students will express their attitudes about death using open-ended statements.

MATERIALS

1. Funeral home director as a speaker.
2. Visit to cemetery.

Method

○ □

Suggested Introductory Activities

As an introduction to the discussion of death, the students can watch seeds sprout or observe a caterpillar becoming a butterfly.

Observing a Caterpillar Become a Butterfly

To watch what was a crawling caterpillar emerge from its chrysalis a beautiful, four-winged butterfly is an exciting and inspiring experience. It is well worth the weeks of waiting. The food the caterpillar will need until it forms its chrysalis or cocoon (a butterfly forms a chrysalis, a moth spins a cocoon) will depend upon the kind of caterpillar you choose. The kind of food can be told by the plant upon which the caterpillar is found. The black swallowtail caterpillar (green and black stripes with yellow dots) can be found in gardens where carrots, celery, and parsley are grown; it feeds on the leaves of those plants. The famous monarch is one of the most beautiful butterflies, and interesting to learn about because of its long migrations. The caterpillar (striped like a zebra with gold spots) can be found wherever there are milkweed plants.

Put the caterpillar on the leaf on which it is found and a short stick in a large glass jar;

punch plenty of holes in the lid of the jar to provide good ventilation. See that it has fresh food and occasionally add a few drops of water. If there is not some moisture, the butterfly's wings will be shriveled. Many good illustrated books about this attractive insect can be obtained from your public library (7, p. 116).

For Everything Its Season*

For everything its season, and for
    every activity under heaven its time:
A time to be born and a time to die;
A time to weep and a time to laugh;
A time for mourning and a time for
    dancing;
A time to scatter stones and a time to
    gather them;
A time to embrace and a time to refrain
    from embracing;
A time to keep and a time to throw
    away;
A time for silence and a time for
    speech;
A time to seek and a time to lose.

□ ☆
Questions:

1. What does this poem mean to you?

2. What seasons are there in a calendar year? What changes occur during these seasons?

3. What did you notice about the seeds? How did they change?

4. What happened to the caterpillar?

5. Do people change or go through "seasons"? How? What changes can you see?

○ □
Story

Have the students draw a picture of what it means to be "living." Ask children to

*Adapted from the Bible.

explain their pictures. What does it mean to be alive? Tell the students that you are going to read a story to them about death and life. Ask them to listen very carefully and to stop you if they have a question.

New Clothes for Old*

Charles had a new suit of clothes. It was blue and fitted him exactly.

"What a pretty suit!" everybody said when he wore it the first time. "How well it fits, and how nice Charles looks in it!"

He wore it for a long time. Grandma Sterling, who lived next door, used to say, "I do love Charles in that blue suit!" But it was not the blue suit she loved; it was the boy inside it.

He wore the blue suit a long time, so long that it was like part of Charles and people knew him by his blue suit.

By and by a button came off and another had to be sewn on. Then one day when he was playing, he tore a big three-cornered tear in it.

"Your blue suit can't go out and play for a few days," his mother said. "It's sick and has to go to bed and have the doctor!"

Charles laughed, for he knew that what she meant was that it had to go to the tailor's and be mended.

After a few days, it came back, and it was almost as good as new.

Then the lining of his sleeve ripped, and Charles couldn't tell where to put his arm through. His mother had to mend it. Then two more buttons came off, and the

*This story was originally written by Jeanette Perkins Brown and appeared in *The Pilgrim Elementary Teacher*. It appears as adapted with her permission. The original story had a strong religious element. The story has been changed so that it might be more widely used for classrooms. Used and adapted by permission of The Pilgrim Press, New York.

lining of his cuffs began to look frayed. His mother sewed on some new buttons and put new pieces in the cuffs. Then a hole came in the knee of his trousers, and his mother had to patch them.

He did not play all the time now. He worked and helped his mother. He could run faster and do her errands, for his legs were longer. He could lift heavy things for her, because his shoulders were broader and his arms were stronger. Once, in carrying an armful of wood, he stretched his suit so that it split up the back.

"Charles has outgrown his blue suit," said his father. "He needs another."

When Grandma Sterling heard he was to have a new suit, she said, "I shall be sorry to see his blue suit go; I always liked it." But it was not the suit she liked; it was the boy inside the suit. For when the new suit was bought—a brown one this time—she said, "What a pretty suit that is! I thought I liked him in blue, but I love him in brown!"

One day Grandma Sterling was quite sick. A doctor came. She was often sick, and the doctor came and made her well for a while, then something would be the matter again. One day he could not make her well. Charles came running into the house.

"Mother," he cried. "Betty says Grandma Sterling is dead. She's not alive any more, and they're going to carry her away!"

His mother said, "The Grandma Sterling you loved is dead. We will miss her very much."

Then his mother went and opened the drawer where his old blue suit lay.

"Remember how Grandma Sterling used to say that she loved you in that blue suit?" she asked. "But it wasn't the suit she liked. That is all worn out now.

She loved the little boy inside it, and he is the same no matter what suit he has on."

"It was only Grandma Sterling's body that they carried away," she said. "It was old and worn out. It kept getting out of order, and the doctor had to keep patching it up, and mending it, just as I had to keep patching up and mending your blue suit. By and by it couldn't be mended any more, just as your suit couldn't be."

"Grandma Sterling is dead. Her body does not move. She does not breathe. Her heart does not beat. She does not feel any hurt or pain. We cannot bring her back to life because she is dead. We will miss her very much, Charles. We loved her and she loved us. We will remember the fun times we had with Grandma."

"I feel sad because I miss Grandma," mother said. "How do you feel, Charles?"

Questions

1. How do you think Charles feels? Why?
2. Can Grandma still get better?
3. Do you think Charles has questions to ask his mother?
4. What questions would you ask?
5. Has anyone close to you ever died?
6. How did you feel?
7. How did you show your feelings?
8. How do people help each other with their feelings?
9. Can a person live in your memory?
10. What memories do you think Charles has?

FUNERAL HOME AND CEMETERY VISIT

The preceding story and question-and-answer session have prepared the students for the following two questions:

1. What happens when someone dies? What does the family do?

2. What happens to the body?

□ ☆

Ask a funeral home director to come and talk to the students or arrange for a visit to a funeral home. Before the visit, ask the students what they would like to know.

□ ☆

After the visit to the funeral home, arrange a visit to a cemetery. If it is difficult to visit a gravesite, use slides or pictures of a cemetery.

Have the students look at the epitaphs on the grave markers. Talk about these markings and what is found on them. (Name, age at death, birth date, date of death). Each student might sketch an epitaph that was of particular interest. The students also might make a grave rubbing.

○ □ ☆

Grave Rubbing

Make a grave rubbing of one of the more interesting markers. Do this by:

A. Laying or taping a sheet of soft paper on the face of the marker.

B. Using the side of a piece of charcoal, crayon, chalk, or pastel, stroke evenly across the paper.

C. Dark colors work best.

D. Rub until the underside of the marker shows through on the paper.

E. Use your imagination to achieve different effects. Try different color combinations, different textures, different pressures, or overlapping designs.

F. Apply a spray fixative to prevent smudging (1, pp. 34–35).

Evaluation

LIFESTYLE CONTENT

○ □

After the teacher reads each of the following statements, students will raise their arm if the statement is true, hold their arm out straight if they cannot answer, or put their arm down if the statement is not true.

1. All living things die.

2. When you die, you are dead.

3. We can bring a dead person back to life.

4. We miss a dead person whom we loved.

5. A cemetery has graves where bodies of dead people are buried.

6. The body can still breathe after death.

7. We can show we miss someone by crying.

8. A funeral helps us to show that we cared for someone.

9. Playing dead is not the same as dying.

10. It may take a while to feel better after someone we know dies.

Lifestyle Value

□ ☆

Each student will complete the following open-ended statements:

1. When I think about death _____ .

2. A funeral _____ .

3. Dying is _____ .

4. Talking about death _____ .

5. When I went to the cemetery ____ .

☆

Depending on the maturity of the students, the teacher could have each student construct a tombstone out of construction paper and write an epitaph.

REFERENCES

1. David W. Berg and George G. Daugherty, *Perspectives on Death: Student Activity Book* (Baltimore: Waverly, 1972).

2. John Burt and Linda Brower Meeks, *Education for Sexuality: Concepts and Programs for Teaching* (Philadelphia: Saunders, 1975).

3. Erich Fromm, *The Art of Loving* (New York: Harper, 1956).

4. Lois I. Greenberg, "Therapeutic Grief Work with Children," *Social Casework* (July 1975).

5. Sam Levenson, *Sex and the Single Child* (New York: Simon & Schuster, 1969).

6. Diane E. Papalia and Sally Wendkos Olds, *A Child's World,* 2d ed. (New York: McGraw-Hill, 1977).

7. Elizabeth L. Reed, *Helping Children with the Mystery of Death* (New York: Abingdon, 1970). Used by permission.

8. Sugar, M. "Children of Divorce," *Pediatrics* 46 (1970).

9. Marlo Thomas, Gloria Steinem, Mary Rodgers, and Letty Cottin Pogrebin, *Free To Be You and Me,* New York: McGraw-Hill, 1974).

10. Linda Jane Vogel, *Helping a Child Understand Death* (Boston: Fortress, 1975).

CHAPTER 7

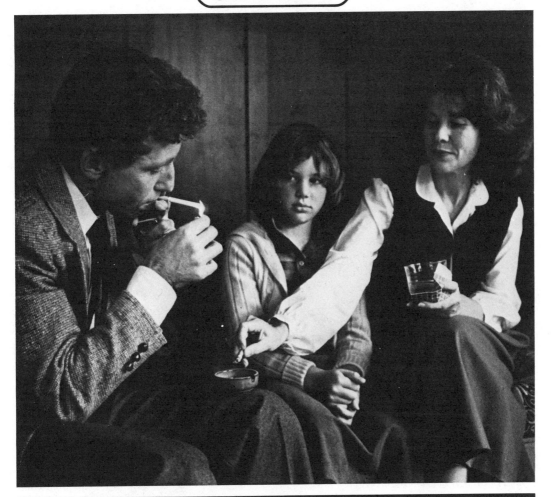

PART A: DRUGS, ALCOHOL, AND TOBACCO

It is difficult to imagine a lifestyle completely devoid of drugs, those chemical or biological agents that have the ability to change the composition or the functioning of the human body. From the first drops of silver nitrate dropped into our newly opened eyes to the drugs urgently administered to sustain our ebbing lives, we medicate ourselves.

Typical ten-year-olds have ingested without question many prescribed pills —both drugs and vitamins. They have received injections for illness, tetanus/diptheria, and polio. They have seen and heard television and radio commercials that offer drugs as a panacea, and they have witnessed their parents and friends using drugs. These are the children we are asked to "drug educate."

While we may hear more about drug use and misuse today, people have always searched for and used drugs in the alleviation of pain and the prevention, treatment, and eradication of disease. For thousands of years humans have also used drugs during religious and social events to enhance the moment or the meaning of the occasion as well as to reduce or escape from psychological pain and discomfort.

A definitive discussion of the use and abuse of drugs is beyond the scope of this text. The discussion has been generally limited to the most widely used substances: tobacco, alcohol, and marijuana. Some background information has been provided on such substances as LSD, peyote, mescaline, psilocybin, caffeine, nicotine, amphetamines, cocaine, barbiturates, and heroin.

DEFINITION OF TERMS

To understand drug use, it is necessary to begin with a definition of some standard terms:

Because of their nature and because of human nature, drugs are frequently used improperly. The healthy or *proper use* of a drug occurs when the choice of the drug meets and fulfills the occasion and the need, that is, when it is taken in the proper amount and at the proper time, and when necessary precautions are observed.

It is apparent that drug *misuse* can and does take place in a number of different ways, the most common being that of taking the drug for a purpose or need that the drug is incapable of meeting. Consequently, relaxing with a cigarette and increasing one's sexual prowess with Vitamin E constitute drug misuse, because these agents simply cannot fulfill those purposes. The common practices of sharing another's medication for similar symptoms, taking twice the amount of wonder drug required, discontinuing a medication as soon as the symptoms abate, and drowning one's sorrow in alcohol also constitute drug misuse.

If a substance is misused to the degree that it results in impaired mental, physical, or social function, drug *abuse* has occurred. Chronic drug abuse has serious implications. It may produce one or both of two different types of dependencies: psychological and physical.

Those persons who feel an overwhelming or compelling emotional need to continue the use of a chemical agent to promote or maintain their well-being are said to be *psychologically dependent*.

Abstinence or *withdrawal* of the drug from a psychologically dependent person may produce such sumptoms as irritability or anxiety, but it does not produce physical symptoms. Psychological dependence or habituation may be associated with the use of any drug, including tobacco, caffeine, diet aids, laxatives, and illicit drugs.

Physical dependence indicates an alteration in the physiological makeup, or cellular state, so that the body acquires a need for the substance to be able to maintain its new homeostatic state. Generally, it takes at least six weeks of repeated abuse to develop such an altered state. Physical dependence is only manifested when the drug is withheld, at which time the abstinence syndrome appears.

The *abstinence syndrome*, or *withdrawal*, is a symptom complex that depends on the nature of the drug and, very often, on the nature and personality of the individual. Withdrawal from some drugs is similar to a severe flu attack, while for others, it can be life threatening and may require close medical supervision. In some cases, death can result from complications experienced during withdrawal, breathing difficulties and self-inflicted injury being among the most frequent causes.

Another phenomenon associated with chronic drug abuse, particularly with the depressants, is that of *tolerance*. While the mechanism involved is not fully understood, the body adapts and adjusts to the agent in such a way that it requires increasingly larger doses to produce the same effect ordinarily achieved with smaller doses. The body has an absolute limit on all foreign substances, but up to that limit, the person who has developed drug tolerance is able to take exceptionally large doses—amounts that would be life threatening without tolerance.

THE DRUG-TAKING MODEL

Our profound encouragement of, and dependence on, chemical agents and cure-alls may have a direct effect on the magnitude of the drug problem in the United States today—especially among youth. Children get their cues from the adult world; the home and the media are the message. The typical home of today has over thirty drugs in it. In addition, most magazines and radio and television compete with each other in an effort to add even more chemicals to our shelves. Without explicitly stating what the agent will do *to* us, that is, how it truly acts, we are told what it will do *for* us. The instant gratification message is always the same.

Even without media bombardment, the human being is an inquisitive creature. Although this wonderful quality is sometimes trampled on or snuffed out by the time adulthood is reached, enough of it remains in some people to cause them to experiment with drugs.

In fact, it appears that this is the motive most frequently involved in drug use and abuse. A parent or teacher should look at the experimenting child as entirely different from an established drug user and abuser, since after having tried a drug a few times, the child's curiosity is often satisfied and the behavior stops. The person who continues to misuse drugs does so in an attempt to fulfill other needs, such as the need to escape.

THE DRUG EXPERIENCE

It is difficult, and less than accurate, to describe the effects of any type of drug or drug experience as being consistent or absolute, because the outcome of each drug encounter depends on three equally important variables: the drug, the user, and the environment. Such factors as the type of drug; the amount, purity, route of administration, and metabolism; the site of action; and the mind set of the individual—including expectations, emotional and physical stability, and conditions under which the drug is taken, for example, company present, physical surroundings, and audio-visual stimulation—all combine to affect the response.

Just as these are variables and can never be present in precisely the same combination again, no two drug experiences will ever be quite the same. Keeping this in mind, as well as the research findings that teaching the effects of drugs by itself may actually do very little to change behavior, the following information is included as reference material.

Hallucinogenic Drugs

An *hallucination* is a false perception that has no relation to reality and cannot be accounted for by any external stimuli. It often indicates a severe mental or physical disorder and may manifest itself through any, or more than one, of the senses.

Hallucinogenic drugs are so called because they are capable of producing bizarre aberrations similar to those experienced during a psychotic hallucinatory episode, with two important distinctions:

1. The drug user is generally able to recognize that he or she is hallucinating while the psychotic individual is not.
2. The drug-induced experience is a temporary one while the psychotic hallucination may occur repeatedly and is not bound by time or drug.

One of the dangers of certain of the hallucinogens, or psychedelics, however, is that they may, on rare occasions, cause hallucinations that persist or recur repeatedly beyond the normal time limit, thus precipitating a psychotic episode. While the reason for this is not known, it is thought to be a function of a transitory or long-term instability or susceptibility within the individual.

Although their popularity shifts with time and location, the psychedelic agents most commonly used in the United States are LSD, mescaline, peyote, and psilocybin. The psychoactive substance marijuana will also be discussed with this category of drugs.

LSD

LSD-25 is an abbreviation for lysergic acid diethylamide tartrate 25. It is derived from lysergic acid and is readily synthesized in the laboratory through processes of freezing and fractional distillation.

Because it is a semisynthetic that lends itself to adaptive techniques, and because it is very strictly controlled, LSD is frequently made in the home or clandestine laboratory. This is not done without a significant compromise in the integrity of the drug, however.

PEYOTE

Peyote is a small brown cactus with tiny buttons on it. These buttons are either chewed raw or dried, or converted into a liquid form. The taste is quite bitter and unpleasant, which may account in part for the intense nausea and vomiting that frequently accompany the use of this drug.

Of the many active alkaloids in peyote, the agent responsible for inducing hallucinations is mescaline.

MESCALINE

Mescaline is now manufactured synthetically and, in its pure form, is more potent than peyote and produces fewer unpleasant side effects, such as nausea and vomiting.

Mescaline comes in powder, capsule, and liquid form and may be taken orally—the most common method—intravenously, or by inhalation.

PSILOCYBIN

History reveals that psilocybe Mexicana, a mushroom, has been a vehicle for hallucinogenic religious experiences in much the same way as peyote. The hallucinogenic alkaloid psilocybin is now synthesized in the laboratory and can be dispensed in powder and liquid form. In the body, it is converted to psilocin.

MARIJUANA

The Indian hemp, cannabis sativa, has been used throughout the centuries for its mood modifying properties. Although it produces best in temperate and tropical zones, the plant is cultivated and used around the world, thereby achieving a standing second only to alcohol as a universal mind-altering agent.

The psychoactive ingredient in cannabis is a class of chemicals called tetrahydrocannabinol, or THC. The origin, method of cultivation, variety, and part of the plant used influence the concentration or potency among its many preparations. The resin contains the strongest concentration of THC, followed by the flowers and the leaves.

Marijuana is usually smoked in cigarette form, although many prefer to use simple or elaborate water pipes, or to consume it in food or drink.

In low doses, such as are contained in the average of one or two American cigarettes, "joints," or "reefers," it produces effects similar to both the sedatives and the stimulants, along with unique properties of its own. Only at very high dosages does the user experience effects similar to those of LSD.

Marijuana causes an increase in heart rate and blood pressure, dizziness progressing to unsteadiness and lack of coordination, dryness of the mouth and throat, and a cough, which is probably caused by the very harsh smoke. The fact that marijuana also causes dilation of certain blood vessels accounts for the bloodshot eyes that are a hallmark of this drug experience. Another very characteristic symptom is hunger, particularly a craving for sweets.

The initial psychological effects include a sense of apprehension, followed by alterations of sensory perception and disjointed thought processes, which may affect ego concepts, producing many moods and effecting many types of behavior. Reactions include euphoria and bursts of giggling, relaxation and release of social inhibitions, distortion of spatial and temporal perceptions, detachment from self or the environment, increased sensual and introspective awareness, and a disturbance in the sense of structural boundaries.

A marijuana user may encounter none, a few, or all of these sensations, depending on the variables. Some people find these reactions exciting or perceive them as a growth experience. Others find them boring or unpleasant.

Although research efforts are hindered and the reports conflicting, it appears that the acute and long-term complications of marijuana are minimal. Panic reactions and psychoses are rare.

The concept of marijuana use leading to use of other more potent and dangerous drugs is probably best put in the same perspective as that of social drinking leading to alcoholism. For susceptible individuals, the possibility exists, but the large majority of marijuana users do not use narcotics, just as the large majority of alcohol users do not become alcoholics. Furthermore, it is estimated that only 2 percent of current marijuana users abuse the drug heavily, smoking as many as eight or ten cigarettes a day.

Stimulant Drugs

The human nervous system may be powerfully stimulated by stress or a category of drugs known as stimulants.

The response under stress allows people in danger to call on the body's resources immediately to cope with the danger or extricate themselves from the scene. (This has given rise to the popularly used descriptive term, "fight or flight" response.)

Because the body is unable to discriminate between the stimulation of a charging lion and the stimulation of an angry boss, a lighted cigarette, a cup of coffee, or an amphetamine diet agent, the stress response, although modified in degree, is always the same. The caveman and our more recent ancestors worked through the stress response and in doing so, alleviated the psychological and physiological byproducts. The opposite holds true for the modern individual, whose life is filled with stress and inactivity.

Stimulants involve the mobilization of mental and physical processes through the use of a chemically induced stress response.

CAFFEINE

Caffeine is found in coffee, tea, cocoa, and cola drinks as well as most nonprescription agents available to counteract fatigue and drowsiness. Consequently, it is the most widely used psychoactive agent in the United States. Because it is a comparatively mild stimulant, caffeine produces a stress response and mental and physical energization of a lesser degree than the amphetamines.

Abuse of caffeine, that is, more than four to six cups of coffee or cola, results in irritability and insomnia. Because of the induced stress response, individuals with cardiovascular diseases and peptic ulcers are generally advised to refrain from using caffeine and all stimulating agents.

NICOTINE

Nicotine is one of over 1,200 different compounds to be identified in tobacco smoke. Besides being a stimulant, it is a highly toxic substance responsible for a number of reported cases of poisoning. See the tobacco and smoking section below for additional information.

AMPHETAMINES

The amphetamines are a class of synthetic compounds frequently called "uppers." The most commonly used and abused, in order of increasing potency, are Benzedrine (Bennies), Methedrine (Meth or Speed), and Dexedrine (Dexies).

COCAINE

Cocaine is derived from the leaves of the coca bush grown in Java, Bolivia, and Peru. Most of the illicit cocaine in the United States comes from these countries.

Cocaine comes as a white crystalline powder and is generally sniffed, because it loses its potency when taken by mouth. This method takes its toll by destroying the mucous membrane and, after a long period of heavy abuse, even the nasal bone.

TOBACCO AND SMOKING

Throughout history the use of tobacco has been as controversial as that of many of the other equally dangerous drugs. At different places and times, tobacco users have been encouraged, discouraged, punished, tolerated, and ignored. As with other types of behavior, smoking probably results from the perception that it mitigates or fulfills physiological and psychosocial needs.

The tobacco plant is a member of the nightshade family, and like most plants, its leaves are composed of a myriad of proteins, carbohydrates, and other hydrocarbons. As a result of burning, these substances are converted into volatilized compounds, gases, and particulate matter.

Nicotine is perhaps the most familiar tobacco component. This substance appears in widely varying amounts due to naturally occurring factors (relative position of leaf on stalk, area where it is grown) and technological factors (special strains and special treatment with steam or solvents).

In order to avoid a false sense of security, it should be understood that the term *denicotinized* implies only that the present nicotine concentration may be as much as half that found in standard cigarettes, and this is true only in some, not all of the so-called denicotinized brands. Low nicotine brands contain another compound, not naturally occurring in tobacco, that is less toxic.

Just as the amount of nicotine inherent in the tobacco depends on a number of variables, so does the amount that is absorbed by the body. The greatest amount is ingested through the use of snuff, a smaller amount is absorbed by chewing, and the smallest amount is obtained through cigarette smoking.

Some people believe that filters will protect them. Filters have been recessed, triple air filtered, treated with special chemicals, tipped, and elongated, but the truth of the matter is that many filters offer no more protection against the harmful ingredients of cigarette smoke than the identical length of tobacco would.

The ingredients or small particles suspended with the gases of the smoke are called tars. They consist of many acids, alcohols, and irritating chemicals. Most important, they contain many hydrocarbons that are known to be carcinogenic, or cancer causing.

To further complicate this already dangerous situation, tars also contain phenols. Besides being toxic to the cilia, phenols are believed to have the capacity to promote tumor activity, either by inciting dormant cancer cells or by accelerating the activity of cancer cells already present.

Among the gases to be found in smoke are carbon monoxide, which combines with hemoglobin in the red blood cell, thereby decreasing the oxygen-carrying capacity of the blood; carbon dioxide: a waste product of metabolism and respiration; and other toxic compounds, such as acetaldehyde, ammonia, formaldehyde, and hydrogen cyanide, which impair the function—particularly the mechanical defense mechanism—of the lungs.

The gases and tar attack and damage the respiratory system in a number of ways. The respiratory passageways are covered with a protective layer of mucus and cilia, tiny hairlike structures. The mucus acts as a shield to preserve the integrity of the structures underneath as well as to trap any foreign particles that might enter the lungs. The constantly beating cilia lift these trapped particles and excess mucus up the passageway to be either expectorated or swallowed.

Smoking impairs or shuts down this operation. The gases from a cigarette may immobilize the cilia for about four hours. Since most people do not wait four hours between cigarettes, this does not allow for a recovery period, except at night. Hence, the smoker's cough develops. It is first noticeable on rising, then as more and more insult and injury are accrued, it becomes continuous throughout the day and night.

It should be remembered that in these high risk days of auto and industrial emissions and poor air quality, the body needs every defense it has. The end result of constant insult to the structure and function of the respiratory system is to leave the individual highly susceptible to respiratory infections, bronchitis, emphysema, cancer, and other lung diseases and dysfunctions.

Bronchitis is an inflammation of the cells lining the bronchi and bronchioles —the tubes that lead to the microscopic air sacs (alveoli) where the actual exchange of gases takes place.

In *emphysema*, the plastic property of the alveoli is lost. Gradually the walls of the alveoli become distended; some rupture and are replaced with scar tissue. This not only decreases the surface area necessary for the exchange of gases with the blood capillaries, but also leads to accumulation of stale air and the debris not removed by the impaired cilia.

In an effort to compensate, the chest cage enlarges, reducing the efficiency of the primary and accessory muscles of respiration. Eventually, these overstretched and overworked muscles cannot function adequately and breathing becomes a labor instead of a function. This puts an extra load on the heart and may lead to heart failure. Although there still is no cure for emphysema, modern medicine can usually slow down the progress of emphysema and help patients live more comfortably.

The leading cause of cancer deaths in the United States today is *lung cancer*. For smokers, this represents the second leading cause of excess deaths; 90 percent of all lung cancers occur among those who smoke.

The symptoms of lung cancer are persistent cough, blood in the sputum, and a lingering infection of the lung or pain in the chest; however, by the time these have appeared, the disease has usually progressed too far to be cured. The National Cancer Institute reports only about 10 percent of patients found to have lung cancer now survive for three years.

There is an immediate consequence of smoking that should be of concern to all pregnant women. According to the Public Health Service, pregnant women who smoke increase their risk for miscarriage by 20 percent over their nonsmoking counterparts. There is also a significant relationship between smoking during pregnancy and both neonatal mortality and lowered birth weight.

As with every situation in life, not everyone who is exposed to disease or injury succumbs. While there are many reasons proposed for this, the important fact remains that these conditions associated with smoking are risks, not certainties.

For years, educators have been teaching about the risks and effects of smoking, but these reports indicate that something more or something different needs to be done. Perhaps the answer lies in doing something different, such as copying the techniques of the adversary, the multimillion-dollar tobacco industry.

In studying cigarette ads carefully, one notes that there is very little said about the cigarettes themselves. The subtle implications are that smoking is associated with and achieves other desirable things: relief, gratification, and the enjoyment of nature, companionship, and social activities.

It is important that the public be made aware of the risks of smoking; these should be included in any educational program at any age level. However, youth do not frighten easily, and the risks seem so far away as to be unreal.

What is needed, then, is positive advertising for the highest level, fullest quality lifestyle. By borrowing and capitalizing on the techniques of the adversary, the value systems emerging in youth, or already strongly in action, may be put to good use.

For example, youth should know that smoking gives them bad breath—a condition that can be detected in intimate situations despite gum, mints, or toothpaste. "Whiter teeth and fresh breath" do not go hand in hand with smoking.

Although smoking has never been proven to cause pimples, it does permeate the skin, hair, and clothes. Those who wish to smell "as clean as all outdoors" must refrain not only from smoking themselves, but also from being closeted with those who do—a positive use of peer pressure.

This kind of education touches youth in the areas where they are most concerned, and thus may be effective. For youth at this age, personal appearance and social construct are extremely important—important enough to give up smoking for those who realize they cannot have it both ways.

Because rebellion is one of the reasons frequently cited for beginning or continuing to smoke, it is important when educating youth about the use of tobacco not be overly negative or prejudiced, for this feeds directly into the syndrome of defiance. A nonjudgmental attitude allows students to develop their own system of values. Also, it is very difficult to rebel against something for which there is no moral standard or set of prescribed behaviors.

Depressants

Drugs that depress the activity of the nervous system may have effects ranging from simple decreased acuity of sensation and inhibitions, to drowsiness and sleep, to coma and death. By and large, these reactions depend on the nature of the drug and its specific site of action. Equally important is the dosage.

Of the many types of depressants, the following, because of their particularly desirous effects, have become subject to misuse and abuse:

Alcohol, the universally used depressant

Sedative hypnotics, which produce rest and sleep

Analgesics, which relieve pain

Certain anesthetics, which may produce loss of sensation and/or loss of consciousness

In the present chapter only alcohol, sedative hypnotics, and heroin will be discussed.

ALCOHOL

Studies reveal that most of what people "know" about alcohol is mythical or misunderstood. Education about alcohol should begin in the primary grades, for even in this country use begins at an early age—for some as early as the toddler stage.

Alcohol is a drug. As such, it has the potential to be used in a pleasant, positive manner or in a dangerous and destructive way. Education can help make the difference.

Ethyl alcohol, or *ethanol*, is so predominant in our society that it is universally understood to be alcohol. It is the common ingredient in beer, wine, and liquor. Pure ethanol is a colorless, inflammable liquid with a burning taste. It is about one-fifth lighter than water, hence, the need to stir mixed drinks.

Contrary to popular belief, alcohol is a depressant drug with far-reaching effects throughout the body. Although it has no nutritional value, ethanol is classified as a food, because it provides seven calories per gram (carbohydrate and protein provide 4 cal/g.; fat provides 9 cal/g.).

The same process that makes bread rise produces alcohol. Using different sources of sugar in the fermentation process produces alcoholic beverages. Beer and ale, for example, are made from malt and cereal grains and contain 2.5 to 6 percent alcohol. Hops are often added to alcohol; their only effect is to give it a bitter taste. They do not induce sleep, as is commonly thought.

Beer contains the least amount of alcohol per unit volume, but the amount consumed is often larger, thereby making the total consumption of alcohol comparable to that consumed in the average highball made with ½ ounce of alcohol. For example, the average twelve-ounce American beer, containing 4.5 percent alcohol by volume, results in the consumption of just over ½ (0.54) ounce of alcohol. It also yields about 150 calories, a significant number.

Wine is made from the fermentation of grapes, berries, or other fruit. Ordinary table wines contain 10 to 14 percent alcohol by volume, while the dessert wines, such as port and sherry, may contain 17 to 21 percent alcohol.

Consequently, three ounces of a sherry that is 20 percent alcohol produces 0.6 ounces of alcohol, or roughly that of the average American beer or cocktail. It would take five ounces of a 12 percent table wine to yield the same amount. A glass of California red wine contains about 85 calories while an equivalent amount of Madeira contains 158 calories.

As a foodstuff, alcohol has unique properties: it does not have to be digested before it is absorbed—in fact, as much as one-fifth of it is absorbed directly through the walls of the stomach. The remainder is passed into the small intestine and is taken up so quickly by a vast network of blood vessels that it may appear in the bloodstream only five minutes after ingestion. Many factors influence absorption, including the nature of the beverage, the presence or absence of food in the stomach and intestines, and the rate of ingestion. Once absorbed, the alcohol is carried by the bloodstream to all the tissues of the body.

Since alcohol cannot be used in its absorbed state, it is recognized by the body as a toxin that should be removed. About 10 percent of the alcohol absorbed will be directly eliminated through the lungs and kidneys. As a result, the strength of the alcohol to be found in the breath and urine is in direct proportion to that found in the blood. This is the basis for the tests used to diagnose levels of intoxication. The remaining alcohol, about 90 percent, is metabolized in the liver. This metabolism takes place at a constant, ongoing rate of one-quarter to one-half ounce per hour until the supply is diminished.

Since this rate is influenced only by the size and state of the liver, as well as by some rare drug reactions, other measures such as drinking coffee, taking cold showers, or exercising will not help a person to sober up more quickly. For those who must perform skills involving judgment and dexterity, such as driving, this hourly metabolic rate to sobriety is a very important concept.

The end product of this first phase of metabolism is acetaldehyde, a toxic substance. The excessive accumulation of this compound is associated with the gastritis, headache, dizziness, and other symptoms of a hangover. Therefore, the practice of consuming more alcohol to cure a hangover makes little sense. The second phase of alcohol metabolism may occur in the liver as well as other organs. The end products of complete metabolism are energy, carbon dioxide, and water.

Metabolic factors make methyl alcohol (wood alcohol) very dangerous, even though it is not by nature more intoxicating than ethanol. *Methanol* is oxidized or destroyed very slowly. Therefore accumulation becomes a significant risk factor. Furthermore, the end product of oxidation is not carbon dioxide and water, but formic acid, a poison that can severely damage the optic nerves and cause blindness.

Physical Effects of Alcohol

While alcohol is used as a food, it is experienced as a depressant drug. It is for this drug experience that most people drink.

The first area of the brain to be affected is the cerebral cortex, the area housing the higher learning centers. One of the first learned behaviors to be depressed is that of personal and social inhibition. As the blood alcohol level increases, the amount of inhibition decreases, causing social or antisocial behavior that would normally be held in check.

The depression of the brain is progressive and is in direct relationship to the blood alcohol level. Following impairment of the cerebral cortex is a disturbance in those areas of the brain that control speech, hearing, and visual discrimination. This accounts for the rise in noise level at cocktail parties as drinking progresses.

Following impairment of the senses comes a marked disturbance in coordination and balance. A continued rise in the blood alcohol level results in marked exaggeration of all symptoms and progressively leads toward unconsciousness, coma, and death. In the United States, deaths due to extreme intoxication alone number about 1,000 each year.

Table 7A-1 shows the relationship between the amount of alcohol consumed, the blood alcohol level, and the effects that can be expected.

TABLE 7A-1 RELATIONSHIP BETWEEN AMOUNT OF ALCOHOL CONSUMED, BLOOD ALCOHOL LEVEL, AND EXPECTED EFFECTS

Approximate Amount of Ethanol	Blood Alcohol Level	Expected Effects
½–¾ ounce or one drink	0.03%	Slight changes in feelings and inhibitions.
1–1½ ounces or two drinks	0.06%	Some impairment in memory, judgment, restraint and fine muscle coordination. Feeling of mental relaxation and well being.
1½–2¼ ounces or three drinks	0.09%	Exaggeration of feelings and behavioral changes. Slightly longer reaction time.

TABLE 7A-1 (cont.)

Approximate Amount of Ethanol	Blood Alcohol Level	Expected Effects
2–3 ounces or four drinks	0.12%	Emotional stability and mental faculties noticeably impaired; moderate difficulty with motor coordination and balance.
2½–3¾ oz. or five drinks	0.15%	Legal intoxication in all states. Loss of control over gross bodily functions and mental faculties. Impaired speech and hearing and visual discrepancy.
3½–3¼ oz. or seven drinks	0.21%	Marked depression of motor areas accompanied by staggering or prostration. Exaggerated and inappropriate emotional behavior.
5–8½ oz. or 10 drinks	0.30%	Depression of primitive perceptive areas. Confusion; often stupor.
8–12 oz. or 16 drinks	0.48%	Unaware of environment. Coma.
10–15 oz. or 20 drinks	0.60%	Depression of medulla. Death from respiratory failure.

In small amounts, alcohol is an effective appetizer, stimulating mild muscular contractions and the secretion of gastric juices. In large amounts, alcohol dulls the appetite. This helps account for the generally poor health of the alcohol abuser, because alcohol, while furnishing a high number of calories, provides no vitamins, minerals, or other nutritional elements.

In stronger solutions, ethanol acts as an irritant on the lining of the upper gastrointestinal tract. With chronic abuse, particularly in the absence of proper nutrition, the lining of these structures may erode, producing serious consequences. Because of its burning properties, people with inflammation of the upper gastrointestinal tract, that is, esophagitis, gastritis, and peptic ulcer, are strongly advised to refrain from consuming alcohol.

The liver is an extremely resilient organ and able to cope quite adequately with short-term abuse. However, a number of debilitating conditions result from many years of alcohol abuse, including fatty liver, hepatitis, and cirrhosis.

About one in every ten alcoholics develops cirrhosis, a disease in which there is irreversible and progressive destruction of viable liver tissue and impairment of many of its vital functions. If drinking ceases, the condition often improves, although the structural damage already done is irreversible. If heavy drinking continues, the risk of death is markedly increased. In New York City, the third leading cause of death for persons aged twenty-five to sixty-five is cirrhosis of the liver.

The concept that alcohol enhances body warmth is not correct. The depressant nature of the drug causes a dilation of the peripheral blood vessels promoting a loss of heat from the body and often provoking sweating and flushing of the skin. Concurrently, there is an increase in the rate and oxygen consumption of the heart and a decrease in blood pressure.

Under normal circumstances, the effects of mild to moderate drinking are not detrimental, but intoxicating amounts tax the mechanical efficiency of the heart. It is not yet known whether this is a direct causative factor in alcoholic heart disease, but it is a decided hazard for the person already suffering a heart ailment.

Because alcohol crosses the placental barrier, a pregnant woman's drinking directly affects the fetus. If the woman is drunk, the fetus is drunk—and decidedly disadvantaged since the fetus is not equipped with the same detoxifying capabilities as the mother.

If the mother is addicted to alcohol, the fetus is also and will need to be treated for withdrawal after birth. Whether or not this constitutes a predisposition to future alcoholism is presently being studied. Regardless, it has long been recognized that the newborn of alcoholic mothers are less healthy and well developed than those of nonalcoholic mothers.

Cancers of the mouth, pharynx, larynx, and esophagus appear to have a definite relationship to heavy alcohol ingestion. Moreover, in cancers of the mouth, pharynx, and larynx, research reveals that combining alcohol and tobacco, as is often the case, produces not only an additive effect, but possibly a synergistic risk as well. Evidence also indicates that there is a relationship between alcohol and cancer of the pancreas, prostate, and liver.

Alcoholism

The word *alcoholic* has been in use since 1856, but the condition has existed throughout the ages. Despite modern technology and increasing research efforts, the cause and cure for alcoholism remain elusive.

Alcoholism is described and defined in terms of the vantage point. Therefore, it means different things to the individual concerned; to the family; to the law officer, employer, or innocent victim of an alcohol-related accident; and to the biochemist, teacher, psychologist, social worker, or physician. Directly or indirectly, the alcoholic generally ends up in contact with all of these people. As a result, it is not possible to find a consistent definition of the terms related to alcohol abuse. (Even the legal definition of intoxication differs among states.)

Such terms as *alcohol abuser, heavy drinker, near alcoholic,* and *problem drinker* have arisen, perhaps in attempts to help define the problem. Often, however, they are merely a source of confusion. On the other hand, the many precise definitions of *alcoholism* render it a somewhat amorphous term. We shall hold to the three concepts that seem to run as a common thread through most definitions: continuity, control, and conflict.

Alcoholism exists when there is a continued or repeated drinking pattern that both results from and further supports a lack of control over the drinking occasion. This eventually results in discord and conflict in a significant area of the person's lifestyle or life space, be it the home, school, community, or place of employment. Accordingly, alcoholism is best not defined in terms of volume or time, as they differ with each individual, but by the effects it has on the individual.

What separates the 10 million individuals who have lost control over alcohol from the 85 million drinkers who still retain it? While the cause of alcoholism is not known, there are a number of theories based on physiological, psychological, and sociocultural factors that have been promoted as predisposing or etiological agents. The large number of theories and the presence of individual differences within the population using and abusing alcohol indicate that there is probably not a single causative agent but rather, a complex of factors that in the proper combination, promote the development of alcoholism.

The only factor that alcohol abusers truly have in common is their abuse of alcohol. Therefore, there are a number of treatment programs and agencies designed to meet the different needs and resources of the individual alcoholic, including individual and group therapy and organizations such as Alcoholics Anonymous. The goal of these agencies is to modify attitudes and behavior in a purposeful manner.

Alcoholics Anonymous functions on a fellowship basis; it has no professional staff, no annual dues, and no membership requirements. It is a self-help organization that believes that alcoholism is a disease involving the loss of the ability to control alcohol.

Al-Anon is an organization for family members of the alcoholic. It attempts to develop understanding and insight into the problems that have developed before, during, and after the alcoholic is ill.

Alateen is an outgrowth of Al-Anon with the same purpose and function. It is designed for the children of alcoholics (ages thirteen to twenty).

In this country, the person who abstains from alcohol is in the minority. Since alcohol is obviously a part of many lifestyles, responsible attitudes toward its use and abuse must be developed early in life, in the home, school, and community.

SEDATIVES AND HYPNOTICS

The difference between a sedative and a hypnotic is one of degree. Sedatives produce a calming, quieting effect and are usually given once or several times a day in a reduced dosage. Hypnotics produce sleep and are given full strength at bedtime.

Barbiturates

The barbiturates are the most widely used sedative drugs. Barbiturates are classified according to the speed with which they act and disappear from the body. They range from the very rapidly acting sodium pentothal through the intermediate, and most frequently abused, group—including Seconal, Nembutal, Butisol Sodium, and Amytal—to the slowly acting Luminal. Although barbiturates are injectable, they are most frequently taken orally.

Barbiturates are desirable because small doses are effective in relieving tension and anxiety without causing excessive drowsiness; however, chronic high-dose abuse creates a psychological and physical dependence.

Tolerance to barbiturates does develop with continued use, but this does not significantly alter the lethal dose, which varies with individuals. This makes them a very dangerous type of drug since abusers will, of necessity, increase their dosage to obtain the desired effect.

Barbiturates are also cross-tolerant with alcohol and increase in potency when combined with alcohol. Used singly or in combination with alcohol, barbiturates are among the leading instruments of intentional and accidental suicide. Because the desired effect of the depressants is primarily escape, it is difficult to know which of these suicides are accidental.

A drug that creates physical dependence produces a syndrome known as withdrawal when the drug is removed for any given period of time. Withdrawal from barbiturates produces symptoms that are even more profound than those produced by heroin withdrawal and closely resemble those produced by alcohol withdrawal. The first symptom is anxiety, which progresses after two or three days to a psychosis with delirium, hallucinations, and paranoid delusions, frequently lasting as long as two weeks.

Heroin

Heroin is an opiate derivative sold in the form of a bitter-tasting white powder. In its pure form, it is 2½ to 3 times more potent than morphine. It is usually mixed with a liquid and taken intravenously (mainlined).

Immediately after injection, heroin produces a sense of pleasure so passionate and powerful that it is likened to orgasm or death. Paradoxically, it depresses the basic drives, including sex. Heroin produces both tolerance and dependence.

DRUG EDUCATION

Hopefully, the preceding reference material will make the teacher more comfortable about discussing drugs, as well as more open and honest in discussing any situation the students might bring up.

The following significant points should be remembered:

1. Knowledge by itself will not prevent drug abuse.

2. Turning to drugs is turning away from life and from the obligation we all have to find life's meaning.

3. One of the more basic tasks of adolescence is to form a stable self-concept or self-definition. Adolescence is a time for experimentation with a multitude of roles and choices, a time to recognize capabilities and weaknesses.

4. A good drug abuse program is a program that teaches decision making. Of course, in order for a student to be able to make decisions, he or she must have developed a sense of self-worth.

5. The teacher should be curious about what need the student is trying to satisfy. Besides drugs, people turn to institutions to satisfy their needs—family, friends, sport, exercise, dance, sleep, music, nature, poetry, food, religion, useful work, and so on. The teacher should help students consider the alternatives.

6. The teacher should encourage each student to explore his or her uniqueness; to strengthen the self that offers the promise of individuality and liberation, the self that society needs but may not recognize until it has been actualized.

FURTHER READINGS

L. Bogert, G. Briggs, D. Calloway, *Nutrition and Physical Fitness*, 10th ed. (Philadelphia: Saunders, 1979).

E. M. Breecher, *Licit and Illicit Drugs* (Boston: Little, Brown, 1972).

J. Fort, *The Pleasure Seekers* (Indianapolis: Bobbs-Merrill, 1969).

D. A. Girdano, and D. D. Girdano, *Drug Education, Content and Methods*, 2d ed. (Reading, Mass.: Addison-Wesley, 1976).

L. Grinspoon and P. Hedblom, *The Speed Culture: Amphetamine Use and Abuse in America* (Cambridge, Mass.: Harvard University Press, 1975).

Herman Krimmel, *Alcoholism: Challenge for Social Work Education* (New York: Council on Social Work Education, 1971).

K. Lamott, *Escape from Stress* (New York: Putnam, 1975).

E. Lichenstein, "How to Quit Smoking," *Psychology Today*, January 1971, pp. 42, 44, 45.

S. Oakley, *Drugs, Society and Human Behavior* (St. Louis: Mosby, 1972).

U.S. Department of H.E.W., *Alcohol and Health* (Washington, D.C., U.S. Gov't Printing Office, 1974).

————. *Smoking and Health* (Washington, D.C., U.S. Gov't Printing Office, 1974).

ADDITIONAL SOURCES OF INFORMATION

Alcoholics Anonymous, P.O. Box 429, Grand Central Annex, New York, N.Y. 10017. (Contact your local chapter first)

American Lung Association, 51 Sleeper Street, Boston, Ma. 02210. (Contact your local chapter first)

American Medical Association, Department of Health Education, 535 North Dearborn Street, Chicago, Il. 60610.

National Coordinating Council on Drug Abuse, P.O. Box 19400, Washington, D.C. 20036.

National Council on Alcoholism, 2 Park Avenue, New York, N.Y. 10016.

National Interagency on Smoking and Health, P.O. Box 3654, Central Station, Arlington, Va. 22203.

Rutgers Center of Alcohol Studies, Rutgers, The State University, New Brunswick, N.J. 08903.

PART B: TEACHING ABOUT DRUGS, ALCOHOL, AND TOBACCO

Most successful drug educators are completely honest with their students and have established an atmosphere of love, security, and trust in their classrooms. They create this environment or climate by establishing a working democratic classroom where students have certain amounts of responsibility, times for sharing with others, times for reflection, and times to converse with the teacher individually as well as in groups.

Effective drug education programs seem to have several things in common.

1. They are *preventive*. Drug education efforts should begin in kindergarten or first grade, when adult influence is still greater than peer pressure.

2. They are based on a *healthy model* rather than a sick model. (They begin with happy, healthy children and try to keep them that way!)

3. They are *realistic*. The program must contain factual information that is kept in perspective. Students have many other things on their minds besides taking drugs!

4. They are *student oriented* rather than teacher oriented.

5. They are *decisions-oriented*. They help students explore the process of arriving at a decision and emphasize problem solving.

6. They involve more than just factual *drug information*. The Ohio Drug, Al-

cohol, Tobacco and Human Behavior program called "A World to Grow In" explores dealing with authority, developing positive personal relationships, developing a positive self-concept, and exploring the student's environment.

7. They offer the student *alternatives* to drug taking. (See Unit V.)

In a country where we spend millions of dollars promoting so-called good drugs and fighting so-called bad drugs, how can we help students determine the appropriate place of drugs in their life-styles?

1. Students need to appreciate the physical and psychological well-being that comes from a healthy body. (See Chapter 8.)

2. Students need to understand that medicines and drugs may be helpful when properly used.

3. Students need to recognize that everything that makes contact with the human body or enters it has an effect on it.

4. Students need to realize that the body and mind are interrelated.

5. Students need to learn that medicines and drugs may be harmful when used improperly.

6. Students need to know that they are important and worthwhile.

UNIT I: OVER-THE-COUNTER AND PRESCRIPTION DRUGS

Factual drug education units are often more effective when they are taught at

Appropriate grade levels are suggested for each teaching strategy and appear as ○, □, ☆ in the left-hand column:

○ = most suited for the primary grades;
□ = most suited for the intermediate grades;
☆ = most suited for the upper elementary grades.

the end of the school year, because by then the students have received a physical and mental health background. This provides a basis for understanding how drugs are a part of most people's life-styles. The teacher has had many months to get to know each student and create a climate of security and trust. Furthermore, by providing each student with support, successful experiences, and responsibility, the teacher may have already helped to prevent the abuse of drugs.

OBJECTIVES

1. After participating in classroom demonstrations, each student will be able to explain that nothing is all good or bad; the effect a thing has depends on how it is used.

2. The students will be able to name at least four ways that drugs-medicines are helpful when properly used. They will also be able to give an example of proper or improper use of a medicine.

3. The students will help make and stock a medicine cabinet for the classroom that will be used in various ways. The students will be able to differentiate between prescription and nonprescription drugs.

4. The students will devise a display that shows how medicines and household substances may sometimes look like candy and explain what they should do to avoid harming themselves.

MATERIALS

1. Thirteen excellent drug transparencies can be made from *Katy's Coloring Book About Drugs and Health.**

*Available for a nominal charge from Contemporary Design, P.O. Box 262, Campbell, CA 95008, or Supt. of Documents, U.S. Government Printing Office, Washington, D.C. 20025.

2. Old medicine cabinet, or materials to make a medicine cabinet, empty prescription and nonprescription medicine bottles, other objects commonly found in a medicine cabinet.

3. Salt, sugar, cold cream, baby powder, matches, cosmetics, bottle of medicine capsules.

4. Bulletin board space, construction paper, magazines, paste, scissors, and optional materials listed with various activities.

5. Atlas Figure 1, Mother Monkey Reads the Label and Follows the Directions.

Methods

It is helpful for your students to understand that the body and mind (including personality) are interrelated. Explain that if you are in pain, your behavior changes. If you are hungry, your mood is affected. An introductory lesson might include the following demonstration to support the idea that everything that makes contact with the human body or enters it has an effect on it.

○ □
Demonstrations

1. Show the students some food. Discuss how food is needed to nourish the body and mind and sustain life. Can food be harmful? Yes, when used in excess, or if it is spoiled. You may want to show the class salt and sugar. Let a student identify each substance and explain how a little is good, but too much can hurt us.

2. Ask your class if air is good or bad. How is it good? How is it bad? (Show a picture of polluted air.)

3. Rub some cold cream on the hand of a volunteer. What effect did it have on the skin? (Cool, wet, or sticky?) What effect does baby powder have on the skin? (Dries skin, etc.)

4. If you have a container of tear gas, show it to the class, and ask them if they think it is good or bad. (Perhaps good if you're being attacked by a mad dog, but bad, if you are the dog!)

5. Strike a match. What effect does fire have? (Good—cooks food, keeps us warm, etc. Bad—burns people and property.)

6. What effect do cosmetics have on people? Show some cosmetics. They may help us look more attractive, but may also cause an allergic reaction.

7. If the sun is shining ask the students to look out the window and explain what kind of effect the sun has on us. (Sun rays are needed for growing food. Give us a suntan. May also give us sunburn or sunstroke if we are in the sun too long.)

8. Show a real X-ray or a picture of an X-ray. What effect do they have on us? (May help cure cancer, or may cause cancer, depending on how they are used.) The number of examples you use will depend on the age of your class. When the students realize that nothing is all good or all bad, and that the effect a thing has depends on how it is used, you can use a bottle of medicine capsules as your last example.

9. Without telling the class what kind of medicine you are showing them, pour a large number of capsules into your hand and ask them if they think you could take that many without harm. Gradually reduce the number of capsules you are holding until someone says that you are holding the correct amount. Lead into a discussion of how medicine may help you when you are ill if it is given in the proper amount, but that an overdose of medicine that is not right for you can make you ill or even kill you. Ask the

students if the doctor would probably prescribe the same amount of medicine for them that he would for an adult? Why not? (Talk about body weight.)

○ □ ☆

Medicines and Drugs Are Helpful When Used Properly

A series of pictures or slides can be used to illustrate the following examples:*

1. Used in the eyes of newborn infants to prevent possible blindness from disease organisms

2. Used in immunizations to protect us

3. Used in the treatment and prevention of infections

4. Used in the prevention, control, and treatment of illness and disease

5. Used to prevent and relieve discomfort and pain

6. Used in the treatment of mental illness. Drugs can alter a person's mood and combat depression

7. Used to make surgery safer and less painful

8. Used in prolonging life

○ □ ☆

What Are The Four Chief Uses of Drugs?

Use a bulletin board, pictures, research reports, and the following information to discuss this question.

1. Fight diseases. Drugs destroy harmful bacteria. These drugs are called antibiotics and sulfanilamides. Ask the students to find out how the body itself tries to fight disease, how antibiotics work, where we can get antibiotics, and what illnesses they have had that have re-

*Helpful pictures can be found in the booklet, *Drugs and Your Safety*, by Elenore T. Pounds (Glenview, Ill.: Scott, Foresman, 1973).

quired antibiotics. Have the students grow mold and test for antibiotics.

2. Prevent diseases. Vaccines, serums, vitamins, and other drugs are sometimes used to keep us healthy. Ask the students: What is a vaccine and how is it made? How are vaccines given? How does the body react? What kind of vaccines have you been given for protection? Have students report on Dr. Jonas Salk, Dr. Albert Sabin, Walter Reed, Edward Jenner, Louis Pasteur, Robert Koch, and Emil Von Behring.

3. Relieve pain. Tell the students to think of the most pain they have ever felt and ask: Can you make another person understand what you felt? What made the pain go away? What situations can you think of that require a pain-relieving drug? Can you name some pain relievers? Where do these pain relieving drugs come from? Have the students report on famous people in this area, such as W. T. G. Morton, Sir James Simpson, Humphrey Davy, Horace Wells, Crawford Long, or George Crile.

4. Help the body work. Some drugs help the body to work correctly. Doctors use insulin in treating a disease known as diabetes. Epilepsy may be treated with drugs such as dilantin, zarontin, or phenobarbital, to control or prevent epileptic seizures. Our bodies need both red and white blood cells. When a person has anemia he does not produce enough red blood cells. The doctor may prescribe certain drugs and vitamins to correct this condition.

○ □

Drawing Activity

Have students draw pictures of people they think are qualified to recommend the use of drugs to them. Ask them why they chose these people.

□ ☆
Field Trip

Discuss the role of the doctor and pharmacist—their training and duties. Explain that drugs can help us get well when they are prescribed by a doctor, measured and bought from a pharmacist, and given to us by our parents. See if you can arrange a field trip to a drugstore to learn what goes on behind the scenes (pharmacist at work).

Medicines and Drugs Are Like Other Instruments Used by Physicians and Dentists to Protect or Restore Health

Medical Instruments

Use transparencies in the Atlas as you discuss various medical instruments and how they are used.

□ ☆
Scrapbook

Have the students draw and collect pictures for a scrapbook of medical instruments. They should label each instrument and write a short explanation of its use.

○ □
Drug Administration Collage

Discuss how drugs are taken. Why are there so many different ways to take medicines? Have the students make a collage showing the various ways medicines are sometimes administered.

1. Medicines that are solids (pills), powders (capsules), and liquids (syrup) are usually swallowed. These drugs go to the stomach first.

2. Some drugs are in a liquid form that must be injected into the blood.

3. Some drugs are inhaled into the lungs, such as sprays, mists, and gases. (Example: ammonia ampule)

4. Some drugs are liquids that must be dropped into the nose, eyes, or ears.

5. Some drugs are ointments, creams, and salves that are applied directly to the skin.

Prescription and Nonprescription Drugs

○ □
Medicine Cabinet

Have the students make and stock a medicine cabinet for the classroom. Begin with an old, discarded medicine cabinet, or a box with a couple of cardboard shelves and a cardboard door with aluminum foil on the front to simulate a mirror. A very nice medicine cabinet can be made from some of the wood curio or "nature" boxes that are available commercially. Encourage the students to bring in empty medicine containers that have been discarded. (Remind them to ask their parents for permission.)

On one piece of construction paper write *Prescription Medicine* and define it as a medicine that is prescribed by a doctor's written order, according to individual need. Explain that while prescribed amounts may be helpful, overdoses can be harmful and underdoses can be ineffective. The students should understand that a prescription drug should be used only by the person for whom it was ordered.

On another piece of paper write *Nonprescription Medicine* and explain that it can be bought without a doctor's written order. Many nonprescription drugs carry a warning label telling the purchaser to

120

discontinue use and see a doctor if the condition for which it was purchased persists. It is important to read the label of "over-the-counter" (o.t.c.) drugs so one may be guided in their proper use and learn of possible dangers.

○ □

Let the students take drugs from the medicine cabinet and place them on the appropriate piece of paper, or have the students match labels that have been cut off medicine boxes and bottles with the appropriate category.

□

Compare and Design Labels

Compare labels of prescription medicines and nonprescription medicines. Ask the students to design a label for each kind of medicine.

○

Poison Label

Show the students a label on a bottle of poison and explain what it means. Compare the old "skull and crossbones" symbol with the newer "Mr. Yuk" symbol.

Read the following story to primary classes and follow with a discussion about the safe storing and disposal of medicines. (Use transparency of Atlas Figure 1.)

Smart Mother Monkey

Once upon a time there lived a very smart mother monkey who knew how to do all the right things. When she got up in the morning she would see to it that her family had a good breakfast before they left for work or school. She would wash their clothes every week and remind them to take baths so they would smell sweet and clean.

However, one day Junior became ill. He started to wheeze and cough. Mother monkey decided she had better call the doctor. "Doctor Ape," she said, "Junior is coughing and doesn't seem to feel well. Could you swing over?"

A few hours later Dr. Ape arrived. He looked into Junior's eyes, which were usually bright and shiny. Now they were dull and droopy. Next, he made Junior stick out his tongue and say "ahh." "My goodness," said Dr. Ape, "your throat really is red and swollen. We must give you a special medicine to make you feel better."

After scribbling something on a piece of paper, he handed it to Mother monkey and explained, "This is a note for your pharmacist. It will tell him what kind of medicine he should give you and how often Junior should take it. This medicine is only for Junior, and nobody else," warned Doctor Ape before he left.

Father monkey was able to buy the right medicine for Junior very quickly, just by handing the pharmacist the prescription Dr. Ape had left.

Mother monkey, who as you remember, was very smart and always tried to do the right thing, carefully read the label on the medicine bottle. It said to give Junior one teaspoon of medicine every eight hours, for the next five days. "I must remember to give you the right amount," she said. So she found a piece of paper and wrote down each time when she gave Junior his medicine.

After receiving his medicine, Junior was curious why his mother always locked it back up in the medicine cabinet. "I know better than to take medicines when I don't need them," said Junior. "I know," said Mother monkey, "but Baby monkey is a very good climber, and he has not yet learned that taking the wrong medicine or too much medicine could hurt him."

"This medicine looks a lot like the candy that Baby monkey likes," said Junior, who was also very smart, "and it smells good too. I wonder if medicines should be made to taste and smell so good?" Junior was suddenly too sleepy to think or talk anymore, and he fell fast asleep . . . probably dreaming he was king of a banana plantation.

○ □
Discussion Questions

If you were coughing and wanted some cough medicine, would you take it by yourself? What would you do?

Where should medicines be stored if there are young children in the house?

How should old medicines be destroyed?

Why is it important for all medicines to be well labeled and used only in the amount ordered?

Can you think of some special directions that may be given for certain medicines? (Store in refrigerator; take with milk or food; do not take more than four times a day, etc.)

○
Story: Snow White

Read the story of Snow White to the class and discuss.

○ □
Look-Alike Products

Have the students devise a display that shows how medicines sometimes look like candy and explain what they should know and do to avoid harming themselves. This may be expanded to include other household products; for example, compare Spic and Span to bluish Pixie

Stix candy; Aspergum to orange Chicklet chewing gum; red vitamins to red M & M candies and red cold tablets.

Evaluation
LIFESTYLE CONTENT
□

Have the students each create an original poster illustrating something they have learned about common household medicines and substances that can be dangerous if used improperly.

○ □
Felt Board

Using a felt board and felt cutouts of people, medicine, house, etc., let the students create stories about the proper and improper use of medicines and household products.

□ ☆
Labeling Quiz

Using the Table 7B-1, see if the students can match the information that is *required* by law to appear on the labels of prescription and over-the-counter drugs by placing an X in the appropriate column.

LIFESTYLE VALUE
□ ☆

Have the students list the medicines they think they need to be healthy. What medicines were listed most often? Determine what percentage of the class has taken certain medicines at one time or another.

□ ☆

Ask the students what they would do if their little sister or brother put a strange substance into her or his mouth?

TABLE 7B-1 INFORMATION REQUIRED BY LAW TO APPEAR ON PRESCRIPTION AND OVER-THE-COUNTER DRUG LABELS

Information	Prescription Label	Over-the-Counter Label
1. The patient's name	X	___
2. Name of the medicine	___ (Name of the drug will appear if requested by doctor.)	X
3. Name of all active ingredients and certain other ingredients	___	X
4. The doctor's name	X	___
5. The pharmacy name, address, and telephone number	X	___
6. Specific warning if the drug may be habit-forming	X	X
7. Printed cautions or warnings	___	X
8. Direction for safe use for each purpose for which the drug is intended.	___	X
9. Instructions for using the drug	X	___
10. The prescription number given by the pharmacy	X	___
11. Exact measurement of the package contents	___	X
12. Name and address of the manufacturer	___	X

○ □ ☆

Ask the students if they think all medicines should be made to look, taste, and smell good. If they say yes, remind them that many children have been accidentally poisoned because they thought they were eating candy. If they say no, remind them of what it would be like to be sick and have to take a bad tasting medicine for a long time.

□ ☆

Ask students: If we have drugs available that will relieve pain, do you think they should *always* be used? If you had a headache would you always ask for aspirin? What else can you think of that might make you feel better? (Hot water bottle, hot bath, taking a nap, back rub, talking to someone about a problem that is worrying you, etc.)

DRUG UNIT II: HARMFUL USE OF DRUGS

Scientists have found evidence of drug production over 8,000 years ago, and some of the earliest mind-affecting substances are still known today. For instance, archaeologists have discovered that opium, hashish, and cocaine were used as far back as the Stone Age. Indeed, there are records of drug use and abuse in all parts of the world.

Arab political leaders tried to ban coffee 600 years ago. Chinese leaders attempted to stop the importing of opium, which resulted in the Opium War from 1840 to 1842 between China and Great Britain. Neither attempt was successful. Narcotic addiction in the United States was probably twice as bad in 1900 as it is today, but we hear more about it now.

The harmful use of drugs includes not only the purchase of illegal drugs, but also the combination of legal drugs. Many people are allergic to certain drugs and can be harmed by them. Legal drugs can result in either a physical or psychological dependency that is difficult to break. Although some drugs have the potential for greater harm, no drug is completely safe.

OBJECTIVES

1. After playing a golf game on the number one course of Hi-Lo Memorial Golf Courses, students will have sufficient drug knowledge to complete successfully the number two course.

2. The number one golf course will permit students to differentiate between narcotics, sedatives, stimulants, hallucinogens, and volatile substances in a nonthreatening situation and will give them sufficient knowledge to complete a drug crossword puzzle.

3. The number two golf course will encourage the development of positive self-concept and decision-making skills and will serve as an evaluation of drug knowledge.

4. After completing the Hi-Lo Memorial Golf Course Drug Education Game, students will be able to name at least three situations that make them feel high (happy) and three situations that could make them feel low (unhappy).

5. After participating in a class experiment, the students will learn that certain drugs can distort their senses much in the way that wearing a glove changes their perception of small objects, and they will be able to define *hallucinogen*.

MATERIALS

1. Atlas Figure 61, The Hi-Lo Memorial Golf Course Drug Education Game and Feeling High and Feeling Low game-cards.

2. One sheet of cardboard or poster board (17″ × 22″), scissors, game markers, one die.

3. Glove, blindfold, small objects.

4. A large doll, wigstand, discarded mannequin, or outline of a person drawn on brown butcher paper.

5. Atlas Figure 62, Drug Abuse Crossword Puzzle.

Methods

□ ☆

Hi-Lo Drug Game

The Hi-Lo Memorial Golf Course Drug Education Game can be used by a single student without markers for review purposes. It can also be played by two to four students at one time. A knowledge of drug information is not needed to play on the number one golf course. The number two golf course is more advanced and requires at least the drug knowledge gained from course one.

Preparation of Game   Tape the four game sheets found in the Atlas together and attach to cardboard for more support. You may want to color each golf course a different color with broad felt-tipped markers. Glue the Feeling High sheet to yellow construction paper and the Feeling Low sheet to blue paper; cut individual cards from sheets in the Atlas.

To Play the Game   Determine who will go first. Throw one die and move your marker the appropriate number of spaces. Read what is written on your space to the rest of the players and follow any directions on your space to the rest of the players and follow any directions that may be given. If you land on a space marked *Draw a Hazard Card* this means you must draw a blue, Feeling Low card and follow its directions. If you land on a space marked with a flag, draw a yellow, Feeling High card and follow the directions. The winner is the first person to reach hole 18. (No Feeling High card is drawn at hole 18.)

The number two golf course game is played in much the same way except that an answer must be given for each space or a direction followed. If an incorrect answer is given, it may be challenged by another player who must prove she or he knows the correct answer. This may be done by referring to a book or an appropriate square from game one. If the challenger is correct, he or she may take an extra turn. Many of the questions in game two have no one right answer and can be answered in many different ways.

After the students have had an opportunity to play the golf course drug game, they may want to make additional Feeling High and Feeling Low game cards that can be added to the game.

□ ☆

Devise Original Drug Education Games

Divide the students into small groups and let each group devise an original drug education game and explain it to the rest of the class.

☆

Drug Display

Various pills and capsules can be safely preserved and displayed by embedding them in clear polyester casting resin. The resin hardens at room temperature when a catalyst is added to it.

Materials needed: Polyethylene molds (designed primarily for resin casting); all-purpose clear polyester casting resin; catalyst (hardener); toothpicks and disposable plastic spoons; level table; adequate ventilation; various pills and capsules to be embedded.

A policeman or pharmacist may be able to help you obtain drugs that you are unable to find on your own. They can also help you simulate illegal drugs for display purposes.

After you have embedded the drugs and removed the molds, label each specimen appropriately. A label maker that punches letters into colored tape is very good for this purpose and the tape will adhere to the polyester castings. (We suggest red tape for stimulants, blue tape for depressants, green tape for hallucinogens, and black tape for narcotics.)

The various drugs, in their clear casts, can be mounted in a wood curio cabinet lined with colored felt. A small, empty liquor bottle, cigarette, spoon, plastic marijuana leaf, matches, eye dropper, and marijuana pipe might also be included in the display cabinet.

○ □ ☆

Make a Medicine Man

Using a large discarded doll, wigstand, discarded mannequin, or outline of a person drawn on brown butcher paper, have the students tape drug labels all over it to represent the various drugs that are often consumed in our society. Lead into a discussion about drug advertising.

☆

Slide Show

Create a slide show presenting various aspects of the drug scene. Ask students: When you hear about the "drug problem" what do you think of?

Scene one: Show slides of the *stereo-*

typed drug abuse scene, i.e., skid row, the derelict, the shoplifter, pill poppers, obviously angry family scene, the runaway, a rock band, a motorcycle gang, tough kids, hospital, etc.

Scene two: Show slides of the *socially acceptable drug use scene.* This may include a cocktail party, singles bar, beer bottles, smoke-filled rooms, business lunch with empty martini glasses, pill ads—diet, Darvon, sleeping pills, pep pills, etc.—a pipe and good scotch, happy drunk with laughing onlookers.

Scene three: Show slides of *chemicals for life or emotional support.* Morton's lite salt, aspirin, insulin, kids being vaccinated, a happy family dinner with wine, Schlitz beer commercial in the midst of adventure, Kojak's lollipop, cosmetics, baby with its "formula," "enriched bread," etc.

☆

After presenting a visual definition of the drug scene, discuss how the following organizations might define the term *drug scene:*

1. Women's Christian Temperance Union
2. The Surgeon General's Office of the United States Government.
3. The Friendly Association of Organic Gardeners
4. The National Institute on Alcoholism
5. The Advertising Council of America
6. The R. J. Reynolds Tobacco Company
7. The National Association of Natural Food Store Owners
8. The National Organization for the Reform of Marijuana Laws
9. The Diabetes Association of America

10. The Waukeshaw Thank God It's Friday Conviviality Club

Discuss how all groups, like individuals, define terms to push their own point, or to highlight some real or apparent danger, and often ignore other facts.

□

Hallucinogen Demonstrations

Show your students three sugar cubes. Ask them which one of the cubes contains enough LSD to cause serious mental changes in a person. How can you tell? (You can't.) Explain that the effects of hallucinogens are commonly called a "trip." Some of the effects are called hallucinations, which are sights, sounds, or feelings that are not real.

○ □

Blindfold some of the students and let them try to identify several small objects. Let them try to identify the objects while wearing a glove. Is it more difficult? Why? The glove has distorted their sense of touch as drugs can sometimes distort the senses. Drugs may make common objects appear fuzzy or different.

☆

Drug Literature

Compile drug literature and display it. Which pamphlets seem to be the best? Compile the names and addresses of agencies in your community that are concerned with drug education.

□ ☆

Essays

Have the students write a paper on how friends influence their choice of activities and feelings.

Present the following situation to your students. Allow them to think about it silently for a few minutes and then write down their thoughts about what the sentence means.

"A little five-year-old boy, who had been bombed out of his home and evacuated to another country, said, 'Now I am nobody's nothing.'"

What makes a person "somebody?"

Evaluation

LIFESTYLE CONTENT

☆

Duplicate enough copies of the Drug Abuse Crossword Puzzle in the Atlas for the students in your class or make a transparency of the puzzle for class review.

Answers

ACROSS: 1. Tranquilizers 2. Marijuana 3. Stimulants 4. Hepatitis 5. Depression 6. Methadone 7. Death 8. LSD 9. Alcohol 10. Eye 11. Communicable 12. Potency 13. Heroin 14. Misuser 15. Pharmacist 16. Cannabis 17. Nausea 18. Experimenters 19. Narcotics 20. Intoxication 21. Cocaine 22. Caffeine 23. Prescription 24. Opium Poppy
DOWN: 1. Pusher 2. Barbiturates 3. Drugs 4. Opium 5. Morphine 6. Anesthetic 7. Psychological 8. Dose 9. Inhalant 10. Thalidomide 11. Allergy 12. Hashish 13. Euphoria 14. Bloodstream 15. Hallucinations 16. Tolerance 17. Penicillin 18. Antihistamines)

The number two golf course also serves as an evaluation of drug knowledge.

LIFESTYLE VALUE

☐ ☆

Divide the class into small discussion groups of six to discuss the following topics:

1. If you learned that a friend of yours was taking drugs, which of the following actions would you take?
a. Say nothing
b. Talk to your friend
c. Tell your friend's parents
d. Tell someone else
2. If you saw a person selling drugs to a young child in a school yard, which of the following actions would you take?
a. Report the incident to the police
b. Report the incident to the principal or teacher
c. Report the incident to someone else
d. Do nothing
3. If you had a problem with drugs, which of the following people would you go to for help?
a. Parents
b. Teachers
c. Doctor or minister
d. Police

☐ ☆

Place an X on the value continuums below that best represents your position.

Leader	All Alone
Larry	Arnold

Being a Member of a Group

Tell-me-what-	Independent
to-do Tina	Ima

Dependency

Breaking	Perfect
Bill	Pam

Obeying Laws

UNIT III: ALCOHOL

Every state in the union requires some instruction about alcohol in the curriculum. The late Raymond G. McCarthy of the Rutgers Center of Alcohol Studies pioneered in urging that this education should be relevant to those who will drink as well as to those who will not. Our philosophy about education in this area is similar: We are not providing education to drink, but education about alcohol; the decision to drink or not to drink is always a matter for individual judgment.

The activities in this unit encourage student involvement and the opportunity for students to teach one another. The results are likely to be more exciting and longer lasting than dull, formal reports and lectures.

OBJECTIVES

1. The students will create a bulletin board showing the uses of alcohol and the effects of its ingestion in the human body.

2. The students will demonstrate their understanding of how alcohol affects the body systems and organs by drawing and labeling a figure, showing at least five organs or parts that are affected.

3. During class discussion, the students will distinguish between acceptable and unacceptable drinking patterns and behavior and create a cartoon showing reasons why some people drink.

4. The students will increase their awareness of social and cultural factors that influence their decision to drink or not to drink through group discussion and collecting and analyzing advertisements for alcoholic beverages.

5. Through role playing the students will develop skills and understanding needed for handling social situations where alcoholic beverages will be served. They will also make a recipe scrapbook of nonalcoholic drinks that could be served at a party.

6. The students will give up something they really like for three weeks—keeping track of their progress—and relate this experience to the alcoholic's dilemma of giving up drinking.

MATERIALS

1. Atlas Figures 2 and 10, Physical and Emotional Effects of Alcohol and The Brain.

2. Atlas Figure 63, Methyl/Ethyl Gameboard and Game Cards.

3. Magazine pictures, scissors, paste, and construction paper.

4. Empty display bottles of products containing a form of alcohol. *Ethyl* alcohol is found in alcoholic beverages: beer, wine, whiskey; *methyl* alcohol is highly poisonous and has benzenes or camphor added to make it unfit as a beverage; shaving lotions, vanilla extract, cough medicine, iodine, hair tonic, antifreeze, cleaning solutions, and so on also contain alcohol.

Methods

During your introduction about the study of alcohol, explain that the type of alcohol found in alcoholic beverages is ethyl alcohol. It is clear, colorless, and gives a burning sensation in the mouth. It is made from the fermentation of sugars or starches.

Methyl alcohol is highly poisonous and may cause death if it is accidentally swallowed. It is sometimes called "wood alcohol," since it used to be produced by distilling wood. Denatured alcohol is alcohol that is unfit for drinking because a harmful substance has been added to it, without altering its usefulness for other purposes.

□ ☆

Uses of Alcohol

Have the students create a bulletin board, collage, or mobile illustrating alcohol's various uses. These uses may be

Industrial (antifreeze, ink, fuel, film, solvent in paint and varnishes, plastics, cleaning solutions, explosives, etc.)

Medicinal (preserving agent, antiseptic, to cool the skin, in cough medicine, sedative, relieve pain, etc.)

Social (beverage with meals, reduce tension, religious and ceremonial uses)

Culinary (in flavoring extracts and recipe ingredients).

□ ☆

Transparency

Using a transparency of Atlas Figure 2, Physical and Emotional Effects of Alcohol, discuss how alcohol affects the body systems and organs:

1. Lips, mouth, throat, and esophagus are irritated. Loss of liquids results in a dry mouth.
2. Heart speeds up (pulse rate increases) with first one or two drinks, but then slows down.
3. Blood pressure rises with the first drink.
4. Blood vessels dilate (skin becomes flushed).
5. Body temperature lowers but person perspires.
6. Breathing slows down.
7. Liver begins to digest alcohol.
8. Stomach acid increases—may lead to stomach ulcers.
9. Large and small intestines are inflamed—may cause diarrhea.
10. Urination increases.

□ ☆

Transparency

A transparency of Atlas Figure 10, The Brain, should be used in conjunction with the following information:

Cerebrum (controls voluntary actions):

1. Alcohol hampers rational thought, planning, and memory.
2. Inhibitions are lessened.
3. Alcohol induces personality changes—a shy person may "come alive" or a person may become withdrawn.
4. Speech becomes slurred.
5. Sense of smell increases.
6. Hearing acuity increases.
7. Coordination decreases.
8. Vision may blur; double images may appear; light may seem offensively bright.
9. Reaction time increases.
10. Blood vessels in brain swell, sometimes causing a headache.

Cerebellum (muscle control, reflex center):

1. Alcohol distorts coordination and equilibrium.
2. Reflexes are deadened.

Thalamus (controls sleep): alcohol induces sleep.

Mid-Brain: Constant abuse of alcohol destroys nerve cells in the middle of the brain, causing death.

Pons (transmits messages): Alcohol depresses this function.

Pituitary Gland (directs work of all other endocrine glands):

1. Alcohol affects the coordination of

digestive, circulatory, and excretive systems.

2. Kidney activity speeds up.

Medulla Oblongata (controls many involuntary functions):

1. Controls heart beat, which is slowed down by alcohol after one drink.

2. Alcohol slows breathing.

Spinal Cord: anesthetized by alcohol, resulting in deadening of pain and slower reflex movements.

☆

Writing/Discussion

Have the students write anonymous descriptions of an individual whose feelings or behavior were altered because he or she was drinking. Shuffle the papers and then break the students into small groups for discussion of the effects mentioned. Mass media examples of the effects of drinking can be substituted for personal experiences.

☐ ☆

Pen Pal

If a student has a pen pal in another country or the names of several foreign pen pals can be obtained, initiate correspondence with them primarily on alcohol issues. You may want to ask questions such as: How do you feel about people who get drunk? Are there rules about children's drinking? Is there a safety problem due to alcohol misuse in your country? How is it handled by your government? Why do people drink in your country? Why do others abstain? What kinds of alcohol are most popular?

○ ☐ ☆

Group Discussion

Discuss how families vary in their attitudes toward and use of alcohol.

Does your family use alcohol with meals?

Does your family use alcohol at social gatherings?

Does your family use alcohol in religious ceremonies?

Does your family use alcohol to celebrate? (weddings, anniversaries, etc.)

Does your family use alcohol for medical purposes?

What factors influence a person to drink or not to drink beverages containing alcohol?

How would you define a responsible drinker?

How would you define an irresponsible drinker?

"The phenomenon of the twelve-year-old inebriate," states a recent editorial published in *Patient Care*, "was once a medical curiosity; today it has become a highly visible problem."

The reasons for this alarming new trend are still unclear. Ask students: Why do you think some young children are becoming dependent on alcohol?

☐ ☆

Cartoon

Create a cartoon showing one reason why some people drink.

☐ ☆

Advertisements

Have students collect and analyze advertisements for alcoholic beverages. Discuss how advertisements for alcoholic beverages try to persuade people to drink their brands. Have students count the number of pages of alcoholic beverage advertising in several popular magazines, and ask them if they think advertising has any influence on the consumption of these beverages.

☆

Role Play

Role play some of the following situations:

Your parents do not believe in drinking. You find yourself at a party where alcoholic drinks are being served. You are asked what you would like to drink. What would you do?

One of your parents drinks so much that it is disrupting your family's life. What would you do?

You are at a party with an older boy. He is getting pretty drunk. What would you do? It is time for you to be going home, but you are too young to drive his car.

What would you do if you had never had a "drink," and you wanted to see what an alcoholic beverage tasted like?

☐ ☆

Scrapbook

Have students compile a scrapbook of nonalcoholic beverages.

☐ ☆

Deprivation Experiment

Have each student give up something he or she really likes to eat or do for a period of three weeks (e.g., using salt or sugar, eating candy, using telephone, watching TV, drinking soda pop). Tell them to keep track of their progress. At the end of the three weeks let the students relate how they feel. Could they abstain for a year or the rest of their life? Relate this experience to the alcoholic's dilemma of giving up drinking.

Discuss why alcohol use affects different people differently, or the same person differently at different times (size of person, amount consumed, mental state, fatigue, food eaten, type of beverage consumed, length of drinking time, etc.)

☐ ☆

Analyze Songs

Have the students collect records, lyrics or tape recordings of songs that involve alcohol use. Discuss the attitudes toward alcohol expressed in the songs and the reasons why the people described drink.

☐

Alcohol and Reaction Time

Discuss situations in which students must act so quickly as to make alcohol misuse dangerous (getting out of way of speeding car, putting on brakes of a bicycle, ducking out of the way of a flying object).

☐ ☆

Bumper Stickers/Posters

Have the students create bumper stickers about drinking and driving or develop posters about the effects of alcohol use on traffic safety.

Evaluation

LIFESTYLE CONTENT

☐ ☆

Methyl/Ethyl Game: Let the students play the Methyl/Ethyl game to evaluate their knowledge of the differences between denatured and ethyl alcohol. Materials needed are a gameboard (in Atlas), a set of cards (in Atlas) and a die for every four students.

Break the class into small groups of three or four students and pass out game materials. The first time the game is played, the students will need to cut out their own set of methyl/ethyl cards. Instructions appear on the gameboard.

LIFESTYLE VALUE

☐ ☆

Discuss the following with students:
Suppose a new law has just made it

legal for anyone to drink as much alcohol as they want at any age. Your parents have told you that whether you drink or not and how much you drink is completely up to you. Will you now do any drinking or any more drinking or drink more openly? If you will, why will you? If you won't, why won't you?

Debate the issue of age limits on drinking.

UNIT IV: TOBACCO

Every day more than 4,000 American children begin smoking cigarettes. Reduced life expectancy and increased vulnerability to illness and disability await those youngsters who continue to smoke. We hope the activities in this unit will encourage early individual behavioral commitments to nonsmoking. Although many of the lessons are planned for grades five through eight, primary grade teachers should also work to create an environment supportive of nonsmoking. Our activities call for active involvement of students and use of peer social pressures.

OBJECTIVES

1. Students will draw a picture to illustrate one of the harmful effects of smoking and will be able to complete the cartoon "Smoking cigarettes may cause . . ." by filling in the six smoke puffs with correct answers.

2. The students will work in pairs or small groups to construct a smoking machine.

3. After participating in class experiments and discussion, the students will review their understanding of the effects of smoking on the respiratory system by participating in the "Smoking Classroom" strategy.

4. The students will interview smokers and nonsmokers in an attempt to explain why people begin smoking and usually keep on smoking.

5. After discussing smoking rights and etiquette, the students will express a preference for clean air and ask smokers, politely, to leave or put out their cigarettes when smoking bothers them.

6. After studying and researching basic facts about smoking, the students will create a bulletin board showing attractive and unattractive features of cigarette smoking and other information they have gathered.

MATERIALS

1. Materials for a smoking machine, depending on which one is made, may include: plastic bottle (including cap), quarter-inch tubing, glue, cotton, and cigarettes.

2. Copies of Atlas Figure 3, Smoking Cigarettes May Cause. . . .

3. Felt board, felt, cardboard, colored markers, and glue.

4. A variety of materials for bulletin board project, i.e., glue, construction paper, magazine pictures, etc.

Methods

The following two experiments are suggested in the curriculum guide developed at Smoking Research in San Diego, California, by Ralph Grawunder, Ed.D(3).

○ □ ☆

Experiment 1: Tar Stain (May be done by student at home)

To demonstrate how much of the inhaled tars in cigarette smoke stay in the lungs, you will need 1 lighted cigarette, 1 clean handkerchief, and 1 cooperating smoker.

Have the smoker take in a big puff of

smoke (without inhaling) and immediately blow it out slowly through pursed lips into a clean handkerchief stretched across the lips. Then have the smoker take the same size puff this time inhaling deeply into the lungs and again blow it through a clean spot on the handkerchief. Compare stains. Why is the second stain lighter? Where are the tars from the second puff? What are these tars doing to the air passages in the lungs?

□ ☆
Experiment 2: Heart Rate

To demonstrate the effect of smoking on the heart rate, you will need 1 watch with sweep second hand, 1 cigarette, and 1 cooperating smoker who has not exercised or had a cigarette for two hours.

Before smoking, count the subject's pulse or heart beats for one minute and record the number. Have the smoker light up and take four deep puffs, one after another. Count the heart beats for another minute and record the number. Continue counting heart beats in a minute every five minutes and record each count. How long does it take for the heart beat to return to its precigarette resting rate? Chart the data collected on a graph. What does this mean in terms of heart functioning and of wear and tear from continual overwork from smoking?

□ ☆
The Smoking Classroom

S. Eugene Barnes, associate professor of health, University of Southern Mississippi, has developed the "Smoking Classroom" as a strategy for reinforcing and enhancing discussions of eight points related to the human respiratory system and how tobacco smoking affects it (1):

1. The respiratory system is absolutely essential to human life.
2. The respiratory system has a natural cleansing mechanism. (Discuss ciliary functions and mucus transport system.)
3. Tobacco smoke paralyzes the normal cleansing function of the respiratory system.

4. Much of the inhaled tars of tobacco smoke remain in the mucus coating of the respiratory system after one exhales.
5. Tobacco smoke tars irritate the respiratory system, producing a cough and a mucus buildup problem.
6. Inhaled tobacco smoke causes restricted air flow capacity in the tubules of the respiratory system.
7. Tobacco smoke tars are malodorous.
8. Many social factors encourage and even coerce one to "become fashionable by becoming habituated to tobacco smoking" in spite of the unpleasant and sometimes aggravating nature of smoke for human life.

Although this strategy takes time to discuss and implement, it is well worth the effort. See *Health Education* for complete details (1). The construction of a simple smoking machine is recommended before using this strategy.

○ □ ☆
Simple Smoking Machine

A simple smoking machine (2, p. 15) can be made by making a hole in the cap of an empty plastic bottle. Place a piece of quarter-inch tubing into the hole, and seal shut with glue. Fill tubing with loosely packed cotton. Insert cigarette into the tubing. Squeeze the bottle firmly to remove all the air. Light the cigarette and continue to squeeze bottle. Remove cotton from tubing to see how much tar has collected. (See Figure 7B-1.)

□ ☆
Interview

Have students interview smokers and nonsmokers using questions such as:

Why did or didn't you start smoking?

How old were you when you started smoking?

Why did you stop smoking? How did you stop smoking?

Do you wish you had never started smoking?

FIGURE 7B-1 Simple smoking machine

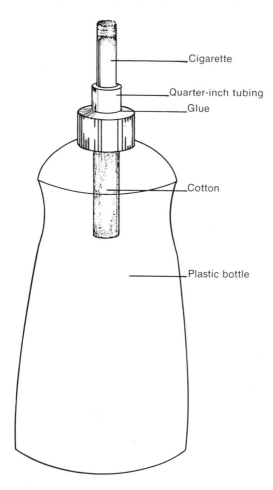

Cigarette

Quarter-inch tubing

Glue

Cotton

Plastic bottle

Would you like to stop smoking?

Have you ever tried to stop smoking?

How do you feel about the possible health hazards involved with smoking?

□ ☆

Smoking Rights and Etiquette

Have students role play the following situations:

1. Ask those around you if you may smoke.

2. If smoking bothers you, politely ask the smoker to put out his cigarette.

3. Demonstrate ways of smoking that might not annoy other people, e.g., smoke by open window, use ashtrays.

4. Problem of smoking in a closed space with nonsmokers present.

□ ☆

Advertising

Have the students collect pictures of cigarette advertising. Do they see a pattern in the kind of image each company is trying to promote: glamour and romance; adventure; pleasure and success; implied safety; "macho" or "womanly," etc.?

Have each student write an essay about the persuasive techniques used in cigarette advertising.

Evaluation

LIFESTYLE CONTENT

○ □ ☆

Let the students design and create a bulletin board showing attractive and unattractive features of cigarette smoking and other information they have gathered.

□

Make enough copies of the cartoon (in Atlas), Smoking Cigarettes May Cause . . . for the students in your class, and ask them to fill in the six smoke puffs with possible answers.

LIFESTYLE VALUE

○ □ ☆

Values Voting: Have the students raise their hand if they agree with the following statements, turn thumbs down if they disagree, and cross their arms if they do not know.

How many of you:

Think cigarettes can be harmful to the body in any amount?

134

Think driving a car on a holiday weekend is more of a threat to your life than smoking two packs of cigarettes a day?

Think you will smoke cigarettes someday?

Would ask your parents to stop smoking?

Think cigarette ads should include health warnings?

Think cigarettes should be taxed to pay for smoking education on television?

UNIT V: GET HIGH ON LIFE!

We believe there is a connection between serious drug misuse and lack of self-esteem. Therefore, all the activities suggested in this book that influence students toward a healthy lifestyle and a greater sense of self-worth may also benefit them by reducing their need for chemical substances.

Although drug use is here to stay, partly because of an increasing need on the part of people to escape the pressures of a complex world, the importance of education about alternatives should not be overlooked.

This unit is intended to help teachers and students understand how their own needs and feelings cause them and others to act the way they do. It emphasizes attitudes, values, and decision-making skills and suggests alternatives to drug use.

OBJECTIVES

1. Students will be able to list five physical and emotional needs and explain how they can influence behavior.

2. Students will develop helpful ways to deal with anger and frustration, as shown by their ability to (a) talk about their own feelings of anger and how they

deal with them, (b) discuss possible causes and consequences of angry reactions, and (c) describe several helpful ways of handling angry feelings.

3. Through participating in various classroom activities, the students will grow more secure, as shown by their ability to identify possible causes of security and insecurity and suggest possible ways to feel more secure.

4. The students will (a) identify their feelings of achievement—that they "count for something," (b) identify feelings of boredom or frustration, and (c) suggest and participate in constructive work and play.

MATERIALS

1. Atlas Figures 64 and 65, In Touch with Feelings Crossword Puzzle and Study Sheet: Need + Blocking = Anger.

2. Atlas Figures 4 and 5, Maslow's Basic Needs Hierarchy and Decision-Making.

3. Old magazines for pictures.

4. Tape recorder or record player, camera (optional).

Methods

Hi-Lo Drug Game

The Hi-Lo Memorial Golf Course Drug Education Game described in Unit II aids in the development of positive self-concept and decision-making skills. The yellow Feeling High cards are actually alternative activities to taking drugs and are intended to increase self-worth and provide positive experiences that the students can relate to.

○ □ ☆

Transparency

Make a transparency of Maslow's Basic Needs Hierarchy (in Atlas). Let the class discuss why people act the way they do.

What needs are they trying to satisfy? How are people alike and not alike?

Explain that all people have the same basic needs and feelings to satisfy, but may use different methods to try to satisfy their needs. We use different methods because each of us has learned different things; we have different resources. Some people have learned to fight very well, perhaps because they needed to know how to fight in order to protect themselves. Other people may never learn to fight, because they have no need to know how. Sometimes the methods we learn to use to meet a need are not the only methods available, and maybe they are not the best; but if we do not know any other methods, then we keep on using them. Therefore, it is important to develop new resources.

The "needs equation" is a way of summarizing behavior:

Basic needs that cause us to act (need for food, rest, activity, security, wanting to count for something), plus

Our own individual resources (physical makeup and abilities, past experiences, opportunities to learn skills, influence of important people, our values and ideas).

Lead to: Effects on ourselves and other people.

Now that you understand these things, it is not quite so easy to say "She's so stupid! She doesn't even know how to play softball." Instead, you may think, "I wonder if she ever had the chance to learn or practice softball?"

○ □ ☆
Bulletin Board

Make a list of human needs on the blackboard that are brought out in class discussion. Let the students make a bulletin board display of pictures and words describing needs.

□ ☆
Study Sheet

Discuss Atlas Figure 65 Study Sheet: Need + Blocking = Anger (4, Student Book, Grade Five, p. 75).

○ □
Open-ended Statements

Let the students respond to some of the following open-ended statements:

Things at school that make me angry are _____ .

My face looks like this when I am angry _____ .

When I get angry I usually _____ .

○ □ ☆
Music and Pictures May Express Anger

Show students pictures and ask them what may have caused the angry reaction portrayed. You can do the same with musical selections, such as, *Night on Bald Mountain* by Moussorgsky, *Finlandia* by Sibelius, the first movement of Beethoven's *Fifth Symphony*, and the *1812 Overture* by Tchaikovsky.

○ □
Role Play

Let the students role play some ways they show anger. Follow up with a discussion of helpful and nonhelpful ways to deal with angry feelings.

Current Anger

Identify a current situation involving angry feelings and discuss the causes and effects of the behaviors involved.

Explain that people may direct their anger toward the thing or person that is blocking a need, but this often does no good. Sometimes, however, people do not realize they are hurting someone and discussion will help.

Can you think of a time when you took your anger out on something or someone that had nothing to do with the situation?

When someone gets angry with us it is often helpful if we:

1. Get things under control.

2. Try to think of reasons why the person might act that way.

3. Try to see if we have found the real reason for the person's behavior.

4. If we are still puzzled, talk the problem over with a parent, a teacher, or someone we think can help.

○ □
Stories

Help make students aware of other's feelings. Read stories from *What Makes Me Feel This Way?* by Eda LeShan.

□ ☆
Pictures

Let each student find one magazine picture that illustrates security and one that illustrates insecurity. Have students assemble a collage for each feeling and create an interesting bulletin board.

☆
Group Discussion

Divide class into small groups, and have them list examples of situations in which students feel secure and insecure, identifying reasons in each case and describing ways to change insecure situations.

□ ☆
Trust Walk

Students can better understand the terms *security* and *insecurity* by taking a "trust walk." Volunteers should be grouped in pairs. One student closes his or her eyes or is blindfolded. He or she is led around the room for a short while by a partner. Switch roles and repeat the experience. Ask the students if they liked leading or being led better and why? If the leaders allow their partners to run into an obstacle it will increase feelings of insecurity.

□
Draw/Write

Let the students draw (or creatively write about) what to them is the "scariest thing" or the "scariest place."

○
Role Play

Provide opportunities for the students to role play and discuss current events that are causing fear or worry. The discussion may be based on magazine or newspaper pictures that the students have brought in.

○ □ ☆
Decision Making

Someone once said, "Life is finding solutions to a series of problems." Discuss with students the following ways of making a decision:

1. I do the first thing that pops into my head, without any other thought.

2. I decide what would be the most fun or the easiest thing to do.

3. I think not only of what I would like to happen right now, but also consider what the results will be later.

4. I consider what effect my decision will have on myself and other people.

○ □ ☆
Transparency

Make a transparency of Atlas Figure 5, Decision-Making, and discuss it with the class. Ask them if they followed these steps, do they think it would help solve problems? Apply methods of decision making to current situations in the class or on the playground.

○ □ ☆

Three Column Activity Chart

Teachers need to help their students learn how to find long-range methods of feeling worthwhile. The third grade teacher manual of *A World to Grow In* (4, p. 127) suggests that pupils list activities in which they can achieve (hobbies, sports, schoolwork); activities that make them feel bored or frustrated; and activities that they need, or would like, to improve.

Next to each item, have pupils list possible ways they might improve themselves or help someone else improve. (This will give the teacher an indication of the pupils' knowledge of the resources available to them.)

□ ☆

Minicourses

If you find that some members of your class have special skills, they can offer minicourses that may involve three or four special sessions. Discuss with your class which courses they would like offered and establish a behavioral objective for each course.

If interest continues, various sessions throughout the year would give many students a chance to teach a minicourse.

○ □ ☆

A similar activity requires students to make a list of activities that would provide them with satisfactory alternatives to the use of drugs. After completing the list, the students should select three activities they each would like to accomplish within the next twelve months. From this list, one activity should be chosen that can be started within the next month. It should be one that holds great interest for the student and is practical in terms of expense and availability of materials or instruction.

Two other activities that build self-concept are a Pupil of the Week bulletin board and asking the students to write a sentence each day answering the question, "What did you do yesterday that you are proud of?"

○ □ ☆

Pupil of the Week

At the beginning of the school year, let the students each draw a number. The number indicates which week they will be featured as pupil of the week. The pupil and other class members can then design a special bulletin board using pictures, stories, and other objects that describe the pupil's identity, achievements, and interests. It may include family pictures, hobbies, travels, and past history such as baby pictures. Perhaps each member of the class can write a sentence describing something he or she likes about the pupil of the week.

□ ☆

Film

Show the film "Get High on Life" by Dana Productions. It is ten minutes long and describes a positive approach to life. You may also want to write for the lyrics of the song "Get High on Life" and create a slide show of class members having a good time.

Evaluation

LIFESTYLE CONTENT

□ ☆

List five physical or emotional needs (e.g., need for food, need for rest, need for activity, need to feel you "count for something," need to feel safe, need to belong, i.e., be a part of some group) and explain how they can influence behavior.

☐
Puzzle

Duplicate enough copies of the In Touch with Feelings Crossword Puzzle for the students in your class (in Atlas).

(Answers to crossword puzzle: DOWN: 1. happy 2. love 3. bravely 4. curious 5. silly 6. anger 7. sober 8. feel 9. sad ACROSS: 10. see 11. jealousy 12. any 13. so 14. dare)

LIFESTYLE VALUE

Values are the standards by which we make our decisions. Each of us has to decide what set of values we want as our own. We learn values from our parents and other important people in our lives.

A few years ago, Ann Landers printed a short essay written by Nadine Stair of Louisville, Kentucky. Stair wrote the story that follows when she was eighty-five years old.

☆
Story About Values

If I Had My Life to Live Over*
I'd dare to make more mistakes next time. I'd relax. I would limber up. I would be sillier than I have been this trip. I would take fewer things seriously. I would take more chances. I would take more trips. I would climb more mountains and swim more rivers. I would eat more ice cream and less beans. I would perhaps have more actual troubles, but I'd have fewer imaginary ones.

You see, I'm one of those people who live sensibly and sanely hour after hour, day after day. Oh, I've had my moments and if I had it to do over again, I'd have more of them. In fact, I'd try to have nothing else. Just mo-

*From Association for Humanistic Psychology, *Newsletter* (July 1975).

ments, one after another, instead of living so many years ahead of each day. I've been one of those persons who never goes anywhere without a thermometer, a hot water bottle, a raincoat, and a parachute. If I had to do it again, I would travel lighter than I have.

If I had my life to live over, I would start barefoot earlier in the spring and stay that way later in the fall. I would go to more dances. I would ride more merry-go-rounds. I would pick more daisies.

What do you think Nadine Stair values? What is not important to her anymore? Do you value the same things she does? Would you rather be serious or playful? Do you enjoy learning new skills even though you may at first appear clumsy or silly to other people?

REFERENCES

1. S. Eugene Barnes, "The Smoking Classroom," *Health Education* (March/April 1976). The American Alliance for Health, Physical Education and Recreation, 1201 16th Street, N.W., Washington, D.C. 20036.

2. Norman W. Houser, *About You and Smoking* (Glenview, Ill.: Scott, Foresman, 1971).

3. Ohio Education Program on Smoking and Health, "Smoking and Health—A Guide for School Action, Grades 1–12" (June 1968). Adapted from the curriculum guide developed by Smoking Research in San Diego, California, by Ralph Grawunder, Ed.D.

4. *A World to Grow In.* Part of a K–12 Drug, Alcohol, Tobacco & Human Behavior Program by the Educational Research Council of America and participating school systems in Dayton and Lima, Ohio, under a grant from the Ohio Department of Education, 1972.

ADDITIONAL SOURCES OF INFORMATION

Pamphlets About Alcohol may be obtained from many sources including Alcoholics Anonymous, American Medical Association,

National Council on Alcoholism, National Institute of Mental Health, National Institute on Alcohol Abuse, and the U.S. Government Printing Office.

Pamphlets About Drugs may be obtained from many sources, including American Medical Association, National Coordinating Council on Drug Abuse, U.S. Public Health Service, National Institute of Mental Health, Food and Drug Administration, Smith, Kline and French Laboratories, and the Metropolitan Life Insurance Company.

Pamphlets About Smoking may be obtained from many sources including the American Cancer Society, American Lung Association, American Heart Association, National Clearinghouse for Smoking and Health, and the U.S. Public Health Service.

Contact your state health department to obtain free pamphlets and borrow films.

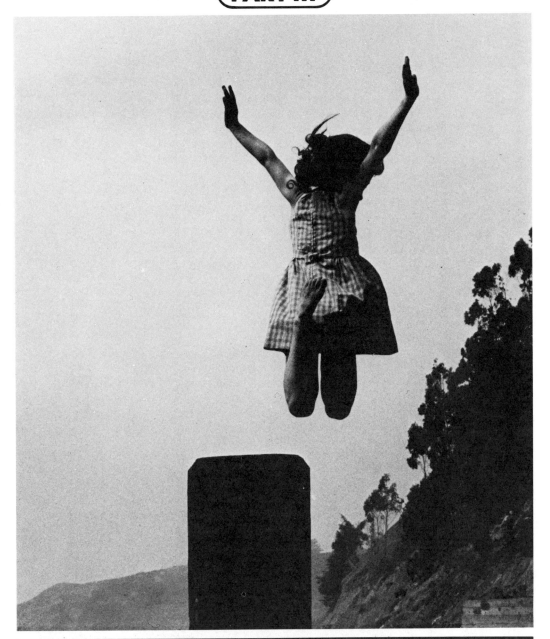

PART III

TOWARD A HEALTHY BODY

CHAPTER 8

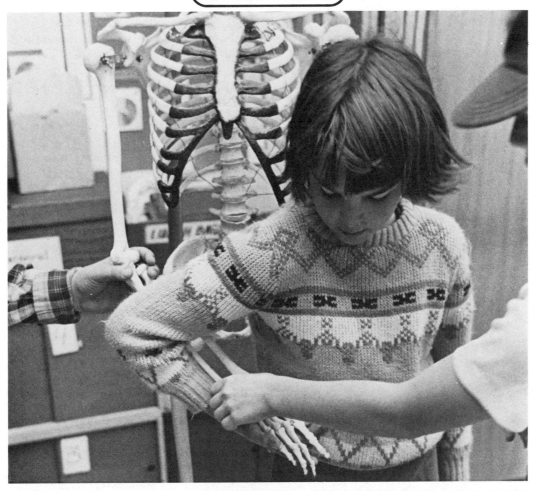

PART A:
THE HUMAN BODY

Most elementary students are eager to learn more about their bodies. The teacher must be careful, however, not to overwhelm them with details of anatomy and physiology. The discussion should be limited to important concepts and implications for planning one's lifestyle. To facilitate this approach, we have only highlighted facts that are covered more definitively in other textbooks.

THE DIGESTIVE SYSTEM

This section will focus on the name and location of the various parts of the food canal and any lifestyle implications that stem from the study of this canal.

Mouth

The entrance to the mouth consists of soft muscular lips that close the entrance to the alimentary canal. The lips are also important to infants for nursing and to lovers for kissing. The lips contain no mucus-producing glands and thus dry or "chap" when they are not constantly moistened with the tongue. Hence, on cold days when one is reluctant to open the mouth, one's lips often dry and split. In such situations it is important to protect the lips with agents that prevent drying.

The tongue contains special cells that react to the chemical nature of foods. These cells are responsible for the sensation of taste and are known as *taste buds*. Taste sensations are primarily a blending of four tastes: sweet, sour, bitter, and salty. Sweetness and saltiness are detected mainly by taste buds at the tip of the tongue. Sourness is detected by the sides of the tongue and bitterness by the back. In addition to its digestive function, the tongue is essential to speech.

Deficiencies of the various B vitamins may produce severe inflammation of the tongue. For this reason, careful attention to diet selection should be considered.

Saliva, a fluid consisting of secretions produced by glands that discharge into the mouth, is a necessary component in the process of digestion. Although it is about 98 percent water, it also contains an enzyme known as *ptyalin* (ty'uh-lin), which initiates the digestion of starches.

Most elementary students become aware of the salivary glands when they are infected with the virus that causes mumps.

Esophagus

Leaving the mouth, food proceeds down the esophagus, a muscular tube about ten inches long and less than an inch wide. Slowly, sequential muscles contract to push food downward. Food does not simply pass to the stomach by the force of gravity. Indeed, it is possible to swallow while standing on one's head or under conditions of free fall.

Stomach

The stomach is located at the level of the lowermost ribs, and not, as most people think, at the level of the navel. Although thought of as a storage bin for food waiting to be digested, the stomach also plays an important role in the digestion of proteins. The lining of the stomach contains many tiny glands that produce fluids called *gastric* (stomach) *juice*. These juices contain about 0.5 percent hydrochloric acid, which accelerates the digestion of both proteins and carbohydrates.

The stomach also contains an enzyme known as *rennin*, which acts to curdle milk in the alkali of the infant stomach where curdling is important. Curdling milk means that the protein portion is removed from solution. In this situation, the protein part is known as *curds* and the liquid from which it was removed is known as *whey*.

Curds and whey can be produced outside the body by adding a preparation of calf stomach to milk. This mixture is what Little Miss Muffet was eating, much to the confusion of most youngsters today. Pepsin is a second enzyme produced by the stomach. Its primary action is the digestion of protein.

After food enters the stomach, the entrance is closed behind it, and the food is trapped. The stomach then contracts, producing a churning of food that assures a thorough mixing with digestive juices. Because gases are also trapped in the stomach, the churning action produces a gurgling sound. Most of the gases in the stomach are nitrogen and oxygen derived from swallowing air.

After the stomach has been empty for a time, the contractions start again. This time, without the presence of food, the gurgling is much louder. The gas trapped in the stomach applies pressure to the walls of the stomach, producing "hunger pangs." Occasionally, the stomach produces too much acid (hyperacidity), which causes additional gases to form. These gases, in turn, apply pressure to the stomach wall and cause pain. In time, relief may occur when some of this gas escapes through the esophagus and mouth. Occasionally, a gas bubble will also take some acid into the esophagus. Unlike the stomach, which is resistant to acid, the esophagus is very sensitive. Hence, this escape of acid into the esophagus often produces pain, generally called *heartburn*. Sometimes the lining of the stomach becomes susceptible to attack by stomach acids. This attack may produce a small break in the stomach lining and a destruction of tissue, known as *gastric* or *stomach ulcer*.

Could we live without a stomach? Yes, but in the absence of this storage compartment it would be necessary to eat smaller meals more frequently.

Small Intestine

Contrary to popular belief, most human digestion occurs in the small intestine, an organ about two inches in diameter and approximately twenty feet long. It begins at the lower end of the stomach and extends to the large intestine.

DUODENUM

The first ten or twelve inches of the small intestine is known as the *duodenum* (doo'oh-dee'num) and serves as a transitional stage between the stomach and the rest of the digestive system. One major function is to neutralize the acid contents that are emptied from the stomach. Because of this function the duodenum is especially susceptible to ulcers. To neutralize the acid and initiate further digestion, two important glands pour their contents into the duodenum: the pancreas and the liver.

PANCREAS

The pancreas is the second largest gland in the body. It is carrot shaped and about six inches long and is nestled behind the lower portion of the stomach. Each day pancreatic juices containing enzymes suitable for the digestion of fats, carbohydrates, and proteins are delivered to the duodenum.

LIVER

To locate your liver, place your left hand over the lowermost rib on the right side of your chest. In this position, your hand directly covers your liver. The liver weighs approximately three to four pounds and is absolutely indispensable to human life. Its major functions are:

1. Storage
2. Filtration of blood
3. Bile secretion
4. Metabolism of foodstuffs

The liver has the capacity to store a number of important substances. It can store enough Vitamin A for two years and enough Vitamin D and B12 for three to four months. The liver also stores iron and small amounts of blood. The liver helps regulate blood sugar by removing and storing it when the supply is high and returning it when the blood sugar is low.

All the chemical substances that get into the body and cannot be broken down for energy are likely to end up in the liver. This includes old red blood cells, drugs, hormonal substances, and poisons. Hence, the liver operates as a kind of detoxification center for the body. For this reason, one must always be careful not to ingest substances that will damage liver cells as they attempt to detoxify the body. Such substances include carbon tetrachloride (a nonflammable dry cleaner), excessive alcohol, and a number of drugs taken in excess.

The liver also produces a yellowish secretion commonly known as *bile*. Bile is important because it contains substances (bile salts) that have a detergent action, without which most of the fat we eat would remain undigested. Bile is secreted into the small intestine.

Did you ever wonder about the color of various substances in the body? Secretions of the liver lend color to several substances in the body, because of the fact that aged red blood cells are broken down by the liver. It happens this way: the oxygen-carrying portions of the red blood cell (hemoglobin molecules) are broken down by the liver, and the iron is removed. The remaining portion is known as a *bile pigment* because of its color (red, orange, or green). In turn, the bile pigments may be traced through the body because of their color. For example, once food comes in contact with bile in the small intestine, it takes on the color of these pigments and is still reddish brown when eliminated from the body. A small amount of bile pigment is absorbed into the circulatory system and eliminated in the urine. This pigment is responsible for the light yellow color of plasma (fluid part of blood) and urine.

When too many bile pigments are produced and get into the circulation, they may show up in the skin and whites of the eyes. This condition is known as jaundice and may result from:

1. Increased destruction of red blood cells
2. Obstruction of the ducts through which bile flows
3. Damage to live cells

Ancient man considered the liver (largest organ in the body) to be the seat of life. There is a striking similarity between the terms *liver* and *live*.

The liver is essential to protein metabolism, and loss of this organ would result in death in a day or two. Among other protein substances, the liver is responsible for the production of many of the factors necessary for blood to clot and is important in the metabolism of carbohydrates and fats.

GALL BLADDER

The gall bladder, located just beneath the liver, stores up to a one-day supply of bile produced by the liver. Bile contains a high concentration of cholesterol. In some people this cholesterol precipitates into crystals known as *gallstones*. The amount of cholesterol in bile is determined principally by the quantity of fat that a person eats. Thus, people on a high-fat diet over a period of many years are prone to develop gallstones. Gallstones may become painful and necessitate removal of the gall bladder, which is not necessary for survival.

JEJUNUM AND ILEUM

The duodenum empties into the jejunum (jee-joo'num). This part of the small intestine is about eight feet long and empties into the ileum (il'ee-um). The ileum, in turn, is about twelve feet long and joins the large intestine. It is in these two portions of the small intestine that final digestion and absorption occur. It is possible to live with nine-tenths of the small intestine removed.

Large Intestine

The large intestine is about five feet long and usually receives food about three hours after it enters the small intestine. Since the large intestine is also known as the *colon*, an inflammation of the large intestine is known as *colitis*, and a painful distention of this area due to accumulation of gas is known as *colic*. Attached to the lower end of the large intestine is a two- to four-inch structure known as the appendix. Occasionally some by-product of digestion finds its way into this blind alley and causes an inflammation that may require removal of the appendix.

Almost no digestion occurs in the large intestine; its main function is to absorb water. Usually by the time the waste product of digestion reaches the end of the colon, it is solid. The last four- or five-inch portion of the colon is known as the *rectum*, and the final opening is called the *anus*. The solid contents eliminated by the anus are known as *feces*. When the colon fails to absorb the usual amounts of water, diarrhea occurs. When feces remain too long in the colon, additional amounts of water may be absorbed, resulting in constipation. When feces become exceptionally hard, elimination may occur only with great difficulty. Regular exercise, adequate fluid intake, and the addition of roughage or bran to the diet help counteract constipation.

THE CIRCULATORY SYSTEM

Living cells require a constant source of oxygen and nutrition and removal of waste products. In the human body the circulatory system provides these "pickup and delivery" services. The importance of these circulatory services is obvious from the fact that malfunctions may result in immediate death. On the other hand, the relationship between one's lifestyle and the health of the circulatory system is not so obvious. For this reason, the present section examines the circulatory system with a view toward suggested lifestyle implications.

Heart

Your heart is located beneath the breastbone and between the lungs and is approximately the size of your fist. Functionally, the heart is a four-chamber, muscular pump. The two upper chambers are known as atria (right and left atrium). Their main function is to receive blood that is returned to the heart. The two lower chambers of the heart are known as ventricles. Their main function is to pump blood.

The flow of blood through the heart is regulated by four valves or control doors. The four valves, however, operate in pairs. The first pair, located between the atria and ventricles, are known as *cuspid valves*. The name stems from the fact that the underside of these valves have small cusps that look like small upside-down cups. The cusps make this a pair of one-way valves. That is, blood passes freely from the atria to the ventricles, but when the ventricles contract, the upside-down cups (beneath the valves) fill with blood and cause the valves to slam shut. Thus, the cusps prevent backflow and allow the blood to flow in only one direction. The valve located between the right atrium and the right ventricle is known as the *tricuspid valve*, because it has three cusps on its underside. On the left, the corresponding valve has two cusps and is known as the *bicuspid valve*. This valve is also known as the *mitral valve*.

Blood passing through the first set of valves enters the ventricles. The ventricles contain a much greater muscle mass than the atria and are capable of contracting with great force. In athletes, the ventricles have an even greater muscle mass because of extensive exercise. This increased strength makes the trained heart more efficient. When the ventricles contract, blood is forced out of the heart: from the right ventricle it is pumped to the lungs and from the left ventricle it is pumped to all parts of the body. In each case, however, blood must pass through a valve before it leaves the heart.

Blood going to the lungs is pumped first into an artery called the *pulmonary artery*. The entrance to this artery is regulated by the pulmonary valve. After blood has entered this artery, the valve closes to prevent backflow.

Blood leaving the left ventricle is pumped through the aortic valve into a very large artery called the *aorta*. Closure of the aortic valve also prevents backflow. The pulmonary and aortic valves open and close at approximately the same time, so they, too, work as a pair.

If you listen to the heart by placing your ear against someone's chest, you will hear two sounds: "lub-dub." The sounds are caused by the slamming shut of the heart valves. The first pair (cuspid) of valves produce the "lub" sound and the second pair produce the "dub"

sound. "Lub-dub" constitutes one heart beat and occurs approximately seventy times per minute.

Sometimes, as a result of diseases like rheumatic fever, the valves do not close properly and blood may flow back through the partly closed valve. A trained physician using a stethoscope can hear this backflow of blood, which is called a *murmur* (abnormal heart sound). Another type of murmur results when the valve becomes abnormally narrow and blood is forced through a small opening. Not all murmurs are unhealthy. Some people exhibit an unusual heart sound, but it does not disturb the flow of blood. This is called a *functional murmur*.

One important precaution for elementary children relates to rheumatic fever. Rheumatic fever is a delayed reaction to streptococcal infection such as "strep" throat, tonsillitis, or middle ear infection. Therefore, it is very important that any persistent sore throat or other lively "strep" infection be properly treated. Suspected cases should be reported to the child's physician. Rheumatic fever can cause serious damage to the valves of the heart.

To understand the heart better, let us trace a drop of blood through its four chambers and four valves. A drop of blood returning from the leg, for example, first enters the right atrium. At this time, it is "oxygen poor," having just delivered a load of oxygen to a leg muscle. This drop, together with blood from all other parts of the body, immediately passes through the tricuspid valve to the right ventricle.

When the right ventricle is filled, the muscular walls of the chamber start to squeeze in on the blood, forcing some of it upward. The upward flow slams the tricuspid valve shut, and we have the first heart sound, "lub." As the pressure increases in the right ventricle, the pulmonary valve opens, and the drop of blood is pumped to the lungs to pick up oxygen. Having successfully passed through the pulmonary valve, the drop of blood is prevented from falling back into the heart by closure of this valve, producing the second heart sound, "dub."

Returning through the pulmonary veins, the drop of blood now enters the left atrium. The blood in the left atrium is "oxygen rich" as a result of its recent trip through one of the lungs. From the left atrium, blood passes through the biscuspid (mitral) valve and flows immediately to the left ventricle.

After filling, the left ventricle starts to contract, causing the biscuspid (mitral) valve to slam shut ("lub"). As the pressure continues to build, the aortic valve opens and blood is pumped to all parts of the body. Immediately after blood is ejected from the left ventricle, the aortic valve slams shut ("dub"). Our drop of blood thus completes its trip through the heart.

Coronary Arteries

As blood leaves the left ventricle, it begins a series of deliveries to a long list of waiting cells, but the first delivery is to the heart itself. This is necessary because:

1. The heart is a working muscle that requires a constant blood supply.

2. None of the blood within the heart can be used directly by the heart muscle. Hence, a delivery system, consisting of two coronary arteries, is necessary.

The coronary arteries are the first arteries to branch from the large artery (aorta) that conducts blood away from the heart. Any malfunction in the coronary delivery system is known as a *coronary*. Such malfunctions occur because something blocks the flow of blood through the artery.

Blockage or reduction of blood flow through the coronary arteries results in sharp pains in the chest. Medically, these are labeled *angina pectoris*. The pains of angina pectoris may be relieved by drugs that cause the coronary arteries to open wide and deliver more blood to the working heart muscle. Nitroglycerin is the best known of this class of drugs.

Blood clots are the usual causes of blocks in the coronary arteries. Since the term for clot is *thrombus*, the condition is usually termed *coronary thrombosis*. Coronary thrombosis usually occurs only after the coronary arteries have become rough and hard. This latter condition is known as *arteriosclerosis*. At present, the exact cause of arteriosclerosis is unknown. However, it is associated with certain patterns of living or lifestyles. A lifestyle that appears to be associated with healthy hearts includes a reduced intake of saturated fats and sugars, regular exercise, adequate rest and relaxation, and no cigarette smoking.

Cerebral Arteries

Like the heart, the brain requires a constant blood supply. Any interruption of blood flow to the brain is known as a *stroke*. This may result from blood clots or a rupture in the cerebral arteries that carry blood to the brain.

Blood Pressure

Because the circulatory system is a closed system, the fluids within it are maintained under pressure. Consequently, blood will spurt out of an artery that is cut.

As in any closed system that increases or decreases in the volume of circulating fluids, there are corresponding changes in pressure. For example, excessive intake of salt draws fluid from the cells into the circulatory system and results in increased blood pressure. Each time the heart contracts and pumps blood into the arteries, there is an increase in blood pressure. When it relaxes, there is a decrease. The difference between this high and low blood pressure is what enables you to feel your pulse. That is, with each change in pressure you are able to detect a pulse.

Suppose that a physician records your blood pressure as 120 over 80. In this case, the 120 represents your blood pressure at the time of heart contraction. This is known as the *systolic pressure*. The 80 represents the pressure when the heart is relaxing and is called the *diastolic pressure*. Blood pressure is measured with a device known as a *sphygmomanometer* (sfig'moh-ma-nom'i-ter).

The size of your arteries and veins is subject to immediate change, and such changes directly modify your blood pressure. For example, placing your hand in ice water causes an immediate increase in blood pressure, because coldness causes blood vessels to constrict. The constriction increases the pressure within the circulatory system. Conversely, on a very hot day the blood vessels open up and decrease the blood pressure. Indeed, if you suddenly stand after being seated in a hot room, you may feel faint. Sudden excitement may also cause the blood vessels to open up, which may result in fainting.

Unfortunately, high blood pressure is a major health problem in the United States today. The condition is termed *hy-pertension*, because of the extra stretching that occurs in the blood vessels when the pressure is high. Hypertension is dangerous, because it places undue strain on the heart and arteries. Blood pressure is often a key to the health of the entire body, and it should be checked on a regular basis.

Blood must sometimes be returned to the heart against the force of gravity, and this may cause overdistention of the veins. Fortunately, the veins contain one-way valves that assist in the return process; muscle contractions force blood toward the heart, and valves in the veins prevent it from flowing backward. If these valves are damaged in any way, the return of blood is inefficient. Occasionally, blood may collect in the veins, causing them to distend to four or five times their usual size. This condition is known as *varicose veins*. In some cases it even becomes necessary to remove these veins. Several factors may be involved in the development of varicose veins, but from the standpoint of lifestyles, it should be noted that lifestyles that involve continuous standing and little activity may cause or aggravate varicose veins.

Blood

What makes up the blood that is constantly flowing through our arteries and veins? Blood is composed primarily of water and red blood cells or erythrocytes (i-rith'ro-sites). These special cells contain a substance known as *hemoglobin* that gives them their red color and allows them to carry oxygen. A deficiency of hemoglobin is known as *anemia*. Although a number of diseases result in anemia, from a lifestyle viewpoint it is important to be sure that iron and vitamin B_{12} are included in the diet.

150

In addition to water and red cells, the blood contains at least five different types of white blood cells or leukocytes (loo'ko-sites). The white cell is different from the red cell in appearance, number, and function. White cells have no definite shape, but they are larger than red cells and fewer in number. There is approximately one white cell for every 600 or 700 red cells in the blood. White blood cells serve mainly to assist the body in fighting infection and toxic agents.

Platelets are another element in the blood. They combine with other substances to prevent excessive bleeding during an injury by aiding in the formation of clots. Clotting, however, is not always a good thing. We have already seen how clots in the coronary arteries cause coronary thrombosis and how clots in cerebral arteries can cause strokes.

THE LYMPHATIC SYSTEM

Outside the circulatory system and between the various cells are very thin-walled capillaries and connecting tubes that drain into the circulatory system. These tubes make up the lymphatic system. Scattered along the lymphatic system especially at the angle of the jaw, in the armpit, and in the groin, are beanlike masses known as *lymph nodes*. Occasionally, these nodes become swollen and sore. This usually means that the lymph nodes are fighting a foreign agent of some type.

THE NERVOUS SYSTEM

Responding to an endless number of stimuli both inside and outside the body, the human nervous system coordinates all of the activities of the body. Conducting nerve impulses at a speed of nearly 350 feet per second, it moves the body quickly away from impending danger. Working through its involuntary divisions, it activates glands, smooth muscles, and cardiac muscle to maintain normal physiological functioning. At a higher level, it enables us to carry out functions possible only to human beings: complex thought, creative work in the arts and sciences, and control of speech.

The nervous system is divided into two major parts: the central nervous system and the peripheral nervous system. The central nervous system consists of the brain and spinal cord. The peripheral nervous system consists of twelve cranial nerves, thirty-one pairs of spinal nerves, and the autonomic (involuntary) nervous system. The autonomic nervous system is not a separate entity, but a grouping of special nerve components that travel within certain spinal and cranial nerves and activate smooth muscles, cardiac muscles, and glands.

The brain is the headquarters of the nervous system and regulates its activities. Because of its central impor'ance, the brain is carefully protected. This amazing three-pound structure is protected by a bony skull and is encased in fluids and "floats" to absorb traumatic shocks. Although the brain is effectively protected, people must do their part. This involves careful attention to recognized safeguards associated with automobile travel, bicycle riding, boxing, football, diving, and a variety of chemical hazards. A head injury that causes jarring of the brain and, usually, unconsciousness is called a *concussion*. In most cases, recovery is spontaneous and does not require treatment. However, anyone who suffers a concussion should be carefully observed for a few days. Unusual drowsiness or weakness of the limbs suggests that there may be hemorrhage in the skull. Such symptoms should be reported to the victim's physician at once.

In many ways, the nervous system resembles a large electrical network. The electrical impulses generated by the brain can be recorded by a machine known as an *electroencephalograph*. These brain wave recordings help the physician diagnose abnormal conditions, such as epilepsy, tumors, infections, and hemorrhages of the brain.

THE RESPIRATORY SYSTEM

The work of the human body requires a constant supply of oxygen and removal of carbon dioxide. This process of transporting oxygen from the atmosphere to the cells of the body and carbon dioxide back to the atmosphere is called *respiration*. Respiration is possible because during the last billion years the earth's atmosphere has contained approximately 21 percent oxygen. Man draws on this supply approximately every five seconds, combining it with nutrients to produce energy and sustain life.

The respiratory system represents a direct link with the outside world. For this reason, there are certain inherent dangers associated with the inhalation of infectious agents and a variety of toxic substances. In addition, there may be a shocking difference between temperature of air inside and outside the body. Fortunately, the respiratory system is not defenseless against would-be invaders and drastic differences in temperature.

Nose

To begin with, the entrance to the nose is partially blocked by hairs that filter out large objects. Secondly, the nasal passageway is lined with a sticky mucus that entangles any particles that make contact with it.

The nasal passages are also moistened by liquid that drains from hollows in the bones of the head. These hollows are known as *sinuses*. In four-footed animals these sinuses all drain downhill, but in man they may take a horizontal or even uphill position. Drainage, therefore, is often inefficient and may even be blocked during a cold. Blockage of a sinus allows fluid to accumulate, and the associated pressure may result in excruciating headaches.

The nasal passages also contain small hairlike projections (cilia) that are constantly moving countercurrent to the flow of air. Thus, the cilia serve as an additional protection against invasion from the outside.

A collection of impurities on the nasal lining may produce a sneeze, which helps to clear the passageway. Finally, the nasal passages serve to warm and moisten the entering air. It is possible to breathe through the mouth, but the mouth has no air purification system, and it is better to breathe through the nose when possible.

Pharynx

Air that enters through either the nose or mouth moves directly to the pharynx (far′inks). It is at this level that a slight anatomical problem arises. The pharynx exhibits two openings to the lower body. First, there is the esophagus leading to the stomach. Then there is the windpipe leading to the lungs. This creates a hazardous junction for both food and air, either of which may go the wrong way.

The opening of the air passage is

called the *glottis*, and it is located below and behind the tongue. Just above the glottis is a flap of cartilage that attaches to the root of the tongue called the *epiglottis*. In swallowing, the glottis moves under the epiglottis, closing the air passage and forcing food to take the road that leads to the stomach. Also at the instant of swallowing, the vocal cords, which stretch across the air passage, come together. This also prevents food from entering the lungs.

Vocal Cords

The vocal cords are two folds of tissue that stretch across the entrance to the air tube or trachea. Expelling air past the vocal cords causes sound and makes speech possible. Controlling the length of the vocal cords produces variations in the pitch of the voice. In general, short cords produce higher tones and long cords produce deeper tones. The high-pitched voices of children stem from the shortness of their vocal cords. When these suddenly increase at the beginning of adolescence in the male, the voice changes. The growth in the length of cords in males may be so rapid that they experience difficulty with the muscular movements that control tension of the cords. Thus, the male may speak in ludicrous bursts of baritone and tenor—a major embarrassment of early teens.

Anatomically, the vocal cords and cartilage that surrounds them are known as the *larynx* or *voice box*. The larynx represents the entrance to a passage leading to the lungs. When the inner lining of the larynx is infected, the condition is known as *laryngitis*, and speech may be reduced to a whisper. To whisper does not require use of the vocal cords.

Trachea and Bronchi

The larynx opens into a small tube about an inch in diameter known as the *trachea* (tray'kee-uh) or *windpipe*. This is a strong tube held open at all times by cartilage. At the bottom of the neck the trachea divides into two branches known as *bronchi* (bron'keye). One branch goes to each lung. Each bronchus, in turn, subdivides into many divisions like the branches of a tree. In fact, the structure is known as the *bronchial tree*. The bronchial tree continues to divide into smaller branches, finally terminating in tiny air sacs that resemble a bunch of grapes. The air sacs end in air cells known as *alveoli* (al-vee'oh-leye). It is here that the exchange of gases between the blood and lungs occurs.

In the normal adult, respiration occurs at a rate of twelve to fourteen times per minute. Breathing may be under either voluntary or involuntary control. That is, we can breathe at whatever rate we like, or we can hold our breath. On the other hand, if we do not think about it at all, respiration goes on at a normal rate. Children who threaten suicide by breath-holding are never successful; if they become unconscious, involuntary breathing takes over.

THE SENSE ORGANS

The human body has a number of highly refined organs with which it is able to perceive the external world. Through the eyes, ears, skin, nose, and mouth, people receive a detailed report of the world and many of its characteristics. They may also possess yet another source of information presently referred to as extrasensory perception. The importance of the various senses and the perceptions that they bring are attested to by the fact that when people are deprived of the external world they are unable to tolerate the effect; they become terrified and later hallucinate the world they need.

Smell

Among the various senses, smell is the least well understood. This is because smell is mainly a subjective phenomenon that is rather poorly developed in people.

The first cranial nerve (olfactory) extends across the top of the nasal cavity, where it is covered by a thin membrane. This membrane is covered by a thin film of mucus in which small hairlike projections wave back and forth. When air is sniffed, the vapors are trapped and dissolved in the mucus. In turn, the hairs of the olfactory nerve are stimulated, and a signal is sent to the brain. This signal is registered as a smell.

Smell is known to contribute significantly to the sense of taste or, perhaps, be confused with it. People who have a cold often say that they cannot taste anything, but tests reveal that there is nothing wrong with their sense of taste. This demonstrates that much of what we call taste is actually smell.

Taste

Taste is a function of taste buds located in the mouth. The taste buds allow a person or animal to select food in accordance with desires and needs of the body. For example, animals who have had their parathyroid gland removed and thus need calcium, automatically select drinking water containing calcium. Activities related to the sensations of taste,

touch, smell, hearing, and sight are suggested in Chapter 8B.

THE MUSCULAR SYSTEM

Human beings are capable of a wide range of movements that include running, jumping, throwing, kicking, lifting, and swimming. All of these movements are made possible by muscles known as *skeletal muscles*. In addition, the body contains many muscles that are not generally under voluntary control. These muscles regulate movement of food through the digestive system, the secretion of some glands, and the size of blood vessels. This type of muscle is known as *smooth muscle*. Finally, the heart is mainly muscle. This type of muscle tissue provides for continuous pumping of blood and is known as *cardiac muscle*. In this section we shall discuss all three types of muscles.

Skeletal Muscle

There are more than 650 skeletal muscles in the human body, most of which occur in pairs. These muscles are responsible for all of our voluntary movements. Collectively, they make up 30 to 40 percent of the total body weight. In general, the size and strength of muscles increase when they are used and decrease when they are not used. There is a close connection between muscles and nerves, and cutting the nerve to a muscle causes it to waste away. Muscles sometimes cramp when we work under conditions of high temperature. This can usually be avoided by adequate replacement of salt.

The most serious threats to muscles are

from agents outside the body. One such threat is the tetanus bacteria. This bacteria may enter the body through any break in the skin. Once inside the body, it produces and releases a deadly toxin. Death occurs because the tetanus toxin causes the muscles to contract and remain contracted. Since the jaws are one of the first muscle groups to be affected, this disorder has also been called *lockjaw*. Fortunately, this fatal condition can be prevented by keeping one's tetanus shots up-to-date. These shots cause the body to produce antibodies against the tetanus toxins.

Smooth Muscle

Almost every organ in the body contains smooth muscles. These muscles are generally under involuntary control, but they are very important to health. Smooth muscles in blood vessels allow us to adjust to hot and cold by controlling the flow of blood to the skin. It is the relaxation of smooth muscles in the blood vessels of the face that causes blushing. Smooth muscles are very important to the movement of food through the digestive system—something we accomplish without even thinking about it.

Cardiac Muscle

The heart is a muscular pump that is able to contract rhythmically due to its special type of muscle tissue known as *cardiac muscle*. The heart is actually made up of three types of cardiac muscle: atrial muscle, ventricular muscle, and specialized muscle fibers that, like nerves, can be excited and will conduct impulses. The cells of cardiac muscle are so tightly bound that when one is excited they all become excited. This provides for the forceful contractions that are capable of pumping blood.

The right atrium of the heart contains a very specialized strip of muscle tissue known as the *pacemaker* (sinoatrial node). The strip of muscle sends out a regular signal that causes the atria of the heart to contract. Other specialized muscle cells in the ventricles pick up this signal from the pacemaker and cause the ventricles to contract. The impulse that is sent out through the atria and ventricles may be picked up and recorded by a machine known as an electrocardiograph. The recording, known as an *electrocardiogram*, assists trained physicians in determining the health of the cardiac muscle.

THE SKELETAL SYSTEM

The skeletal system consists of more than 300 bones at birth, but many of these bones fuse, and the adult skeleton is left with approximately 206 bones. Occasionally, people exhibit an extra bone in some part of the body. For example, one person in twenty has an extra rib. However, except for minor anomalies, the skeletons of different people are very similar.

The skull is made up of twenty-two bones that grow together in sawtoothed joints during adult life. The primary function of the skull is to protect the brain and associated sense organs.

The vertebral column consists of thirty-three individual bones called *vertebrae*. These bones provide a pivot for support and movement of the head; provide a structural base for the arms and legs; protect the spinal cord; and afford the body flexibility.

The thorax is located between the neck and the diaphragm. It consists of the sternum, ribs, and a section of the vertebral column. The twelve pairs of ribs are like bony ribbons that enclose such important structures as the heart and lungs.

The arms and legs contain thirty bones apiece, most of which are concentrated in the hands and feet. These and other bones protect and support the body and provide highly efficient movement patterns. Additionally, the bone marrow manufactures red and white blood cells.

THE ENDOCRINE SYSTEM

The endocrine glands determine what "metabolic tune" is to be played by the body, how loud or soft, how vigorous or quiet. They set the rate, the mood, and the harmony among the organs and tissues of the body. Indeed, the endocrine glands have often been compared with an orchestra of which the pituitary gland is the conductor. All the other endocrine glands, although extremely important, play harmoniously under the direction of the leader.

Pituitary Gland

The pituitary gland is rightfully called the *master gland*. Its functions include regulating growth, controlling the adrenal glands, regulating the thyroid gland, determining sexual development and function by acting on the testes and ovaries, stimulating production of milk in the breasts, and regulating the amount of urine.

Adrenal Glands

The adrenal glands are divided into two parts, each with separate functions: the medulla and the cortex. The medulla se-

cretes a hormone commonly called *adrenaline*. It is released when you are angry, fearful, or excited. Adrenaline causes the heart to beat faster and prepares the body for action. The cortex regulates the salt and water content of the body and helps control sugar and protein metabolism.

Pancreas

Diabetes is probably the most familiar of the diseases caused by endocrine failure. The pancreas produces a hormone called *insulin*, which enables the cells to use glucose. In the absence of insulin, glucose accumulates in the blood, causing excessive urination and thirst. Fortunately, the hormone can be injected when the body fails to produce it.

Thyroid Gland

The thyroid gland is extremely important in maintaining the all-around health of the body, because it regulates the rate at which the body uses oxygen. The thyroid gland needs iodine to function properly, and it is important that iodine be included in the diet. The use of iodized table salt is usually sufficient.

Parathyroid Glands

The parathyroid glands are tiny glands embedded near the base of the thyroid. The parathyroid glands are essential, because they regulate the supply, distribution, and metabolism of calcium and phosphate, which are needed by all cells.

Gonads

The gonads consist of testes in men and ovaries in women. The gonads are responsible for the production of sperm or ova. Additionally, they produce hormones that trigger the development of male and female characteristics and regulate the reproductive systems.

Unclear Functions

The thymus gland appears to be related mainly to the immune mechanism of the body; it is not clear whether the thymus has an endocrine function. The pineal body may have an effect on the gonads in early life, but at present, its actual function is disputed.

THE RETICULOENDOTHELIAL SYSTEM

The human body is constantly attacked by infectious agents through the mouth, respiratory passageways, the eyes, the colon, and the urinary tract. But before an invading organism can enter the core of the body and attack unprotected individual cells, it must evade a highly organized system of defense known as the reticuloendothelial system. This system is hard to locate exactly, but it is best described as being made up of certain watchdog cells located throughout the body.

The basis of the system that provides the body with its resistance to disease is the reticulum cell. These cells are located in the spleen, liver, lymph nodes, and many of the vascular and lymph channels of the body. At each of these locations, reticulum cells have the ability to ingest and destroy foreign organisms. Additionally, reticulum cells at any part of the body may produce the plasma cells in which nearly all of our antibodies are formed.

Antibody Formation

To protect the body from foreign invaders, an elaborate security guard of antibodies is established at an early age. The thymus gland initially contains the cells capable of forming antibodies. Its job is to distinguish between "insiders" and "outsiders" and thus avoid the unfortunate situation in which the body produces antibodies against itself, often with fatal results. One example of this is myasthenia gravis, in which antibodies against one's own muscle tissues are produced.

To avoid self-immunity, the thymus gland attempts to identify all the proteins that are a regular part of our bodies. Then all the cells that are capable of producing antibodies against our personal cells are destroyed at a very early age. This provides us with a special defense system that will produce antibodies against all outsiders (other proteins).

This system, however, is a mixed blessing. On the one hand, it allows us to develop antibodies against diseases like smallpox, polio, diphtheria, yellow fever, and influenza, and in childhood this is of great value. In later life, however, when some of our organs wear out, and we attempt to transplant donor organs, we have a serious problem. The defense system treats the proteins of the donor organs like unwanted invaders and in time destroys them.

Allergy

Allergic reactions occur when a person is only mildly immunized against outside invaders. Thus, a baby is likely to become temporarily allergic to many substances, including egg albumin and many meat extracts. But as more immunity develops, the allergy usually disappears. There is, however, an inherited tendency to produce incomplete antibodies. About one tenth of the population suffers with lifelong allergies.

Asthma results when foreign substances (e.g., ragweed pollen or horse dander) are inhaled and an allergic reaction occurs within the tubes that bring air to the lungs. The allergic reaction causes a constriction of these air tubes and makes it difficult to breathe.

Most of the antibodies produced by the body are released to wander around and fight invaders wherever they are found. The invaders are attacked before they can enter our cells. Some antibodies, however, remain within the cells, and the fight begins only when the invaders enter the cell. The result is "delayed reaction allergies," which include contact dermatitis, such as the reaction to poison ivy.

Since allergies occur because the body is only weakly immunized to a foreign substance, it is often possible to treat allergies by making a person more completely immune to the substance. This process, called desensitization, involves collecting the substance that causes the allergic reaction, sterilizing it, and injecting it into the allergic person in small but progressively larger amounts. In time, such an individual becomes completely immune and no longer exhibits an allergic reaction.

THE URINARY SYSTEM

In many ways the burning of carbohydrates, fats, and proteins by the cells is like the burning of wood or coal in your home; the burning process results in heat, gas, and ashes (waste). When the cells burn carbohydrates and fats, they are reduced to carbon dioxide and water. The carbon dioxide is mainly eliminated by the lungs. But when protein is burned it is another story. The cells cannot use all the by-products of protein metabolism. Hence, there is a remainder—like the ashes of a home fire. In the case of cells, the remaining ash is primarily nitrogen. Waste nitrogen is converted to a soluble solid substance called *urea* (yoo-ree'uh), which must be emptied from the body. Urea and a few other metabolic waste products are extracted from the blood by the kidney.

In addition to removing cellular waste, the kidney also regulates the concentration of most of the substances contained in body fluids. Hence, the kidney collects and eliminates the waste products from the blood that are not volatile and cannot be eliminated by the respiratory system. A number of organs and passageways assist the kidney with this excreting function. The kidney and these associated structures are collectively termed the *urinary system*.

The urinary system consists of the following structures:

1. Two kidneys
2. Two ureters (to take urine to the bladder)
3. A urinary bladder (to store the urine)
4. A urethra (to eliminate the urine)

The main solid substance contained in urine is urea. But almost any substance found in excess in the body is likely to find its way into the urine, including glucose when the individual suffers from diabetes.

ADDITIONAL SOURCES OF INFORMATION

The following organizations provide free or inexpensive materials and information about some aspect of the human body:

American Academy of Pediatrics, 1801 Hinman Avenue, P.O. Box 1034, Evanston, Ill. 60204

American Cancer Society, 219 E. 42nd Street, New York, N.Y. 10017

American Dental Association, Bureau of Dental Health Education, 211 Chicago Avenue, Chicago, Ill. 60611

American Diabetes Association, Inc., 600 Fifth Av., New York, N.Y. 10020

American Heart Association, National Center, 7320 Greenville Avenue, Dallas, Tex. 75231 (Write for "Putting Your Heart into the Curriculum," 1978)

American Lung Association, 1740 Broadway, New York, N.Y. 10019

American Medical Association, Department of Health Education, 535 N. Dearborn Street, Chicago, Ill. 60610

American Optometric Association, Department of Public Affairs, 243 N. Lindbergh Blvd., St. Louis, Mo. 63141

American Podiatry Association, 20 Chevy Chase Circle, N.W., Washington, D.C. 20015 (Foot care)

Arthritis Foundation, 3400 Peach Tree Rd., Atlanta, Ga. 30326

Colgate-Palmolive Company, 300 Park Avenue, New York, N.Y. 10010

Epilepsy Foundation of America, 733 15th Street, N.W., Washington, D.C. 20005

Kimberly-Clark Corporation, Life Cycle Center, Neenah, Wi. 54956

Muscular Dystrophy Association of America, 1790 Broadway, New York, N.Y. 10019

National Institutes of Health, Department of Health, Education and Welfare, U.S. Public Health Service, Building 8, Room 100, Bethesda, Md. 20014

National Kidney Foundation, 116 E. 27th Street, New York, N.Y. 10016

National Multiple Sclerosis Society, 257 Park Avenue South, New York, N.Y. 10010

National Society to Prevent Blindness, 79 Madison Avenue, New York, N.Y. 10016

Public Affairs Committee, 381 Park Avenue South, New York, N.Y. 10016

PART B: TEACHING ABOUT THE HUMAN BODY

We believe that an understanding of the function and structure of the body systems will lead students to a greater appreciation of the body's complexity and will help them understand other areas of health.

Before exploring the body systems with the class, discuss how all people are alike. How are all people different? (Even identical twins have differences.) Our individuality begins in our *cells*—extremely complex building blocks that independently carry on their own essential processes of respiration, digestion, and reproduction. Blood flows through the body delivering nourishment to the cells and removing their wastes. To keep the cells healthy, blood must do its work at the right speed all the time.

Cells vary in size and shape (see Atlas Figure 6, Your Body Is Made of Millions of Tiny Cells), according to the work they do. When a group of muscle cells combine, they make a muscle *tissue*. A group of nerve cells make nerve tissue and transmit impulses back and forth from the brain to other parts of the body. Tissues may also combine to perform a particular kind of work as an *organ* in the body. For instance, the eye is an organ that performs the function of seeing. The eye has many parts, and each part is made of a particular kind of tissue.

Organs work together in systems, to perform special functions. This chapter includes classroom activities for the skeletal system, muscular system, circulatory system, respiratory system, digestive and excretory systems, sensory and nervous system, and growth and reproductive systems, as well as a unit about grooming.

All of the body systems work together so we can live a healthy life. If one tissue or organ in the body is damaged, it affects the rest of the body in some way. You may want to read Robert Campbell's "The Life-Giving Balancing Act," and look at the accompanying paintings by Arthur Lidov (4). The article dramatically illustrates the chemical reactions that take place in the human body.

How can we motivate students to value their bodies and want to take care of them?

1. Students need to recognize that there are many ways they can help themselves stay healthy.

2. Students need to appreciate the physical and psychological well-being that comes from a healthy body.

3. Students need to understand that a long life expectancy has much to do with habits developed as a young person.

4. Students need to discover some of the fascinating secrets of their personal inner world.

UNIT I: THE SKELETAL SYSTEM

Students like to learn about bones. They often bring a bone into the classroom and ask what it came from. This unit encourages natural curiosity by engaging students in interdisciplinary activities that involve investigation and problem solving.*

The student may cut out and assemble their own human skeleton; identify mystery bones; make skeletons from animals; investigate joints; and participate in games, songs, and other activities.

OBJECTIVES

1. After assembling their own human skeleton, the students will be familiar with a variety of bones and be able to explain that bones provide:

    a. support

    b. protection

    c. movement (along with the muscle system)

2. By handling various bones and possibly helping to make a real animal skeleton from bones they have prepared themselves, the students will:

    a. observe that bones are very hard, yet light in weight

    b. view how a bone is constructed

Appropriate grade levels are suggested for each teaching strategy and appear as ○, □, ☆ in the left-hand column.

    ○ = most suited for the primary grades;

    □ = most suited for the intermediate grades;

    ☆ = most suited for the upper elementary grades.

*The authors wish to thank Doris Utgard, Sharon Heit, Linda Taylor, Barb Guertal, Charlotte McGrath, and Jeannie Hufschmitt for their assistance in developing this unit and successfully implementing the ideas in their classrooms.

and recognize similarities and differences among the bones

   c. be able to identify various kinds of bones

3. The students will learn how bones aid in movement by dissecting some joints and examining their structure. They will also compare the movement of their own bones with that of familiar mechanical joints.

MATERIALS

1. Atlas Figure 66, Human Skeleton Pattern (three pages); cardboard or old manila folders; glue; scissors or X-acto knife; tiny metal fasteners; and Atlas Figure 67, Study Sheet: Comparison of Bone Names.

2. X-rays, fresh chicken wings or legs, sharp knife, magnifying glasses, and music for the songs "Dry Bones" and "Looby Loo."

Methods

Begin this unit by duplicating enough copies of the Atlas Figure 66, Human Skeleton Pattern, for every student in your class.

□ ☆

Skeleton Construction Instructions

1. Have the students carefully and smoothly glue their patterns to a piece of cardboard or old manila folder for extra strength.

2. The students may wish to outline the skeleton bones with colored ink before cutting them out.

3. Have the students cut out all of the bones, using scissors or an X-acto knife.

4. See if the students can figure out how to assemble their skeletons by con-

necting the bones with tiny metal fasteners. (The numbers correspond with the bones listed on Atlas Figure 67, Study Sheet: Comparison of Bone Names, which may be used as a handout).

5. The skull may be assembled in two different ways (see Figure 8B-1). *Easier Method*: Cut the skull out as one piece. Insert fastener in chin to connect skull with vertebra and ribs. Cut holes for eye sockets (optional). *Advanced Method*: Cut the skull out separate from the mandible (jaw bone). Cut out the pattern that looks like a black square. Attach the upper part of the black square to the back of the skull with a dab of glue. One metal fastener will be inserted in the bottom of the black square to connect the skull with the vertebra and ribs. Another metal fastener should be used to hinge the jawbone and skull. The lower jaw will open and close (showing black in the mouth) if properly assembled. (Note: If you want the mouth to open, do not make a hole in the chin as you did in the easy method.)

Learning Center

Display an assortment of bones from different animals brought into class by you and your students. You may want to mix real bones with plastic bones. Permit the students to examine and try to identify the bones during their free time. If the students cannot figure out what animal a bone came from, encourage them to use resource books for help and to establish the approximate size of the animal.

The learning center should also contain X-rays, a magnifying glass, and pictures of bones.

○ □

Have the students compare the shape and size of the bones to pictures and to the

FIGURE 8B-1 Easy and advanced methods of assembling skull

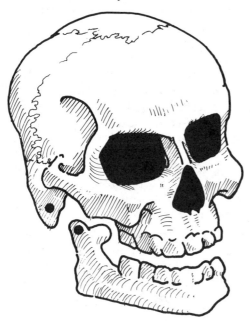 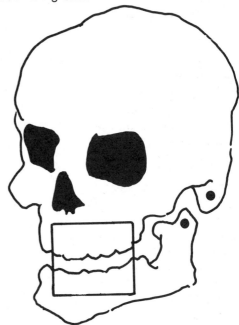

bones that they can feel in their own bodies.

○ □ ☆

Dissect a Joint

To see the true construction of joints, dissect a raw joint (fresh chicken wing or leg, leg of lamb or beef). Using a sharp knife, cut into the joint and expose the ligaments that cover the entire joint. Under the ligaments the students will be able to see a smooth layer of cartilage covering the ends of the bones. There is also a membrane that secretes a fluid and makes the joints moist and able to move smoothly. The joints in our bodies need lubrication just like moving parts in machinery.

○ □

Importance of Joints

Ask the students why they are able to move their bodies in different ways. Have

them walk like tin soldiers. What did they look like? Can they remain in a tin soldier position and write their name, see behind them, chew gum, or give their name and address?

○ □ ☆

Hinge Joints

Have the students find examples of hinge joints in the classroom. (Doors, crayon boxes, lunch boxes, eyeglasses, books, etc.) Ask them to name a hinge joint in the body. (Jaw, elbow, knee, fingers, toes). Hinge joints allow movement in one direction.

○ □ ☆

Ball-and-Socket Joints

Ask the students where in the body they have a ball-and-socket joint. Have them stick out their arm and move it in a circle, feeling the movement with their other hand. Ask what they feel. Besides

162

our shoulders, these joints are found in our hips, a TV antenna, a shower nozzle, and a car visor. They provide the widest range of movements.

Fixed Joints

We also have fixed joints that "give" but do not move very much. Most of these joints are located in the skull.

☆

X-rays and Fracture

Have the students study some X-rays and observe fracture. Discuss first aid for simple or closed fracture, compound or open fracture, and complex fracture—where the bone is broken in more than one place. In a greenstick fracture the bone splits part of the way down its long axis. The objective in treating a fracture is to keep the broken bone ends and the adjacent joints quiet.

○ □

Make an "X-ray"

To make an animal "X-ray," let each student choose an animal skeleton to draw on a sheet of black construction paper using white chalk or ink. Then have them trace the outline of the animal on a sheet of transparent paper. Next have the students cut out the outline and paste the top edge of the transparent paper cutout over the skeleton or simply paste the entire transparent sheet to the top edge of the black construction paper skeleton.

□

Other Art Activities

Other art activities might include assembling imaginary animals out of various bones; making bony caricatures and labeling their parts; and constructing small, jointed marionettes.

○ □

Music

Teach students the song "Dry Bones"* and have them point to their own bones as they sing. If the students know the scientific names for bones (see Study Sheet in Atlas) they may want to sing "Phalanges connected to de metatarsals" instead of "Toe bone connected to de foot bone," and so on.

Have the students join hands and form a circle. As they sing "Looby Loo" they should march around acting out the words. The teacher or another student may give the directions.

> I put my right humerus [or arm] in,
> I put my right humerus out,
> I give my right humerus a shake,
>   shake, shake
> And turn myself about.

□ ☆

Careers

Research careers in anthropology, archaeology, and orthopedic surgery.

Evaluation

LIFESTYLE CONTENT

□ ☆

Game: Skeleton Concentration

Materials: twenty large cards cut out of poster board, pictures of various bones.

Preparation: Glue pictures of various bones on the front of ten cards; print names (to match pictures) of bones on the front of ten cards; shuffle cards and ar-

---

*The words to this song may be found in *Bones—Teacher's Guide* (New York, N.Y.: Webster/McGraw-Hill, 1965), pp. 4–6, along with many other excellent activities.

range on the floor face down. Object: The object of the game is to match the picture with its correct label and form a pair. Another turn may be taken when a correct match is made. The winning player or team is the one to accumulate the most cards.

○ □ ☆

Skeleton Questions

A variation of this game is to draw a skeleton on a large piece of poster board and then cut the poster board into twenty squares. On the back of each square is a question. If the student correctly answers the question (which may involve pointing to a particular bone on his body or at the learning center table), the student keeps the card and gets another turn. Otherwise, the card is turned question side down again. The student with the most squares at the end of the game wins.

○ □

Simon Says

Play the familiar game, Simon Says, using such statements as, "Simon says touch your jawbone," etc. The leader may point to another part of the body and try to get other students to follow. Gradually switch to scientific names, such as, "Simon says touch your mandible."

LIFESTYLE VALUE

□ ☆

Divide the class into pairs and have one student tie yardsticks to the other student's legs and rulers to his arms, while he is in a sitting position. Ask the student to get up. Was it difficult? Can the student run, skip, or jump rope? Have the students switch roles. After all the students have had the experience of immobilized elbow and knee joints, ask them to write how they felt about the experience. This is a perfect time to lead into a discussion about arthritis.

UNIT II: THE MUSCULAR SYSTEM

What do you, Mighty Mouse, and Popeye all depend on? The answer is muscles. More than 600 skeletal muscles are fastened to our bones by tendons and make movement possible. Muscles help hold our bones in place and our bodies straight. They help blood return to the heart; in fact, the heart is a muscle that pumps our blood. Muscles focus the lenses of our eyes and draw air into our lungs; they push food along the digestive tract and provide us with facial expressions.

This unit deals with the vital role that muscles play in our everyday lives and why we should try to strengthen our muscles.

OBJECTIVES

1. Students will be able to make a model of a skeletal muscle and explain how it works.

2. Students will be able to locate their bicep and tricep muscles and explain that skeletal muscles work in pairs.

3. After class discussion, students will be able to give at least five reasons for exercising their muscles and a minimum of three precautions that should be taken regarding exercise.

MATERIALS

1. Pictures of muscles and how they are connected to the bones.

2. Atlas Figure 7, Muscle Types.

3. Cardboard tubes (from wax paper, toilet paper, etc.), string, scissors, rulers,

rubber bands, and stopwatch with second hand.

4. Atlas Figure 68, What's Your Muscle Power? Crossword Puzzle and Questions.

Methods

○ □

Introduction

Begin a class discussion by asking the students if they have ever watched a high school boy or girl playing ball and said to themselves, "I wish I could throw a ball as well as that." Have they ever had a younger boy or girl say to them, "I wish I could throw a ball the way you can"?

Ask students why they can throw a ball farther and better than boys and girls younger than themselves. The students may mention their muscles at this point. Point out that if your muscles are large and well trained, you can throw a ball a long distance. As you grow older, your muscles grow larger. As you practice throwing a ball, you improve the way you throw it, so the ball will go further.

○ □ ☆

Marionette

Show the students a marionette. What makes the puppet move? What makes people move? Do you have "strings" inside of you?

○ □ ☆

Locate Tendons

Encourage the students to feel their own arms, legs, chest, and face. Help them locate the tendons in their heels, behind their knees, in their hands, and in the inner bend of their arms.

Our "strings" are called *muscles* and *tendons*. If it is possible to obtain a foot from a chicken, duck, or turkey, expose the tendon that controls the movement of the bird's toes. Pulling the tendon will cause visible movement in the foot. Why does this happen? Actually, a bird walks on its toes, and its heel is where the feathers start. The tendon extends over the heel, just as it does in a human foot.

☆

Read About Achilles

Have the students feel the tendon of Achilles just above their heel. As muscles in the calf contract, they pull this tendon, which moves the heel and foot. Perhaps some of the students would like to read the story of Achilles in a mythology book.

○ □

Discovery Exercise

Ask if any students can wiggle their ears. The use of many of our muscles is learned. We must learn how to control our muscles before we can write. The tongue is a muscle. We have to teach our tongue how to move so we can talk. When we move our eyes, we use many muscles. Since we have over 600 muscles, we can move different parts of our body at the same time. Experiment: Have the students try to pat the top of their head with one hand and rub their abdomen with the other hand.

○ □ ☆

Transparency: Muscle Types

Make a transparency of Atlas Figure 7, Muscle Types, and give examples of using skeletal muscles. The skeletal muscles are attached to bones and can be commanded to move with nerve impulses from our brain. We call these muscles *voluntary*. When the skeletal muscles work, the bones move. Ask students, Did you notice that some of you could pat your head and rub your abdomen right away while others of you still cannot do it? Explain that there are many reasons for this—the kinds of muscles you inherit from your families and the amount of skill you can develop have certain limitations. Regardless of how much you practice, you may never have muscles as large or skillful as some other students. Usually those who are not physically skillful have some other characteristics that are admired and bring them recognition. Most of us, however, can greatly develop our muscles with exercise and good food. Exercise actually enlarges the fibers that make up our muscles, but they must be built up slowly. Ask students, Do you remember what it feels like when you have not exercised much, and then you suddenly do a whole lot of exercise? Do you feel sore? If we do not use our muscles very much over the winter they lose their "tone" or readiness for use. A muscle without tone is flabby and tires easily. Sudden, vigorous exercise can strain, stretch, or tear muscle fibers, which makes us feel sore.

○ □ ☆

Exercise Precautions

How can we prevent damage to our muscles?

1. Warm up gradually before strenuous exercise.

2. Participate in strenuous games only when properly conditioned.

3. Do not exercise to the point of exhaustion, just until somewhat tired.

4. Do not always confine exercise to indoor activities.

5. Cool off gradually after becoming perspired.

6. If possible, take a warm shower after exercising. Warmth increases the circulation of the blood and helps relieve sore muscles.

□ ☆

Some of the benefits of exercise include:

1. Increased circulation of the blood

2. Increased muscle tone, endurance, skill, and coordination of mind and muscle

3. Increased air to the lungs

4. Relief from tension and an improved outlook on life

5. Enjoyment of activities and physical well-being

6. An opportunity to develop good sportsmanship and friendship

7. Increased perspiration, which opens pores and gives the heat-regulating mechanism a workout

8. Indirect aid to digestion

○ □ ☆

Demonstration: Muscles Work in Pairs

Have the students stand and repeat the actions as you perform the following experiment:

With your arm down at your side, hold the book with your fingertips, palm facing out. Lift the book. Now place your other hand on the muscle on the front of your arm. Lift the book again. What happens to the muscle as you lift the book? Place your hand on the back of your arm. What happens to that muscle when you lift the book? Muscles work in pairs. They are attached to the bones by tendons and the muscles contract and relax. When your muscles get shorter and thicker, they are contracting.

The ends of the muscles are like tough cords. These cords are called tendons. Lift the book up and down and feel the bicep muscle getting shorter and thicker. It is the muscle on the front of the upper arm. The tricep muscle, on the back of the arm, gets longer and thinner. When the book is lifted, the muscle on the front of the upper arm bears the weight and pulls up the forearm. The muscle contracts and becomes thicker. The muscle at the back of the arm relaxes and expands. It becomes longer and thinner.

Can you feel your tendon on the inside of your elbow? Place the palm of your left hand on the muscle on the back of your upper arm. Move your arm up and down. The muscle moves. The tendons of the muscle are attached to bones. The muscle pulls the forearm downward. When it is pulling, it is contracting.

○ □

Model of Skeletal Arm Muscle

Have students make a model to show the way muscles and bones work. Provide bones of the arm or rulers or cardboard tubes. Each arm model will require two "bones." Also provide string, balloons, or rubber bands for "muscles." Have the students made a model according to Figure 8B-2 and demonstrate that when we pull string A and make it shorter, it lifts up the bone C. When we pull string B, it brings the bone back down.

FIGURE 8B-2 Model of muscles and bones

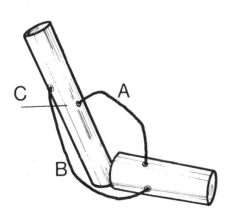

○ □ ☆

Discovery Exercises

Explain that when muscles contract, they pull on bones and make parts of the skeleton move. This is how a person can move from one chair to another. Have students find the leg muscle that helps them rise from a chair and the ones that help them sit down.

Have students capture a large grasshopper and a fly, and measure and compare:

1. The legs of the insects to the size of their bodies.
2. These measurements with the students' own leg measurements.
3. The distance a grasshopper jumps with the proportional distance the students can jump.

Our bones and muscles are in some ways like simple machines that do work when they move objects. Energy is used to make machines work. Food and oxygen in a muscle are chemically changed to release energy. These chemical changes also produce waste products in the muscle. Carbon dioxide is one of these waste products.

When the supply of food and oxygen has been used, the muscle becomes tired because no more energy is available. The muscle must rest until the circulatory system takes away the carbon dioxide and brings new supplies of food and oxygen.

Lift a book as many times as you can without stopping. How does the bicep muscle move as it tires? Fatigue is a safeguard against muscle strain.

Some muscles, such as our hearts or those in the walls of our stomach and intestines, work by chemical action and do not rely on our conscious control. These are called *involuntary* muscles.

Evaluation

LIFESTYLE CONTENT

☐ ☆

Duplicate enough copies of Atlas Figure 68, What's Your Muscle Power?, for every student in the class. Let them work individually or in small groups to complete the puzzle.

Answers

DOWN: 1. Skeletal, 2. Voluntary, 3. Food, 4. Carbon Dioxide, 5. Fatigue, 6. Movement, 7. Exercise, 8. No, 9. Warm, 10. Achilles, 11. Sore, 12. Flabby.
ACROSS: 1. Muscles, 2. Tendon, 3. Bicep, 4. Energy   5. Contracting,   6. Bone, 7. Sprain, 8. Oxygen, 9. Heart, 10. Strain, 11. Involuntary, 12. Tricep, 13. Circulatory, 14. Relaxed, 15. Pairs

LIFESTYLE VALUE

○ ☐

Have the students rank order the following activities as to their importance in building strong muscles (number one most important).

_____ Get plenty of fresh air.
_____ Exercise every day.
_____ Eat a balanced diet, with foods from all the food groups.
_____ Get plenty of rest.
_____ Drink lots of water.
_____ Gradually increase the amount of exercise you do.

☐ ☆

Have students rank order the benefits that exercise provides.

_____ Increased circulation of the blood
_____ Increased muscle tone and endurance
_____ Increased skill and coordination
_____ Relief from tension
_____ Improved health
_____ Opportunity to develop new friendships
_____ Opportunity to develop good sportsmanship

☐ ☆

Thought question: Hippocrates was a Greek physician, known as the father of medicine. He said, "Exercise strengthens and inactivity wastes." Ask students what they think he meant.

UNIT III: THE CIRCULATORY SYSTEM

If your heart could talk, it might tell you that it weighed between nine and eleven ounces, was reddish brown in color, and had an unimpressive shape. Actually, it is a powerful muscle that pumps blood loaded with carbon dioxide waste from the body into the lungs to be cleansed. The blood picks up fresh oxygen and returns to the heart, which pushes it through the arteries to all the body tissues.

The activities in this unit are designed to acquaint the students with their heart, arteries, veins, capillaries, and blood and to encourage behavior that will strengthen the heart.

OBJECTIVES

1. Students will demonstrate an understanding of the circulatory system by identifying its basic components (heart, arteries, veins, capillaries, blood) and their respective functions.

2. Given an outline of the human heart, the students will correctly label the four chambers and valves and indicate the direction of blood flow.

3. Each student will construct a

"model" of blood, including red blood cells, white blood cells, platelets, and plasma, and will describe the purpose of each component.

4. The students will be able to locate a pulse in two different places on the body (e.g., wrist and side of neck).

MATERIALS

1. Atlas Figure 8, Animal Hearts.

2. Atlas Figure 69, Worksheet: Inside the Human Heart.

3. Chicken heart and other animal hearts, if possible.

4. Paper, crayons, watch with second hand, eight ounce glass, four or five gallon jugs, water gun or turkey baster, basketball, tennis ball, empty egg shell (make a hole on both ends and blow out the contents), music for the song "If I Only Had a Heart" from *The Wizard of Oz*.

5. Jar, water, red and white paper.

Methods

○ □ ☆

Have students clench their fist, open it, then close it, for as long as they can at a rate of little more than once every second. Point out that in a few minutes their hand muscles will be tired but their heart muscle will still be contracting and dilating at a rate of 72 times a minute, or about 100,000 times a day.

Imagine an organ so strong that it could contract nearly 40 million times a year and only rest a fraction of a second between contractions. "The work done by your heart is about equal to the work you would perform if you lifted a ten pound weight three feet off the ground and repeated this task every minute for a lifetime. One scientist has figured that

heart muscles work twice as hard as the leg muscles of a person who is running" (2, p. 18).

○

Powerful Pump

The heart is a powerful pump that can pump four to five gallons of blood each minute. Demonstrate this concept by bringing in an eight-ounce glass and four or five gallon jugs. Let the students count out loud how many glasses of blood are pumped by the heart each minute (3).

○

Draw Your Heart

Ask the students to draw a picture of what they think their heart looks like and where it is located.

○ □

Simple Pumps

Show some different kinds of pumps, for example, a water gun, a turkey baster, and a toy that moves by squeezing a rubber bulb.

○ □ ☆

Locate Your Pulse

Have the students try to find their pulse (the throbbing of the arteries caused by contractions of the heart). One pulse location is on the wrist directly below the thumb. Another pulse can be felt on the side of the neck, under the jawbone.

○ □

Record Pulse Rate

Have the students count how many times their pulse beats in thirty seconds and multiply by two. Have them do ten jumping-jacks and count their pulse again. Did it increase? Why? Usually a small heart beats faster than a large one. In children, the heart beats about 100 to

120 times a minute. In adults, it beats about 70 to 90 times a minute. An elephant's heart beats only 25 times a minute, but the heart of a mouse beats about 700 times a minute!

○ □

Animal Hearts

Let students examine a model of a heart. A human heart is a little larger than a person's fist. Show a transparency of Atlas Figure 8, Animal Hearts. A rabbit has a heart about the size of an egg (hold up an egg). A giraffe has a heart the size of a basketball. A dog has a heart about the size of a tennis ball, and a mouse has a heart the size of a small raspberry (3)!

○ □ ☆

Transparency

Show a transparency of Atlas Figure 69, Worksheet: Inside the Human Heart. Explain to the students that the heart is really two pumps that work together.

Review circulatory system content in Chapter 8A and then trace a drop of blood through the heart using a heart model or outline of the human heart.

Film

Show the film "Your Heart and How It Works," or "The Work of the Heart," available through your local branch of the American Heart Association. Another excellent film is "Hemo, the Magnificent."

○

Examine a Leaf

Examine the network of veins in a leaf. This may help reinforce the students' mental image of their own network of blood vessels.

Review: Ask the students why the blood from an artery is brighter in color than blood from a vein.

○ □

Circulatory Man

Request "Circulatory Man" from your local heart chapter to present an overview of the relationships between the arteries, veins, and capillaries, or, have a student lie down on a large piece of brown paper and have another student trace his or her outline on the paper. Draw the heart in its proper position and glue red and blue yarn from the heart to the arms and legs to represent arteries and veins.

Explain to the students that arteries are blood vessels that carry food and oxygen to every part of the body. Veins are blood vessels that return blood to the heart and carry waste products from every part of the body to the kidneys, lungs, and other organs for elimination from the body. Capillaries are very small blood vessels that bridge the gap between the arteries and veins. The exchange of food and waste and oxygen products takes place through the walls of the capillaries.

○ □ ☆

Model of Blood

Let each student construct a model of "blood," using a jar as a small section of artery.

Red Blood Cells   The special cells that carry food, oxygen, and other materials through the arteries to different parts of the body are called *red blood cells*. These cells contain a material called *hemoglobin*, which gives them their red color and allows them to pick up oxygen and carry it along. Have the students cut circles of red paper to represent the red blood cells and put them into their arteries (jars). Review what red blood cells do.

Red blood cells make up 45 percent of the blood but are so small that a large drop of blood will contain more than 250 million of them. Red blood cells only live about 120 days, so they must be replaced continuously. They are formed within the marrow of some bones.

White Blood Cells   Our blood has another type of cell that fights off and destroys the germs that make us sick. These special cells are called *white blood cells*. Have the students cut irregular shapes of white paper to represent white blood cells.

White blood cells are larger than red ones and fewer in number. There is only one white cell for approximately every 650 red cells. White blood cells have no definite shape and move by changing their shape. They only live eight to ten days.

Platelets   A cut bleeds for awhile, but then the blood automatically stops. What has happened? *Platelets*, combined with other substances, prevent excessive bleeding by aiding in the formation of clots. When we cut outselves the platelets rush to the cut and clump together to stop the blood from running out. Have the students cut small circles of white paper to represent platelets. Platelets are believed to live only three to four days.

Plasma

The last part of our blood is a very watery fluid and is important because the cells need a liquid to carry them through the body. This liquid is called *plasma*, and it carries water (92 percent), proteins (7 percent), minerals (1 percent), sugar, vitamins, hormones, and enzymes. Have the students add water to their jars to represent plasma.

Contact your local heart association to obtain the *Heart Project* (3), "Your Heart and How It Works" handouts, and for further information.

Evaluation

LIFESTYLE CONTENT

☐ ☆

Duplicate enough copies of Atlas Figure 69, Worksheet: Inside the Human Heart, for each student in the class. After they have identified the correct parts of the heart (1. Right Atrium, 2. Tricuspid valve, 3. Right Ventricle, 4. Pulmonary valve, 5. Left Atrium, 6. Mitral valve, 7. Left Ventricle, 8. Aortic valve), have them indicate the direction of blood flow.

○ ☐

Game

Draw a large chalk outline of a heart on the pavement outdoors. Have the students stand on the lines and form chambers and valves. Let several students at a time run through the large heart as if they were drops of blood.

☐ ☆

Happy Heart Quiz

Cover a rectangular piece of cardboard with red felt or Velcro for the background (see Figure 8B-3). (If you want to make this visual aid more permanent, use lightweight wood instead of cardboard and attach a handle to the top.) Title the game "Happy Heart" and draw a little cartoon figure of Super Heart Muscle. Attach a small box to the middle of the board to hold question cards, for example, "The great trunk artery that carries blood from the heart to all parts of the body is the __ __ __ __ __ (Aorta)." To show that the answer has five letters, you may want to attach five small white circles to the board. Divide the class into teams and have them take turns guessing a letter. If a correct letter is chosen, the team may take another turn. If the correct word is identified, the team gets a point

FIGURE 8B-3 Happy heart quiz

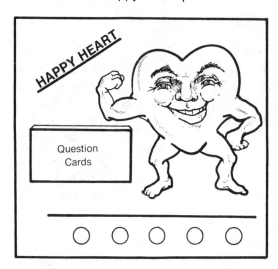

and selects one of their members to draw the next card and attach letters as they are identified for the new word. Another way of scoring is to see which team can spell HEART first; identifying the correct word is rewarded with one letter.

LIFESTYLE VALUE

○ □

Teach the students the song "If I Only Had a Heart" from *The Wizard of Oz*. Why do they think he wanted a heart? What does the word *heart* mean to different people?

UNIT IV: THE RESPIRATORY SYSTEM

Mankind has been sucking in and expelling invisible air for a long time—some people believe since "the Lord God formed man of the dust of the ground, and breathed into his nostrils the breath of life" (Genesis).

This nothingness, which is plainly something, travels through hairy nostrils and smooth pharynx, larynx, and trachea, to the branching bronchi and cavernous lungs. Enroute, it is cleansed, moistened, and warmed in preparation for its trip around the body.

The human breathing system is of fundamental importance. We hope that the following activities will help students grasp its workings, convince them not to start smoking, and encourage them to support programs to clean up the air.

OBJECTIVES

1. Given an outline of the respiratory system, the students will correctly trace the passage of air into the lungs and label the various parts.

2. The students will explain why we need to breathe and why we breathe faster after vigorous exercise.

3. The students will help make a model breathing apparatus and participate in three tests to determine the adequacy of their lung power.

4. The students will actively participate in a variety of experiments designed to show how breathing is controlled.

MATERIALS

1. Atlas Figure 70, Worksheet: Trace the Passage of Air into the Lungs, which may be used as a handout or transparency or for evaluation.

2. Model breathing apparatus requires jar with bottom cut off (or bell jar), Y-tube, two small balloons, one large balloon. Alternate method requires a straight rubber tube, Y-tube, two small balloons, bell jar, and rubber stopper with a hole through the center.

3. Watch with second hand, wooden matches, tape measure, small birthday cake candles, toy accordion, paper bag, balloons, scented liquid perfume, onion juice, and other odor sources.

Methods

○ □

Introduction

One day while on the playground, have the students run relays until they appear to be breathing hard. Ask them what they thought caused them to be breathing faster.

When you go back to the classroom, give the students the following pretest:

○ □

Pretest

1. I carry air from your nose to your lungs. Who am I? (Windpipe or trachea)

2. We get larger when filled with air. Who are we? (Lungs)

3. My name begins with the letter O and I make up a very important part of the air that you breathe into your body. Who am I? (Oxygen)

4. If you breathe correctly, you first take air through me and into your windpipe. Who am I? (Nose)

5. We both begin with the letter E and we can make you breathe more rapidly. Who do you think we are? (Exercise and Emotion)

Ask the students, Can you think of something that you have been doing while taking this test? Of course, you have been breathing. You keep breathing all the time. Your body may use five quarts of air a minute, when you are not exercising. When you are strenuously exercising as you were a few minutes ago, your body may use twenty or thirty times as much oxygen as it does at rest.

You are constantly breathing in oxygen and breathing out wastes. One of these wastes is carbon dioxide. We can detect carbon dioxide with the simple demonstration below.

○ □

Experiment

Obtain a jar of phenolphthalein solution and ask a student to exhale into it. The red liquid will change to a clear liquid, indicating that a weak carbonic acid is being formed. We know from this and other experiments that the material being exhaled and causing the color change is carbon dioxide.

A large illustration of the respiratory system (obtained from your local branch of the Lung Association) can be used as you explain the following material:

○ □ ☆

When you breathe in, the large muscle that divides the chest and the abdomen, called the *diaphragm*, contracts downward causing the chest to expand and the ribs to move upward and outward. This produces a partial vacuum in the lungs. Since the pressure of the air outside the body is now greater than the pressure in the lungs, air rushes into the nose, down the windpipe (trachea), and into the lungs. When you breathe out, the diaphragm goes up to its original position, and the air leaves your lungs.

○ □ ☆

Simulate Diaphragm and Lungs

To make a model that will show how the diaphragm and lungs work together:

1. Obtain a bell jar or cut the bottom off a jar.

2. Cut the bottom off a large balloon and fit the balloon securely over the bottom of the jar. (You may need to tie a piece of string around the jar to help secure the balloon.)

3. Tie a knot in the balloon mouthpiece so that no air can pass through.

4. Fit small balloons on branches of Y-tube.

FIGURE 8B-4 Model of respiratory system

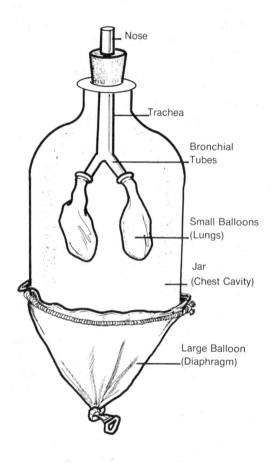

Nose

Trachea

Bronchial Tubes

Small Balloons (Lungs)

Jar (Chest Cavity)

Large Balloon (Diaphragm)

5. Put the stem of the Y-tube through the rubber stopper in the top of the bell jar.

6. Pull downward on the mouthpiece of the large balloon and see what happens!

A similar model can be made with an ordinary jar, Y-tube, two balloons, and a rubber stopper. Since this version does not have a diaphragm, you must blow through a small rubber tube connected to the end of the Y-tube to inflate the balloons (lungs).

How are the gases (oxygen and carbon dioxide) actually transferred from the alveoli to the bloodstream?

□ ☆

Diffusion of Gases

You can demonstrate diffusion of gases with the following experiment (14, p. 14):

Place a drop of scented liquid in a balloon. Blow up the balloon and tie securely. Place balloon firmly in mouth of large jar, sealing well, and let stand 15–20 minutes. Remove balloon and sniff air in the jar. Use with different liquids: perfume, onion juice, etc.

This demonstration shows that not all walls are airtight or gastight; they may be *semipermeable*. In other words, they may hold some molecules in and let others out. The walls of a balloon should be able to hold every drop of water that was put into it a week ago, but it will not be able to hold all the air that was blown into it a week ago. The walls of all the cells in our body are semipermeable. They let molecules of oxygen and carbon dioxide through very quickly, while holding other molecules back.

Most of us take fourteen to eighteen shallow breaths a minute when we should be taking about eight deep ones. This results in our using only one-sixth of our lung capacity.

○ □ ☆

Discovery Exercises

To prove this, have the students open their mouths and exhale all they can. Then have them purse their lips and blow. There is air left in the lungs, and what is left is stagnant. The stagnant gases fill lung spaces and cheat the tissues out of oxygen. Lungs will hold six pints of air, yet with each breath desk workers inhale only about one pint is consumed. This means that five-sixths of their lung capacity lies idle.

□ ☆

Drawing the shoulder blades together immediately opens up the chest cavity. Let the students take a good breath and see how far they can read in a book on one breath. They can try it again each day and see if they can gradually increase the number of lines they can read without inhaling.

□ ☆

Dr. Thomas L. Petty, Professor of Medicine at the University of Colorado Medical Center, suggests the following three tests to provide a good indication of one's lung power (11, p. 52):

1. *Speed of expiration:* For this you'll need a watch or clock with a second-hand. Take a large breath and blow out as hard and as fast as you can with your mouth wide open, watching to see how long it takes you.

Normally it takes about three to four seconds, depending on the size and age of the individual (slightly longer for older persons, and less for younger persons). A longer time —say, six to eight seconds—indicates obstructed airflow, which might suggest emphysema, chronic bronchitis, or asthma.

2. *Blowing out a match:* Take a standard wooden kitchen match, and place it, lit, eight inches in front of your open mouth. Now exhale quickly with your mouth wide open (do not purse your lips). If you extinguish the flame, your lungs are probably in good shape; however, if the match remains lit, it may mean trouble.

3. *Chest expansion:* A more old-fashioned and yet reliable way of gauging your lung power is through the tape-measure test. Wrap a tape measure around your chest (if you're female, just under your breasts; if male, across the nipple line).

Breathe out as far as you can and then measure the expansion of your chest as you take a deep breath. Expansion should be well over 1½ inches, and probably more than 2 inches (once again, this depends on the size and the age of the individual). If it is less, this may mean some form of lung restriction.

If one has any trouble passing these tests, it would be a good idea to see a doctor for more elaborate tests.

Although we can alter our natural breathing rhythm for a short time, our breathing will automatically adjust itself to insure a steady flow of air. The booklet, *Breathing . . . What You Need to Know,* suggests the following two activities (1, p. 34):

○ □ ☆

Breathing Patterns

Try inhaling very slowly, only four or five times a minute. Notice how you automatically begin to take much deeper breaths. Try inhaling 30 or more times a minute; each breath will be much shallower. Either pattern of breathing will deliver just about as much air a minute to your alveoli.

Inhale and exhale as deeply and quickly as you can half a dozen times in a row, sending your alveoli far more air than they need. Relax. Your subsequent breathing is somewhat slower and shallower than usual.

Have the students breathe into a paper bag for three minutes and notice the increase in their rate of breathing. What is happening?

○ □ ☆

Have the class exercise and try to maintain a constant rate of breathing.

□ ☆

Invite a music teacher to discuss and show the breathing techniques used when singing or playing a wind instrument.

Evaluation

LIFESTYLE CONTENT

□ ☆

Give each student an outline of the respiratory system (Atlas Figure 70, Worksheet: Trace the Passage of Air into the Lungs) and ask them to trace the passage of air through the body to the lungs. Label each part.

Check each student to see if he or she met the stated objectives:

_____ can orally explain why we need to breathe and why we breathe faster after vigorous exercise.

_____ helped construct model breathing apparatus.

_____ participated in tests of lung power and other breathing exercises.

□ ☆

Show the students a real or toy accordion. Pull the two ends apart and see if the students can relate it to breathing. (Air rushes into the accordion when the ends are pulled apart and there is space for it. When the space is squeezed smaller, the air is pushed out again.) How does an accordion that is squeezed small relate to our breathing?

LIFESTYLE VALUE

○ □ ☆

Ask the students what they think could be done to make air better to breathe.

○ □

Ask the students what they would do if they saw children playing in places where there might not be enough air. (Hiding in old, discarded refrigerators, boxes, or chests, etc.)

○

Ask the students if they think it is sometimes safe to put a plastic bag over their head.

UNIT V: THE DIGESTIVE AND EXCRETORY SYSTEMS

In a zoo at midnight, a good-sized live pig was pushed inside the door of the bachelor apartment of the python. The pig was nervous. After the conventional preliminaries that began with squeezing the holy breath of life out of the pig, the python dislocated his jaw, which is part of the ritual for any of his better meals, and in went the pig, slowly. Whereupon at his upper end the python bulged. Next morning he bulged less and farther down. The pig was melting. Life was making life out of life as the pig advanced through the great snake's digestive tube.

Man gets in his pig without dislocating his jaw and next morning does not bulge, not much. Man also makes life out of life (8, p. 199).

The purpose of this unit is to follow the food we eat through various tubes until it dissolves through the walls of the small intestines into the bloodstream or, in the case of materials that cannot be digested, moves through the large intestine and out of the body.

Through playing the Digestion Game, constructing Digestion Danny, and participating in experiments, the students will continue to develop an appreciation of their bodies.

OBJECTIVES

1. After playing the Digestion Game and completing the other activities in this unit, students will be able to label the digestive organs, describe their function, and trace a piece of food through the body.

2. Students will be able to explain the importance of correct eating habits and the influence their emotions have on digestion.

3. Each student will assist in the construction of Digestion Danny and experiments that illustrate the digestive system.

4. The students will be able to relate the excretory system to digestion and explain that their kidneys filter wastes from the blood and maintain fluid balance.

MATERIALS

1. Atlas Figure 71, Digestion Game and game cards.

2. Sheet of brown or white paper five to six feet long, set of artificial teeth, construction paper, scissors, glue, needle and thread, rubber tubing of various lengths, marble, balloons, and crayons or felt-tip markers.

3. Bread, sugar cubes; other foods, depending on which experiments you select.

4. Felt board and felt pieces (head, torso, mouth, small intestine, large intestine, rectum; accessory organs include liver, gall bladder, and pancreas).

5. Atlas Figure 72, Worksheet: Outline of the Digestive System, that may be used as a study sheet or for evaluation; transparency Atlas Figure 9, Front View of Urinary Organs.

Methods

(You may want to follow the unit on nutrition in Chapter 10B with this lesson on digestion.)

○ □ ☆

Introduction

Ask the students to think about the dinner they had last night. Point out that after they finished eating, their body was just beginning to work and change the food they ate into food that could be used by the cells of their body.

Digestion begins in the mouth. Ask the students: Have you ever heard anyone say, "It smells so good it makes my mouth water?" What do you think that means?

○ □

Pass out cookies or some other treat to the students. Have them look at the cookie, think about eating it, and smell it. Ask if they can feel anything happening in their mouths. (If your mouth "waters" it is because you are producing more saliva. Saliva is a digestive juice that helps break food down chemically.)

○ □

What else do we have in our mouths that helps make digestion easier? Show the students a set of false teeth. Teeth help us cut, tear, crush, and grind our food into small pieces. (Let the students chew and swallow their cookie.) Do you think the cookie would have been hard to swallow if it had not been softened by saliva and broken into small pieces with the teeth?

○ □

Give each student a piece of bread. Have them chew it for about a minute before swallowing it. What happens? Does the "feel" of it change? Does the taste change? The bread begins to break down immediately as the teeth go to work on it. The taste changes from starchy to sweet due to the action of the digestive juices.

○ □ ☆

Test for Starch

1. Prepare a fresh iodine solution by adding ½ tsp. iodine to ½ cup water. Stir.

2. Control—cornstarch

a. Mix 2 tablespoons cornstarch with ½ cup water.

b. Add a few drops of the iodine solution to the cornstarch solution. A purple color will develop. The purple color is a positive indication that starch is present.

c. Set test tube aside for comparison with foods to be tested.

3. Add several drops of the iodine solution to foods such as bread, cookie, potato, milk, hot dog, cheese, orange, and nuts.

4. Record results on a data sheet (6).

○ □ ☆

Test for Sugar

1. Control—corn syrup

a. Put 1 teaspoon corn syrup in a test tube.

b. Add 2 full droppers of Benedict solution (which can be purchased at a pharmacy).

c. Heat, making sure to hold open end of test tube away from you while heating. Wait for blue color to change to red orange. The red orange color is a positive indication that sugar is present.

d. Set test tube aside for comparison with foods to be tested.

2. Try this test with other foods. Put a small piece of food in a test tube, add about one ounce (or two full droppers) of Benedict solution, heat, and wait for the color change. Some foods that contain sugar are oranges, cookies, and ripe bananas. Foods that do not contain sugar are meat, cheese, and nuts.

3. Record results on a data sheet (6).

○ □ ☆

Test for Protein

1. Control—feather

a. Smell a burning feather. The odor of burning protein is distinctive. This odor is a positive indication that protein is present.

2. Burn various foods to determine those that contain protein and record the results on a data sheet. Most foods can be put on a piece of aluminum foil and placed on a hot plate; one or two drops of milk can be burned in a test tube. Foods that contain protein include meat, beans, cheese, and eggs. Some foods that do not contain protein are tomatoes, oranges, and celery. Meat must be tested raw (6).

○ □ ☆

Test for Fat

1. Control—butter

a. Rub some butter on wrapping paper (butcher paper). The grease spot is a positive indication that fat is present.

b. Some foods that contain fat are cheese, nuts, and hamburger or hot dogs. Some foods that do not contain fat are oranges, tomatoes, and celery.

c. Allow liquids to dry before recording results. Hold each sheet up to sunlight or a lamp and compare with the grease spot control (6).

○ □

Digestion Danny

By building Digestion Danny, students can find out more about the digestive system.

Have one student trace the body of another student on a sheet of brown or white paper. Another student can cut the form out and attach it to a bulletin board or sturdy cardboard backing. Another student should color eyes and a nose on Danny. Hair may be drawn or made out of yarn. Attach a set of artificial teeth or draw a mouth with teeth showing.

Remind the students that the food we

eat is the source of our energy. Ask them if we could get energy from eating paper or straw. Tell them that our system will not digest these materials, and therefore we would get no energy from them.

What are some of the organs that are used for digestion? (Mouth, esophagus, stomach, small intestine, large intestine; accessory organs include the rectum, liver, gall bladder, and pancreas.)

Where does the food go once it has been swallowed? (Down the esophagus.) The *esophagus* is a long, muscular tube leading from the mouth to the stomach. It is lined with glands to keep it wet and slippery.

How do you think food moves through the esophagus? Give each group of students a piece of rubber tubing and a marble that is only slightly larger than the tubing. The students will soon discover how to push the marble through the tubing by squeezing the tubing behind the marble.

Attach a piece of rubber tubing about ten inches long to Digestion Danny, so that he has an esophagus.

Where does food go next? (Stomach) Ask the students to describe what they think the stomach looks like. (The stomach is a swollen bag that is hollow and has two small openings at opposite ends. It is made up of muscle and lined with glands that manufacture hydrochloric acid, which aids digestion.)

Give Digestion Danny a stomach by attaching the end of a large balloon to the tube representing his esophagus.

Divide the students into groups and let them discover how the stomach works on food. Put some bread chunks and water into a balloon. Inflate it slightly. Ask the students to get the bread broken down. When they think they have succeeded, let them pour the contents of the balloon

into a container. What does the mixture look like? What does the water represent in this activity? (Stomach acids)

Where does the food go after it is broken down? (Small intestine) Most of digestion takes place in the small intestine.

There are three organs that aid in the process of digestion although no food ever passes through them. The liver, pancreas, and gall bladder secrete digestive juices to help break down the fats, carbohydrates, and proteins. These juices enter the small intestine.

Ask the students to describe the small intestine. It is a long, coiled tube, at least four times as long as you are tall.

Give Digestion Danny a small intestine by cutting a hole in the other end of the balloon and attaching about twenty-two feet of rubber tubing. It must coil around and around to fit into a relatively small area. (The students may want to look at some pictures to see what the intestine looks like.)

Digested food passes through the capillaries found in the walls of the small intestine and moves into the bloodstream on its way to the cells.

Is all food able to be dissolved? (No) What happens to food that is not digested? (This undigested food, in a fluid state, passes into the large intestine.)

Ask the students to describe the large intestine. The large intestine is much wider than the small intestine (about three inches in diameter) and about five feet long. It begins at the small intestine and moves up the right side of the body, under the liver and stomach, and down the left side of the body to connect with the rectum.

Give Danny a large intestine by connecting about five feet of larger rubber tubing to the small intestine with glue or needle and thread.

Since the undigested food is in a fluid state, the large intestine absorbs most of the liquid, leaving a soft, solid waste material.

The rectum is actually a part of the excretory system, but it is at the end of the digestive process. The rectum gets rid of undigested waste materials.

Give Danny a rectum by adding another piece of tubing about five inches long and attaching it to the large intestine. (A discussion of how to avoid constipation may be interjected at this point.)

☐ ☆

Digestion Drag Track

To review the lesson on digestion let the students play the Digestion Drag Track* game (Atlas Figure 71).

Materials The game board consists of two pages that should be taped together on the back side and then securely glued to sturdy cardboard or poster board. The game may be covered with contact paper for longer use. Each player needs a marker. Small cardboard models of food or other objects may be used. To prepare playing cards, attach the two sheets of questions (in Atlas) to the appropriate color of construction paper and cut the cards out.

Instructions Players take turns answering questions on the cards they have selected. They may move their markers forward for a correct answer: two spaces for a gold card; four spaces for a pink card; and six spaces for a blue card. Mark-

*Adapted from the comic book, *Mulligan Stew,* with permission of Extension, 4H, U.S. Dept. of Agriculture in cooperation with State Extension Services of the Land Grant Universities; and from *Health and Growth,* Book 5, Teacher's Edition, by Julius B. Richmond, et al. Copyright © 1971 by Scott, Foresman & Co. Reprinted by permission.

ers must be moved back for a wrong answer: one space for a gold card; two spaces for a pink card; and three spaces for a blue card. The first player to reach the end is the winner.

All players begin at the mouth. Stack the cards so the questions cannot be seen. Provide a separate pile for each color. Twenty question cards have been provided for each color, plus four cards that can be made any color. You may want to make up additional cards of your own.

The first player selects a card and gives it to the next player to read out loud. If the first player gives the correct answer, he may move his marker the number of spaces indicated by the color of card chosen. After a question has been answered, the student should put that card on the bottom of the pile.

○ ☐ ☆

Supplementary Activities for the Digestion System

Write a play or puppet script, using characters such as Vickie Vitamin and Mickey Mineral, for the students to perform. These characters could tell about their adventures in the body, who they meet, and where they go.

☐

Have the students make flash cards of the new vocabulary words they learned in this lesson. (Vocabulary word on one side and the definition on the reverse side.) This activity develops dictionary and spelling skills.

We have discussed how the large intestine and rectum get rid of solid waste materials that cannot be digested, but we also produce liquid waste material that must be removed.

1. Some of the water (along with salts and wastes) is removed through the pores in our skin when we perspire.

2. A small amount of water is lost each time we breathe out.

3. We lose some water through the large intestine along with undigested food.

4. But most of our waste water is removed through the kidneys. Have students point to where they think their kidneys are located. Ask them what they think the kidneys look like. We have two kidneys located high in our back, and they are bean shaped. They contain thousands of little filtering tubes that remove excess water and wastes from our blood.

Waste material that cannot be reabsorbed in the kidneys is known as *urine*. Urine flows through a small tube from each kidney into a muscular bag called the *urinary bladder*. This is where our urine is stored until we urinate.

If our kidneys are healthy they:

1. Remove wastes from the blood
2. Regulate the internal chemistry of the body
3. Regulate the amount of water in the body
4. Help regulate blood pressure
5. Help control red blood cell production

(Make use of a transparency of Atlas Figure 9, Front View of Urinary Organs, while discussing this material.)

Evaluation

LIFESTYLE CONTENT

○ □

Evaluate the student's knowledge of the digestive system by using a felt board with a felt head and torso already attached. Ask the students to trace a piece of food throughout the body. (Have felt pieces of a mouth, small intestine, large intestine, esophagus, stomach, rectum, and perhaps liver, gall bladder, and pancreas already cut out.) Ask the students to identify the various organs and place them on the felt board in the correct position. Have them describe the function of each organ.

□ ☆

Duplicate enough copies of Atlas Figure 72, Worksheet: Outline of the Digestive System for every member of your class and ask them to complete it.

Ask the students to explain how their emotions can influence their digestion.

LIFESTYLE VALUE

○ □ ☆

Ask the students the following questions:

How do you feel about the statement, "The more you eat, the better you feel." Do you agree or disagree? Why?

Do you feel that it is important to avoid constipation? Why or why not?

Why is it better to be happy and relaxed when eating? What can you do to make mealtime more pleasant in your home?

UNIT VI: THE SENSORY AND NERVOUS SYSTEM

Billions of cells in our brain make it possible for us to read and understand, remember the past, and dream of the future. Hippocrates, a famous Greek physician who lived over 2,000 years ago, was probably the first man to try to explain how the brain helps us see, hear, smell, touch, and taste. He also believed that the brain was responsible for our memories, emotions, and ability to think.

The purpose of this unit is to stimulate interest in some of the fascinating things the brain can do and to give students a basic understanding of our wonderful sensory and nervous system.

OBJECTIVES

1. After completing the activities in this unit, the students will be able to complete the nervous system worksheet found in the Atlas.

2. The students will successfully complete the Brain Maze activity in the Atlas.

3. The students will participate in class activities involving the senses of seeing, hearing, smelling, tasting, and touching and will be able to explain that this is how they learn about their surroundings.

4. The students will be able to list at least ten ways that their senses may contribute to their personal safety.

MATERIALS

1. A lifesize model of the human brain; chart showing a cross-section of the brain (see Atlas Figure 10, The Brain and Its Functions, showing its major parts and various functions.)

2. Atlas Figure, Worksheet: The Nervous System.

3. Calf or pig brain for dissection.

4. Hairpins and rulers; empty pie tin; paper or aluminum foil; handkerchief for use as blindfold.

5. Transparency of Atlas Figure 11, Nerve Cell/Reflex Action.

6. Straws; various liquids (e.g., milk, soft drink, tea, salted water, vinegar); bag full of familiar objects; other materials needed for sensory experiments will be listed with each method.

Methods

○ □ ☆

Introduce this unit by asking the students if they know someone who is the boss in a factory or an office. Explain that a boss oversees others, makes sure everyone is doing the work properly, and tells people what to do. The nervous system is a kind of boss over the other systems.

□ ☆

Model: Parts of the Brain

Using a model of the brain, charts, or a transparency of Atlas Figure 10, describe the various parts of the central nervous system. The brain is made up of the largest mass of nervous tissue in the body and weighs about three pounds when it is fully grown. (At birth, the brain weighs about twelve ounces and possesses virtually all the neurons or nerve cells it will ever have.)

The brain and spinal cord are directly connected. Have the students feel their backbone. The spinal cord is about eighteen inches long and is protected by vertebrae, small circular bones that make up the backbone.

As you name each part of the brain and explain its function, write the name on the blackboard.

Cerebrum The cerebrum is where thinking takes place and the control of all the voluntary actions. Emotions, reason, judgment, and speech have their home base here. This is where memories are.

□ ☆

The cerebrum makes up about 85 percent of the total brain. Ask a student to measure and draw a square on the blackboard that is two feet by two feet. Tell the class that this square represents the amount of space that the cerebrum would take up if it were unfolded.

A wrinkled brain has more room for brain cells than a smooth brain would have. To demonstrate this, have a student line an empty pie plate with unwrinkled aluminum foil or paper. Have another student crumple up paper or foil and see how much is needed to line it.

Cerebellum The cerebellum controls our muscles so that they will work together; it is responsible for our reflexes and is about the size of a clenched fist. The cerebellum plays a big role in controlling our posture, balance, and movement.

Medulla Oblongata The medulla is located on top of the spinal cord at the base of the head. It is about three-fourths of an inch to one inch long and consists of nerve tracts passing into other areas of the brain. The medulla controls swallowing, vomiting, breathing, digestion, metabolism, and the beating of the heart. This is the area where many depressant drugs have their effect.

□ ☆

Dissection

Let the students observe the brain structure of a pig or cow; cut off a section of the cerebrum and see if they can see both gray matter and white matter, the nerve fibers that carry messages.

□ ☆

Transparency

Show a transparency of Atlas Figure 11, Nerve Cell/Reflex Action. Draw a nerve cell on the chalkboard if you do not use the transparency and label it *neuron*. Explain that cells that make up the nerve tissue are different from other cells in the body because they do not multiply. We have nearly the same number of nerve cells all of our lives. (An older person actually has fewer because when brain cells die, as a result of drug overdose, age, or lack of oxygen, they are not replaced.)

It has been estimated that we are born with over 10 billion neurons, or nerve cells, which consume one-fourth of the body's oxygen supply. Each of these tiny neurons consists of a cell body and a number of fibers. The fibers connect the cell body with other cells. At birth, we may have very few connections between the cell bodies, but as we grow older and increase in intelligence, many more connections appear.

○ □

Neuron Messages

Each neuron receives messages and passes these messages to the next neuron. The messages travel across the ends of the neurons' fibers. Neurons actually form chains, which we can think of as wires along which messages move. Have the students get in a circle and sit down. Whisper a message to one student and have him or her repeat the message to the next student, or have the students hold hands and send a message by squeezing their hands.

Explain that we have two different kinds of nerves:

1. Sensory nerves carry signals from various parts of the body (eyes, ears, skin, etc.) through the spinal cord to the brain. They keep the brain informed about what is happening inside and outside the body.

2. Motor nerves carry orders from the brain and spinal cord to the muscles.

Touch a pin to the back of a student's hand, and brush cotton against the skin to demonstrate two sensations that do not feel the same. The nervous system is responsible for these different sensations.

☆

We have learned that a neuron has a cell body, including a nucleus. (Use transparency) *Dendrites* are nerve endings with many branches. They carry messages from the skin to the nerve cell. A nerve cell also has an *axon*. The axon does not have many branches. It carries messages away from the nerve cell. After the axon and dendrite leave the nerve cell they are called *nerve fibers*. Nerves are nourished by the blood. They need food and oxygen to live. Signals flash through neurons, but they are not wires.

□ ☆

Story

One day Mary was sitting at her desk in school when she accidentally knocked her pencil to the floor. If she was looking at the blackboard at the time, how did she know that her pencil had fallen? (The sound was heard by her ears.) The sound of the falling pencil caused electrical impulses to move from her ears along auditory nerves to her brain. What main part of the brain do you think received the electrical impulses from the ears? (Cerebrum)

The cerebrum received the impulses as sound and passed this information on to another part of the cerebrum that is concerned with recognition. This part of the brain called on the part that stores information—the memory. Mary had heard a pencil fall to the floor before, so her memory recognized the sound. Her brain decided to pick the pencil up.

Electrical impulses shot from her brain to the muscles in her eyes. Why? (She needed to move her eyes around to bring the pencil into view.) When Mary's eyes found the pencil, electrical impulses flashed back to her cerebrum again to recognize and identify the pencil. Now the cerebrum sent out hundreds of electrical impulses along nerves to the many muscles that would be needed to help Mary bend over, reach out her arm, close

her fingers around the pencil, and straighten up again. What kind of nerves made this possible? (Motor nerves) If she noticed that the pencil was wet, what kind of nerves would have carried this information to the brain for recognition? (Sensory nerves)

□ ☆

Reflex actions are automatic movements that help protect us. Demonstrate a reflex action by sitting comfortably in a chair with your right leg crossed over the upper part of your left leg. Feel around just below the kneecap of your right leg for a tendon and tap it with the edge of your hand. Ask the students what happened.

□ ☆

Have the students think of a situation in which a reflex action is involved and draw a picture showing the situation. Draw arrows depicting the paths of the messages that are sent along the sensory and motor nerves. (See picture in Atlas for an example.)

Since the nervous system is responsible for the many sensations we have, engage the students in some of the following activities:

○

Sense of Touch

Set up an independent learning center that contains a large envelope holding such objects as a sponge, popcorn, smooth cardboard, and sandpaper, each mounted on pieces of construction paper. Clipped to the outside of the envelope should be the names of the objects' textures, such as rough, bumpy, smooth, and so on. Instruct the student to match the object to its description. (Answers could be written on the back of the construction paper.) This activity encourages awareness of the sense of touch and uses language art skills.

○ □

Blindfold students and let them reach into a box and identify items or describe what they feel like. Items may include silk, SOS pad, sandpaper, cotton, stuffed animal, cooked spaghetti, brush, nut, eraser, leaf, dish, stone, key, and thimble.

□ ☆

Other Activities

Introduce the Braille system. Integrate the sense of touch with other cultures—for example, Indians standing in a freezing river to prove their manhood and courage. In math class use geometric shapes, an abacus, and other objects to enhance learning. Also help the students realize that the touch sensation is not just in the fingertips (tight belt, cold wind against the face, etc.).

○ □

Sense of Smell

Have students identify items by their sense of smell—for example, incense, fruit-scented shampoo, old tennis shoes, perfume, sour milk, vinegar, honey, lemon juice, onions, peppermint, flowers, and mothballs.

○

Let the students use scratch-and-sniff books.

□

Discuss how animals use their sense of smell to find food and for protection. Ask students to write a story about an animal and how its sense of smell aids in its protection.

○ □ ☆

Put various objects to be smelled into baby food jars (or soak a piece of cotton with the odor-producing substance and put it into the jar). Let the students wave the odor toward their noses and try to sort and classify the smells. Make a chart of "smell" words.

After the students have experimented with their sense of smell read "Foods Have Different Odors" (8).

○ □ ☆

Discuss ways our sense of smell makes life more enjoyable.

○ □

Sense of Taste

Let the students blindfold themselves, sample various foods (sugar, bittersweet chocolate, butter, salt, pure lemon juice, lettuce), and try to identify the item or describe it.

○ □ ☆

Try to map the taste areas of the tongue. Dip clean cotton swabs in honey or sugar water, lemon juice, salt water, and cold black coffee, then touch them to various areas of the tongue. Have the students make charts of their results and compare them with charts of other classmates (or with Figure 8B-5).

○ □

Let the students draw their idea of a taste bud holding a corresponding food, giving the taste bud expression and character.

○ □ ☆

Have a tasting party to taste unusual foods or foods from other countries.

○ □

Sense of Hearing

Introduce the sense of hearing with the book *The Listening Walk* by Paul Showers (13). Then take a walk around the neighborhood and see how many differ-

FIGURE 8B-5 Taste areas of the tongue

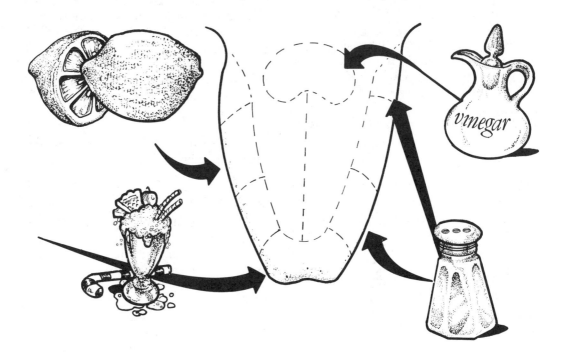

ent sounds you can hear. Make a tape recording of the sounds. Before going on the walk, discuss with the students the sounds they expect to hear. After returning to school, compare what they expected to hear with what was actually heard. (A tape recording of sounds may also be made before class and used instead.)

○

Have the students take turns creating sounds for the class to identify (drop a pencil, crush a peanut shell, crackle some cellophane, shut a door, snap a twig, make an animal sound).

□ ☆

Discuss how life is safer and more pleasant with a good sense of hearing.

□ ☆

Investigate how some insects are able to hear and to make sounds.

○ □ ☆

Sense of Sight

See if the students can answer these questions about someone in their family: What color hair does the person have? Is the hair parted? Which side? What length? What color eyes does the person have? Can you describe the person well enough that an artist could draw her or him?

○ □

Have students work with a partner and decide on a color. Have them write down as many things as they can that are the same color or find as many different

186

things as they can and make a display. They should consider such questions as, How does color make you feel? How does the color taste?

○ □ ☆

Artists often see things differently from other people. Have the students look at pictures of paintings by different artists and ask them, Which artist seems to see things closest to how you see them?

□ ☆

What is an optical illusion? Show the students a book like *The World of M. C. Escher* (9).

○ □

Play a recall game where students view a table of objects for a few minutes and then try to name as many as they can, or blindfold the students and let them explore your desk top. The students can then describe or draw a picture of what they think it looks like.

○

Multisensory Experiences

Have the students collect pictures showing various senses. Write the names of the five senses on the chalkboard, and let the students come up and draw a picture from a sack or box. Have the students explain what sense their picture represents and place the picture on the chalk tray below the appropriate sense.

○ □ ☆

Hide a popcorn popper somewhere in the room and turn it on right before the students come in from recess. How is it discovered? With only a popcorn popper, popcorn, a little bit of oil, salt, and butter, you can involve all five senses. The stu-

dents will hear the corn popping, smell it, see it, feel it, and finally taste it.

After taking a nature walk or during it, have the students record their observations and sensations:

Seeing—an ant carrying a blade of grass
Hearing—a bee buzzing
Feeling—a smooth stone
Smelling—pine needles
Tasting—mint leaves

Evaluation

LIFESTYLE CONTENT

☆

Give each student a copy of Atlas Figure 73, The Brain Maze, and set a time limit for its completion.

□ ☆

Atlas Figure 74, Worksheet: The Nervous System, can be completed as a quiz to determine whether the students have learned the various structures and functions of the nervous system.

○ □ ☆

Have the students list at least ten ways that their senses may contribute to their personal safety (seeing traffic signals, smelling smoke or gas, smelling or tasting spoiled food, seeing and hearing trains or automobiles coming, feeling heat from objects too hot to touch, etc.).

LIFESTYLE VALUE

○ □ ☆

Ask the students to write or tell what they think people would miss if one or more of their senses were not working. Which sense is most important to them?

187

UNIT VII: EYE AND EAR CARE

Americans with defective vision now outnumber those with normal vision, and one out of every ten schoolchildren is handicapped by some hearing impairment.

Contributing to this situation is the fact that millions of people neglect the health of their eyes and ears. They may not know what to do to safeguard their vision and hearing. Even worse, they may know the fundamentals of good eye and ear care but ignore them until it is too late. Unfortunately, many people believe they know the basic facts but actually have certain misconceptions that confuse and sometimes harm them.

For these reasons, we believe that it is necessary to teach not only the fundamentals of vision and hearing, but also how to care for our eyes and ears and detect possible disorders.

OBJECTIVES

1. Given a model or diagram of the eye and ear, the students will be able to name the major parts and

   a. Explain the structures that light rays pass through beginning with the cornea and ending with the brain

   b. Explain the structures that air vibrations pass through beginning with the pinnap (outer ear) and ending with the brain

2. After playing *Bullseye* and *Ear-Opener*, participating in classroom experiments, dissection, and discussion, the students will be able to discuss and demonstrate

   a. The relationship of adequate vision to their appearance, safety, and good grades

   b. Good eye and ear health practices, including professional care, personal care, and protection from possible injury and infection

3. The students will develop greater understanding of people who are blind or deaf by participating in several experiments, inviting a handicapped person to their class, and researching one of the following topics: a local school for the blind or the deaf; lip reading; sign language; total communication (which attempts to combine oralism and sign); braille; talking books; Pilot Dogs, Inc. (625 Town Street, Columbus, Ohio 43215); Eye Dog Foundation (P. O. Box 815, Beaumont, California); or any voluntary agency with relevant information about eyes and blindness or ears and deafness.

4. After completing the activities in this unit the students will know what to expect when they have their eyes or ears examined; they will be able to identify an eye chart, an ophthalmoscope, a machine used for prescribing eyeglasses, an otoscope, a tuning fork, and an audiometer.

MATERIALS

1. Atlas Figures 48 and 49, Otoscope and Audiometer; 51, 52, and 53, Ophthalmoscope, Eye Chart, and Refractor Machine Used for Prescribing Eyeglasses and Examining Eyes; and 57, 58, and 59, Structure of the Human Ear, Function of the Lens and Brain, and Structure of the Eye.

2. Atlas Figures 75 and 76, Sample Cards for Bull's-Eye and Ear-Opener Games.

3. Models of eye and ear if possible; record player and records.*

*See if you can use *The Science of Sound* by Bell Telephone Laboratories, which includes How We Hear, Frequency, Pitch, Intensity, and many examples of sound. You may also want to request the record album *Getting Through*, from Zenith Radio Corporation, 6501 West Grand Ave., Chicago, Ill. 60635, ($1.00).

4. Pictures of children wearing glasses and hearing aids. Pictures that show children seeing and hearing. Scissors, glue, cardboard, construction paper, shoebox, masking tape, stapler.

Methods

Introduction

To help the students understand the importance of good vision and hearing, introduce this lesson with the question, How do we learn? Do not immediately attempt to answer the question, but lead into the following pirate patch activity.

○ □

Pirate Patches

Materials: Scissors, black cloth, elastic banding or string, pencils, and paper.

Help the students construct "Pirate Patches" to cover both of their eyes. After they have made the patches, have them cover their eyes and imagine that they have to work, study, play, and go to school under these conditions. Next, have the students place their palms tightly over their ears so that their hearing is minimal, if present at all. For a third effect, have the students cover both their eyes and ears.

○ □

A Record Without Sound

A version of this same theme is to tell the students that you have a brand new record that you know they will enjoy. When you "play" the record for them, turn the volume down all the way so that nothing can be heard. Then sit back and act as though you can hear it and are enjoying it immensely. Ask the students what they thought of the record. Why didn't they enjoy the record? If you have access to a television, you can turn to an interesting show and let the students view it without sound.

Now if you ask the question, How do we learn? the students will probably respond that much of their learning is achieved through vision and hearing. Indeed, we may receive more than 80 percent of our knowledge through our eyes.

□ ☆

Writing Activity

To follow this activity, ask the students to write short paragraphs entitled "A World Without Eyes" or "A World Without Ears."

Once you have the students interested in learning more about their precious eyes and ears, they may want to know how they are able to see and hear. Depending on the age of your students, several of the following activities may be applicable.

○ □ ☆

Transparency

Have an inflated balloon hidden somewhere in the classroom. Tell the class to shut their eyes. Break the balloon and ask the class what happened and how did they know? Using a transparency of Atlas Figure 57, Structure of the Human Ear, explain that the outer ear (the part that we see) picked up the air vibrations and passed them through the middle and inner ear until they reached the eighth nerve (hearing nerve), which carried them to the brain.

○ □

Tin Can and Balloon Ear Drum

An eardrum can be represented with a tin can and a balloon. Cut both ends of the can out. Stretch the balloon across one end of the can, and fasten it with a rubber band. Put several pieces of dry cereal on the stretched balloon. Hold the tin can (eardrum) up to demonstrate vibrations. Have someone say "boom-boom-boom" underneath it. What happens to the cereal? What do sound vibrations do to the stretched balloon? (Make it move) If we touch the balloon, what do we feel?

Supplementary Information About Sound

Sound is a form of energy that is produced by a vibrating object. Energy is the capacity to do work. *Vibrate* means to go back and forth. The hum given out by a plucked rubber band is due to the back and forth motions of the band.

○ □ ☆

Experiments with a Tuning Fork

1. Strike a tuning fork on the table and hold it to a student's ear. We can *hear* air vibrations.

2. Strike the tuning fork again and gently touch one of the prongs to a student's finger. We can *feel* air vibrations.

3. Strike the tuning fork and lower it into a glass of water. We can *see* the result of air vibrations.

The students may wonder how you can hear the back and forth movements of a vibrating object. Air serves as the go-between to bring the vibrations from the object to your ears. Many other materials will conduct sound as well as or better than air.

○ □ ☆

Sound Conduction Experiments

Place a watch on a bare wooden table and have the students press their ears to the other end of the table. Wood, a solid, will enable them to hear the ticking of the watch.

Sound vibrations usually travel faster in liquids and solids than in air or other gases. If there is no medium to carry the vibrating waves, there is no sound.

Experiments to Determine Sound

What determines sound? Stretch a rubber band until it is taut, then pluck it. Ask the students, What kind of sound did you hear? Does it sound the same as the sound you get from a short rubber band? Length must have something to do with sound.

When we speak our vocal cords vibrate. These cords are controlled by muscles. During speech the cords stretch, and the air from the lungs causes the cords to vibrate. These vibrations produce sound waves in the air that moves outward from the mouth.

□ ☆

Bring Musical Instruments to School

Ask some of your students who play musical instruments to bring their instruments to class. Discuss pitch (a change in vibrations) and how pitch is determined with various instruments.

○ □ ☆

Locate Structures on a Model

We have learned that after sound vibrations in the air reach the outer ear, they pass through a tube about one inch long that is lined with hairs and glands that secrete wax. This is the *auditory canal*. The sound waves are guided to the *eardrum*, which we have illustrated with a sheet of rubber. The eardrum conducts vibrations to three little bones that are the smallest in the whole body. These *hammer, anvil,* and *stirrup* bones conduct vibrations to the inner ear. In the inner ear, the hearing portion is known as the *cochlea*. It looks like a bony snail and is able to "feel" the movements of the sound waves. It analyzes the vibrations and sends the results to the brain through the auditory nerve.

Ask the students:

What happens when we put our fingers over our ears? (There are fewer vibrations so we cannot hear as well.)

If our eardrums are broken, can we still hear? (Yes, but not as well.) Demonstrate by making a hole in the tin can eardrum.

○ □ ☆

Record Sounds

Pass out pencils and paper. Have the class write down all the sounds they can hear in two minutes. What kind of sounds did you hear? (Soft, scratchy, etc.) From what source? (Furnace, bell, etc.)

○ □ ☆

Where Am I?

Blindfold several students one at a time and seat them at the front of the room. In stocking feet, move silently to the left, right, front, behind, and overhead, making noises with a clicker. Have the student try to identify where the sound is coming from. The other students can keep score of correct identifications. Ask the participating student to name the positions that were the easiest to locate. Hardest? Why?

○ □ ☆

Model of Semicircular Canals

Show your class the inner ear and semicircular canals on the model. Explain how we keep our balance. Ask the students, Why do we get dizzy? Does riding in a car or spinning around ever make you sick? Do you feel wrong or funny if you bend down or stand on your head?

Look at Your Face In a Mirror

Let the students look at themselves in mirrors. Ask them, What do you see on your face? (Hair, eyebrows, eyes, eyelashes, nose, etc.) How do you see these things? We need *eyes*, *light* to see by, and a *brain* to interpret what we have seen. Light must strike an object for us to see it. Light rays are reflected from the object to our eyes. Each eye sees a slightly different image, so our brain fuses both images into a single, sharp picture.

□ ☆

Eye Dissection

Dissect the eye from a steer and use a model of the human eye for comparison. (Cattle see in black and white.)

1. Cut around the side of the eye to see the *choroid*, which contains the blood vessels. This will involve cutting the *sclera*, or outside layer of the eye. It is made up of tough white connective tissue.

2. Make an incision through the *cornea*, which is like a clear glass window that protects the inside of the eye but lets light into it. A colorless liquid will spurt out. This is the *aqueous humor*.

3. Remove the *iris*, or colored part of the eye. The black *ciliary muscle* can now be seen on both sides of the iris. It is responsible for controlling the iris, which controls the amount of light entering the eye by controlling the size of the pupil. The *pupil* is simply a hole in the center of the iris. In strong light the pupil becomes smaller, and in dim light it becomes larger.

4. It is now possible to "pop" the crystalline *lens* through the incision. It is like clear hard jelly and will magnify print if you place it on a piece of paper.

5. A little more cutting will expose more liquid; this time it will be black in color. This jellylike mass is called the *vit-*

reous *humor* and fills the cavity between the lens and the retina.

6. Reverse the eyeball and show the students the inner layer of the eye: the *retina*. In the steer it is a beautiful bluish green color. (In people, it is red. The retina contains nerves and blood vessels as well as rods and cones that are sensitive to light.)

7. It will also be possible to see the *optic nerve* and possibly where the *blind spot* is. The optic nerve carries messages from the retina to the brain. The blind spot or optic disc marks the entrance to the optic nerve into the eye. Since there are no rods or cones in this spot, the area is insensitive to light.

Transparencies

You may want to review the structures of the eye with the transparencies made from the following Atlas Figures.

○ □ ☆

Atlas Figure 58, Function of the Lens and Brain

Helps explain how the lens is responsible for turning images upside down on the back of the eye. It also explains that the optic nerve carries messages to the brain. The brain receives the messages and turns them right side up.

□ ☆

Atlas Figure 59, Structure of the Eye

   A. Canal of Schlemm
   B. Cornea
   C. Aqueous humor
   D. Pupil
   E. Iris
   F. Lens
   G. Suspensory ligament
   H. Ciliary muscle
   I. Vitreous humor
   J. Retina
   K. Choroid
   L. Sclera
   M. Fovea (where only cones are found; place of clearest vision)
   N. Optic disc or blind spot (no rods or cones)
   O. Optic nerve

Accommodation

The normal eye is at rest when it is focusing on a distant object. We must make an effort to focus on an object nearby; this is called *accommodation*. The distance to the nearest object that is focused on the retina is called the *near point* of vision and the distance to the point that the eye can see without accommodation is called the *far point*. The far point is infinity, for the normal eye.

Experiment to Locate Near Point

Our near point changes with age. If you were to try the following experiment with an infant, adult, and elderly person, you would see a difference in your results. As age increases, the near point of vision moves further away.

○ □ ☆

Have the students focus one eye on a pin, held upright at arm's length. Then have them gradually bring the pin closer to the eye, continuing to focus on it. Measure the distance to the point where the pin can no longer be seen sharply—the near point.

Visual Acuity Tests

To test distance acuity, a lighted twenty-foot Snellen chart, using *E*'s, pictures, or letters, is recommended. (Available from the Society for the Prevention of Blindness.) Students may also be tested with a near visual acuity card and for color deficiency.

○
Light Reflex

Face a light with your eyes closed. After thirty seconds, shield one eye from the light and open your eyes. Have the students observe the pupillary changes in each eye. What happens to the pupil when you remove the cover?

○ □
Eye Dominance

Have the students choose partners. Play catch, using lightweight balls. Have another person record each time the ball is caught, fumbled, or dropped. After a short amount of time have the students each close one eye and continue to play catch. Compare the record of catches with one eye and two eyes. Why are there seldom one-eyed players in major league baseball?

○ □ ☆
Peripheral Vision

Have the students stand up with their arms straight in front of them. Tell them to start moving their arms to each side while wiggling their fingers. Without turning their heads, and keeping their eyes straight forward, how far back can they move their hands before their hands disappear?

○ □

Look at pictures of various animals. Where are their eyes located in comparison to ours? How far back do you think a camel could see without turning its head?

□ ☆
Transparencies

Show transparencies of Atlas Figures 51, 53, 48, and 49—Ophthalmoscope, Refractor Machine Used for Prescribing Eye-glasses and Examining Eyes, Otoscope, and Audiometer. Explain what each instrument is used for.

□ ☆
Real Instruments

If possible, borrow several of these instruments so the students can see the real thing, or have the school nurse demonstrate how an audiometer or ophthalmoscope works.

Explain how a hearing aid can help some people hear better, just as glasses help some people see better.

○
Eye Chart

A similar demonstration can be done for a lesson on sight. Prepare a blurred reading chart and a clear normal eye chart that can be placed near the appropriate doll models.

○ □
Correcting Amblyopia (Lazy Eye)

Place a patch over one eye of a doll. Explain that sometimes one eye is stronger than the other eye. The weak eye may turn in or out; it may not learn how to look at objects. Treatment may involve patching the better eye so that the weaker eye is forced to work. If treatment is delayed until the child reaches age seven or eight, very little can be done to improve the child's vision.

RESEARCH

□ ☆

Encourage your students to research schools for the blind or deaf; lipreading; sign language; total communication; braille; talking books; guide dogs; and voluntary health organizations concerned with these handicaps.

193

An easy way of teaching the names of eye and ear specialists, as well as good personal eye and ear health practices, is through the use of the Bull's-Eye and Ear-Opener Games. Cards for these games can be found in the Atlas (Figures 75 and 76). Simply make another copy of each page and glue the question sheets to construction paper. Cut the cards out and select those that you feel are the most appropriate.

□ ☆
Games: Bull's-Eye and Ear-Opener

Bull's-Eye and *Ear-Opener* can each be played with two to four players at one time. Deal the whole deck of cards. The object is to make the most pairs. The first player draws a card from the person on his left. If the card matches one of his cards he puts the pair down in front of him and takes another turn.

□ ☆
Review Cards

The game cards can also be used by individual students for review purposes.

□ ☆

Another way the cards can be used is to role play the statement, answer the question, or carry out the request. Students can each draw a card and take turns playing.

Evaluation

LIFESTYLE CONTENT

Duplicate copies of "Hike Through the Eye" (10, p. 32) for your students to read and complete.

Encourage students to write their own "Hike Through the Eye (or Ear)" stories. See the example below:

□ ☆
Hike Through the Ear

Choose your answers from the following possible answers listed below:

Audiologist	Eustachean
Otologist	Tinnitus
Otoscope	Otosclerosis
Auditory canal	Audiometer
Auditory nerve	Wax
Semicircular canals	Bones
Eardrum	Dry
Wet	Cochlea

We will begin our hike through the ear by climbing aboard our microscopic shuttle craft as it awaits us on a protruding flap of the outer ear. This is going to be an extremely hazardous journey, partly because of the many sound vibrations that will be jarring our craft almost constantly. We fasten our seatbelts as our craft silently begins to glide through a long passageway known as the (a) _____. Looking out our window we can see tall stalks of hair and globs of yellow sticky-looking stuff that seem to have trapped particles of dust. We hold our breath, hoping that our small craft will not get stuck. The large accumulations of yellow (b) _____ seem to be responsible for the ringing sound we hear in the ear. Suddenly, our craft comes to an abrupt halt. There is something that looks like a delicate, circular membrane that is blocking our passage to the middle ear. We recognize that this is the (c) _____ and because we are so small we can bore a hole through it without impairing this person's hearing. On the other side of the membrane we take a rest break to study our surroundings. To one side we see three tiny (d) _____. (The hammer, anvil, and

194

stirrup.) We see the hammer picking up vibrations and striking the anvil. The anvil is trying to move the stirrup, but for some reason new bone has started to grow in the middle ear. This condition is known as (e) _____, and is one of the most common causes of middle ear deafness in adults. If this continues, the stirrup will become unable to move at all. The wonderful sounds that this person should be hearing will not be able to get through unless the stirrup is surgically removed and replaced with a stainless steel wire. A few years ago we were in the ear of a soldier who had his eardrum and middle ear destroyed by the concussion from a land mine. A surgeon was able to reconstruct the whole chain of bones plus eardrum (by tympanoplasty) to restore his hearing. It was a wonderful experience to see the dramatic results of modern ear surgery. Well, that's enough daydreaming. At the lower portion of the middle ear we spy the (f) _____ tube, which leads into the throat and connects it with the nose. This tube serves as a channel for equalizing air pressure between the middle ear cavity and the auditory canal. This middle ear is (g) _____, so that means the tube is working normally. Often we will find that the tube has become infected and a highway for germs. When infected adenoids or tonsils, colds, allergies, or sinus infection interfere with the normal opening and closing of this tube, a person's hearing is impaired. It is getting dark as we glide into the fluid of the inner ear. Packed in a tiny space are organs of balance known as the (h) _____ and 20 thousand to 30 thousand hairs connected to nerve fibers. A variety of things can damage these sensitive nerve endings and produce nerve deafness. Next we circle the hearing portion of the inner ear, known as the (i) _____. We think it looks something like a snail. Ahead of us is a long narrow tube branching to connect the two major structures of the inner ear. It is called the (j) _____ and will lead to the brain. We would like to send a message to the brain asking this person to see an (k) _____ (ear physician), so his middle ear trouble can be diagnosed and treated. The doctor would probably use an (l) _____ to light up the ear and an (m) _____to test his hearing, during the examination.

(ANSWERS: (a) *Auditory canal;* (b) *Wax;* (c) *Eardrum;* (d) *Bones;* (e) *Otosclerosis;* (f) *Eustachean;* (g) *Dry;* (h) *Semicircular canals;* (i) *Cochlea;* (j) *Auditory nerve;* (k) *Otologist;* (l) *Otoscope;* (m) *Audiometer*)

○ □

What Is Your "Eye-Q?"

Duplicate enough copies of Atlas Figure 102, *What Is Your Eye-Q?,* for each student in the class. Have them answer the questions, or use it as a transparency for class discussion and review purposes.

LIFESTYLE VALUE

○ □ ☆

Have the students write a story telling about a time when their sight or hearing could have been harmed and what they did or could have done to protect themselves.

○

The Story of Johnny M. Voy

Read *The Story of Johnny M. Voy* to the class and then ask:

Why do you think Johnny got mad and started to cause problems when he liked the teacher and other children at first?

How did Johnny behave that made you think he was hard of hearing?

What made Johnny a happy boy again?

Would you rather play a game that you know you are good at or learn a new game?

How would you feel about having a blind or deaf student as your best friend?

The Story of Johnny M. Voy*

This is the story of Johnny M. Voy
A likeable, natural, ornery boy.

He got himself born the usual way,
And just kept on growing day after
    day.

He did all the things boys do as a rule,
'Til proudly his folks headed John off to
    school.

John liked the teacher and each of the
    kids,
But he didn't quite catch all the things
    that they did.

The teacher would smile and her lips
    would move so,
But whatever she said, little John
    didn't know!

Everyone else knew just what to do!
John's face was red and he felt so blue!

So he'd watch all the kids with a shy
    little look,
To see if they reached for their hats or
    a book.

*By Ruth Withrow Bacon, Former Hearing Consultant of Health, 246 North High, Columbus, Ohio 43215.

This might have gone on for a year and
    an age—
Had Johnny been able to guess the
    right page.

But after some failures, alack and alas!
John found he was grouped with the
    slowest in class.

This business of guessing the right
    thing to do
Made him so mad he was mad through
    and through.

He couldn't make friends with "smart"
    boys and girls
So he tromped a few toes and he
    pulled a few curls!

The teacher was worried about Johnny
    Voy.
"He's gotten to be such a problem boy.
He won't pay attention and leaves me
    no choice.
John only will listen when I raise my
    voice."

"His speech is so loud it comes out as
    a scream,
Whenever he's quiet, he seems lost in a
    dream."

One day when Johnny had been pretty
    bad,
And was perched in the corner,
    unusually sad,
He saw the school nurse come in
    through the door.
He knew it was her by the dress that
    she wore.

John liked her deep voice—
    but her smile was the best,
Say! Maybe she came for
    another eye test.

Johnny liked eye tests 'cause he knew
  what to do—
The nurse thought that HE was a real
  smart boy too.

The nurse and the teacher talked for
  awhile,
Then the nurse looked at Johnny and
  gave him that smile.
—"Another test—but here's a surprise,
This time it's your ears, instead of your
  eyes!"

"Put on these earphones—just like
  pilots do,
And quick as a wink the test will be
  through.
If you listen and listen, girls and boys,
For the tiniest, littlest, beeping noise,
As soon as you hear it put your hands
  up to stay
Until the time the sound goes away."

John waited and watched and soon
  took his place,
Then a real funny look came over his
  face.
The other kids' hands had gone up
  with a bound,
But try as he did, John could not hear a
  sound.

After the test, the nurse smiled her
  smile,
"You can go on out and play for
  awhile."
The nurse told the teacher that she
  thought she would
Visit John's mother as soon as she
  could.

The nurse talked to Mrs. Voy one
  afternoon.
She suggested that John see an ear
  doctor soon.

John saw the doctor each week or two,
And soon he was hearing, and happier,
  too!

After a few months this Johnny Voy
Turned out to be such a different boy.

He was moved from the back of the
  room with the V's,
And put right smack up in front with
  the B's.

Now he liked the kids and he knew all
  their names,
And he had a good time when he
  played all their games.

UNIT VIII: THE GROWTH AND REPRODUCTIVE SYSTEMS

In Chapter 6 we discussed the importance of interpersonal relationships and family life education. We learned that family life education is about love as well as the creation of new life. The purpose of this unit is to explore growth and development.

Students need to accept their bodies and to recognize individual differences in growth and maturation. They need to learn that their endocrine glands secrete hormones that influence their growth and maturity, the replacement of tissues, and the development of sexual characteristics. The human male and female reproductive systems (including menstruation) will be discussed in this chapter.

OBJECTIVES

1. The students will learn about individual differences in growth by making an outline of their body and participating in classroom experiments including mea-

suring and simulating various endocrine glands to paste on the body outline.

2. While viewing a demonstration by the teacher where male and female reproductive systems are simulated using inexpensive materials, the students will participate in class discussion and be ·able to play *Fertilization—A Game of Chance* after the lesson is completed.

3. After completing this lesson, the students will be able to differentiate between the male and female reproductive organs pictured in the Atlas and successfully assemble the puzzle pieces in their proper order.

MATERIALS

1. Atlas Figures 12 through 15 The Endocrine Glands, Male Secondary Sex Characteristics, Female Secondary Sex Characteristics, and Inserting the Tampon.

2. Gameboard and game cards for Fertilization: A Game of Chance, Atlas Figure 77.

3. Roll of brown or white paper, crayons, scissors, construction paper, and glue.

4. Other materials listed with demonstrations.

Methods

○ □

Ask the students to bring in magazine photographs of children, teenagers, and adults. Place these around the room and relate them to growth. You may also want to read some stories from the book *Very Special People* (7).

Explain that our endocrine glands are very important. They secrete chemical substances called *hormones* into our bloodstream. Hormones affect our entire body: they influence growth, the repair and replacement of tissues, the development of sexual characteristics, and the use of sugar, and they can sometimes temporarily provide superstrength.

□ ☆

Transparencies

Using a transparency of Atlas Figure 12, The Endocrine Glands, identify the pineal, pituitary, thyroid, parathyroid, thymus, adrenal, pancreas, ovaries, and testes.

Pituitary

Which gland directs and regulates growth? (Pituitary) Display pictures of a giant and a dwarf. The tallest man on record was Robert Pershing Wadlow, who grew to be 8 feet, 11.1 inches and was still growing when he died at the age of twenty-two. Most cases of giantism are due to a pea-sized gland located at the base of the brain: the pituitary. If it secretes too much of a certain hormone while the person is still a child and the long bones are still growing, then the person will grow to a great height. Sometimes this person can be treated with surgery on the pituitary or irradiation.

If the pituitary does not produce enough growth hormone, the person is likely to be a midget. Charles Sherwood Stratton was better known as Tom Thumb, the most famous midget in history. He grew to a height of three feet four inches and weighed seventy pounds. General Mite, at age fourteen, was only twenty-two inches tall!

As with giantism, there are other causes of dwarfism besides a faulty pituitary gland. Not all dwarfs are perfectly formed either. They may have a normal-sized torso but short arms and legs.

Dwarfs are becoming scarcer as we learn more about the endocrine glands and how to treat such disorders. In fact, there is a prominent clinic for the treatment of dwarfism at Harbor General Hospital, which is operated by the University of California at Los Angeles.

○ □ ☆

Ask the students what they think it would be like to be a giant or midget all of their lives. What kinds of problems would they have?

○ □

Have the students divide into pairs and trace each other's outline on a large sheet of paper. Is everyone the same height? Why not? The children may want to record their measurements—height, weight, length of arm, etc.—on the back of their outline with the date they were taken. At the end of the school year, the children can measure themselves again and see if they have grown.

□

Have the students color the *pituitary* gland in its correct location on their body outlines or cut it out of construction paper and glue it in place.

The pituitary gland also stimulates milk-producing glands, adrenal glands, and sex glands and causes arteries to contract. It is called the *master gland*, because it directs the work of all other endocrine glands.

Thyroid

The *thyroid* is our energy gland. It is a small, butterfly-shaped gland in the neck that produces a hormone that sets the energy level for the body. Have the students color the thyroid gland on their outlines. The thyroid also influences our growth as well as our metabolism. If the thyroid is overactive the heart beats faster, and we are likely to be irritable and underweight. This can be treated with medicines or surgery.

If the thyroid does not produce enough of a certain hormone, our body uses food more slowly, and we gain weight. The heart beats slower and the mind may become dull. Prescribed doses of pure Thyroxin may be given as treatment.

A lack of iodine in our diet may cause a goiter, or swelling, in the neck. This is because our thyroid has become enlarged. By using iodized salt we can prevent a goiter from occurring.

Adrenal Glands

How can some people lift extremely heavy objects when they are very excited? You may think of your *adrenal* glands as "Superman" glands. The adrenal glands are like little caps on the top of each of our kidneys. (Have the students color the adrenal glands on their outlines.) The outer portion produces hormones, including cortisone, that we need to live. The cortisone reduces swelling in the skin and joints and regulates salt and water balance. The inner portions of our adrenal glands produce adrenin (often called adrenaline), one of the quickest acting and most powerful of the hormones. Adrenal glands respond to feelings of fear and bring about body changes that make it possible for us to react quickly, including the release of more sugar into the blood for energy, enlargement of arteries to the big muscles, increased beating of the heart, and contraction of arteries to digestive organs.

Pancreas

What is a gland within a gland that makes insulin? (Islets of Langerhans).

The *pancreas* is called the *sweetbread* in animals. When we were studying the digestive system we learned that the pancreas lies below the stomach. (Have the students color the pancreas on their outlines.) The pancreas is a gland that contains islets of Langerhans—small clusters of endocrine gland cells that are responsible for the metabolism of sugar. They secrete the hormone insulin, which regulates the body's use of sugar. Insulin enables the body to use sugar and starch and directs the liver to store sugar. If a person does not produce enough insulin what condition does he have? (Diabetes—see Chapter 14B for more information.)

Thymus

You have a mysterious organ located behind the breastbone. It produces certain types of white blood cells and may be involved with antibody formation. It grows during childhood and shrivels as you grow older; it may even disappear. This gland is called the *thymus*. Have the students draw and color this gland on their outlines. You may also want to have them color four *parathyroids* or small glands inside the thyroid. They enable the body to use calcium.

Reproductive Glands

The only glands that are different in men and women are the reproductive glands. The hormones secreted by *ovaries* in women and *testes* in men produce our physical sexual characteristics. Testes manufacture testosterone in a boy and cause his voice to deepen, his muscles to grow rapidly and strengthen, and his beard to grow. (Have the boys draw two testes on their outlines.)

The ovaries produce estrogen and progesterone in girls. They cause the breasts to mature, the hips to broaden, and menstruation to begin. (Have the girls draw two ovaries on their outlines.)

REPRODUCTIVE INFORMATION

○ ☐

There are many ways to present additional information regarding reproduction to students. Many teachers incubate fertilized chicken eggs in a corner of their classroom. Detailed instructions for this activity may be found in Burt and Meeks, *Education for Sexuality* (4, chap. 15).

○ ☐

You may want to show one or two films such as "Human and Animal Beginnings" (Henk Newenhouse Inc., 13 min. color); "Fertilization and Birth" (Henk Newenhouse Inc., 10 min. color); "Kittens: Birth and Growth" (Bailey Films, black-and-white and color, 11 min.); "The Story of Birth" (Bailey Films, filmstrip and record).

If possible, take slides from the Book *A Child Is Born* (15) and develop a slide show for the class.

Burt and Meeks suggest the following lesson in their textbook *Education for Sexuality* (4) when you wish to discuss the male and female reproductive systems in greater detail.

☐ ☆

Male Reproductive System

Assemble the following materials:

1. One small cellophane lunch bag for the scrotum.

2. Two Ping-Pong balls for the testes.

3. Red coil of yarn on top of the testes represents the epididymis.

4. Yellow yarn leading up into the body is the vas deferens.

5. Two small uninflated balloons for the seminal vesicles.

6. Green yarn leading through a paper cup for ejaculatory duct.

7. Small paper cup for the prostate gland.

8. Blue yarn leading out of paper cup for the urethra.

9. Two small balls of clay attached to the blue yarn for the Cowper's glands (or round buttons with a hole in them sewn to the yarn).

10. Cardboard on which to draw an outline of a man and attach the reproductive organs.

11. A marble attached to the cardboard outline to show the location of the pituitary gland.

Review where the male and female reproductive cells are made and the changes that occur in the body during puberty. (Use transparencies of Atlas Figures 13 and 14, Male and Female Secondary Sex Characteristics.) These changes are necessary before a boy can produce sperm and before immature eggs in the girl's body begin to mature.

A sperm must fertilize an egg for new life to begin. When a boy is about eleven or twelve years old, the pituitary gland in his brain sends a hormone (FSH) to the *testes*. The hormone tells the testes to begin working to make many sperms. These sperms must be made at the right temperature, so boys have a little sac between the legs called the *scrotum*. The scrotum helps the testes to make sperms by keeping the testes at just the right temperature.

After the sperms are made, they travel to the *epididymis*, where they rest and grow. A sperm has a head and a tail just like a tadpole. It swims, too.

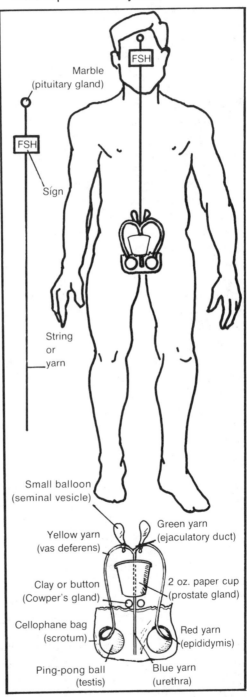

FIGURE 8B-6 Demonstration guidelines —male reproductive system

FSH

Marble
(pituitary gland)

FSH

Sign

String
or
yarn

Small balloon
(seminal vesicle)

Green yarn
(ejaculatory duct)

Yellow yarn
(vas deferens)

Clay or button
(Cowper's gland)

2 oz. paper cup
(prostate gland)

Cellophane bag
(scrotum)

Red yarn
(epididymis)

Ping-pong ball
(testis)

Blue yarn
(urethra)

The sperm wait in a long tube that winds its way up into the body. This tube is called the *vas deferens*. When it is time for the sperm to be used, they travel through the vas deferens and receive sugar (for energy) from the *seminal vesicle*. Then they travel over a very short path called the *ejaculatory duct*, which is right in the middle of a milk and water storage tank. This tank is called the *prostate gland*, and it empties some milky-sugary liquid called *semen* into the ejaculatory duct.

The final stage of the trip is through the penis in a tube called the *urethra*. Urine also leaves the body through this tube, but they never travel together.

The semen with sperm in it makes sure that there is no urine in the tube. Beside the urethra are two cleaning stations called the *Cowper's glands* that squirt fluid on the urethra to clean the road for the semen. The tube is now clear for the semen.

Remember that we said the urethra is a long tube inside the penis. The father can use his penis to place the semen inside the mother. The penis is usually very soft and hangs down between the father's legs, but when semen is going to come out of it the penis becomes very hard. This makes it easier for the father to put his penis into the mother's vagina. When the penis is inside the vagina the semen comes out and the sperms begin to swim about looking for an egg.

Boys may notice an occasional discharge of clear, sticky fluid from the penis. This is semen that is beginning to form and often overflows at night. Sometimes this overflowing of semen is accompanied by a dream about girls or about growing up. Some people call this a *wet dream*. Scientists call it a *nocturnal emission*. It is a normal part of growing up and nothing to be afraid of.

Review the male reproductive system thoroughly before beginning the female reproductive system. You may wish to make individual copies of Atlas Figure 77, Fertilization: A Game of Chance, so that each student can better visualize the reproductive systems.

☐ ☆

Female Reproductive System

Assemble the following materials:

1. Cardboard with an outline of a woman.
2. A marble to represent the pituitary gland.
3. FSH sign with string attached (leading from pituitary to ovary and representing the hormone signal for growth).
4. Two Ping-Pong balls for ovaries.
5. Two four-inch straws to represent fallopian tubes.
6. One three-inch straw to represent the vagina.
7. A paper cup for the uterus.
8. Aluminum foil shaped to line the paper cup and represent the inner lining (endometrium) of the uterus.
9. Pieces of clear plastic stapled together with an opening left at the bottom to place a small rubber doll in to show pregnancy.
10. Yarn attached at one end to the navel of the doll (by attaching it to a rubber band at the doll's waist) and at the other end to the uterus to represent the umbilical cord.

An egg must be fertilized for new life to begin. The egg cells are made in the *ovaries*. Girls have thousands of egg cells in each ovary waiting for the pituitary gland to send out its FSH signal. (You may want to use a transparency of Atlas Figure 14, Female Secondary Sex Characteristics, at this point.) This may happen as early as nine or ten, and when the sig-

FIGURE 8B-7 Demonstration guidelines—female reproductive system

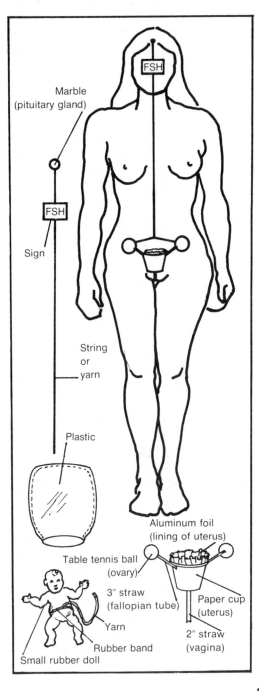

Marble (pituitary gland)

FSH

Sign

String or yarn

Plastic

Aluminum foil (lining of uterus)

Table tennis ball (ovary)

3" straw (fallopian tube)

Paper cup (uterus)

Yarn

2" straw (vagina)

Rubber band

Small rubber doll

nal comes a girl begins having a *menstrual cycle.*

After the FSH signals the eggs in the ovary, some of the eggs begin to grow. Only one of these eggs matures completely and is ready for fertilization. The mature egg leaves the ovary and travels through a long passageway called the *fallopian tube.*

If any sperms are in the fallopian tube, they begin to swim toward the egg. When a sperm enters the egg this is called *fertilization.* Fertilization is a partnership where each partner gives part of what it knows to form a new baby. The sperm cell and the egg cell join to form one cell. From this one cell a new baby will grow.

Since the cell needs a comfortable place in which to grow, it journeys through the rest of the fallopian tube until it reaches the uterus. The uterus has a soft lining of blood and food, and the cell attaches itself to that lining. The cell is smaller than the tiniest grain of sand and has a lot of growing to do!

The uterus keeps getting bigger as the cell grows into a baby. A baby never grows in a mother's stomach, only in her uterus.

The *umbilical cord* is a special cord that connects the baby to the mother and supplies the baby with food. After the baby has grown for about nine months, it is old enough to be born. It usually comes head first down through the tunnel between the mother's legs. We call this tunnel the *vagina.* After a baby is born it no longer needs to be connected to its mother, so the doctor ties the cord and cuts it. The mark that is left on the baby from this cord is called the *belly button* or *navel.*

Menstrual Cycle

The menstrual cycle is another way of saying that a girl's body is preparing each month to have a baby. If no sperm meets the egg in the fallopian tube, the egg and the blood lining of the uterus are not needed, and they leave the uterus and come down the vaginal tunnel out of the body. This is called *menstrual flow* or *menstruation*, and it happens about every twenty-eight days and lasts about three to five days. During the menstrual flow, a girl has to wear something to collect and absorb the blood.

☐

Fifth-grade boys and girls should be familiar at this age with menstrual hygiene products. Show the class a sanitary napkin and belt, and a tampon. Give a simple and factual explanation:

A sanitary napkin is a soft disposable pad used to absorb the menstrual flow. It is held in place with a narrow elastic sanitary belt.

The tampon is another easy way of absorbing the menstrual flow. It is worn inside the vagina and inserted through the same opening by which the menstrual fluid leaves the body. A tampon works something like a blotter. It absorbs the blood as it flows from the uterus into the vagina.

A girl will only need to wear some type of sanitary protection for the three to five days of her menstrual cycle each month when unneeded blood flows out. After the menstrual flow is over, her body begins to prepare her uterus again. This preparation occurs over and over again, every month for years and years.

These changes begin to happen in our bodies long before we are ready to marry and have children, because it takes many years to adjust to these changes and many years to learn about ourselves and others. These years of learning and growing are important in having a good marriage and in becoming good parents in the future.

You may want to present another lesson about menstrual hygiene to just the girls. Excellent pamphlets that may be distributed to the girls for reading and discussion with their mothers include:

Growing Up and Liking It and *Strictly Feminine* (Director of Education, Personal Products Company, Box SS-6, Milltown, N.J. 08850).

It's Time You Knew (Educational Director, Tampax Incorporated, 161 East 42nd Street, New York, N.Y. 10017).

World of a Girl (Scott Paper Company, International Airport, Philadelphia, Pa. 19113).

Your Years of Self Discovery (The Life Cycle Center, Kimberly Clark Corporation, Box 551, Neenah, Wis. 54956).

This lesson may include information about personal hygiene, amount of menstrual flow, or mistaken ideas. You may want to use a transparency of Atlas Figure 15, Inserting the Tampon.

Evaluation

LIFESTYLE CONTENT

Game: Pin the Gland on the Body

Let each student draw an endocrine gland or label from a paper bag and pin or tape it to a paper cutout body. (You may repeat this game so everyone in the class has a chance to participate.)

Fertilization: A Game of Chance

Make a large drawing of Fertilization: A Game of Chance, using an opaque projector and poster board, or use the drawing in the Atlas and make individual copies for the students to use in pairs.

Markers may be made of construction paper cut to look like sperm.

Up to four players may play Fertilization using a large board. Players begin at the starred (*) spaces in the seminiferous tubules and flip a die to see who goes first (largest number). If identical numbers come up, they should flip again.

Players take turns moving the number of squares shown as they flip one die. If a player lands on a ⬤ space, the player draws a Sperm Card and hands it to the next player to read. If the player does not answer the question correctly, the player's next turn is forfeited.

If a player lands on "Risk Card," the player draws a Risk Card and follows its directions. If a player lands on "you must take path to the left," the player must continue to the left ovary and then retrace some of the journey to the other fallopian tube where an egg is waiting to be fertilized.

If a player overshoots the fertilization space by one, two, or three spaces, the player is still in the game and may backtrack to try to land on the correct space. However, if the next toss turns up a number that will send the player past the ovary, that player is out of the game.

Sample Sperm Cards and Risk Cards can be found in the Atlas (Atlas Figure 77). Simply glue them to construction paper and cut out or make up a set of your own cards.

□ ☆

Duplicate enough copies of the male and female reproductive systems pattern in the Atlas (Atlas Figures 78 and 79) for every student in your class, or glue the original pattern to posterboard for extra strength, cut out pieces, and use as a puzzle for optional use in a learning center environment.

LIFESTYLE VALUE

□ ☆

After the students have studied all their body systems, ask them to complete a handout of Atlas Figure 80, Worksheet: This Is Me! Encourage the students to think about their answers and be specific. For example, older students may complete the sentence, "I like using my EYES to _____" with *read adventure books* or *view sunsets*, rather than simply writing *see.*

This handout should be used for discussion rather than graded. It will, however, give you a good idea of what your students know, and how they feel about health.

UNIT IX: GOOD GROOMING

Consistent and proper grooming is a must for a healthy lifestyle. If students are encouraged to care for their personal appearance and health, it will nurture a desire to care for their immediate surroundings, and in a wider application, their environment. If students do not care about themselves and the way they look and feel, how can they possibly care for their environment?

It is well known that habits are difficult to break. This is true of good habits as well as bad. The following activities were developed to help students acquire good grooming habits. Once instilled, these grooming habits become second nature rather than boring, often frustrating routine.

OBJECTIVES

1. After the Grooming Rally, students will be able to discuss the importance of: diet, sleep, exercise, bathing, washing the face, hairstyle, shampoo, brushing the hair, deodorant, cologne, fresh breath, brushing the teeth, foot powder, clipping toenails, clean socks, fashions, manners.

2. Students will use the Grooming Grand Prix Checklist to evaluate their grooming habits for one day.

3. Through television drama, students will be able to explain the importance of one item found in the Body Tune-up Box.

4. During the game "I'm Going on a Trip," students will name at least five good grooming items.

5. Students will place themselves on a personal grooming continuum to indicate their behavior and habits in four situations.

MATERIALS

1. Booklet, "Avon's Grooming Rally" from Avon.

2. A very large duplicate of Atlas Figure 81, Grooming Rally gameboard illustrated in the Atlas.

3. Model car to use with Grooming Rally game.

4. Several flags made of construction paper or cloth.

5. Copies of Grooming Grand Prix Checklist, Atlas Figure 82.

6. Large decorated Body Tune-up Box and Atlas Figure 83, Worksheet: Body Tune-up.

7. Toothbrush, toothpaste, dental floss, bar of soap, washcloth, shampoo, brush, comb, fingernail file, toenail clippers, Kleenex, Q-tips, deodorant, toilet paper.

8. Large cardboard box for a "TV" and aluminum foil antenna.

Methods

○ □ ☆

Grooming Rally Bulletin Board and Lecture*

The following information on grooming is presented in the form of an analogy to a Grand Prix or car rally. To present the material, redraw the racetrack illustration in the Atlas on a large sheet of poster board. Place a model car at the starting line on the board. Have a flag for each aspect of grooming (see illustration).

As you discuss each grooming tip, wave a flag giving the model car the go-ahead to move one space on the board. When you have completed the grooming tips, the car will be at the finish line. The analogy: The human body should be a winning car with all the finishing touches for success.

YOUR GROOMING RALLY

A Grand Prix is a championship race of Formula I cars. The term is used loosely to describe any big race. For people entering their first race, it may have all the excitement of a Grand Prix.

Whatever the category, one of the big questions is, What makes a winning car? Some say engine design; others say brakes, body material, rear-end design, or visual sportiness. Actually, a winning car cannot be judged by what it is; it can only be judged by what it does. And what every winner must do—whether in a rally or a Grand Prix—is perform well on the road.

The same rules apply when looking at

*This method of presenting grooming is adapted from the booklet "Avon's Grooming Rally," which was written for teens. The authors have adapted the material for elementary level and have designed the Grooming Rally Game in cooperation with Avon, Nine West Fifty-Seventh Street, New York, N.Y. 10019. Avon is an excellent resource for educational materials on grooming.

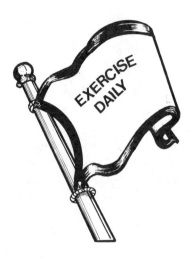

the human body as a winning car—one that is designed to carry us successfully through life.

Keeping Your Engine In Tune

When handling a car, the engine must be kept in tune at all times. The same is true of your personal engine, your body. To keep it in tune, you must make sure it has a proper diet, adequate sleep, and reasonable exercise.

Diet: The Fuel Nourishing meals should include foods from each of the four basic groups daily: milk and milk products, breads and cereals, fruits and vegetables, meats and fish.

Sleep: The Pit Stop A simple measure of the amount of rest or sleep you require is the Night's Rest test. If, after a night's sleep, you feel refreshed and ready for another day of equal activity, the previous day's activities were not excessive. But, if after a good night's sleep, you are not fully refreshed, your activities have been too strenuous, and you should scale them down.

Sleep is essential to provide rest for a number of bodily functions. But more important, while the body's engines are

not being used to perform and work, they repair. Skin cells, for example, which must be produced continually, divide more rapidly by night than by day.

Exercise: The Staging Exercise results in a body with an engine that is in fine running order. It can start and stop regardless of extra strain.

Concours D'Elegance

The Concours D'Elegance is a test in which cars are judged on maintenance, cleanliness, and taste. The winner is the one whose owners have taken just a little more time to make an appearance that shows a little "extra."

Bathe Daily Sure, you take a bath every day, and you probably are clean. But what about those grimy nails and problem skin? Just a little extra body buff can help. (Demonstrate how to cut fingernails and toenails.)

License Plates: Wash Your Face Your face is your license plate. It is one of a kind and identifies only *you*. So, added care here is a must. You should wash your face at least twice a day—always after gym class or exercise. Using a good skin soap, work up a lather and massage the face with your fingertips to free dirt particles and aid circulation. Rinse well!

Headlights: Clean Hair Headlight hairlights get a great deal of attention these days. Hairstyles for boys and girls are lots of fun. However, rule number one is: keep your hair clean. Hair should be washed at least twice a week. If you exercise strenuously or if you have oily hair, you may need to wash your hair more often.

No matter what shampoo you use, use your fingertips to rub and scrub your scalp briskly. Rinse well and lather a second time. Rinsing is important. Shampoo that stays in your hair will make it dull.

Brush your hair daily to remove surface dirt. This brushing will also improve circulation and help your hair shine.

Safeguards: Deodorant—Cologne Safeguards serve a double purpose. They eliminate bodily odors and make us more agreeable to others. Safeguards include deodorants, antiperspirants, toothpaste, mouthwash, and colognes.

Grillwork: Brush Your Teeth If you take care of your teeth, you will have a brighter, healthier smile. You have learned the importance of daily care at home and of visiting the dentist at least twice a year. Keep up this practice so your teeth will last a lifetime.

Tires: Foot Powder, Clip Toenails, Clean Socks A little attention to your hard-working feet will improve your footwork. For itchy, flaky, or calloused feet, use a smoothing cream. A spray can help feet that smell. Powder will help keep the feet dry.

Nail clipping is important in proper foot care. You should clip your nails straight across in order to help prevent ingrown toenails. Clean socks daily and properly fitted shoes are a must for total foot comfort.

The Flag Station (Signals to Sensible Styles)

In racing, many things can happen. A flag station is on the roadway in a place where the flagman can see the whole road. The flagman uses different colored flags to signal the drivers. For instance, a green flag means to go ahead. A white flag means that there is an emergency car on the path. A yellow flag means danger, be ready to stop.

Someone may be waving a flag at you—a fad flag, telling you what to wear. When it comes to choosing clothing, be your own flagman. No style is best for everyone.

Rules of the Road (Etiquette—The Finishing Line)

In a race, how well you compete within the rules determines the extent of respect you receive from your fellow drivers. This mutual courtesy eliminates unnecessary hazards, adds to the excitement of competition, gives meaning to victory, and even contributes dignity and style to losing!

Off the track, in everyday life, courtesy makes everyone a winner. Courtesy is contagious. What you give is generally what you get.

And You?

The human body should be a winning car, with all the finishing touches for success. How do you rate? Where do you finish in the Grooming Grand Prix?

○ □

The follow-up lesson on the Grooming Grand Prix uses the Grooming Grand Prix checksheet found in the Atlas. Instruct students to place a check next to the grooming habits they have taken care of that day.

□ ☆

Decorate a large box with pictures of health products. Place the following items in the box: toothbrush, toothpaste, dental floss, bar of soap, washcloth, shampoo, brush, comb, fingernail file, toenail clippers, Kleenex, Q-tips, deodorant, toilet paper, etc. Explain that there are many things in the Body Tune-up Box that help keep the body in good running order. Ask each student to select one object that he or she feels is important for a good body tune-up and complete the worksheet on Body Tune-up found in the Atlas. Allow time for class discussion.

○ □

Grooming Game

What things are really important to have in the Body Tune-up Box? The students can play "I'm going on a trip and I'm going to take _____ ." The first student says, "I'm going on a trip and I'm going to take (a toothbrush to brush my teeth)." The next student completes the same sentence and adds a grooming item that he or she will take. Each student must be able to name all the preceding grooming items in order. Any student who misses is out of the game. The last student remaining in the game is the winner.

Evaluation

LIFESTYLE CONTENT

○

Give each student a small piece of heavy paper with a picture on it. This picture should represent a basic hygiene activity, such as washing the face, brushing hair, cleaning fingernails. The activities may be represented by a symbol as simple as a picture of a brush and comb, a bar of soap, or a toothbrush.

To represent a television set, cut a large, rounded-off square out of one side of a large cardboard box, and glue buttons or old knobs across the lower edge of the "screen." The students will each have a turn inside the "TV set" to act out the health practice they were given. The teacher may evaluate the student doing the demonstration in the television. Does

he or she explain the health practice correctly? The teacher may evaluate the students watching the TV show by using values voting, i.e., by asking, Do you want to practice this health habit every day?

LIFESTYLE VALUE

○ □

The students can place themselves on the personal appearance continuum below.

REFERENCES

1. *Breathing ... What You Need to Know* (New York: American Lung Association, 1968).

2. *The Wonderful Human Machine* (Chicago, Il: American Medical Association, 1971).

3. Donald Brown, *Heart Project, Levels A, B, C* (American Heart Association, Central Ohio Chapter, 200 East Rich Street, Columbus, Ohio 43215).

4. John J. Burt, and Linda Brower Meeks, *Education for Sexuality* (Philadelphia, Pa.: Saunders, 1975).

5. Robert Campbell, "The Life-Giving Balancing Act," *Life*, 8 November 1963.

6. Dairy Council of California, "Nutrients from Food" (1970).

7. Frederic Drimmer, *Very Special People* (New York: Amjon, 1973).

8. Gustav Eckstein, *The Body Has a Head* (New York: Harper & Row, 1969).

9. M. C. Escher and J. L. Locher, *The World of M. C. Escher* (New York: Abrams, 1971).

10. "Hike Through the Eye," *Current Health* (November 1975), p. 32.

11. Thomas L. Petty, "Test Your Lung Power," *Family Health* (December 1975).

12. Illa Podendorf, "Foods Have Different Odors," *Food Is for Eating* (Chicago: Children's Press, 1970).

13. Paul Showers, *The Listening Walk* (New York: Crowell, 1961).

14. *Teachers' Resource Guide for "Breathing . . . What You Need to Know"* (Ad Hoc Committee on Courses of Study in Respiratory Health, National Tuberculosis and Respiratory Diseases Association, 1968).

15. C. Wirsen, and Lennart Nilsson, *A Child Is Born* (New York: Delacorte, 1965).

FIGURE 8B-8 Personal appearance continuum

CHAPTER 9

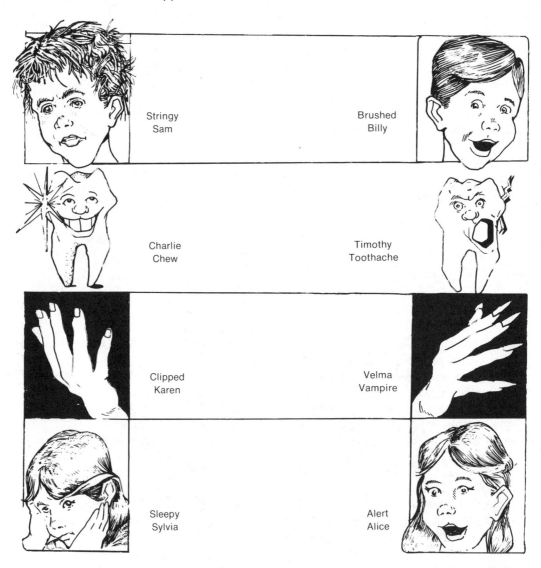

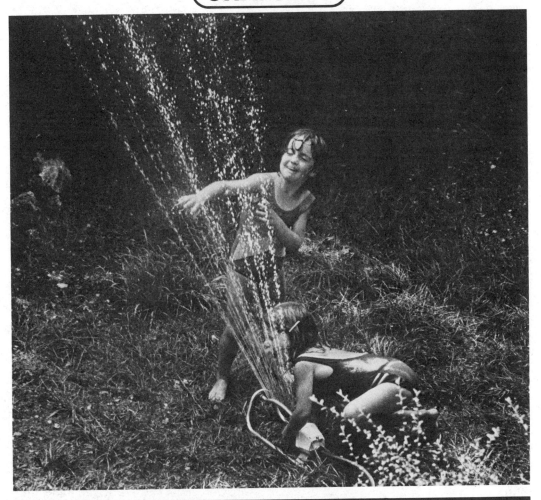

PART A: EXERCISE, REST, AND RELAXATION

The long journey of the human race up and out of the caves and jungles into a modern push-button society is a tribute to the magnificent advances in science and technology. Yet these advances are responsible for a decrease in physical fitness in an ever increasing portion of the American population. In turn, this country's sedentary way of life has had detrimental effects on the health of the nation. Medical science warns that people who do not exercise are more likely to suffer from coronary heart disease, diabetes, duodenal ulcer, and low back pain. The American Medical Association has published this statement in its journal:

The successful use of physical activity in the medical management of patients indicates the beneficial effects of exercise in preventing or delaying organic disease and degeneration—obesity, muscle atrophy, cardiovascular inefficiency, joint stiffness, and impairment of various metabolic functions are possible effects of prolonged inactivity.

In view of the health consequences of a sedentary lifestyle, it is important that elementary school students become acquainted with the values of exercise and establish early patterns of regular exercise. In addition to activity, students should also learn the values of inactivity and rest. The present chapter discusses both ends of an important continuum—exercise and rest.

EXERCISE AND THE HEALTH OF THE CARDIOVASCULAR SYSTEM

While the rest of the body sleeps each night, the heart accomplishes a work load roughly equivalent to carrying a 30-pound pack to the top of the 102-story Empire State Building. However, when a person neglects his or her physical fitness, this highly efficient pump loses some of its efficiency.

People who undergo three weeks of bed rest experience an acceleration in resting heart rate; that is, their hearts must work harder to pump the same amount of blood. Conversely, it has been amply demonstrated that the resting heart rate can be lowered with training. Distance runners have been found to have

heart rates 50 percent slower than the average person.

It is also established that wild animals have a far lower heart rate than domestic animals. The tame rabbit, for example, has a heart rate of approximately 200 beats per minute, whereas the wild rabbit has a rate close to 64 beats per minute. It therefore appears to be generally established that physical exercise increases the efficiency of the heart.

Coronary Artery Disease

Many scientists now think that exercise may reduce the tendency to develop arteriosclerosis, or hardening of the arteries, a process that may even start in childhood. One theory offered to explain arteriosclerosis suggests that lipids (fatty materials) are deposited in the arterial wall. It has been observed that persons suffering from coronary artery disease take longer to clear lipid materials from their circulating blood than do healthy people. The belief that exercise is beneficial stems from the fact that several studies indicate exercise following a meal will reduce the level of fats in the blood. A second theory suggests that arteriosclerosis is caused by the deposition of fibrin (formed by the coagulation of blood) on the arterial wall. Since it has been observed that exercise greatly activates the destruction of circulating fibrin, it would appear that exercise might play a significant role in the prevention of arteriosclerosis.

EXERCISE AND WEIGHT CONTROL

The American Medical Association states, "There is no longer any doubt but that the level of physical activity does play a major role in weight control."

To be sure, the importance of exercise as a factor in weight control has been recognized since antiquity. The practice of penning livestock to fatten them has been employed for many years, and the lean hunter or soldier has always been contrasted with the fat merchant. Additional studies of children have revealed a direct relationship between obesity and inactivity.

According to research by Dr. Jean Mayer of Harvard University, a physically active animal or person automatically adjusts food intake to the level of energy requirements. Consequently, the weight remains constant unless the activity is extremely prolonged or intense, in which case he or she may lose weight. Dr. Mayer found, however, that in habitual inactivity this relationship between food intake and energy requirements no longer holds true. Hence, inactive people are likely to eat more than they need and put on extra pounds.

If one remains active, it is relatively easy to maintain a constant weight; once overweight, it is difficult to get rid of extra pounds. It is therefore advisable to follow a program of active exercise that will help maintain proper weight throughout one's life.

There are several reasons why exercise is in some respects a more desirable method of losing weight than dieting (although a combination of dieting and exercise usually is the most successful approach). First, participation in sports is enjoyable for most people; dieting is not. Second, moderate exercise actually may reduce one's appetite and thus produce the two-way benefit of increased caloric expenditure and decreased caloric intake. Finally, weight reduction through exercise tends to cause the loss of more fat and less protein than an equivalent weight reduction by diet. For example, in animal studies leading to a 21 percent weight loss, it has been reported that when exercise was the method for weight reduction, 78 percent of the weight loss was fat and only 5 percent was protein. When a diet was used, 62 percent of the weight loss was fat and 11 percent was protein.

In addition, weight reduction by diet was accompanied by a loss in heart weight (and, presumably, a loss in functional capacity); whereas heart weights of the exercised animals, who lost the same amount of body weight, did not change. If one must choose between exercise and dieting for weight control, exercise seems to be the best method from a physiological point of view.

EXERCISE AND THE RELIEF OF NERVOUS TENSION

Living a sane life in a complex environment requires a keen insight into the problem of handling anxieties. In this connection, a joint statement by the American Medical Association and the American Association for Health, Physical Education, and Recreation states:

The relationship of physical activity to mental health should not be overlooked; from this standpoint, the ability to be engrossed in play is basic. Pleasurable exercise relieves tension and encourages habits of continued activity. In fact, muscular effort is probably one of the best antidotes for emotional stress. Fortunately, such a variety of activities is available that everyone should be able to find some from which he gains pleasure as well as exercise.

To fully appreciate the tranquilizing effect of exercise, it is necessary to understand some of the physiology of stress. When a person becomes angry, the autonomic nervous system is strongly stimulated. As a result, the heart beats faster, respiration increases, the blood sugar level increases, and blood clots faster. These are but a few of the physiological changes intended to prepare the body for "fight and flight." At one time in the evolutionary development, such responses were essential to the preservation of life. However, fight and flight are no longer acceptable responses to the stresses of modern life. Unfortunately, the human body has not fully adapted to this change in lifestyle and hence continues to respond in the classic way. Meanwhile, "civilized" people attempt to compensate with millions of dollars worth of tranquilizers each year.

A more effective way to handle stress is to engage in regular exercise. The additive effects of one full day of stressful situations may be dissipated by an hour of physical activity at the end of the day. Another effect of exercise on the nervous system is that a certain amount of exercise seems to be required for deep, restful sleep. Studies on cats show that either too little or too much exercise results in wakefulness.

To maintain healthy muscle tone, one must engage in some kind of regular exercise. Digestive processes also are aided by exercise. Frequently, vigorous sports and other exercise eliminate constipation by increasing the tone and strength of the abdominal muscles and enhancing completely normal movement of the digestive organs.

Good muscle tone is also helpful in promoting good circulation of the blood. Strong abdominal muscles aid the diaphragm in pumping blood to the heart. In the legs, well-toned muscles press the blood through the veins, preventing stasis and clotting.

As a rule, a healthy person with good muscle tone automatically assumes a comfortable, attractive posture. Pride and poise are reflective of good postural training, but they are difficult to maintain if physical conditioning is neglected.

Regular activity has a beneficial effect on the bones. This probably can best be understood by witnessing the decrease in bone density that occurs in bedridden patients or in people who have limbs immobilized in casts. When a minimal amount of exercise is not performed, calcium leaves its storage sites in the bones and is excreted in the urine. The mechanism by which exercise stimulates bone growth remains uncertain but may involve compression forces achieved by standing, walking, or running; twisting forces at the bone surfaces (caused by muscles pulling on the bones); or increased blood flow to bone cells as a result of a massaging action of muscles.

Scientists have also demonstrated in laboratory animals that physical training improves the strength of ligaments around joints. Such training becomes especially important in weight-bearing sports activities, such as skiing, in which tremendous twisting forces can be developed in knees and ankles. It is also important in the rehabilitation of injured joints, in which case it may be wise either to avoid putting casts on damaged joints altogether or at least to remove casts as soon as possible to prevent loss of ligamentous strength through lack of exercise.

Chronic Fatigue

One of the most common complaints among modern men and women is chronic fatigue. Too many people come to the end of the workday completely exhausted, even when they have performed very little physical work. They are tense and irritable, unable to enjoy the fruits of their work, and frequently unable to sleep.

Many cures have been proposed for this rundown feeling, especially through television commercials. Unfortunately, most are of no value; in fact, doctors frequently are unable to find any physical cause of chronic fatigue. Recently, emphasis has been placed on prevention. It has been proven that fatigue can be prevented simply by exercising more on stressful days, and tests in research laboratories confirm that exercise reduces tension.

EXERCISE AND SCHOLASTIC ACHIEVEMENT

The results of good physical fitness show up in a variety of areas, some of them unexpected. For example, there appears to be a definite relationship between physical fitness and academic achievement, according to a study conducted on first-year males at the State University of Iowa. This study showed that, in general, good grades accompanied good physical fitness. The results of the study were partially confirmed by a study of the first-year male students dismissed from Syracuse University because of low grades.

The famous psychologist L. M. Terman has stated after many years of studying the intellectually gifted that:

The results of the physical measurements and the medical examinations provide a striking contrast to the popular stereotype of the child prodigy, so commonly depicted as a pathetic creature, over serious, undersized,

sickly, hollow-chested, nervously tense and bespectacled. There are gifted children who bear some resemblance to this stereotype, but the truth is that almost every element in the picture, except the last, is less characteristic of the gifted child than of the mentally average (2, p. 24).

SPECIAL CONSIDERATIONS IN EXERCISE

For a long time it was believed that athletes, especially children, could permanently damage their hearts by strenuous exercise. There is absolutely no experimental evidence to support this myth of the pathological athlete's heart. Strenuous exercise does not injure a normal heart in any way. The fact that this also holds true for older age groups has been demonstrated by a Miami heart specialist, Dr. E. Sterling Nichol, who indicated no adverse changes in the electrocardiograms of men aged sixty-five to eighty-one years following participation in singles tennis matches. However, older persons would be advised to have a physical examination, including an electrocardiogram administered during exercise, and to increase their exposures to exercise gradually before undertaking strenuous athletic competition or strenuous exercise of any kind.

Exercise in Heat

Fatigue sets in much earlier while working in the heat, because the blood supply must be divided between the working muscles and the skin. During work, most of the blood is delivered to the muscles to sustain performance. However, when the temperature becomes very high, a large portion of the blood must be diverted to the skin to eliminate heat. Because the muscles are thus robbed of a large portion of their normal blood supply, they may tire easily.

If exercise is prolonged before a person becomes acclimated to the heat, the combined needs of the skin and muscles for blood may exceed the capacity of the heart to pump blood, which leads to a type of circulatory shock that is not qualitatively different from that suffered in hemorrhage and usually results in fainting, which obviously terminates the exercise. This condition, known as heat exhaustion, is not serious, and recovery usually follows a period of inactivity. Secondarily, this circulatory inadequacy may lead to a breakdown in the heat regulatory mechanism (heat stroke), a serious condition in which the body stops sweating. Untreated victims can die.

People should take every precaution to prevent heat-related conditions. The first step is to achieve heat acclimatization. Given time, the body will adjust to heat, allowing one to work with a lower body temperature and heart rate. This process takes four to seven days. During this period, an hour-long exercise program of gradually increased effort should be undertaken. Simply living in a hot environment does not prepare the body for work in heat.

Fluid Replacement

Replacement of fluids and salts lost through normal perspiration is also important. Water should be replaced at least each hour; salt may be replaced at mealtime. Failure to replace salt leads to heat cramps. Water and salt balance are basic to normal body function.

There are a number of popular misconceptions about water replacement. One is that withholding water from an athlete makes him or her tough or better able to do without water. This is not true and furthermore may result in heat stroke.

A second misconception is that drinking water before exercise impairs performance, and a number of studies have disproved this theory. In one study, thirty-three college track men were given one pint of water just prior to running 220-yard time trials. The water had no effect on their times. In a further study, drinking more than a quart of water just prior to exercise had no effect on the ability of college students to run on a treadmill.

A third misconception is that the more one drinks, the more one perspires. In the absence of severe dehydration, drinking more water does not affect the rate of perspiration. It is important to drink freely when working or exercising in the heat. One's intake of water should be equal to the amount lost through perspiration if one is to maintain maximum physiological efficiency. If water is properly replaced, heat stroke is unlikely.

Menstruation

There is little agreement among physicians about the effect of menstruation on athletic performance. Studies made some years ago indicated that a woman's strength decreases suddenly a few days before menstruation begins and remains at this lowered level during the menstrual period.

Another study, however, involving 111 athletic women participating in track and field events, indicated that 55 percent showed no decrease in performance during the menstrual period, and some women actually improved. The other 45 percent turned in a poorer performance than usual during or just before the menstrual flow.

There is no convincing evidence that physical activity (including swimming) during menstruation is harmful, that it affects the menstrual flow adversely, or that it causes menstrual pain.

Pregnancy

Pregnant women are often advised to give up strenuous athletic competition during the second and third trimesters of pregnancy. Particular caution is directed toward horseback riding, high jumping, and skating, because a fall might cause malposition of the fetus. There are very good indications, however, that the better abdominal development of women engaged in regular exercise (and muscular training during pregnancy in general) may shorten the course of labor or reduce the pain.

Miscarriage

There is no scientific evidence to support the belief that overexertion is a cause of miscarriage. Based on a study of the records of 250,000 pregnancies and deliveries in New York City, Dr. Carl Javert concluded:

It is the lack of physical and mental activity in our modern civilization, rather than overactivity per se, that is responsible for spontaneous abortion.

Premature Aging

As early as the fifteenth century, the artist-scientist Leonardo da Vinci sug- gested that premature aging was due to lack of exercise. Physically active people often appear to be much younger than their chronological age.

If a person continues to exercise regularly through the years, she or he will be able to enjoy many of the active sports in later life. The key is regularity. Once sedentary habits develop, it is difficult to get back into regular exercise. Motivation in middle age is low, whereas the process of rationalization is highly efficient. The athletic performance of men in the older age brackets, however, is often astounding. Among runners in a recent marathon race of 26 miles, one was sixty-three years old and five were over fifty.

Undoubtedly, a number of persons scorn exercise and yet live to a ripe old age. Indeed, some have contempt for all the commonsense rules of health and yet live far beyond the average life expectancy. Sir Winston Churchill is a notable example. In addition to indulging in brandy and cigars before breakfast, he was famous for his physical laziness.

Although individual cases may provide solace to those who have uncontrolled appetites and habits, one must be cautious about statistics that result from a small sample. The critical person does not ignore the hazards of tobacco on the grounds that an uncle who was a heavy smoker lived to be ninety-five. Nor would that person dispute the value of the polio vaccine because his or her nonimmunized grandmother never had polio or ignore the hazards of obesity because an overweight in-law is celebrating her or his ninety-second birthday. Nor should the critical person neglect exercise: its obvious benefits and fundamental values in normal body physiology and development are not theoretical; they are medical facts.

FATIGUE, SLEEP, AND REST

Thus far this chapter has emphasized the importance only of physical exercise; but inactivity and rest are of equal importance. In fact, every living organism, from the simplest amoeba to human beings, shows alternating periods of activity and inactivity in the daily cycle. People can feel very lively at certain times of the day and listless and fatigued at others; everybody seems to have a characteristic cycle.

Generally, a person can easily tell when this cycle has been disrupted. The much discussed jet lag experienced by travelers crossing many time zones is a good example. The average person may take up to two weeks to adjust completely to a new sleep/work cycle.

As yet, the many causes of fatigue are not fully understood. But, whatever its origin, it is Nature's cry for rest and diversion. Unlike mechanical machines, human machines must regularly slow down and rest.

The fatigue that develops after intense or prolonged physical activity or lack of sleep is a normal and natural phenomenon. However, a person who constantly feels fatigued even when he or she should be rested and relaxed should suspect some illness or emotional disturbance and consult a doctor.

In strenuous exercise, the body has a certain limit of endurance, past which it is warned by a sensation of actual pain that fatigue has set in. The pain is probably caused by a metabolic disturbance resulting from a lack of oxygen in the overworked muscles.

Sometimes, when fatigue has not reached too extreme a level, the body succeeds in making the necessary adjustments in time to take care of immediate and pressing needs. Because of these physiological adjustments, athletes who feel they are ready to drop often succeed in making the "gears re-mesh" and obtain the energy needed to finish grueling contests.

Sleep

The amount of sleep necessary to maintain good health varies tremendously from person to person. Eight hours appears to be the average, but some individuals require more and others less. Thomas Edison, for example, apparently managed on only five hours of sleep a night.

In a study conducted at the University of California School of Medicine, a college student slept for only four hours a day for a period of one year. He slept from 4:00 A.M. to 6:00 A.M. and again from 4:00 P.M. to 6:00 P.M. Although this schedule appeared sufficient for the student, it obviously cannot be generally recommended until the long-range health effects of such a regimen are fully investigated.

Sleep requirements are greatest at birth and decline progressively with the years. A newborn infant may sleep twenty to twenty-two hours a day, although some do well on as little as fifteen hours. Between the ages of one and four, about half the day is spent in sleep. For children four to twelve years old, about ten hours of sleep are required. Adolescents usually need eight to ten hours, while adults require seven to nine hours. College students tend to sleep, on the average, a little less than eight hours. However, it is important to remember that anyone who is easily fatigued or who engages in strenuous athletics needs more sleep than the average person.

Insufficient Sleep

The tremendous need of the human mechanism for a daily period of rest from the strain and fatigue of everyday life is obvious. Insufficient sleep probably means incomplete repair and restoration of body cells, resulting in less than maximum efficiency the following day and perhaps nervousness and irritability. Fatigue from inadequate sleep causes many automobile accidents at night. Far too many people fall asleep while driving on long trips and may awaken only when the crash occurs. Some never awaken.

200 HOURS WITHOUT SLEEP

The following reactions were reported from the study of a New York disc jockey who stayed awake for 200 hours (1).

By 100 hours, tests requiring minimal mental agility had become unbearable to him, and the psychologist testing later recalled:*

Here was a competent New York disc jockey trying vainly to find his way through the alphabet.... By 110 hours there were signs of delirium.... From his later statements, his curious utterances and behavior at the time, it became clear Tripp's visual world had grown grotesque. A doctor walked into the recruiting booth in a tweed suit that Tripp saw as a suit of furry worms. A nurse appeared to drip saliva. A scientist's tie kept jumping.... Around 120 hours, he opened a bureau drawer in the hotel and rushed out calling help. It seemed to be spurting flames.... By about 150 hours he became disoriented, not realizing where he was, and wondering who he was.... On the final morning ... Tripp ... came to the morbid conclusion that the man (a neurologist who was examining him) was ac-

*From *Sleep* by G. G. Luce and Julius Segal, copyright 1966 by Coward, McCann & Geoghegan. Reprinted by permission.

tually an undertaker, there for the purpose of burying him alive. With this gruesome insight, Tripp leaped for the door with several doctors in pursuit ... following an hour of tests, he sank into sleep for 13 hours. When he awakened, the terrors, ghoulish illusions, and mental agony had vanished.

Snoring

Everybody jokes about snoring, but the various unpleasant noises made by 21 million snorers can be seriously disturbing to their unhappy listeners:

Laugh and the world laughs with you.
Snore and you sleep alone.

Approximately one out of eight Americans, women as often as men, makes some kind of unmusical sound nightly. It may take the form of a grunt, hiss, snort, gurgle, or an assortment of noises, and it sometimes assumes a surprising intensity. To indicate the nuisance value of this problem, the United States Patent Office has on file patents for more than 300 snore-curbing devices.

Snoring is caused by vibrations in the soft palate and other soft structures of the throat when they come in contact with inflowing and outflowing air. The position of the tongue, enlarged tonsils or adenoids, a blocked nose, a bent or twisted nasal septum, and nasal polyps or growths can all be responsible. Other common causes are allergic conditions or colds which cause swelling of the mucus linings of the nose and induce mouth breathing, excessive smoking, fatigue, overwork, and general poor health.

Fortunately, many of these conditions can be corrected, either surgically or medically. For example, removal of enlarged tonsils and adenoids or of nasal polyps may give enormous relief. Certain drugs—antibiotics to reduce an infection, antihistaminics to shrink the nasal membranes, and steroid hormones—often clear up extreme nasal congestion.

Most people snore only when lying on their backs, and an enforced change in position to prevent the tongue from falling back will prevent the snoring. An old remedy, dating from the eighteenth century, stopped the snorer from sleeping on the back by sewing a hairbrush to the back of the nightshirt.

THE ACTIVE LIFESTYLE

Physical exercise and carefully planned programs of physical education are important during the years that a student attends elementary school. Unfortunately, many elementary schools are unable to have special physical education teachers. Hence, much of the responsibility for the students' understanding the value of an active lifestyle remains with the teacher.

This is a critical responsibility, because it has been clearly demonstrated that the activity patterns established during the elementary years greatly affect future lifestyles. At least three factors deserve the careful consideration of those responsible for the elementary curriculum:

1. There is an immediate health need for physical exercise during childhood.

2. Developing or failing to develop recreational sports skills at an early age usually determines future activity patterns.

3. The benefits of exercise need to be learned and appreciated at an early age.

REFERENCES

1. G. G. Luce and Julius Segal, *Sleep* (New York: Coward, McCann & Geoghegan 1966).

2. L. M. Terman, ed., *Genetic Studies of Genius*, *IV*, "The Gifted Child Grows Up" (Stanford, Calif.: Stanford University Press, 1947).

FURTHER READINGS

The following articles are from *Family Health* magazine, Portland Place, Boulder, CO 80302, beginning with the most recent.

"Get Moving," Dalma Heyn, January 1979 (rhythmic movements).

"You Should Be Dancin'!", Maryann Brinley, November 1978 (disco).

"Mommy, Can I Leave the Lights On?", V. Thomas Mawhinney, October 1978.

"Biking!", Hank Herman, September 1978.

"Exercises You Can Take Lying Down," Nicholas Kounovsky, August 1978.

"Do You Dream (Perchance) of Sleeping?", Carol Kahn, September 1977.

"Easy Isometrics," Robert R. Spackman, Jr., May 1977.

"Exercise—It Ain't Watcha Do, It's the Way That Ya Do It," Bill Maness, April 1977.

· "Put on Those Jogging Shoes and Run for Your Life," Barbara Ribakove, February 1977.

"Eight Ways to Stop Snoring—Sometimes," Robert Smith, January 1977.

"Flipping over Gymnastics," Penelope Lemov, November 1976.

"Plan Now for a Bon Voyage," Ruth Winter, May 1976.

"Get Set for Tennis," Ernest M. Vandeweghe, April 1976.

"How the Famous Stay Fit," Neal Ashby, April 1976.

"When Your Dreams Turn into Nightmares," Richard Trubo, March 1976.

"Exercise—Do It Right!", part of a special section on building yourself a better heart, February 1976.

"Touch Away Tension," Anne Kent Rush, December 1975 (massage).

"Winter Sports—Don't Start Them Cold," Suzy Prudden and Jeffrey Sussman, September 1975.

"The Weekend Athlete's Way to a Pain-Free Monday," Hyman Jampol, May 1974.

"Everybody, Sleep!", Senator William Proxmire, October 1973.

PART B: TEACHING ABOUT EXERCISE, REST, AND RELAXATION

Most young people do not get enough exercise on their own. Statistics show that children spend a large proportion of their free time engaged in sedentary activities such as television, bus riding, studying and idle socializing. The schools can play an important part in meeting physical development needs of children if they provide a daily period of physical activity. Now, more than ever, the school should continue providing the physical education that all children need to prepare them for an adult society that is continually reducing the need for physical tasks and in so doing, is promoting the increase of diseases associated with inactivity (3, p. 14).

In view of the health consequences of a sedentary lifestyle, it is important that elementary schoolchildren become acquainted with the values of adequate exercise and rest.

1. The student needs to understand the importance of a good night's rest.
2. The student needs to cooperate with his or her parents in establishing a regular bedtime.
3. The student needs to learn to balance periods of activity with rest.
4. The student needs to develop the habit of regular daily exercise.
5. The student needs to know the health benefits of exercise and the health hazards of a sedentary life.
6. The student needs to develop good posture and the desire to have good posture.
7. The student needs to value physical fitness as a lifestyle component.

UNIT I: WHY EXERCISE?

What are the lifestyle benefits to the child who develops a regular program of exercise? What program of exercise should the elementary child follow? When should the program begin? The preceding questions are asked by the teacher who is careful in planning a curriculum that will have long-lasting as well as immediate benefits to the child.

To summarize one important benefit:

After comparing superior and inferior third-grade pupils in motor proficiency, Rarick and McKee concluded that children in the superior group were judged by their teachers to be active, calm, resourceful, attentive, and cooperative, whereas children in the inferior group were more frequently judged as showing negative traits and were more often indicated as being shy, retiring, and tense (4, p. 142).

The long-range benefits of exercise are the focus of the lesson Why Exercise? The student learns ten reasons to exercise and participates in an exercise program for his or her age group designed by the President's Council on Fitness. Through

Appropriate grade levels are suggested for each teaching strategy and appear as ○, □, ☆ in the left-hand column.

○ = most suited for the primary grades;

□ = most suited for the intermediate grades;

☆ = most suited for the upper elementary grades.

221

a valuing activity, the students can examine the extent to which exercise has become a part of their lifestyles.

OBJECTIVES

1. The student will be able to identify at least ten reasons for exercising while participating in the Happy Health Walk.

2. The student will be able to identify exercises for the arms, legs, and heart and for flexibility while participating in the dart board exercise.

3. The students will express a desire for a daily exercise program in their telegrams to themselves and will evaluate their plans on the exercise value continuum.

MATERIALS

1. Why Exercise? posters.
2. Atlas Figures 84 and 85.
3. Dart board.

Methods

WHY EXERCISE?

Make ten posters to use to discuss the question Why exercise? Draw or paste magazine pictures on posterboard to depict various healthful exercises. Place the ten posters around the room. Give the students five minutes to examine the pictures. Ask the students to name the health benefit of the exercise depicted in each picture. Use the following outline of discussion and activities to discuss their answers.

Heart Rate

(Poster No. 1, Picture of Child Running) "The normal heart pumps more than 4,000 quarts of blood each day, resting only between beats."

Demonstrating Heart Rate

To demonstrate the beating heart, clench your fist and beat on a desktop. Explain to the children the two sounds they hear—the beat and the rest. Next demonstrate how hearts beat differently. First, beat quickly on the desk. Then beat forcefully on the desk with longer pauses.

"You have just listened to two hearts. The first heart was beating quickly. The heart muscle was weak and the heart needed to beat more often to get blood to the body. The second heart was very strong and could pump more blood with each beat, while resting between beats."

Atherosclerosis

(Poster No. 2, use Atlas Figures 84 and 85, Normal Artery and Abnormal Artery) "Your blood needs paths just as you need highways to travel upon. The blood has a pathway of arteries. The arteries lead away from the heart and carry fresh blood to the body. The flow of the blood in the arteries is controlled by pressure."

Demonstrating Blood Pressure in the Arteries

A garden hose can be used to demonstrate arterial pressure. The hose is the artery, the nozzle is the diameter, and the water is the blood supply. With your garden hose, turn the water on without a nozzle. How does the water flow? Turn on more water. What happens? Now attach a nozzle to the hose. What happens to the outlet of water if the opening is wide open? Turn the opening of the nozzle smaller. How is the pressure of water affected?

"You can see from our experiment that blood pressure is very important in controlling the flow of blood. The arteries are elastic like a rubber band so that they can get larger and smaller to control the flow of blood.

"Sometimes people have habits that make the arteries less elastic. It may change blood flow and blood pressure.

"Let's look at the poster. You can see the normal artery. You can see that there is room for blood to flow and the lining on the inside of the arteries is smooth.

"In the next artery, there is something sticking to the sides of the artery walls. These are fats. Fats are very sticky, especially fats such as butter and gravy. When people eat too many fats, some of the fats stick on the artery wall. Then the artery is no longer smooth. There is not as much room for the blood to flow.

"If people continue to eat sticky fat foods for years and years, the buildup gets very hard on the artery lining. The artery will no longer be elastic like a rubber band.

"The buildup of fat on the artery wall and the hardening of the wall is called atherosclerosis.

"Exercise can help to prevent atherosclerosis by increasing blood circulation and not allowing the fats to stick on the walls of the artery."

Weight Control

(Poster No. 3, Picture of Overweight Person) "Your weight depends upon how much you eat compared to how much you burn up. The measure is done in calories. How do calories relate to you? The following rules apply.

1. If you want to gain weight, you need to eat more calories per day than you will burn up that day.

2. If you want to lose weight, you need to burn up more calories per day than you will eat that day.

3. If you want to maintain your weight (stay the same) you should eat the same number of calories that you will burn up."

(Write "3500 calories = 1 pound" on the blackboard and "Playing tennis one hour = 500 calories.")

"If we work the problem on the blackboard we can learn how exercise affects our weight. How long would it take someone to lose one pound if they played tennis for one hour a day? Yes, it would take one week. If the same person played tennis for one year, how many pounds of calories would be used (52)? You can see that exercise does not cause you to lose weight rapidly, but it helps day by day."

Nervous Tension

(Poster No. 4, Picture of Face Showing Worry or Stress) "I want you to write the alphabet five times. Make the letters as small as you can. After you are done, stand up and stretch, jump up and down three times, and shake your hands.

"Exercise helps us to work off tension. The experiment we just did was a simple way to demonstrate how exercise and movement relieve tension. When you are very worried or down in the dumps, exercise may help you feel much better."

Aging

(Poster No. 5, Pictures of Various Faces) "Let's guess the age of each person on this poster. Sometimes it is hard to guess age, isn't it? That is because all of us look different as we grow older.

"People who exercise seem not to grow old as fast. Through exercise, they keep good circulation throughout their body. They feel younger and many times look younger than their age."

Good Grades

(Poster No. 6, Picture of Student at a Desk) "We have all heard the saying, 'A sound mind—a sound body.' In studies done on boys and girls your age, it has been found that those who exercise regularly get better grades in school. Why do you think this is true? Better circulation helps us to be alert and to concentrate for longer periods of time."

Sleep

(Poster No. 7, Picture of a Child Sleeping) "A certain amount of exercise seems to be required for deep, restful sleep."

Posture

(Poster No. 8, Pictures Depicting Differences in Posture) Have the students put their palms on either side of their body while sitting and press as hard as they can on the chair. Now tell them to relax. This isometric exercise will leave the students in good sitting posture.

"How does it feel to be sitting tall? We have just done an exercise to help you sit tall. It is important to exercise our muscles so that we can stand, walk, and sit with good posture."

Muscle Tone

(Poster No. 9, Picture of an Athlete) "What do you notice about the person in this picture? He (she) has good muscle tone. Through exercise, we can tone our muscles so that they can work very hard for us."

Fatigue

(Poster No. 10, Picture of Someone Who Looks Tired) "Have you ever known someone who was always tired? Without good circulation and body conditioning, we can feel tired all the time."

Evaluation

LIFESTYLE CONTENT

○ □

Happy Healthy Walk

To review the lesson Why Exercise?, use the posters for a Happy Healthy Walk (see Figure 9B-1). Arrange the posters as stepping stones around the classroom. Appoint a tour guide. The guide will lead the students around the room stepping on the posters. While the students are walking, play music. When the music stops, the tour director will ask one tourist on the Happy Healthy Walk how exercise helps his or her stepping stone. If the student answers correctly, he or she becomes the tour director.

LIFESTYLE VALUE

○ □

Animal Exercises

Children in elementary school need to participate in a variety of exercises that involve gross body movement. Select an animal for the children to imitate for each day of the week. Some examples include

1. tortoise and hare
2. bunny hop
3. bear walk
4. frog stand
5. rabbit race

LIFESTYLE CONTENT

○ □

Dart Board

The students form a line. Each student gets to throw a dart at the board. The student leads an exercise to help the part of the body that corresponds to the color hit on the dart board.

FIGURE 9B-1 The happy healthy walk

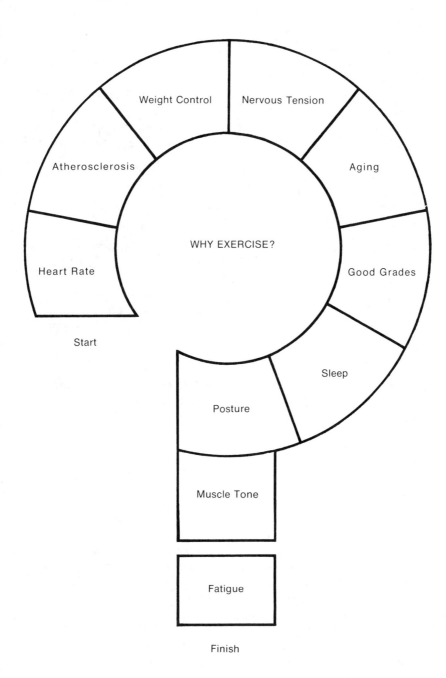

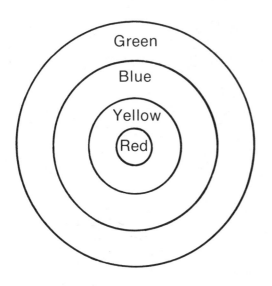

Green: arms

Blue: legs

Yellow: flexibility

Red: heart

Bouncing Betsy (Bill)

Bouncing Betsy is my name
Exercises are my game.
Every morning run in place
Jumping jacks, keep up the pace.

Then a good breakfast for me
To keep physically fit, as you can see.
So keep up the good exercise
And you'll be healthy as well as wise.

Lazy Lucy (Larry)

Lazy Lucy is my name
Sleeping late is my game.
Up just in time to catch the bus
Exercises are such a fuss!

No breakfast, or I'll be late
No exercise, and fat is my fate.
But I feel terrible, as you can see
And to look like this, just be like me.

Exercise Value Continuum: Where are you?

Bouncing Betsy		Lazy Lucy
Bouncing Bill		Lazy Larry

LIFESTYLE VALUE

○ □

Telegram

The students will write telegrams to remind themselves of the exercises they should do daily. The telegrams are put into envelopes addressed to each student. The teacher mails the envelopes in one month. After the students receive their envelopes, they place themselves on the exercise value continuum.

UNIT II: SLEEP AND REST

Many of the lifestyle lessons have focused on the self-actualization process during the waking hours. A critical aspect of lifestyle focuses on the rest and sleep needed to meet day-to-day challenges. Both inactivity and activity are components in the development of a healthy lifestyle.

School-age children vary greatly in the

amount of sleep required for maximum efficiency. In the article "When Bedtime Brings Problems," Dr. Robert W. McCammon, Director of the Child Research Council at the University of Colorado Medical Center, says, "The thing that is strikingly true is the wide variation in sleep needs between healthy and vigorous children" (1, p. 40).

Dr. McCammon continues, "What conditions are conducive to a child's restful sleep? In general, sleep is induced when several conditions exist: (1) fatigue, (2) absence of a strong stimulation, (3) peace of mind, and (4) desire to sleep. A regular bedtime is as important as a regular mealtime" (1, p. 41).

Dreams are also discussed in the article. Dr. Alfred A. Messer, an Atlanta psychiatrist, says that when the stimuli of sound and light are removed, children's imaginations take over (1, p. 41). Night fears and bad dreams are common sleep problems with the preschool and early school-age child.

It is the authors' hope that the lesson on sleep will help the student become more relaxed about bedtime, more desirous of a regular bedtime, and more likely to balance periods of activity with rest.

OBJECTIVES

1. After observing a puppet show featuring Rip Van Winkle and the seven dwarfs, the student will draw his or her favorite dwarf and describe a good night's sleep.

2. The student will write a letter to the sandman telling him what he knows about sleep and rest.

3. The student will express a desire for a regular bedtime in the Stars for Sleep activity.

MATERIALS

1. Eight puppets.

2. Stage for puppet show (cardboard box painted as a forest).

3. Atlas Figure 86, Worksheet: Stars for Sleep.

Methods

○

Puppet Show

To discuss sleep and students' sleeping habits, produce a puppet show. In the puppet show, Rip Van Winkle goes to the forest and he meets several sleepy dwarfs. Each time he meets a dwarf, he stops to ask the dwarf why he is so sleepy. The following list offers reasons the sleepy dwarfs may give:

1. Stayed up too late watching television.

2. Played with toys in bedroom rather than sleeping.

3. Bothered by noises outside bedroom window.

4. Had a frightening dream.

5. Was wide awake; couldn't fall asleep.

6. Didn't want to go to sleep until older brother did.

Rip Van Winkle then meets a bright, alert dwarf. The cheerful, alert dwarf went to bed at a regular time. Rip Van Winkle asks the students the following questions:

What is your bedtime?

Who decides what time you go to bed?

Do you know what reason your parents have for a certain bedtime for you?

What things do you do before you go to bed?

Do you dream when you sleep?

How do you get a restful sleep?

○

Each student can draw a picture of his or her favorite sleepy dwarf. Have the student describe how this sleepy dwarf could be convinced to get a good night's sleep.

○

Storytime

Share some of the following books with young children:

What's That Noise? by Carol Nicklaus
Hildilid's Night, by Cheli Duran Ryan
Sleep, pictures by John Mousedale
The Long Winter Sleep, by Ellen H. Goins
Bedtime! by Beni Montresor
Eugene the Brave, by Ellen Conford
Bedtime for Frances, by Russell Hoban
Dreams, by Ezra Jack Keats
While Susie Sleeps, by Nina Schneider

○ □

Dreams

During sharing time, divide the students into groups of three. Have each student share a dream with the other students in the group. Discuss the following questions:

Why do we dream?
What is a dream?
What is a nightmare?
When do you dream?
Do you like to dream?

○ □

Rest

Have the class perform the following experiment to illustrate why people need to rest after becoming fatigued. Divide the students into three groups. The first group will have three things to do at once. The second group will have a job to do under uncomfortable conditions. The third group will work on a tiring project for 30 minutes without a break. Ask the students the following questions:

How did you feel about your group?
Were you tired?
Did you want to rest?

○ □

Have each student draw a picture showing how they best like to rest. Discuss different ways to rest.

1. Exercise
   a. Sit for several minutes, do not fidget or blink.
   b. Take off shoes and clench toes, then slowly relax them. Do the same with legs, arm muscles, jaws, and mouth.
   c. Stand on tiptoes and stretch, reaching for the ceiling with your fingertips.
   d. Rotate your head gently.
   e. Shrug and relax shoulders.
   f. Rotate arms at shoulders.
2. Breathing
   a. Inhale deeply and raise shoulders.
   b. Exhale slowly and lower shoulders.
3. Massage (long, sweeping hand strokes with palms and fingers, pressing gently)
4. Warm bath (tepid, not hot, water soothes)
5. Naps (cat naps)
6. Music
   a. Lullabyes and quiet music.
   b. Play different records for the students that will help them to relax. Ask them what records are their favorites.

Evaluation

LIFESTYLE CONTENT

○ □

Each student can write a letter to the sandman telling him what she or he learned about sleep and rest.

LIFESTYLE VALUE

○

The students can examine their sleeping habits to see if they value a regular bedtime by using the Stars for Sleep inventory in the Atlas. The student who feels bright and alert in school that morning gets to paste a star in the sky on the sheet. When the sky is full of stars, the student should be praised for her or his good night's sleep habit.

UNIT III: POSTURE

"He really stands tall." "She carries herself with dignity." Often the first impression that people have of someone carries with it many ideas as to how people perceive that person according to their lifestyle. The posture of a person gives people a general impression of the self-image of that person, his or her mood at the time, and his or her general health.

Most elementary children are capable of assuming good posture. For them to maintain good posture depends upon knowledge of the elements of good posture and a willingness to practice these, balanced muscular development, and sufficient stamina (muscle tone) to maintain good alignment. Emotional outlook and physical abnormalities also affect the child's ability to practice good postural habits (2, p. 119).

The lesson on posture is included to help the elementary child maintain good posture and value posture. The teacher should, however, also check the student's posture throughout the school year.

OBJECTIVES

1. After the discussion of good posture, the student will be able to describe good sitting, standing, and walking posture.

2. Through role play, the student will show how emotions and feelings affect posture.

3. The student will evaluate five different pictures for good and bad posture using an evaluation checklist.

4. The student will be able to describe the effect of shoe fashions on foot posture through a shoe store activity.

5. The student will express a desire for good posture by completing three posture exercises each day.

6. The student will express a desire to match his or her value about posture with her or his posture behavior using an evaluative chart.

MATERIALS

1. Atlas Figure 16, Posture.
2. Pipe cleaners.

Methods

□

Riddle

Begin the lesson by having the students guess the answer to the following riddle:

1. Both animal and man have this characteristic.

2. It is habit forming.

3. It involves both your muscles and your bones.

4. You have it when you are walking, standing, sitting.

INTRODUCTION TO POSTURE

"Every child needs to feel when his body is in good postural alignment. One simple way to establish the kinesthetic feeling is to have the child assume proper foot and leg position, tuck the seat under, and lift the rib cage by taking a deep breath. At the same time he stands tall, flattening his abdominal wall, and keeps his head and shoulders in good position. Have him release the air, but maintain the position without tenseness" (2, p. 119).

○ □ ☆

Transparency

Using the posture figure in the Atlas, discuss the following material with the students:

1. What do you think posture is?
    a. Posture is the way that you hold your body as you sit, stand, and move.
    b. When you have good posture, your bones are in the position for which they were constructed and your organs have room to work.
    c. When you have good posture, your body supports your weight.
    d. Good posture becomes a habit.
2. What is good sitting posture?
    a. Head up.
    b. Lower back touching chair.
    c. Back of chair used for support.
    d. Both feet flat on the floor.
3. What is good standing posture?
    a. Head stretching to ceiling.
    b. Breastbone farthest point forward.
    c. Feet parallel with weight on both feet.
    d. Arms hanging comfortably at sides.
4. What is good walking posture?
    a. Feet parallel.
    b. Strong push from toes.

c. Arms swing opposite to feet.
    d. Lead with your knees, not your nose.

○ □ ☆

Pipe Cleaner Activity

Distribute pipe cleaners. Have the students make stick figures. After discussing each of the following deviations, have students make the deviation with their stick figures to illustrate poor posture.

1. Forward Shoulders
    a. Shoulder blades are held to the side of the body instead of close to the spine.
    b. Shoulders roll forward.
    c. Round back.
    d. Angel wings.
2. Swayback
    a. Hips tilt forward.
    b. Lower back hollows.
    c. Strain put on backbone.
    d. Often accompanied by a sagging lower abdomen.
3. Backward Knees
    a. Knees bend in backwards.
    b. Often accompanied by swayback.
4. Knock-knees
    a. Inner sides of knees are brought together.
    b. Often caused by weak ankles which turn in.

○ □ ☆

Role Play

Explain that posture often tells something about one's emotions or feelings. Have the students role play different emotions showing how posture changes by asking the following questions:

How would you sit if you were ashamed of yourself?

How would you stand if you were proud? alert? tired? embarrassed?

How do you walk when you are friendly? happy? down in the dumps? frightened?

○ □ ☆

Shadow Drawings

Have a student stand in front of a sheet of paper hanging on the wall while another student shines a bright light at the first student. The second student can trace around the first student, showing that student's posture. Evaluate with the class.

□ ☆

Picture Evaluation

Have the students evaluate five different pictures according to good or poor posture habits. Have them place a check mark in the correct column on the posture chart in Figure 9B-2.

○ □ ☆

Foot Tracing

Pair off the students. Have one student stand on paper and the other student trace around his or her feet. Have the students trade places. Ask them to note the differences in the foot tracings. Discuss with the class the importance of good foot posture and provide the following information:

1. The normal foot has a strong arch.
2. Flat feet have a weak arch.
3. Toeing in or out contributes to poor posture.
4. The students can notice weight distribution from the foot tracing.

□ ☆

Shoe Store

Have the students bring in shoes for a shoe store. Have them make an advertisement for each pair of shoes describing what is good or bad about each of the following kinds of shoes: tennis shoes, platform shoes, high heels, pointed shoes, sandals, earth shoes.

○ □ ☆

Exercises to Improve Posture

The following three exercises are designed to help students improve their posture. These exercises are taken from Dauer and Pangrazi, whose textbook on elementary physical education is an excellent book for the classroom teacher (2, pp. 125–126).

1. *Tailor Exercise* (Head-Shoulder-Upper Back)

Position: sit tailor fashion (cross-legged) with trunk erect and locked fingers on middle of back of head, elbows out.
Movement: force head and elbows back slowly against pressure. Be sure that there is no change in the erect body position.
Beginning Dosage: ten repetitions.

2. *The Mad Cat* (Abdominal Muscles)

Position: on hands and knees with the back somewhat sagging.
Movement: arch the back as rounded as possible with a forcible contraction of the abdominal muscles. Hold for two counts and return to position.
Beginning Dosage: six repetitions.

3. *Marble Transfer* (Feet)

Position: sitting on a chair or bench. A marble or a wadded piece of paper is needed.
Movement: pick up the marble with the right foot and bring it up to the left hand. Transfer the marble to the right hand and bring up the left foot to put the marble back on the ground.

	Good head position	Poor or fair head position	Shoulders position	Shoulders back	Shoulders forward	Sitting back in chair	Not sitting back in chair	Good walking posture	Good foot posture
Picture One									
Picture Two									
Picture Three									
Picture Four									
Picture Five									

FIGURE 9B-2 Posture Chart

Evaluation

LIFESTYLE CONTENT

□ ☆

Matching Test

Directions: choose the good posture characteristics from the second column and place the letters under 1, 2, or 3.

1. SITTING
   a. head up
   b. shoulder blades near sides of body
   c. shoulders back
   d. hips tilted forward
2. STANDING
   e. lower back touching chair
   f. knees locked into position
   g. knees touching
   h. both feet on floor
   i. toes turning in
3. WALKING
   j. breastbone farthest part forward
   k. arms hanging comfortably at sides
   l. toes turning out
   m. feet parallel
   n. heel touching ground first
   o. leading with knee

LIFESTYLE VALUE

□ ☆

Tell the students that their posture often tells something about their emotions and feelings. Certain postures tell others certain things about people.

Have the students complete the accompanying chart according to the following directions. There are four columns on the chart. The first column represents three different postures. In the second column, write down how you usually sit, stand, or walk. In the third column, write what you think this posture says about you. In the fourth column, write what you would like your posture to say about you.

Examples you may choose from for postures:

Sitting:
   forward or backward
   head in hand
   arms folded
   slouched or straight
Standing:
   weight on one leg
   slouched or straight
   toes in or out
   arms folded or
      hanging to sides
Walking:
   big steps
   little steps
   slowly
   quickly
   swing your arms
      looking down or up

Different things posture can say:

proud
confident
discouraged
excited
lazy
sleepy
alert
relaxed
shoes too tight
peppy
alone
aggressive
sick

How I usually:	What does this say to others?	What do I want it to say?
Sit		
Stand		
Walk		

UNIT IV: AAHPER YOUTH FITNESS TEST

The American Association of Health, Physical Education and Recreation (AAHPER) Youth Fitness List has been officially adopted by the President's Council on Physical Fitness and Sports as part of its motivational and evaluation program. The test consists of a battery of six tests designed to measure various components of physical fitness in girls and boys, ages ten to seventeen. The Youth Fitness Test is the only test for which national norms have been developed.

Because the AAHPER Youth Fitness Test has gained national recognition, the authors suggest that you purchase the *Youth Fitness Test Manual.**

OBJECTIVES

At the end of the AAHPER Youth Fitness Test, the student will have been evaluated on the following test items:

1. Pull-ups (boys); flexed-arm hang (girls)
2. Sit-ups, flexed legs (boys and girls)
3. Shuttle run (boys and girls)
4. Standing long jump (boys and girls)
5. 50-yard dash (boys and girls)
6. 600-yard run (boys and girls)

ADDITIONAL METHODS

□ ☆

If you decide to use the AAHPER Youth Fitness Test, you may want to include the following activities at the same time.

*Available from AAHPER, 1201 Sixteenth Street, N.W., Washington, DC 20036.

1. Invite an athlete to talk to your students about his or her training program. For example, in Columbus, Ohio, teachers have invited Archie Griffin, two-time Heismann Trophy winner.

2. Have the students make a map of the community indicating the different recreational activities available. The students can write reports on the value of participating in those activities to become physically fit.

3. The students can examine famous people's efforts to be physically fit (Eisenhower—golf; Ford—skiing). Have the students determine why these people valued physical fitness and how exercise was worked into their schedules.

4. The class could compile a Book of Athletes. Have each student select an athlete and find out about that person's training program.

REFERENCES

1. James J. Cox, "When Bedtime Brings Problems," *Today's Health* (May 1967).

2. Victor P. Dauer and Robert P. Pangrazi, *Dynamic Physical Education for Elementary School Children* (Minneapolis: Burgess, 1975).

3. President's Council on Physical Fitness and Sports, *Youth Physical Fitness* (Washington, D.C.: U.S. Government Printing Office, 1973).

4. Lawrence Rarick and Robert McKee, "A Study of Twenty Third-Grade Children Exhibiting Extreme Levels of Achievement on Tests of Motor Efficiency," *Research Quarterly* 20, no. 2 (May 1949).

CHAPTER 10

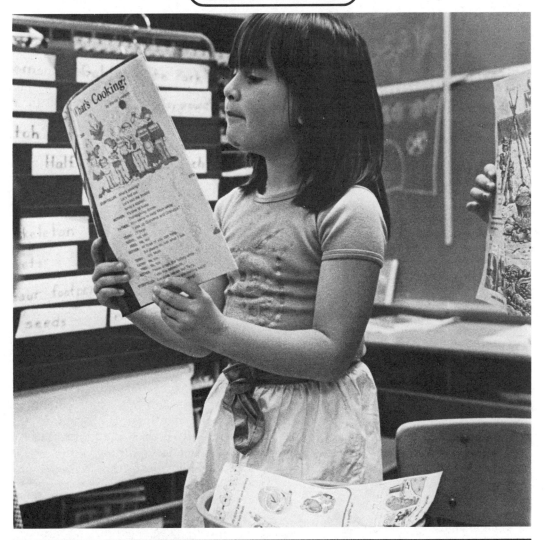

PART A: NUTRITION

Few areas provide as many alternatives in lifestyle as does the area of nutrition. Some of the more common types of eaters include meat eaters, vegetarians, low carbohydrate eaters, sweet eaters, breakfast skippers, lunch skippers, volume eaters, picky eaters, snackers, night eaters, social eaters, nervous eaters, and eaters who wash down their food. Fortunately, many nutritional styles are compatible with good health. A number of styles, however, reduce effectiveness and general health. Hence, what one eats makes a great difference. Indeed, one's nutritional style is a significant factor in:

attaining normal growth and development,
obtaining the energy required for work and play,
maintaining normal body functions,
assuring repair and healing,
preventing disease,
delaying degeneration,
regulating body temperature,
obtaining substances required for certain chemical reactions essential to life,
determining personal appearance.

Obviously, these factors are major considerations in one's total health. But, how can one ever gain knowledge about all of the many foodstuffs that are available for consumption? It would appear impossible to study all of them. Fortunately, the foods we eat may be biologically broken down into seven categories: water, carbohydrates, fats, proteins, vitamins, minerals, and roughage (dietary fiber).

WATER

In general, most people attach little nutritional significance to water. Everyone knows that it relieves thirst, but the nutritional value of water is seldom appreciated. A clue to its real significance should be apparent, however, from the fact that although one can remain alive for several weeks without food, survival without water lasts approximately one week. In view of this, the elementary student should become acquainted not only with the biological significance of

water but with ways and means of maintaining an unpolluted water supply.

The major portion of the human body is composed of water. The nonfat portion (lean body mass) contains 70 to 85 percent water, while fat contains 10 to 20 percent. In the average adult, water accounts for approximately 57 percent of the total weight.

A major function of body water is to serve as a transport system, just as in early American history when products were transported downstream. Nutrients are floated inside the human body to the cells, and cellular waste is floated away. Inside the body, however, materials being transported in fluids are actually dissolved in the water. As waste, the body excretes about 1.4 quarts of urine each day.

As a lubricant, water serves several important functions. In the joints of the body, it serves as a cushion for easy movement. As a major component of saliva, it serves to lubricate food and assist in the swallowing process. In the lower digestive tract, the lubricating nature of water is useful in the prevention of constipation. In fact, digestion cannot occur without water. This does not mean, however, that water must be ingested at mealtime.

The body keeps cool through evaporation of water from the lungs and skin. On a cool day, one does not notice this loss, which is termed insensible sweating. (In science, the terms sweat and sweat glands are preferred over the more euphemistic terms perspiration or perspiration glands.) In a hot environment, however, sweating is very obvious, and the body may eliminate as much as 5 quarts per day.

The amount of water required for

healthy living varies from one individual to another and with the environmental conditions. The average person living but not performing heavy work in a cool environment requires approximately two liters (about two quarts) per day. In a warm environment and with exercise, the requirement may be several quarts per day.

Ordinarily, one's thirst mechanism is a reliable guide to fluid replacement. However, this is not an adequate guide for those individuals who work in the heat, in which case one should ingest more water than one's thirst would indicate is necessary. The onset of summer or travel to hot climates necessitates a change in nutritional style, especially as it relates to greater water and salt intake.

CELLULAR FUEL

In addition to requiring water, the 100 trillion cells of the body, working like small engines, require fuel to perform the work. That is, they require fuel to contract, conduct nerve impulses, secrete, produce needed substances, repair themselves, and grow. To perform their many tasks, the cells require a high-energy fuel—a fuel that can quickly release enough energy to support cellular work. This high-energy fuel is known as ATP (adenosine triphosphate).

If humans could simply fill up a storage area with ATP, nutrition would be a far less complex problem. But as it happens, the cells must produce ATP and then burn it to perform their work. To produce ATP, the cells require raw products, which in turn are refined to produce the high-grade fuel burned by the cells. The raw products essential to the produc-tion of cellular fuel are carbohydrates, fats, and proteins.

CARBOHYDRATES

Carbohydrates are a class of organic substances composed primarily of starches and sugars. Sugars are usually derived from sugar beets, sugarcane, and the sap of the sugar maple. Milk and honey are sources of animal carbohydrate. Starch is found in the cereal products of corn, wheat, rice, barley, rye, and oats and is also widely present in many types of vegetables. Bread, cakes, pies, cookies, waffles, and pancakes may contain both starch and sugars and are thus substantial sources of carbohydrates.

Approximately 80 percent of the by-products of carbohydrate digestion are glucose. When carbohydrates have been digested and absorbed, a substance called insulin aids in getting glucose into the cells to be burned. If the proper amount of insulin is not produced by the body (pancreas), the individual is said to be diabetic. (See Chapter 12B, Unit III, for further information on diabetes.)

In the United States, approximately 45 to 50 percent of the dietary calories are derived from carbohydrates. The major role of carbohydrates in the diet is to provide energy for work and general efficiency. The most important derivative of carbohydrates is glucose, which is utilized by all cells in the body.

Glucose is of major significance to the central nervous system (brain and spinal cord), since (a) the central nervous system can only burn glucose and (b) only small amounts of glucose can be stored in the cells of the central nervous system. Consequently, long periods of low blood sugar can cause permanent brain damage.

FATS

The fats contained in the foods we eat are in the form of an alcohol called glycerol and organic acids known as fatty acids. The type of fat that is stored in the body and the type that we eat is mainly a triglyceride. In this form, three fatty acids are attached to glycerol (Figure 10A-1). When the body requires energy, triglycerides are immediately broken down into glycerol and fatty acids. These components are then converted into the energy which all cells burn.

Fats are a major source of energy for humans. If equal amounts of carbohydrates, fats, and proteins were eaten, the body would derive twice as much energy from fats as from the other two classes of foods. Hence, fat is an efficient way for the body to store energy. Fats also remain in the stomach longer than other foods, thereby producing a greater satisfaction of appetite.

Some of the fatty acids are essential to growth and healthy skin. They cannot be produced by the body and must be taken in via the diet. Vitamins A, D, E, and K require the presence of fat before they can be absorbed from the digestive system. This means that it would be unwise to cut all fats out of the diet. Other vitamins are soluble in water and do not require the presence of fats.

Fatty acids contain varying numbers of hydrogen atoms. In turn, the number of hydrogen atoms held by the fatty acids determines the appearance of fats at room temperature. Fats that hold the greatest possible number of hydrogen atoms are known as saturated fats and are solids at room temperature. Saturated fats are found in the hard fats of land animals, in dairy products, and in vegetable oils that have had hydrogen atoms added (hy-

FIGURE 10A-1 Triglyceride

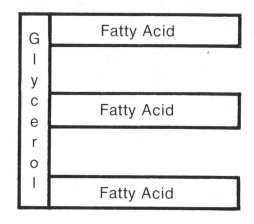

drogenated) to render them solids.

Unsaturated fats contain two fewer hydrogen atoms than maximum, while polyunsaturated fatty acids contain at least four fewer than maximum. The latter types of fatty acids are found in vegetable oils and fish oils and are often called essential fatty acids, since they are necessary to health. Unlike many fatty acids, polyunsaturated fats cannot be produced from other foods.

Cholesterol

The discussion of saturated and unsaturated fatty acids is significant to nutrition because of the relationship between these types of fatty acids and a substance called cholesterol. Cholesterol, in turn, is of great contemporary interest because of its relationship to diseases of the arteries.

Cholesterol is a white, waxlike, solid substance that may be deposited on the walls of the arteries, narrowing them or even completely blocking them. Additionally, this hardening of the arteries may initiate an internal blood clot.

Cholesterol is manufactured by the body and is also consumed in some of the foods we eat. It is now generally recognized that the saturated fats we eat have a marked effect to increase blood cholesterol levels. Unsaturated fats appear not to affect cholesterol levels, whereas polyunsaturated fats actually lower cholesterol levels.

Most nutritionists recommend that not more than 30 to 35 percent of one's total caloric intake should be in the form of fat, with polyunsaturates substituted for other types of fats whenever possible. The ratio of polyunsaturated to saturated fats should be approximately two to one.

PROTEINS

To maintain health, the body requires protein. Proteins are made up of many amino acids linked together in a chemical chain. In a sense, amino acids are similar to an alphabet in which the letters may be used to write various proteins. Proteins are essential to several functions, including:

1. Growing and maintaining body tissues.
2. Producing hormones, enzymes, and antibodies to protect against disease.
3. Providing a source of energy.

For healthy functioning, one should ingest 55 to 65 grams of protein per day, which means from 275 to 325 calories derived from protein.

VITAMINS

Proteins, carbohydrates, fats, and water are not enough to maintain a high level of health. Many years ago it was discovered that animals who were not given vitamins soon exhibited poor health. Today, it is known that the body requires not one but several vitamins.

Vitamins are organic compounds required in very small amounts to promote growth, normal functioning, and reproduction. In order for vitamins to be absorbed from the digestive system, they must become soluble in some substance that is easily picked up and transported by the circulatory system. Presently, vitamins are fat soluble or water soluble, according to the manner in which they are absorbed.

You will recall that the fat soluble vitamins are A, D, E, and K. Water soluble vitamins include B vitamins, thiamin, riboflavin, niacin, biotin, B6, pantothenic acid, folic acid, B12, and C (ascorbic acid). Water soluble vitamins are secreted in body fluids, whereas fat soluble vitamins may be stored with fat in the body. Because they are stored in the body, large quantities of vitamins A and D can actually create a health hazard.

Figure 10A-2 describes the various functions and sources of vitamins and other nutrients.

MINERALS

In addition to needing water, carbohydrates, proteins, fats, and vitamins, the body requires small amounts of inorganic minerals for healthy functioning, including:

blood clotting,
regulation of acid-base balance,
production of hormones and vitamins,
rigidity of skeletal structure,
conduction of nerve impulses and muscular contraction,
catabolism and anabolism of foodstuffs,
control of water balance.

FIGURE 10A-2 Functions of food in nutrition

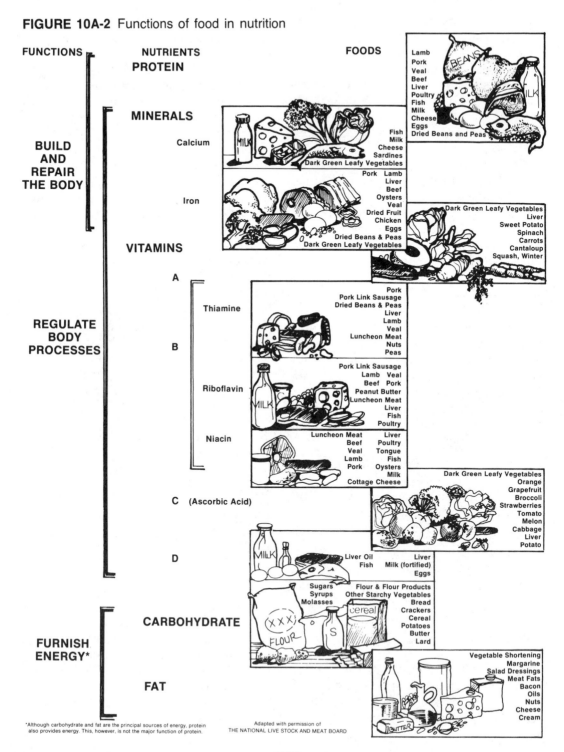

FUNCTIONS   NUTRIENTS   FOODS

PROTEIN

Lamb
Pork
Veal
Beef
Liver
Poultry
Fish
Milk
Cheese
Eggs
Dried Beans and Peas

BUILD AND REPAIR THE BODY

MINERALS

Calcium

Fish
Milk
Cheese
Sardines
Dark Green Leafy Vegetables

Iron

Pork Lamb
Liver
Beef
Oysters
Veal
Dried Fruit
Chicken
Eggs
Dried Beans & Peas
Dark Green Leafy Vegetables

Dark Green Leafy Vegetables
Liver
Sweet Potato
Spinach
Carrots
Cantaloup
Squash, Winter

VITAMINS

A

REGULATE BODY PROCESSES

B

Thiamine

Pork
Pork Link Sausage
Dried Beans & Peas
Liver
Lamb
Veal
Luncheon Meat
Nuts
Peas

Riboflavin

Pork Link Sausage
Lamb Veal
Beef Pork
Peanut Butter
Luncheon Meat
Liver
Fish
Poultry

Niacin

Luncheon Meat Liver
Beef Poultry
Veal Tongue
Lamb Fish
Pork Oysters
Milk
Cottage Cheese

C (Ascorbic Acid)

Dark Green Leafy Vegetables
Orange
Grapefruit
Broccoli
Strawberries
Tomato
Melon
Cabbage
Liver
Potato

D

Liver Oil   Liver
Fish   Milk (fortified)
Eggs

CARBOHYDRATE

Sugars
Syrups
Molasses

Flour & Flour Products
Other Starchy Vegetables
Bread
Crackers
Cereal
Potatoes
Butter
Lard

FURNISH ENERGY*

FAT

Vegetable Shortening
Margarine
Salad Dressings
Meat Fats
Bacon
Oils
Nuts
Cheese
Cream

*Although carbohydrate and fat are the principal sources of energy, protein also provides energy. This, however, is not the major function of protein.

Adapted with permission of
THE NATIONAL LIVE STOCK AND MEAT BOARD

Depending upon the quantity required, minerals are referred to as either macro elements (substantial amounts required) or trace elements (very small amount required). Macro elements include calcium, phosphorus, potassium, sodium, chloride, and magnesium. Trace elements include iron, manganese, copper, iodine, zinc, fluoride, cobalt, selenium.

Calcium

Approximately 2 percent of the total body is calcium, most of which is found in the bones. Calcium is required for blood clotting, muscle contraction, and conduction of nerve impulses. Milk is probably the best single source of calcium. Other sources include collards, kale, broccoli, turnips, and mustard greens.

Fluoride

Fluoride is found in the bones and teeth and is required for maximum resistance to dental caries. The best source of fluoride is drinking water that has fluoride added.

Iron

The body contains only about 4 grams of iron, although iron is a most essential element in normal physiological function. Aside from contributing to other functions, iron is a necessary component of hemoglobin, the portion of red blood cells responsible for the transport of oxygen. Iron deficiency produces an anemia which leaves the body weakened and susceptible to illness. Iron is also needed for release of energy from carbohydrates and fats.

Good sources of iron include meats, clams, oysters, dried fruits, lima beans, spinach, and nuts. Because of the small amount of blood loss during menstruation, the recommended intake of iron is greater in the adult female than for the male.

Sodium

Approximately 0.15 percent of the body is sodium, 30 to 40 percent of which is found in the bones. Sodium is the element in the fluids that bathes the cells. Since it is essential to healthy water balance, the intake should be increased in environments in which sweating is likely to be profuse. Sodium also aids in relaxing muscles and in transmitting nervous impulses. Most Americans, however, take in ten to fifteen times more salt than they need. Besides causing too many fluids to move into the circulation, excess salt may be a factor of high blood pressure. Sodium is found in milk, meat, eggs, and vegetables.

Chloride

Chloride, the other component of salt, helps sodium to balance the acid/base ratio of fluid in the cells. Approximately 0.15 percent of the body is chloride.

ROUGHAGE

In addition to requiring the nutritional value of various foodstuffs, healthy physiological function also requires some roughage in the diet. Known as dietary fiber, roughage has recently been the subject of widespread investigation because of its possible role in preventing with such problems as appendicitis, hiatus hernia, diverticular disease (abnormal outpouching of the colon), constipation, varicose veins, and cancer of the colon.

Although cause-and-effect relationships have not been clearly established, the incidence of all of these conditions is much higher in persons with a low content of dietary fiber, the indigestible part of plant cell walls present in large amounts in grains and cereals and to a lesser degree in fruits and vegetables.

With the advent of modern roller mills, the outer husk of cereal grain kernels is now usually removed to produce refined white flour. As a consequence, fiber content is one-tenth what it was.

Fibrous foods add bulk to the diet. Once inside the intestinal tract, the fiber absorbs water and swells, resulting in softer stools and the prevention of constipation. The straining associated with constipation increases pressure in the colon and may cause diverticular disease. Straining also increases intra-abdominal pressure, which can push the stomach up through the diaphragm, resulting in hiatus hernia with its heartburn, regurgitation of stomach acid back into the esophagus, and a burning sensation behind the breastbone. Increased intra-abdominal pressure may also result in varicose veins and hemorrhoids.

Fiber is beneficial because it accelerates the transit time of a meal through the digestive system. A number of medical scientists now feel that this may explain the lower incidence of cancer of the colon among those populations that still ingest a high percentage of dietary fiber.

Good sources of fiber include whole meal breads, whole meal flour, sesame and sunflower seeds, seed-filled berries (raspberries, blackberries, and loganberries), and raw or slightly cooked fruits and vegetables.

ALTERNATIVES IN NUTRITIONAL STYLE

To this point, the chapter has discussed the needs of the human body for the seven basic types of nutrition. Next comes the task of developing a nutritional style that fits both one's desires for food and one's nutritional needs. One of the healthiest styles appears to involve the daily selection of foods from each of four basic food groups: milk, meats, fruits and vegetables, and breads and cereals (Figure 10A-3).

Breakfast

Breakfast is considered to be the most important meal of the day. It is now generally agreed that work performance is far better on a well-balanced, high-protein breakfast. Medical scientists have shown that a high-protein diet at the beginning of the day provides energy at a more uniform level throughout the morning than do other types of breakfast.

It is significant that the blood sugar does not fluctuate nearly so much after a high-protein breakfast as it does after a high-starch breakfast, since changes in blood sugar affect both the appetite and energy levels. Because the appetite is satisfied for a longer period after a high-protein breakfast, the actual calorie intake later in the day may be reduced, which helps those with weight problems.

A high-protein breakfast would include a selection of eggs, cereal, milk, and meats. Breakfast skippers may feel bv midmorning the effects of low blood sugar—hunger, sensations of dizziness, and even fainting.

FIGURE 10A-3 A guide to good eating (Courtesy of National Dairy Council)

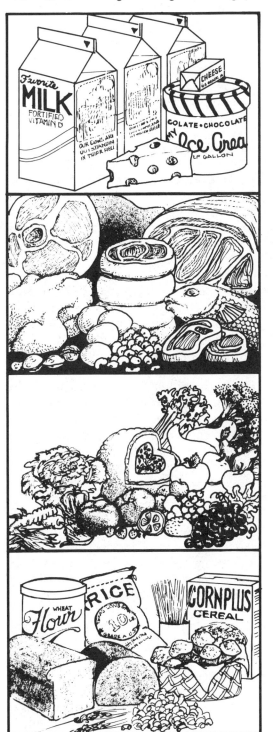

A recommended daily pattern

Milk Group

Calcium
Riboflavin (B₂)
Protein
2 Servings/Adults
4 Servings/Teenagers
3 Servings/Children

Foods made from milk contribute part of the nutrients supplied by a serving of milk.

Meat Group

Protein
Niacin
Iron
Thiamine (B₁)
2 Servings

Dry beans and peas, soy extenders, and nuts combined with animal protein (meat, fish, poultry, eggs, milk, cheese) or grain protein can be substituted for a serving of meat.

Fruit – Vegetable Group

Vitamins A and C
4 Servings

Dark green, leafy, or orange vegetables and fruit are recommended 3 or 4 times weekly for vitamin A. Citrus fruit is recommended daily for vitamin C.

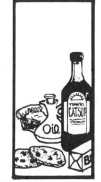

Grain Group

Carbohydrate
Thiamine (B₁)
Iron
Niacin
4 Servings

Whole grain, fortified, or enriched grain products are recommended.

Others

Carbohydrate
Fats

Foods and condiments such as these complement but do not replace foods from the four groups. Amounts should be determined by individual caloric needs.

243

Snacking

Most people have been taught to eat regular meals and avoid snacking. This recommendation stems from the observation that what people eat between meals often consists of sweet foodstuff (carbohydrates, empty calories, or foods that do not represent a nutritional balance). In addition, snacking may spoil the appetite for the next meal and add calories that contribute to obesity.

With these exceptions, however, there is no reason to avoid eating between meals. If a snack consists of nutritious foods, it may actually represent a healthy nutritional style. In a study with animals, it was demonstrated that those who ate many times daily were less likely to develop arteriosclerosis than those eating regular meals. Animals that nibbled all day put on less weight for the same number of calories than animals who ate only one meal daily.

Vegetarian Diets

There are several types of vegetarians:

1. Total vegetarians eat only fruit, vegetables, and nuts.
2. Lacto-vegetarians eat plant foods plus dairy products.
3. Lacto-ovo-vegetarians eat plant foods, dairy products, and eggs.
4. Some vegetarians also eat fish and shellfish.

In general, there is no conclusive evidence that vegetarian diets possess any unique virtues, although the people who adhere to them receive less fats and appear to be more lean, which is usually a good thing. Lacto-ovo-vegetarians who include cheese, nuts, beans, and fish get their recommended daily allowance of protein, vitamins, and carbohydrates while enjoying an infinite variety of flavors, textures, and colors in their food. Strict vegetarian diets, however, do not provide the essential nutrients needed for optimum health.

OVERNUTRITION

The previous discussion has focused totally upon required nutrients. Now let us turn our attention toward a problem of equal concern to good nutrition: overweight.

Anyone who is markedly overweight is suffering from a type of ill health. Obese persons may be subject to one or more of the following: overworked heart and circulation, shortness of breath, tendency to high blood pressure, tendency to diabetes, poor adjustment to hot weather and changes of temperature, increased strain on joints and ligaments, reduced capacity for physical exercise, and personality problems related to poor appearance. Considerable evidence also exists that the longer the waistline, the shorter the lifeline. For example, the mortality from circulatory disorders is 44 percent higher in males who are 5 to 15 percent overweight than in males of normal weight.

With many people there is a direct relationship between food intake and weight gain. But to generalize this to all cases would be somewhat of an oversimplification of a complex problem. For just as some breeds of livestock gain more weight than others from an equal amount of calories, so does it now appear to be true of humans. Indeed, more than 25 physiological and biological differences between obese and normal weight individuals have been discovered. For this reason, anyone who is more than 15 pounds overweight and wishes to markedly reduce would be wise to consult with his or her physician first.

One of the most important factors in weight control is regulating the caloric intake to approximate the energy expenditure. It is truly amazing that so many people are able to maintain their exact weight day after day and year after year.

To understand the process of balancing calories, the term "calorie" must first be defined. A calorie is a unit of measure of heat. In nutrition, it is the amount of heat given off when food is burned. Calories are burned inside the body to accomplish all biological functions. The number actually burned can be judged from the amount of oxygen utilized by the body; that is, the body requires oxygen to burn food, and measuring the amount of oxygen burned by the body is an accurate method of determining how many calories are utilized.

The air that people breathe contains approximately 21 percent oxygen. But the air that they exhale contains less oxygen because, the body is constantly using oxygen. Thus, measuring the oxygen content of expired air provides a way of determining how many calories the body is burning at any given time. Table 10A-1 contains the caloric cost of several common types of activities. Given the fact that one pound of fat is equivalent to approximately 3500 calories, the table can be utilized to determine how much work would be required to burn a pound of fat.

TABLE 10A-1 COST OF VARIOUS ACTIVITIES IN CALORIES PER MINUTE

A. Recreational Activities and Hobbies

Painting, sitting	2.0
Playing piano	2.5
Driving car	2.8
Canoeing (2.5 mph)	3.0
Horseback riding (slow)	3.0
Volleyball	3.5
Bowling	4.4
Golfing	5.0
Swimming (20 yd/min)	5.0
Dancing	5.5
Gardening	5.6
Horseback riding (trotting)	8.0
Spading	8.6
Skiing	9.9
Squash	10.2
Cycling (13 mph)	11.0

B. Industrial Activities

Watch repairing	1.6
Typing	1.8
Armature winding	2.2
Radio assembly	2.7
Bricklaying	4.0
Plastering	4.1
Wheeling barrow (115 lb., 2.5 mph)	5.0
Carpentry	6.8
Mowing lawn by hand	7.3
Felling tree	8.0
Shoveling	8.5
Ascending stairs (17-lb load, 27 ft/min)	9.0
Tending furnace	10.2

C. Household Tasks

Hand sewing	1.4
Sweeping floor	1.7
Machine sewing	1.8
Polishing	2.4
Peeling potatoes	2.9
Scrubbing, standing	2.9
Washing small clothes	3.0
Kneading dough	3.3
Scrubbing floors	3.6
Cleaning windows	3.7
Making beds	3.9
Ironing, standing	4.2
Mopping	4.2
Wringing by hand	4.4
Hanging wash	4.5
Beating carpets	4.9

One of the most important things to learn about weight control is the fact that weight gain and weight loss are generally accomplished gradually. One does not eat an extra 3500 calories at one sitting, nor does one burn off 3500 calories in one bout of exercise. Rather, one usually adds or removes only small amounts at a time.

As an example of the way this works, suppose a person were to eat each day one extra banana containing approximately 85 calories. For a while, he or she would not notice much of a difference simply from eating a banana. But suppose that person did this every day for a year. He or she would have gained approximately nine pounds.

On the other hand, suppose someone decided to swim an extra 15 minutes each day. Since a 15-minute swim burns up approximately 85 calories, not much difference would be noticed after only a few days of swimming. But in a year that person would have burned up approximately nine pounds.

Thus, if someone ate a banana and swam 15 minutes each day, the weight would remain rather constant.

Diets

High-protein diets have attracted some people who want to lose weight, but they should not be used by people with kidney disease or gout or who are pregnant. People on high-protein diets may experience fatigue and possess a foul breath. They would be wise to increase their fluid intake while on the high-protein diet.

Through the years, a number of people have advocated a high-fat diet as a means of losing or controlling weight. The usual suggestion has been that if people cut down on other types of foods (especially carbohydrates), then they can eat all the fat they like. Not only are such diets unscientific, they are potentially dangerous to men and postmenopausal women because of the increased risk of heart disease.

There is much to recommend a low-carbohydrate diet, if certain precautions are observed. If must be remembered that a low-carbohydrate diet is not the same as a zero-carbohydrate diet. With no carbohydrates, one is likely to exhibit extreme fatigue and dizziness.

Many of the advocates of low-carbohydrate diets have not considered fat intake. Although carbohydrates are reduced, careful attention should also be given to the reduction of fats, especially saturated fats.

Low-carbohydrate diets result in increased fluid losses, and when one goes off such a diet, these fluids are soon regained. That is, some of the weight lost on a low-carbohydrate diet is not permanent. It has been shown, however, that most people reduce their total caloric intake by approximately 35 percent when they go on a low-carbohydrate diet.

A number of diets have attracted attention because of emphasis on a single food, such as grapefruit, bananas and milk, ice cream, alcohol, and candy. None of these foodstuffs possess any special power for weight control. Their value is in direct proportion to the amount of other foods included in the diet or to the total number of calories, if the diet is limited to a single food.

On the basis of current evidence, the most prudent diet is a diet high in protein, with no more than 30 percent fat (with a ratio of two parts unsaturated fat to one part saturated), and a minimum of carbohydrates (including very little sugar).

PART B: TEACHING ABOUT NUTRITION

Is a student's selection of a personal nutritional style a matter of heredity, or does the student simply mimic the nutritional style of parents, family, or friends? Is the student's nutritional style mainly a matter of availability of different foodstuffs? Is it a matter of taste or cost? And finally, is the selection of a nutritional style amenable to education intervention?

The elementary school teacher needs to be concerned with these questions when planning lessons. The future lifestyle of students has the greatest potential for being healthy and self-actualizing if the nutrition teaching plan considers the following needs of the elementary school student:

1. The student needs to recognize alternatives in nutritional style and to become acquainted with the facts that speak for and against each alternative.

2. The student needs to try out some of the alternatives in nutritional style.

3. The student needs to develop an overall nutritional style based upon his or her values (e.g., health, pleasure, or cost).

Based on several factors, the student selects and holds to a general nutritional pattern.

Appropriate grade levels are suggested for each teaching strategy and appear as ○, □, ☆ in the left-hand column:
   ○ = most suited for the primary grades;
   □ = most suited for the intermediate grades;
   ☆ = most suited for the upper elementary grades.

UNIT I: WHY PEOPLE EAT AND HOW THEY GROW

Most likely a small child eats because his or her family does, because it is a part of the socialization process, and because he or she likes to eat. Although the child is probably not eating to obtain healthy growth, he or she has undoubtedly heard his or her mother or father mention the relationship between food and healthy growth. It is not uncommon for a child to hear at dinner, "Finish your carrots, they're good for your eyes. You're not getting up from the table until your milk is gone. Don't you want to have nice teeth and a pretty smile?"

Thus, the child has some feeling that food and growth are related by the time he or she reaches elementary school. However, this relationship needs to become obvious to the child if he or she is to decide that eating carefully will be a lifestyle component. During a child's elementary years, the teacher wants the child to learn to value eating for the sake of proper growth in addition to the other reasons mentioned.

OBJECTIVES

1. Through making growth booklets, the students will recognize their growth patterns and will contrast their current size to the size they were as babies.

2. Through the development of a comparative classroom chart, the stu-

dents will conclude that they grow at different rates.

3. After the lesson, the discussion, and the activities, the students will be able to describe why people eat and how eating helps them to grow.

MATERIALS

1. Clothesline, clothespins, sample clothes.

2. Letter to parents.

3. Yarn, scissors, paper stapler, tape nametags, scales, weights.

Methods

○

Attach several examples of small infant clothing to a clothesline before students enter the classroom. After class begins, initiate a discussion about growth and why people's bodies need food.

○

Supplementary activities require parental cooperation. You may wish to write a letter similar to Figure 10B-1 and ask the students to return with the answers the following day.

○

Bulletin Board

Some teachers utilize the information they receive from parents to construct a classroom chart as a bulletin board display. Each student is weighed and measured. This information is recorded on the chart along with their birth weight and length.

Students may also want to lift a weight that is closest to their birth weight and cut strips of yarn representing their present height and their length at birth.

FIGURE 10B-1 Note to parents

Dear Parents:

We are going to be studying growth, and I need some information. Would you please answer the following questions.
What was the weight of your child at birth? _____
What was the length of your child at birth? _____

Also, if you have any clothing your child wore as an infant, would you let us use it for a display? We could also use any drawings of little hands or feet that you might have.

Please do not send us anything of real value to you. We will return all items. Thank you for your cooperation.

○

Display

If the parents have sent in display items, let the students put their items on a table and compare their present size with their size as a baby.

○

Growth Chart and Discussion

The construction of a classroom growth chart may help students conclude that people grow at different rates. This concept may be followed by asking the students What other things are different about us? What else could we put on the classroom chart to show our differences? Use the student's ideas. If none are forthcoming, try eye color, hair color, number of baby teeth, permanent teeth, complexion, etc. After completing the chart ask if the students think being different is good or bad and Why. This is an open-ended value-setting question, but the teacher should guide the discussion to foster the idea of accepting and appreciating differences.

○

Growth Book

Give each student two pieces of construction paper, six sheets of white paper, yarn, scissors with a blunt edge, and tape for the construction of a growth booklet.

Contents of the Book

Give the students the following instructions to complete the books:

1. On the cover put "Meet Me—Tom Jones—Six Years Old." Take yarn and outline a head, ears, nose, and mouth. Draw in the eyes. (The teacher can cut a tiny piece of hair to show hair color.)

2. Cut yarn the same as the height of the student at birth and now. On the first page put "I am _____ inches tall. I was _____ inches long when I was born."

3. The next page can have the weight. "I am _____ pounds. I was _____ pounds when I was born." Make a yarn waist for this page.

4. The next page can be yarn measurements of "My Head," "My Shoulders," "My Neck."

5. Page 4 can be yarn measurements of "My Wrist," "My Knee," "My Ankle."

6. Page 5 can be a length of yarn of "My Arms and Legs."

7. Trace your hands and put fingerprints on page 6.

8. Trace your feet and put footprints on page 7.

Ask the students for additional ideas.

Evaluation

LIFESTYLE CONTENT

○

To evaluate this lesson, the teacher will need to observe the students' comments during the various activities. Since this lesson lasts over a period of days, it would be helpful to have a checklist for each student.

Checklist

____ Is able to name, locate, and measure body parts.

____ Completed the booklet accurately.

____ During discussions compared own growth patterns and physical characteristics with those of classmates.

____ Is beginning to accept self as a unique individual.

____ Is beginning to accept others as unique individuals.

LIFESTYLE VALUE

○

After the students have completed their growth booklets, have them utilize "I Learned Statements" (2). The students should finish such statements as:

I learned that I _____
I was surprised that I _____
I was pleased that I _____
I was displeased that I _____

UNIT II: SELECTING FOODS FOR A HEALTHY BODY

Eating foods from the Basic Four represents a healthy nutritional style. In this approach it is recommended that one select food from each of the following groups: milk, meats, vegetables and fruits, and breads and cereals. To develop a healthy nutritional style, children will need information about each of the food groups and opportunities to develop healthy habits. In addition, children need to examine their snacking habits. Sugar-based foods such as candy and soft drinks afford energy but lack essential nutrients and as a result have been labeled "empty calories." On the other hand, there are many snacks that offer children nutritional value and do not harm the teeth.

The lesson Selecting Foods for a Healthy Body is a compilation of games and activities designed to impart nutritional information to the student. The content evaluation is a timed activity. The timed response of the student will enable the teacher to evaluate whether the student can quickly recall nutritional information. Throughout life, food selections are often made in a hurry. If one is to exemplify a healthy nutritional style, a hurried choice must also be a wise one.

OBJECTIVES

1. The student will be able to identify the four basic food groups.

2. The student will be able to select nutritious snacks.

MATERIALS

1. A Guide to Good Eating chart.*
2. Paper bags, crayons, paints, scissors.
3. Letter to parents.
4. Snacks.
5. Empty cans, wrappers, cartons.
6. Sacks.
7. Cardboard.
8. Iodine.
9. Bread.
10. White potato.

*Available from the National Dairy Council, Chicago, IL 60606. Published in 1964.

Methods

○ □
Grocery Store

Before beginning the unit on nutrition, send a note home to the parents asking them to help their children save empty cans, wrappers, and cartons. Have the students bring them to school. Arrange a mock grocery store. You can correlate this unit with other subjects by having the students do art work to advertise products (art and consumership) and price the foods (math).

By having the students bring things from home, the teacher will be talking about foods eaten in the locality in which he or she is teaching. This helps to consider geographical, social, and economical factors when the foods are discussed.

After the grocery store display is arranged, have the students discuss which foods they like best, least, eat most often, think are good for them, think are not so healthy for them, etc.

□

Food Groups

Use the chart A Guide to Good Eating to explain the Basic Four to the students. The back of the chart explains each food group.

○ □

Divide the class into groups of four. Give each student a paper sack large enough to fit over the head. Each group is to illustrate a food from each of the four food groups. (For example, one student might draw an apple on the sack to show the fruit and vegetable group.) Have the students cut out eyes on each sack. When the groups are finished, each student will have a sack with a picture on it to put over his or her head.

Mix the sacks up so that the student does not have his or her own sack. Have the students close their eyes and then put the sacks over their heads. The students cannot see the sacks on their own heads, although they can see out. Each child asks the class questions to help guess what food she or he is.

○

Have each child bring a snack to class. At an appropriate snack time, the child shows her or his snack to the class. In order to eat the snack, the child must be able to tell the class three reasons why the food is good for her or him.

GAMES

Games can be played to see whether or not the children can place foods into the correct food groups. The following games were developed by Charlene Montonaro, Executive Director, Dairy Council—Mid-Ohio, and are included with her permission.

□ ☆

Nutrition Bingo

Equipment
   1 gameboard per player
   16 food cards per player
   16 cover squares per player

Rules
   To make food cards, each student should:
   1. Divide sixteen cards into four piles (one pile for each food group).
   2. Write one specific food on each card, being careful not to combine food groups such as macaroni and cheese or beef stew.
   3. Think of four different foods for each food group. (Example: whole milk, yogurt, cottage cheese, and buttermilk.)

To make gameboards, each student should write the same foods written on the food cards under the correct food group on the gameboard. (Examples: If card one is whole milk, write whole milk in the first space under the milk group.) Mix all of the food cards together and give to the leader. Each student may keep the gameboard she or he made or exchange it for another.

To Play
   1. The leader calls one card at a time, giving both the food group and the food name.
   2. When the food called by the leader matches the food on a gameboard, the player should cover it with a paper square.

The first player to have four foods covered, either diagonally or horizontally, with one food from each food group, is the winner.

Food"d"ball

Preparation
   Draw a playing field divided into yards on the blackboard or a piece of paper and have a moveable football, drawn with chalk or cut out of construction paper. Select examples of foods from each of the four food groups; make each food worth a specific number of yards.

To Play
   1. Choose sides; toss a coin to decide the team that receives the ball.
   2. The defensive team (team *not* receiving the ball) will name a food (worth a specific number of yards). The offensive team (the team receiving the ball) must name the food group in which this food belongs. If the offensive team answers

251

correctly, it advances that number of yards.

(Example: Defensive team kicks off by asking, "Milk belongs in the _____ group." For 10 yards. The offensive team answers "milk"; this is correct, so they gain 10 yards.)

3. The offensive team continues to advance down the field to score a touchdown so long as they answer *correctly*.

4. When the offensive team answers *incorrectly* they lose the ball. The defensive team then gets the ball and continues until they score a touchdown or answer *incorrectly*.

5. When a team scores a touchdown, it receives six points. The opposing team then "gets the ball."

6. The team with the most points at the end of the game wins.

7. Optional: the team that scores the touchdown could be given another food; if the entire team answers with the correct food group, it earns the extra point after a touchdown.

Basic 4 Baseball

Preparation
1. Draw a baseball diamond on the blackboard or paper.

2. Make symbols for each team to represent the runners. (Example: make four red circles and four blue squares.)

To Play
1. Choose sides; assign team color or symbol.

2. Toss a coin to determine which team will bat first.

3. First player on the pitching team pitches the ball by asking the first player on the batting team which food group a specific food belongs in. (Example: "Milk belongs in the _____ group.")

4. To advance to first base, the first batter must answer *correctly*. If the first bat-

ter answers *incorrectly*, the pitcher must then name the correct food group for the batter to be out. If the batter answers *incorrectly*, and the pitcher also answers *incorrectly*, the batter walks to first base.

5. The batting team continues playing until it has three outs.

6. When a team has three outs, the opposing team comes to bat.

7. The team with the most runs at the end of nine innings wins the game.

Variations
1. Add foods that would score a double, triple, or home run.

2. Students could actually move around designated bases on the diamond instead of using symbols.

Evaluation

LIFESTYLE CONTENT
☐
To evaluate this lesson, the teacher can use a relay in the activity class.

Nutrition Relay

1. Divide the class into two teams.

2. Each team gets a grocery bag with an equal number of sample foods. Each item in the bag belonging to Team No. 1 has "No. 1" marked on it. All items in the Team No. 2 bag have "No. 2" on them.

3. At a point equally distant from both teams are four empty grocery bags, each labeled with one of the four food groups.

4. At the call "Go!" the race begins. The first student of each team grabs an item from the team bag and places the item in the proper food group bag. The student runs back to the team and tags the next person in line, who repeats the action. This continues with both teams until one team finishes first.

5. The first-place team gets fifteen points. The second-place team gets ten

points. In a tie game, each team gets fifteen points.

6. The four food group bags are now checked to be sure the items in them belong there. For each item placed in the wrong bag by a certain team, the other team gets two additional points. Thus, Team No. 1 may have finished first but has three incorrect items. Team No. 2, having no incorrect items, would then get six additional points, giving it a total of sixteen, and they win the game.

7. If each team has an equal number of incorrect items, the teams cancel out and no additional points are given.

LIFESTYLE VALUE

□ ☆

Have the students rank order the following questions, using a 1 for their first or best choice. Have them explain their reasons.

1. You are going on a two-day camping trip and are taking only five different foods. What will you take?

_____ eggs, peanut butter, bread, apples, cereal

_____ cheese, milk, peaches, carrots, fruit juice

_____ peanut butter, bread, cheese, apples, green peppers

2. You skipped lunch and are really hungry about three o'clock in the afternoon. What will you eat?

_____ grilled cheese sandwich

_____ crackers and milk

_____ candy bar

3. You can't stand milk. What will you do?

_____ drink milk anyway

_____ eat cottage cheese

_____ drink chocolate milk

The teacher can make up other rank-order questions to accompany the teaching situation. The important thing is to determine what the students consider when making their choice. Find out if their considerations take into account healthy nutritional habits and if the students are consistent.

UNIT III: CALORIES AND WEIGHT CONTROL

Children who are growing and developing at a fast rate will enjoy eating plenty of food. At this point in their lives, they are developing a good habit, since their bodies can utilize the calories. This habit can have a turnabout, however. One important thing to learn about weight control is that weight gain and weight loss are generally gradual in nature. Often a young person can eat and eat and not gain weight until the adult years when weight suddenly begins to appear around the waistline.

Americans are known to be diet abusers and to fluctuate in weight in adulthood. Nutritionist Jean Mayer refers to those who select a lifestyle with constantly fluctuating weight as being trapped in "the rhythm system of girth control." A healthy adult selects a nutritional style in which an optimal weight is maintained day after day and year after year.

The lesson Calories and Weight Control will help the student determine the number of calories needed per day. It also discusses the wise selection of those calories. Eating patterns last a long time, and the emphasis on a calorie-based plan will lay the foundation for a healthy nutritional style.

OBJECTIVES

1. The student will be able to state how energy in a given food is measured and through experimentation show what is meant by calorie.

2. The student will determine the number of calories he or she needs per day and will make a sample balanced menu with this number of calories for one day.

3. The student will differentiate the caloric needs of the overweight and underweight by developing a chart.

4. The student will express her or his values by making choices on a post-test.

MATERIALS

1. A 3-cup can, black paint, cork, 2-gram Brazil nut or walnut, pin, test tube, candle, centigrade thermometer, matches.

2. Pamphlets showing calories and desirable height/weight charts.

3. Clothes hangers, paste, scissors, string, magazines.

Methods

□ ☆

Calorimeter

Have the student, with the help of the teacher, construct a calorimeter to measure the energy in a given food (1, pp. 232–233).

Directions

A 3-cup can is sprayed with black paint and two openings are cut in it before the class period begins. (One hole is cut in the bottom of the can to hold the test tube, and another hole is cut in the side of the can large enough to hold a cork to which a 2-gram nut (Brazil or walnut) is attached with a pin.

The teacher blackens the end of the test tube in order to cause it to absorb more heat. (A candle could be used.) The tube is then inserted through the hole and the student pours 8 milliliters of water into the test tube.

Using a centigrade thermometer, he measures the temperature of the water and records

it. The thermometer is removed carefully, and the nut is lighted by the student with a match. It is allowed to burn until nothing remains but the ash.

As soon as possible after the nut is consumed by the flames, another reading is taken of the water to measure the heat energy the water absorbed. This reading is recorded and the differences are noted on this chart. For example:

Temperature

1st Reading	2nd Reading	Difference
24°C	44°C	20°C

The child makes his computation by multiplying the water times the increase in heat, i.e., 8 ml(gm) of water $\times$ 20° difference gives the total of 160. Therefore, each gram of nut produced 80 calories of heat.

The child should be able to state that a calorie is the amount of heat required to raise the temperature of 1 gram or ml of water one degree centigrade.

□ ☆

Calorie Counter Mobile

Each student, with the teacher's help, should determine his or her daily caloric needs. The student can then make up a sample menu to show how to nutritionally get the appropriate number of calories by careful selection at breakfast, lunch, and dinner. Have each student create a mobile according to the following directions:

1. Select one meal from the sample menu and cut out pictures of the foods in the meal.

2. Paste the pictures on construction paper and trim off any parts showing around the edges of the picture.

3. Write in ink or crayons the food group the picture represents.

4. Cut string into various lengths.

5. Punch a hole in the top of the picture and tie one of the strings to the picture. Repeat for all pictures.

6. Insert one clothes hanger inside another so that they are at right angles. You may want to tape them or secure them with a rubber band.

7. Tie the remaining ends of the string to the hangers. The pictures should now hang at different lengths.

The students can discuss their mobiles with the class. Each mobile must be correct in its representation of each food group and the mobile must represent a balanced meal.

☐ ☆

Overweight and Underweight

The students can then discuss individual differences. Discuss the caloric needs of the underweight and the overweight.

Have each student divide a sheet of paper in half, and at the top of one side write "Overweight" and at the top of the other side write "Underweight." Have them do the following:

1. Name one food for each group to avoid.

2. Name one food for each group to eat in moderation.

3. Name one food for each group to eat in plenty.

4. Name one food for each group that could be eaten as often as desired.

Evaluation

LIFESTYLE CONTENT

☐ ☆

The student will have completed objectives 1 through 3 through the different activities in the lesson.

LIFESTYLE VALUE

☐ ☆

In order to discuss the students' values, ask the following questions and have the students discuss their choices.

1. You are trying to lose weight by reducing your daily caloric intake. You are with three other people in a snack bar. Everyone else ordered a banana split. What would you do?

a. Order a banana split to go along with the group.

b. Order a glass of milk, since it is lower in calories.

c. Tell them you are not hungry and order nothing.

d. Tell them they should not order banana splits since they are too high in calories.

2. You have just decided that you are overweight and want to lose weight. Which one or ones of the following would you do?

a. Reduce daily caloric intake.

b. Increase daily activities.

c. Go on one of the fad diets, since they are lower in calories.

d. Go without eating for a day or two, since it is not necessary to eat foods every day.

3. When you go home from school and are hungry, which of the following would you eat?

a. A glass of milk and cookies.

b. An apple.

c. A candy bar.

d. A hot dog sandwich.

UNIT IV: LABELING

Coupled with the need to select wise patterns of eating to achieve a healthy nutritional style is the need to be a wise consumer. The lesson on nutrition labeling is designed to help the student learn to select foods that provide good nutrition for every dollar spent. Classroom activities include reading labels and making comparisons based on price and nutritive value.

OBJECTIVES

1. The student will demonstrate a knowledge of nutrition labeling by correctly answering five multiple-choice questions.

2. The student will make a food carton with a nutrition label for a fortified food.

3. The student will demonstrate that he or she can select foods that provide good nutrition for the dollar through a grocery store value-ranking activity.

MATERIALS

Pamphlets for the children: *We Want You to Know About Nutrition Labels on Foods.**

Methods

□ ☆

Have the students bring in empty cartons and containers from their favorite foods. Discuss the following information with the class.

NUTRITION LABELING

Nutrition labeling is a program developed by the Food and Drug Administration. It is required for some foods and optional for others. Since 1975, all foods for which a nutritional claim is made as well as all fortified foods have had nutritional

*Available through U.S. Department of Health, Education and Welfare, Public Health Service, Food and Drug Administration, 5600 Fishers Lane, Rockville, MD 20852. DHEW Publication No. (FDA) 74-2039.

information displayed on their labels. The usual information, such as name, net weight, and ingredients appears, as well as information on calories, protein, carbohydrates, fat, vitamin A, vitamin C, thiamin, riboflavin, niacin, calcium, and iron. This nutrition information appears in a standard format always on the part of the label immediately to the right of the panel. The nutrients are always listed in the same order, so it is easy to make comparisons.

What do you find on the label?

The label gives the size of the serving and tells how many servings are in the container. Also listed on the container are the number of calories; amount of protein, carbohydrate, and fat (in grams); seven vitamins and minerals; and perhaps other vitamins and minerals. A listing of cholesterol, fatty acid, and sodium content is optional.

How do I read grams?

Grams are smaller than ounces, and this smaller measurement is more precise. To give you an idea:

    1 pound = 454 grams (g)
    1 ounce = 28 grams (g)
    1 gram = 1,000 milligrams (mg)
    1 milligram = 1,000 micrograms (mcg)

How do I read RDA?

The U.S. recommended daily allowances (RDA) are the amounts of protein, vitamins, and minerals that are needed daily to be healthy. These are listed by percent on the label.

Why is it important to know about nutrition labeling?

Nutrition labels can help people in several ways to:

1. Plan more nutritious meals.
2. Get more nutrition for the food dollar.
3. Select foods for special diets.
4. Count calories.
5. Compare new foods with familiar ones.

Evaluation

LIFESTYLE CONTENT

☐ ☆

Have the students answer the following questions:

1. Since 1975, the nutrition labels on all fortified foods and on all foods for which a nutrition claim is made have displayed:
  a. net weight and ingredients
  b. number of calories in a serving size
  c. the number of servings per container
  d. Seven vitamins and minerals
  e. all of the above
2. Which of the following is *not* required on the nutrition label?
  a. riboflavin
  b. vitamin C
  c. cholesterol
  d. iron
  e. all of the above.
3. Nutrition labels show amounts in:
  a. grams
  b. ounces
  c. pounds
  d. liters
  e. all of the above
4. What does RDA mean?
  a. regular diet allowance
  b. recommended daily allowances
  c. regular diet averages

  d. recommended differences allowed
  e. all of the above
5. Nutrition labels can be used:
  a. to plan more nutritious meals
  b. to get more nutrition for your food dollar
  c. to count calories
  d. to select foods for special diets
  e. all of the above

LIFESTYLE CONTENT

☐ ☆

Ask each student to design a food carton with a nutrition label for a fortified food. Use the following checklist for evaluation.

1. ____ Name of product
2. ____ Net weight
3. ____ Ingredients
4. ____ Calories
5. ____ Protein
6. ____ Carbohydrate
7. ____ Fat
8. ____ Vitamin A
9. ____ Thiamin
10. ____ Riboflavin
11. ____ Niacin
12. ____ Calcium
13. ____ Iron
14. ____ Information appears on the right of the panel
15. ____ Nutrients listed in the correct order
16. ____ Information is per serving and gives serving size
17. ____ Number of servings in the container
18. ____ Indicates amount in grams
19. ____ U.S. RDA listed by percentage
20. ____ Label neatly done

LIFESTYLE VALUE

○ □ ☆

Evaluating Groceries

Ask the students to take a sheet of paper and do the following. On the left side of your paper, list five foods that your family frequently buys. Go to the store and look for three brands of each of these foods. Determine which brand helps you to get more nutrition for your food dollar. On the right side of the paper, write this brand name first, then your second choice. The brand with the least nutrition for your food dollar will be the third choice.

REFERENCES

1. Edith M. Selberg, Louise A. Neal, and Matthew F., *Discovering Science in the Elementary School* (Reading, Ma.: Addison-Wesley, 1970), pp. 232–233.

2. Sidney B. Simon, Leland W. Howe, and Howard Kirschenbaum, *Values Clarification* (New York: Hart, 1972).

ADDITIONAL NUTRITION RESOURCES

At the Local and State Level:
Contact Public Health nutritionists in state and local health departments; nutritionists in voluntary agencies, such as visiting nurse associations, diet counseling services, diabetes associations; and those in local hospitals and heart associations.

Nutritionists and dieticians are also found in clinics, health centers, and hospitals.

State and local cooperative extension services.

Professional organizations concerned with nutrition include the American Dietetic Association, American Home Economics Association, and American Public Health Association with state or local affiliate chapters.

University and college nutrition and medical faculty members.

Local affiliates of the National Dairy Council.

State and local welfare agencies.

At the National Level:
U.S. Department of Health, Education, and Welfare, 5600 Fishers Lane, Rockville, MD 20857. Health Services Administration/Bureau of Community Health Services, Food and Drug Administration.

U.S. Department of Agriculture, Washington, DC 20250.

National Dairy Council, 6300 North River Road, Rosemont, IL 60018 is probably the best source of nutrition education materials for use in schools.

CHAPTER 11

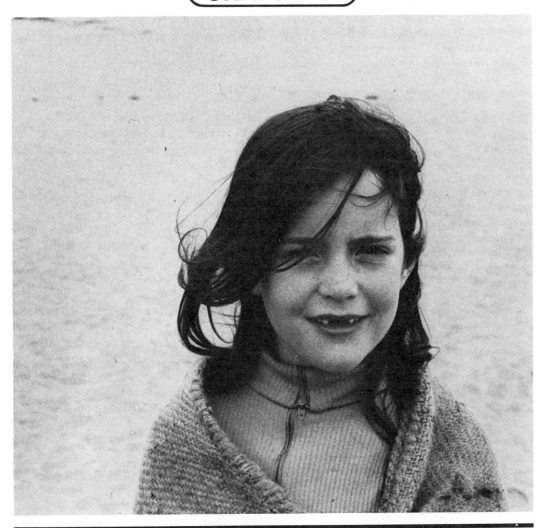

PART A: DENTAL HEALTH *

Dental health education is essential to the person interested in developing a healthy lifestyle. The authors hope that this chapter will present information and methods of translating that information into behavioral changes which will result in prevention of dental disease.

According to Nancy Jane Reynolds, D.D.S.,*

*This chapter was co-authored with Nancy J. Reynolds, D.D.S., Assistant Dean for Auxiliary Programs, College of Dentistry, The Ohio State University, 305 West 12th Avenue, Columbus, OH 43210. Dr. Reynolds is nationally recognized for her work in

259

This country is approaching a national health care crisis and systems must be developed to prevent and correct dental disease. Statistics do very little to motivate action, but it should be stated that dental disease affects more than 95 percent of our population and that only 40 percent of the total population receives any dental treatment. It is a responsibility of those with knowledge and expertise to educate the 60 percent who do not seek or receive dental care to appreciate optimal dental health. The public is becoming more and more aware of the availability of comprehensive health treatment and with third party payment plans, such treatment will become a possibility for more families.

An effort is currently being made to increase the number of dentists and auxiliaries and to improve the efficiency of those presently in practice by delegating many dental procedures to trained auxiliaries; however, the ultimate solution of dental problems lies in the prevention of diseases. Few people are aware that almost all dental problems are preventable and that each individual can control his own dental destiny. Only the individual can prevent dental decay and diseases of the bone and soft tissues (gums) which support and nourish the teeth. Furthermore, it is his responsibility to do so. This, however, involves a prior responsibility on the part of the educators, both school and dental, to provide the individual with the knowledge necessary for prevention (4, Preface).

---

resources, curriculum, and program development in dental health education and has graciously permitted large amounts of material from her publications *Guidelines for a Dental Health Curriculum for Public Schools* (4) and from the publication and *Dental Health Guide for Teachers* (3) which she edited and to which she contributed much material from the above publication to be incorporated into this chapter. Her teaching units have received overwhelming endorsement from Ohio dentists and educators, and the Ohio Dental Association published and distributes the *Dental Health Guide for Teachers.*

THE ROLE OF THE SCHOOL NURSE IN THE DENTAL HEALTH PROGRAM

School nurses in most school systems are more sensitive than anyone else to dental needs and the vast number of children who exhibit total dental neglect. They are frequently concerned but totally frustrated about obtaining assistance for these children. Consequently, they are generally eager allies in planning and implementing a dental health program.

School nurses can assist in the classroom and make personal contacts with parents. If there is a required registration of students, they can perform an invaluable service by taking a health history; checking a child's weight, height, and vision; and by looking into the child's mouth.

THE TEETH AND THEIR FUNCTIONS

A child has twenty primary (deciduous) teeth that begin forming before birth and start to erupt between four and eight months of age. Eight incisors (for cutting), four cuspids (for tearing) and eight molars (for grinding) have usually erupted by the time a child is two and a half years old.

Around age six, shedding begins as the permanent tooth, developing beneath the primary one, exerts pressure on the primary roots causing them to be resorbed. Gradually, the roots disappear, and the remaining crown portion of the tooth loosens as its support is lost. The tooth literally falls out of the mouth.

Permanent Teeth

The permanent tooth now emerges into the mouth. If the permanent anterior teeth erupt prior to the shedding of the corresponding deciduous teeth, the child may appear to have two rows of front teeth, since the permanent anterior tooth position is directly behind the corresponding primary tooth.

Mixed Dentition

At the same time this process is beginning, the first of the permanent molars appear. The period of mixed dentition (primary and permanent teeth in the process of shedding and erupting) lasts until the child approaches the teens. This is a difficult time for a child to practice good oral hygiene, since the process of eruption is sometimes accompanied by inflammation and infection. However, because the newly erupted teeth are highly susceptible to decay, they must be kept scrupulously clean. The child must be impressed with the need for thorough cleaning of the teeth and the tissue surrounding the teeth. He or she must be assured that this can be accomplished with very little discomfort so long as a hard-bristle brush is not used and close attention is paid to what he or she is doing.

The adult has thirty-two permanent teeth, consisting of eight **incisors** (cutting teeth) with single roots; four **cuspids** (or canine teeth), also with single roots; eight **bicuspids** (or premolars) with two raised parts, called cusps, on the crown and single or double roots; and twelve **molars** with ridged surfaces that are effective for grinding food.

WHY THE TEETH ARE IMPORTANT

Teeth give shape and expression to our face and mouth, as they support the lips and the cheeks. They determine the length of the face as they maintain the vertical relationship between the upper and lower jaws (4, p. 42).

Teeth have a direct influence upon the personality. Everybody likes to have pretty teeth, and one might sometimes get the idea that everyone has pretty teeth. Flip through the magazine ads and what do you see? Everyone seems to be smiling and showing their dazzling white teeth. People with bad teeth are often self-conscious about them, while people with good teeth find it easier to relax and be themselves.

Teeth enable people to chew food properly for body nourishment and well-being. The digestive process is facilitated when the teeth reduce food to small particles which are more readily broken down into a form easily assimilated. Teeth aid in enunciation and the sounding of words. Try to make these consonant sounds without involving the teeth: C,D,F,L,N,S,T,V,X,Z.

The loss of a single tooth creates many problems, since a gap causes the teeth to shift their positions in an effort to become stable again. Efficient and healthy functioning depends on the proper distribution of the work load. Teeth that are extruded and tilted receive forces in directions they were not designed to withstand. If the situation is not corrected through orthodontics, more teeth will soon be lost.

In the mouth of a small child, the problems of premature loss of a primary tooth are complicated by the underlying permanent teeth. Each primary tooth not only functions in the ways mentioned, but acts as a maintainer of a space in the mouth for its permanent successor. If a primary tooth is lost prematurely, the space is usually filled in by the drifting of the remaining teeth, and the permanent tooth is unable to erupt into its proper position. If it can erupt at all, it will be crowded out of alignment.

THE ROLE OF THE ELEMENTARY TEACHER IN DENTAL HEALTH EDUCATION

Teachers should ask themselves what the objective of dental health education is. The answer must be the prevention of dental disease. The methods of control which the schools have been teaching have failed in preventing the disease. Tooth decay is occurring among children six times faster than it is being corrected, and approximately 90 percent of all school-age children are in need of dental care. Twenty-four million American children between the ages of six and eleven each have an average of 10-1/2 decayed, missing, or filled teeth. In the United States, children between the ages of five and nine have over 71 million unfilled cavities.

There are not enough professional people available to remedy the damage which has already occurred; help is therefore needed from the classroom teacher to keep the problem from worsening. The classroom teacher is at present the only person who consistently has every child in a situation that adapts itself to mass prevention. She or he alone can play a significant role in this major health area.

Control methods in the prevention of

tooth decay to date have been to encourage regular and thorough cleansing of the teeth, elimination of sweet snacks, regular dental treatment, and an adequate diet. Some of these methods are the responsibility of the parents, who can teach their child how to clean the teeth, what a cavity is, and how to help prevent tooth decay.

THE PROCESS OF DECAY

Before prevention methods can be taught in the schools, both the teacher and the student must understand completely the process of decay. The process is so easily understood when presented correctly that even the kindergarten child can learn about it.

The process of decay is always associated with the presence of a deposit called dental plaque on the tooth. Plaque is a microscopic community of bacteria that also contains the waste products of bacteria; dead cells, which slough off the tongue or cheeks; and thick secretions of the glands which contain a gluelike protein called mucin. The essential portion of this deposit with regard to decay consists of the bacteria. It must be understood that the mouth is full of bacteria.

Except in a completely sterile environment, it would be impossible to free the mouth of organisms. However, those bacteria which are floating about free are not the ones with which we are concerned. Until they have affixed themselves to a tooth and begun to organize plaque, they are of no consequence in tooth decay. If the deposit is on a surface that is brushed regularly, at the next cleaning it will be removed. If it is not removed, the bacteria multiply and the plaque grows larger.

In the case of plaque, the bacteria that

survive are those not easily reached by a toothbrush, dental floss, the tongue, or by harsh foods which might remove the bacteria. Dental plaque *can* be removed by the individual, but since it is closely adherent to the tooth because of the attachment of the bacteria, it is not always easily removed. Built-up plaque is best removed by one's dentist during periodic dental checkups.

In order for bacteria to live and grow and carry on their activities, they must have food, just as people do. One of their chief sources of food is sugar. Saliva, which helps to cleanse the teeth, also helps dissolve food. Unfortunately, there are many refined sugars which are readily dissolved in the saliva and will cover the entire microbial colony with a substance it can readily utilize.

When the bacteria use up the sugars, their digestive processes, like ours, have waste products. Some bacteria (known as acidogenic bacteria) in the mouth produce as one of their products of elimination an acid. In plaque several days old which is composed of many acidogenic organisms, there may be considerable acid produced each time sugar is dissolved and floods the deposit of bacteria on the tooth.

The tooth to which the plaque is attached is vulnerable to acid, as are most things, especially living tissues. Whenever acid is produced on a tooth, some of the minerals that make the tooth hard are dissolved; a hole appears in the tooth and gets larger every time more acid is produced. After decay begins, it is irreversible; it does not heal the way a wound does.

Prevention of decay can begin by making the tooth harder and therefore less vulnerable to the acid through building fluoride into the tooth.

The following information regarding fluoride is adapted from Procter and Gamble's pamphlet *Fluorides—Fact vs. Fiction*.

Fluorides are chemical compounds of the halogen fluorine. They have been known to exist in minerals and have been used industrially for centuries. Their presence in plants, animals, and human tissues has been known for more than 160 years, yet accurate analytical methods for small quantities of fluorides have existed only since 1933.

Fluorides occur naturally in many foods of vegetable and fish origin, and it is almost impossible to select a diet totally free of fluorides.

In 1938, H. T. Dean and his associates proved the decay-inhibitory effects on dental tissue and first suggested a study of adding fluoride to water deficient in the fluoride ion.

Since then, over 50 clinical and 3,000 biological studies have been made and more than 9,000 articles published. Few preventive health measures have received such thorough and widespread approval.

The basic methods of administering fluorides are:

1. Ingestion into the body
   a. fluoridated community water supply
   b. home water fluoridation
   c. fluoride tablets or drops
2. Application to the teeth
   a. topical fluoride application by the dentist after prophylaxis
   b. fluoride prophylaxis paste
   c. effective fluoride toothpaste.

While fluorides do not completely eliminate decay, they significantly reduce it and would therefore partially solve the problem. Even with fluorides, a dirty tooth is simply a harder dirty tooth.

People could eliminate sugar, which would probably solve most decay problems; but it would not solve the problem of disease of the soft tissues or the gingiva (gums).

Although people need carbohydrates in their diets, it would be better for everyone to discourage indulgence in sweet snacks. Nutritionists are also concerned with the resultant diet of a child whose appetite is constantly curbed by sugary food.

The decay process can also be arrested or, better still, prevented by removing the dental plaque thoroughly and regularly before it reaches the quantity necessary for the production of sufficient acid to etch the tooth. Plaque can be cleaned from the teeth by the individual who understands where it is and how to remove it.

Plaque begins to grow back almost immediately after it is removed, but it takes a few hours to grow to maximal size in most mouths. Therefore, even more important than teaching the student to brush within fifteen minutes after eating is teaching that when cleaning the teeth, *every* deposit from *every* tooth must be removed at least once every day. This is not to say teachers should not encourage after-meal brushing. This is good oral hygiene and provides added insurance against decay, but the important battle against decay is waged when the individual has the time to do a complete and thorough cleaning.

HOW TO CLEAN THE TEETH

Disclosing Tablet

It is helpful to discuss with students the fact that just looking at the teeth does not always allow one to see the plaque that bacteria builds. However, a disclosing tablet will stain the bacteria a bright red color and allow students to easily see and thus remove the plaque. The disclosing agent is simply red food coloring, which is perfectly harmless and may be used indiscriminately by all individuals. Since it is in wafer form, it is less troublesome than a liquid, as it will not spill. If clothing is inadvertently stained, ordinary laundry methods will remove the stain.

PROPER USE

Disclosing wafers should not be used in the classroom before the teacher first explains their use and permits the students to clean their mouths thoroughly. (Teachers should also try this method themselves before using it in the classroom.)

The students should chew the wafers, roll the pieces around over all the teeth for about 30 seconds, and either swallow the residue or empty it into a paper cup. When they look into their mouths after using the tablet, they will observe the areas that are not clean, and the plaque will be clearly visible. Almost everyone will have many stained areas the first time the wafer is used, since few people have really clean mouths.

If the students have been properly prepared for this process, they will understand that the mouth is very dirty. If they did not brush their teeth, they will see why they should; if they did brush, they will see that there are many areas they missed or did not clean thoroughly.

The dye will dissipate in a very few minutes, since it is soluble in saliva. There is therefore no need to brush in the classroom if it is not convenient or if time does not permit. The stain will remain on the tongue longer than on the teeth, but this should present no problem.

Staining of the gingiva (gum tissue) indicates that colonies of bacteria lie in those areas and may cause inflammation of the tissues. Gums should be cleaned as thoroughly as the teeth.

Brushing the Teeth

Scientists have found evidence indicating that twigs were used as toothpicks by humans to clean their teeth over 3,000 years ago. The idea was elaborated for centuries until Victorian times, when the well-dressed man carried a gold toothpick.

Tooth cleaning was achieved with sponges and cloths by the 1700's. Pierre Fouchard, the French dentist, wrote careful instructions for cleaning teeth by using a wet sponge with salt water. At the same time, a brush was developed from natural products. Roots of special plants were boiled and cut into 6-inch pieces, and the ends were slit into brushes and dried. To use the brush it was necessary to wet the end and put it into tooth powder. The bristle toothbrush was developed in most European and Oriental countries about 300 years ago. It was not in common usage until about the 1800s, when large quantities of brushes were machine made.

Today, dentists usually recommend using a medium-soft or extra-soft brush.

Advantages of using a medium-soft brush are that:

1. The many bristles more completely cover the surfaces of the teeth.
2. The bristles are soft enough that they can be brushed over the gums and into the grooves.
3. The bristles can be pushed onto the surfaces away from the greater convexities of the teeth and also in between the teeth.

Advantages of using an extra-soft brush are that:

1. It can be used on or under any tissue, hard or soft, healthy or inflamed, and do no damage.

2. The bristles can reach more areas than those of any other brush.

While toothbrushing techniques vary, a definite routine is recommended so that every surface of each tooth is cleaned every time. Most dentists recommend that a person begin on the upper right last tooth. The teacher can help the students establish a beneficial brushing method by teaching them that there are five surfaces of every tooth that need to be cleaned:

A chewing surface with which even the smallest child is familiar.

A facial side (the outside which is seen when one smiles).

A lingual side (towards the tongue).

Two sides which touch the teeth on either side of the tooth. These are the surfaces which are found between the teeth. They are large areas that are particularly susceptible to decay because they are so difficult to clean. Few people ever clean them, yet it is on these areas that most new cavities begin.

Teachers should teach the student that teeth are not flat and brushing up and down will not do the job. A person must brush into those areas that are curved away from the most rounded portion of the tooth. This means pushing the bristles against the tooth with adequate pressure to ensure their finding their way onto every surface.

Flossing

"Generally, the tooth sits very tightly against the one in back of it and the one in front of it. The only way now available for cleaning these surfaces is with dental floss. These surfaces should be cleaned daily" (4, p. 37).

The following directions for flossing

should be observed. "The floss is inserted gently through the contacting parts of two teeth, wrapped around the tooth in back of the space and moved up and down. Repeat this on the tooth in front of the space and then remove the floss in the same way it was inserted, or if this is difficult, simply pull it straight out."

Repeat this procedure between all of the teeth.

"Unwaxed dental floss is excellent for cleaning because it does not leave a sticky residue to which the bacteria may affix themselves and begin forming a fresh plaque."

Toothpaste

"Most toothpastes that are marketed in the United States are safe, but one toothpaste may be better for you than another" (4, p. 38). According to Hamilton B. G. Robinson, D.D.S., the key to the choice lies in the product's polishing power and the nature of one's own teeth.

Every dentifrice contains an abrasive agent designed to polish the teeth. There is no reason generally to believe that the abrasives used in modern dentifrices cause increased vulnerability to tooth decay. No one has presented persuasive scientific evidence of tooth damage caused by dentifrices.

Yet there is a reason for some people to choose their toothpaste or powder with particular care. These people have exposed dentin, the softer material that makes up the exposed root of the tooth. While polishing agents cannot damage enamel, they can wear away dentin. A fairly significant number of Americans have this condition. About 15 percent of people in their early twenties have exposed dentin, and the percentage rises

with age. More than two of every five people in their fifties have it. The right dentifrice for such people is strong enough to keep the teeth free of brown stain but not strong enough to harm exposed dentin. To choose the correct dentifrice, a patient can ask the dentist's help.

For some brushers, such as children, other ingredients influence the choice of a dentifrice. Fluoride, for instance, is recommended for youngsters. Most people buy a toothpaste for taste and to make brushing more pleasant and easier. A thorough cleaning can be accomplished, however, by using a brush with salt or baking soda and flossing or by brushing with water alone and flossing.

"The thorough cleansing that is required to remove all plaque takes time to accomplish and should be done at night after the person has eaten for the last time. Much decay activity occurs at night when salivary flow is diminished. Also, at night the person has more time than during the day" (4, p. 38).

Mouthwash

According to the American Dental Association, the reason for using a mouthwash is to help remove food particles from the teeth and mouth. Drinking water is satisfactory to accomplish this. Some people prefer a diluted solution of common salt (½ teaspoonful to ½ glass of water) or of baking soda (¼ teaspoonful to ½ glass of water).

Medicated mouthwashes should not be used except when prescribed by a dentist. They have no effect on the bacteria in the mouth and are a waste of money and effort in tooth decay prevention.

GINGIVITIS AND OTHER ORAL PROBLEMS

Periodontal diseases are diseases of the soft tissues (gums) and bone which support the teeth. These diseases include gingivitis, an inflammation of the gingiva (correct terminology for gums).

Any inflammation is associated with swelling, redness, heat, and pain and is the body's response to injury. There may be many types of injury to the gums, such as damage from improper toothbrushing.

It could be that the gingiva is abraded or scraped off. Many can undoubtedly recall a tender area that they could trace back to a piece of toast or a slice of pizza. Generally speaking, however, a sore place in the mouth means the presence of infection, which is a condition in which bacteria or other living organisms (germs, viruses, etc.) have entered the body and are living and multiplying.

The ideal conditions for bacterial growth include a place that is protected, warm, moist, and constantly nourished. The gingival crevice could not be better suited. It is a little collar of gingiva that surrounds the tooth and is not tightly attached to the tooth. It is here that bacteria grow luxuriantly.

"Do these bacteria need our food to survive? If we were fed intravenously so no food passed through our mouth, would the bacteria all die? As long as our body was properly nourished, the bacteria would live and grow in numbers, but we would get no decay because there would be no sugar in the mouth. The bacteria would be getting their food from the gingiva.

"The gingiva secretes fluids constantly. These substances are rich in nutrients or foods for the bacteria.

"Bacteria are pretty 'ugly' little fellows.

They have a tendency to destroy everything they come into contact with. While they are going about their business of using up these foodstuffs from our body, they are also giving off certain substances.

"What do these waste products do to the gingiva? The gingiva not only secretes or manufactures and provides nourishment for the bacteria, but it also absorbs or takes in the substances that the bacteria are making. It is at this point that we have problems.

"The products produced by the bacteria are poisonous and injurious to the gingiva. They cause the tissue to be damaged. Immediately, we can have an inflamed red area and soon an infection.

"If the process stopped right here it would be serious enough since there are now areas in the mouth that hurt and bleed. However, this is only the first step" (4, pp. 49, 50).

People can remove the cause of infection. Through the use of disclosing tablets that stain not only plaque but also bacterial accumulations on the gingiva, people can properly clean their mouths.

Pyorrhea

"In the beginning stages, pyorrhea [also called periodontitis] may resemble gingivitis. As it progresses, the gingiva recedes from the tooth and a pocket, filled with bacteria and pus, may be formed. The bony support of the tooth is gradually destroyed and the tooth may be lost.

"Soft and hard deposits around the teeth and beneath the gum margin may lead to pyorrhea. These deposits with their bacterial inhabitants usually cause the initial irritation to the tissues" (3, p. 2). A person who never has gingivitis will never have pyorrhea.

"The best way to prevent this is by thorough and regular toothbrushing and flossing, adequate nutrition, and regular trips to the dentist for necessary treatment including correction of malocclusion, or crowded teeth.

"Periodontal disease, like gingivitis and decay, is the result of bacteria which are out of control in the mouth. This is the most serious and the most prevalent of all adult dental diseases (3, p. 2). (Tooth decay is the most prevalent childhood dental disease, and most of the damage it causes occurs before the age of 35. After that age, the chief cause of tooth loss is periodontal disease.)

There is some evidence which suggests that inadequate nutrition may be a factor in the development of periodontal disease or in a poor response to treatment. An inadequate or unbalanced diet or the inability of the body to make use of food properly may contribute to decreased resistance to periodontal disease.

Malocclusion

According to Thomas M. Graber, D.M.D., Chief of Orthodontics at the University of Chicago Hospitals, orthodontists are going through a period of major reassessment. Orthodontists formerly recommended corrective treatment because of the belief that a bad bite (malocclusion) usually led to tooth decay, gum disease, and other destructive changes in the oral cavity (2). In many cases, there has been no long-term evidence to support this general contention, but people are becoming more aware of the value of orthodontics and are more receptive to this type of treatment. Adult patients are becoming more numerous; today one out of every ten persons seeking orthodontic treatment is an adult, and the trend is increasing.

A recent survey conducted by the National Center for Health Statistics found that 50 percent of both boys and girls be-

tween the ages of twelve and seventeen definitely would like to see a dentist because of crooked teeth. Forty percent of the schoolchildren surveyed revealed that they preferred straight teeth with cavities to crooked teeth that were cavity free.

"The world, unfortunately, is filled with crooked teeth. An estimated 50% of the children in this country need some teeth-straightening work. Estimates of malocclusion problems, on a global scale, range up to 80%.

"Orthodontists agree that the most common treatment is to straighten the teeth that have crowded around a missing tooth so that room can be made for a bridge or partial denture to fill in the gap.

"Other typical procedures are aimed at teeth that are either pushed out too far or pushed in too much. Teeth that are twisted, crooked, spaced too far apart, or crowded too close together also merit correction" (2, p. 24).

Bad Breath

Television repeatedly warns people that they are not kissable because they have "moose breath" making Americans the most breath-conscious people in the world.

"Most of us—even if we practice good oral hygiene—do have mild halitosis at times," according to Howard E. Kessler, D.D.S. "Some of us seem to have chronically bad breath" (1, pp. 55–56).

Frequent sips of water might be the solution, or at least part of it. Dr. Kessler feels that water is the natural enemy of halitosis.

"When the mouth membranes dry out, we have unpleasant breath. This is because food particles decompose more quickly in a dry mouth—and bacteria multiply more quickly. It's the 'backward tide' of saliva that normally washes bacteria down the throat and keeps them from stagnating in the mouth" (1, p. 55).

This explains why most people have morning breath. The salivary functions slow down while people sleep, drying the membranes and causing a person to wake with a distasteful odor, no matter how carefully he or she had cleaned the mouth the night before.

Strong emotions such as fear, anxiety, sorrow, and anger may also contribute to mouth dryness, as can the taking of certain medications, such as tranquilizers and ulcer pills. Chronic dryness can also be a symptom of illness and should be checked by a physician. It is not merely inconvenient; it can be decay producing.

"All halitosis does NOT originate around the teeth. It can just as often come from the throat, nose, lungs, sinuses, and other parts of the body."

"However, it has been proven that bad breath can result from badly decayed and unbrushed teeth, pyorrhea, deep crevices in the tongue which hold decaying food particles, and a number of other oral conditions" (1, p. 56).

MOUTHWASHES

"Mouthwashes, often thought of as the cure-all for bad breath, have come under heavy fire in a preliminary study made by the National Research Council for the Food and Drug Administration.

"The NRC reported: 'There is no convincing evidence that any medicated mouthwash, used as part of a daily hygiene regimen, has any therapeutic advantage over a physiologic saline solution or even water.'"

BREATH FRESHENERS

"Mints, chewing gum, and other breath fresheners may effectively mask breath odor. And, even more, they have the advantage of tending to keep the mouth moist. The sugar in the gums or mints could promote tooth decay, but sugarless ones are now available in different flavors.

"If you are embarrassed by bad breath, visit your dentist and physician for checkups. Ask your dentist about a water-jet device. Brush your teeth carefully after meals. Try to avoid extreme emotions, and don't pass the water faucet without taking a sip" (1, p. 56).

Dental Emergencies

Teachers may be faced with dental problems more serious than bad breath. It is important to know how to handle a student with a toothache, fractured tooth, or a tooth that has been knocked out. The following procedures may be employed if a child is in pain or has had an accident to the teeth or jaws. Both the child's parent and the dentist must be consulted immediately.

1. Toothache
   a. Determine that the pain involves a tooth or teeth.
   b. Call a dentist or a clinic.
   c. Flush out any debris with dental floss and warm water.
   d. If swelling is present, apply cold to the face near the affected tooth.
   e. Do not place aspirin in a cavity or on the gum tissue next to the aching tooth.

2. Fractured Tooth
   a. Cover tooth with sterile gauze pad to protect it.
   b. Apply cold to face near fractured tooth to minimize swelling.
   c. Send child immediately to the dentist.

3. Knocked-Out Tooth
   a. Locate tooth and place it in a glass of water or wrap it in wet towel.
   b. Do not attempt to wash the tooth.
   c. Take tooth and child to the dentist immediately.

THE ROLE OF THE DENTIST—HOW THE DENTIST CAN HELP

"Dental disease can be prevented and the dentist can help prevent it. He can also repair damage that has been done. Everyone should be examined by a dentist at regular intervals. The dentist will determine how frequently to see a patient.

"The dentist or the dental hygienist can clean teeth professionally, removing any deposits, hard deposits which cannot be removed by the individual or soft deposits that are difficult to reach.

"They can help show a person how to do a more thorough cleaning of the mouth at home. They can apply fluorides to the teeth to make the enamel harder.

"The dentist will examine the teeth for cavities. He will take X-rays when it is necessary so that cavities that are on surfaces he cannot see can be repaired before they become extensive and painful.

"He will examine the mouth for infection or inflammation of the soft tissue; for example, the gingiva (gums), the tongue, the lips, and the cheeks. If there is soreness or swelling or bleeding of the soft tissues in the mouth, he will demonstrate what to do to solve this problem" (3, p. 12).

Perhaps the person is not eating enough foods with vitamin C, such as orange juice, grapefruit, or tomatoes. Perhaps the person is not eating enough foods with vitamin A, such as dark green vegetables (broccoli) or dark orange vegetables (carrots). Perhaps the diet does not contain enough protein or vitamin B, which is found in meats. Perhaps it is just that the soft tissues are not clean. This happens when people do not clean the gingiva when they brush their teeth.

If there are cavities, the dentist can restore the tooth to its natural shape and size and function with a filling. If there are problems that require a special dentist to solve, the dentist can refer the patient to someone for specialized service. For example, if the teeth are crooked, the dentist may send a patient to an orthodontist, a dentist who has special training in straightening teeth.

Other specialties recognized by the American Dental Association include:

Pedodontics: children's dentistry; equivalent to pediatrics in medicine.

Periodontics: diagnosis and treatment of periodontal disease which affects the gums and other structures surrounding and supporting the teeth.

Prosthodontics: making of crowns, dentures, and bridges.

Oral Surgery: diagnosis and treatment of oral tumors and lesions.

Oral Pathology: diagnosis of unusual oral conditions.

Endodontics: treatment of tooth pulp or nerve.

NUTRITION AND ORAL HEALTH

"Diet is important in the formation of the teeth, in maintaining the tissues of the mouth, and in the prevention of decay.

"In the formation and care of teeth, food is extremely important. The teeth begin to form before birth and the enamel is still forming until the child is eight years old.

"The body will build teeth no matter if it has the right materials or not. The kind of tooth it builds depends on the foods available to it.

"Every cell that is produced has protein in it—so we need eggs, meat, fish, milk, cheese, etc." (4, pp. 32–33).

Vitamins

"Vitamin A and Vitamin C are important to the formation of teeth and to the maintenance of the soft tissues (the gums, the tongue, the cheeks, etc.), so we need milk, butter, cheese, egg yolks, dark yellow or dark green vegetables or tomatoes for vitamin A; and citrus fruits, tomatoes, potatoes, cabbage or raw greens for Vitamin C" (4, p. 32).

Minerals

"The teeth are not hard when they are first formed, but before they erupt into the mouth, certain minerals are deposited into the tooth to harden it. These minerals are mainly calcium and phosphorus. Therefore, until the child is eight years old, he needs foods that supply these minerals.

"They are both found in milk, cheese, and greens. Phosphorus is found in fish and eggs as well as in meat and dried vegetables.

"Calcium is also necessary later for the development of healthy bones in the face and jaws and the rest of the body. It is essential throughout life for the muscles and the heart. In order for calcium to be used in the body, Vitamin D must be present—so milk with Vitamin D added, fish liver oils, or plenty of sunshine are also important" (4, p. 32).

"As soon as the first tooth appears in the mouth (usually at five to six months of age), dietary considerations involve the process of decay and the maintenance of the tissues. . . . After the age of eight, nutrition no longer involves the formation of the teeth."

Sugar

"The frequency of eating sugar, the form of the sugar, and the kind of sugar consumed are all important factors in the process of decay.

"Ordinary table sugar (sucrose) is the most cariogenic of the carbohydrates. In the foods containing it, the concentration of sugar is usually high enough to penetrate the plaque and provide a suitable diet for the bacteria.

"Each time a food containing table sugar is consumed, if there are plaques on the teeth with acid-forming bacteria, there will be acid on the tooth. This occurs within five minutes, and the acid will remain on the tooth up to thirty minutes. Each exposure to sugar in a

day adds up to thirty minutes of potential decay activity."

"If the sugar is in the form of a sticky, retentive food that may be held against the teeth over a long period of time, the length of time of exposure to acid is increased" (4, p. 33).

Snacks

Sweet snacks are extremely harmful, because they usually contain table sugar and because they are eaten between meals, which adds significantly to the total time of acid formation. However, families can select a lifestyle that substitutes foods which provide better nutrients and which are not a dental hazard. Nuts, fresh fruits, fresh vegetables, and popcorn are preferable to candy, cake, and cookies.

Eating the right foods will not prevent tooth decay, but it will help assure well-formed teeth and contribute to healthy gums and bone structures supporting the teeth. The reduction of sweets (the average American consumes approximately 100 pounds of sugar a year) in the diet will reduce decay.

Other foods to avoid include canned sweetened fruits and juices, cocoa, dates, figs, honey, jams, jellies, soft drinks, raisins, syrups, and all dried fruits. If it tastes sweet, it is probably loaded with sugar.

Heat and Cold

Hot foods and cold drinks may be enjoyable together, but there is evidence that the combination can result in dental damage. University of Utah researchers have found that intensive cycles of heat and cold can cause tiny cracks in tooth enamel, inviting tooth decay and the possibility of tooth fracture.

Heat alone seems to do no harm. Cold

is the villain, and when warm teeth are suddenly exposed to cold, the temperature drop can be shocking. Thus, if after-dinner coffee of 140 degrees is followed by ice cream at 35 degrees, the enamel contracts severely. The inner tooth material, however, retains its normal dimensions. The resulting pressure on the shrinking enamel may make the tooth crack. Repeated exposure to such temperature changes increases the probability of tooth fracture.

Another way to injure teeth is by chewing cracked ice, warns Wayne S. Brown, one of the researchers. The physical pressure from chewing the hard ice combined with the sudden temperature drop subjects teeth to dangerously high levels of stress.

PARENTAL RESPONSIBILITY

The real responsibility for prevention lies with each individual. However, the child must have someone else who will assume the responsibility not only to help teach him the techniques, but also to teach him how to assume his own responsibility.

The parent's responsibility is to:

1. Supervise and assist in regular and thorough cleansing of the mouth.

2. Provide the child with a well-balanced diet and control the consumption of sweet snacks.

3. Provide the child with regular dental treatment.

Ideally, the dentist would initiate preventive education and regular dental treatment both preventive and reparative; the parents would implement the preventive procedures at home and supervise the child until the habits were established. The teacher could reinforce this with a dental health unit in the classroom, and the result would be an effective team approach to preventing dental disease.

The parents must be involved in the preventive program and we must seek ways to involve them. Information for them can be included in P.T.A. meetings. Printed information can be sent home to them and they can be recruited to act as aides in the classroom.

The teacher cannot provide constant daily supervision year in and year out, but the parent can. However, the teacher can provide enough repetition to begin to establish a pattern (4, p. 44).

The teacher can also bring to the parents' attention some basic teaching principles that most parents do not know. Most parents do not know, for example, that children learn by using their hands and that they are eager for adult as well as peer approval.

Most parents are not aware that ther children are seeking behavior patterns and that they have different psychological needs at different ages.

The teacher could help the parent provide home support and reinforcement by educating the parent too. Parents frequently do not understand their role toward their child's learning experiences. They need to know that their role is one of an encouraging, cooperative, and understanding consultant.

The child wants to feel that the parent approves of whatever projects he is involved with. The parent should never exhibit disapproval or derision because it confuses the child. Who is right—the teacher or mother? The child may become resentful of the teacher and this is an effective barrier toward further learning. It may force the child to choose between the parent and the teacher and children do not like to make choices between people they respect.

The parent should be as fully informed as possible about the health program and should be encouraged to set the example at home. Others in the family can and should receive the benefits of a preventive health program. The informed parent can provide supervision and guidance for the entire family.

We need an agreement of goals by the teacher, the parent, and the child, the understanding of the methods of achieving these goals, and their consistent guidance. All of these are essential to the success of an effective health education program. The parent and the teacher must be fully informed and in basic agreement. They can then act as a team to teach and supervise the child (4, p. 45).

CHANGING THE BEHAVIOR PATTERN OF THE CHILD

If we are to be effective with our teaching and realize our goal which is the prevention of dental disease, we must remember that the imparting of factual knowledge does not necessarily result in a change in attitude. We need the change in attitude with a resultant change in behavior.

Information is essential to wise decision-making. However, even though he retains the facts presented to him, a child must be motivated to change a habit.

Dental health must be taught by providing information and building on this base to relate the facts into concepts.

Perception is the capacity for comprehension. We view facts and symbols and patterns begin to form. We begin to perceive relationship among the facts. Ideas emerge and we call these ideas concepts.

Every concept is subject to change and we differentiate and make choices and decisions. There are many choices open to us, but often the choices are not clear (4, p. 46).

It is a teacher's responsibility to help make the choices known and to guide the child in making rational decisions and clarifying his values, keeping in mind that a person chooses values that are relevant to his life.

REFERENCES

1. Howard E. Kessler, "Bad Breath!", *Family Health* (October 1969): 55–56.

2. Ronald Kotulak, "The Old Gray Braces Ain't What They Used to Be," *Today's Health* (January 1976).

3. The Ohio State Dental Association, the Ohio Department of Health, and The Ohio State University, College of Dentistry, *Dental Health Guide for Teachers*, 1973 revised edition, Council on Dental Public Health and Information, Ohio Dental Association, 41 South Third Street, Suite 207, Columbus, OH 43215.

4. Nancy Jane Reynolds, *Guidelines For a Dental Health Curriculum for Public Schools*. Published by the Ohio State University, Columbus, Ohio. Revised February 8, 1974. Copies may be obtained by writing to Dr. Reynolds at 305 West 12th Avenue, Columbus, Ohio 43210.

ADDITIONAL DENTAL HEALTH RESOURCES

American Cancer Society, 219 East 42nd Street, New York, NY 10017. (Pamphlets: Cancer of the Mouth; Cancer of the Larynx; Open Wide; Your Defense Against Cancer of the Mouth)

American Dental Association, Bureau of Dental Health Education, 211 East Chicago Avenue, Chicago, IL 60611. Write for a catalog listing pamphlets, posters, and films.

Amurol Products Company, P.O. Box 300, Naperville, IL 60504. (Pamphlets: The Critical Years of Tooth Decay; Enjoy Good Teeth and Good Times; Guideposts to Better Brushing)

Block Drug Company, Inc., 105 Academy Street, Jersey City, NJ 07302. (Pamphlets, large typdont and toothbrush)

Colgate Palmolive Company, 300 Park Avenue, New York, NY 10022.

Crest, Professional Services Division, Procter and Gamble Company, P.O. Box 171, Cincinnati, OH 45201.

Denoyer-Geppert, 5235 Ravenswood Avenue, Chicago, IL 60601 (films, transparencies, posters, and tooth models).

Johnson and Johnson, Consumer Services, Dental Care, 501 George Street, New Brunswick, NJ 08903 (films, pamphlets, samples of dental floss). For dental floss write to Johnson's Dental Floss, Box 308, Cherry Hill, NJ 08002.

Division of Dental Health, National Institutes of Health, 9000 Rockville Pike, Bethesda, MD 20014 (pamphlets and posters).

PART B: TEACHING ABOUT DENTAL HEALTH

Constant tooth decay seems to be a disease of modern civilization. Some 25 million Americans lose all of their teeth by middle age. Although 90 million Americans have at least eighteen missing, decayed, or filled teeth, only four out of ten Americans are receiving any dental treatment. In contrast, people who live in remote areas of the world under primitive conditions have a lifestyle that is relatively free of tooth decay. When these people adopt the average American lifestyle, their teeth begin to decay immediately.

Although diet is probably a major factor, many questions remain regarding the extraordinary lack of dental decay in some parts of the world. While research continues, there is a great deal that one can personally do to have a healthy mouth and still live in this country. By the daily removal of plaque, people are helping both their teeth and their gums. Dental health units involve students in the process of learning about and practicing such recommended measures as toothbrushing, flossing, selecting orally safe snacks, and visiting the dentist. The students learn how to protect their teeth both from decay and from accidental injury.

Teachers can motivate students to value their oral health and consequently to practice habits which result in the prevention of dental disease by recognizing the students' following needs regarding their dental health:

1. Students need to recognize that to a great extent they are responsible for their dental destiny.

2. Students need to appreciate the physical and psychological value of having healthy teeth.

3. Students need to understand that it is now possible for them to keep their teeth all their lives.

4. Students need to realize that false teeth have special problems and must be given more care than natural teeth.

UNIT I: TEETH TO LOSE AND TEETH TO KEEP

Children are interested in their teeth—how they grow and why they fall out. They are curious about false teeth. The purpose of this unit is to answer their questions and to impress upon them that it is now possible for them to keep their teeth for as long as they live.

OBJECTIVES

1. The student will explain in his or her own words how teeth grow and why they are lost.

2. The student will identify the names of the different teeth and the function of each during the game, What Tooth Am I?

3. The student will be able to describe precautions that will help prevent injuries to the mouth and face and will explain the correct procedure to follow if a tooth is accidentally fractured or knocked out.

Appropriate grade levels are suggested for each teaching strategy and appear as ○, □, ☆ in the left-hand column.
○ = most suited for the primary grades;
□ = most suited for the intermediate grades;
☆ = most suited for the upper elementary grades.

4. The student will express his or her attitude toward his or her teeth through a rank-order activity.

MATERIALS

1. Paper and pencils, 8-by-5-inch index cards.

2. Poster board, glue, and objects such as pencils, hair clips, bobby pins, paper clips, pens, sticks.

3. Atlas Figures 17, 18, and 19: Functions of Teeth, Primary and Permanent Teeth, How Does a Tooth Grow?

4. Poster: Have a Happy, Healthy Smile.*

5. Scissors, pliers, a nutcracker, a mortar and pestle, various foods.

Methods

Introduction

○ □

This unit may be introduced by asking the students to draw pictures of themselves smiling and showing their teeth. Ask the students to describe something that makes them smile. Display the poster Have a Happy, Healthy Smile. After reviewing the dental health content chapter, discuss such questions as Why do you think we need teeth? and Why are they different shapes?

○ □

Functions of Teeth

Using Atlas Figure 17, Functions of Teeth, explain that each tooth has its own special job in helping people chew their food. Demonstrate this concept by permitting the students to use scissors, pliers, a nutcracker, and a mortar and pestle in an effort to break up different kinds of foods while you provide the following information.

*Available from the National Dairy Council.

Incisors (Scissors) The front teeth are called incisors. You can see that they have a flat, rather sharp edge. These are the teeth we use to cut, or incise, our food. They work very much like your pair of scissors that has a flat, rather sharp edge and can cut through an apple.

Cuspids (Pliers) The next teeth are called cuspids. (Some people call them canine teeth or fangs.) The cuspids come to a sharp point, often called a cusp. These teeth tear food apart. Look at the end of the pliers. Can you tear off a piece of licorice using pliers?

Bicuspids (Nutcracker) The teeth next to the cuspids are the bicuspids. As you know, bi means two, as in bicycle, which has two wheels. These teeth are called bicuspids, because they have two points or cusps. The bicuspids help us to tear and crush our food. Although we know we could hurt or chip our teeth if we used them to crack a nut, you may try cracking a nut using a nutcracker to compare the way the bicuspids work.

Molars (Mortar and Pestle) In the very back of the mouth are the molars. There are (or will soon be) two molars on the top and bottom of both sides of the mouth. As you get older, you will probably get still another set of molars. These are called wisdom teeth, because most people do not get them until they are in their twenties and have acquired more knowledge than when they were younger. The molars help to crush and grind food into small pieces. Try to grind or break apart a cracker with a mortar and pestle.

○ □

Primary and Permanent Teeth

Using Atlas Figure 18, Primary and Permanent Teeth, review the various teeth and their functions. This transparency may lead to the observation that there are more permanent teeth than primary teeth. Children are interested in knowing why they lose their baby teeth. Explain that this process occurs as the permanent tooth developing beneath the primary one exerts a pressure on the primary roots, causing them to be resorbed. Gradually, the roots disappear and the remaining crown portion of the tooth loosens and falls out.

○

How Does a Tooth Grow?

Compare a growing tooth to a growing plant by using the following explanation and Atlas Figure 19, developed by Nancy J. Reynolds, D.D.S.:

> Everyone has seen how a plant grows. A seed grows into a plant because there is food and water in the earth. As it grows, the seed changes in size and shape and finally grows up through the ground. The seed has now become a plant.
>
> A tooth grows in much the same way. At first it is very small, like a seed. It does not look like a tooth at all. You cannot see it while it is growing because it is inside the jawbone just as the seed was inside the earth. There is food and water and there are minerals in the body for the growing tooth to use just as there was food and water in the earth for the seed to use. As the tooth grows, it becomes larger and it begins to look like a tooth. Finally, it comes up through the bone and into the mouth. When this happens, we say the tooth has erupted. This means part of it is now in the mouth where we can see it (2, p. 98).

○ □

X-Rays

When available, show X-rays of a child's jaw (showing the permanent teeth embedded in the jawbone and the primary teeth visible) or a jawbone from a calf (cow jawbone) showing teeth in the jawbone that can be seen because the gingiva is not present.

○

Bulletin Board

Divide a bulletin board into two sections. The left side should be devoted to pictures showing the important jobs of primary teeth (for chewing food, helping a child to talk, and reserving space for the permanent teeth forming beneath them). The right side should illustrate ways people sometimes lose their teeth (e.g., bumping someone at the drinking fountain or shoving someone on the playground). Students should be warned about putting objects such as pencils, hair clips, bobby pins, pens, and sticks into their mouths, as they may also cause injury to the teeth and gums. Such items may be glued to poster board for display on a bulletin board.

○ □

Knocked-Out Tooth

Role play a scene showing a child's tooth being knocked out because she or he fell or had a rock thrown at her or him. The tooth should be found, wrapped in a wet cloth (preferably dipped in salt water), and taken with the child to a dentist as fast as possible. A tooth's soft inner pulp cannot survive outside the mouth for more than thirty minutes. The dentist will bathe the tooth in a sodium fluoride solution to help retard the loss of valuable root material, coat the tooth with an antibiotic, and put it back in its socket. The antibiotic stimulates the growth of jawbone around the tooth, thereby securing the tooth in the mouth once again.

Ask the students how old they expect

to be when they have to get false teeth. Impress upon the students that it is not necessary for them ever to lose their teeth.

○ □
False Teeth

Show a set of false teeth to the class, and ask the students if they think false teeth are just as good as their own. If a child answers yes, spend some time discussing appearance, comfort, and care of false teeth.

You might ask the class to locate some pictures of George Washington. Ask if he is smiling or if they can see his teeth. Tell the class about Dr. Reidar Sognnaes, Professor of Anatomy and Oral Biology at UCLA, who has made a scholarly hobby of studying the dental tribulations of George Washington. Sognnaes said the first president of the United States had dental troubles which affected him so severely that not only was his intake of food limited, but he had to avoid *s* sounds in his speech. He said Washington was so sensitive on the subject that when he sought dental care, he instructed his staff that the matter "not be made a parade of." In fact, he once camouflaged his dental bill by paying it as a hat bill.

Sognnaes said the President's dilemma resulted from bad gums rather than tooth decay. By the time he took office at age fifty-seven, Washington had only one of his own teeth left. The professor said the President tried dentures made of wood, lead, gold, and tusks of elephants and walruses. Emphasize to the students that although false teeth are much more comfortable and better looking today than in George Washington's time, they still do not compare favorably to the real thing.

Evaluation

LIFESTYLE CONTENT

○ □
What Tooth Am I?

Arrange players in a semicircle (ten or sixteen students) to represent a row of teeth. (Twenty or thirty-two students could also play—creating two semicircles representing the upper and lower teeth.)

At the start of the game, another player closes her or his eyes and walks by the "teeth," stopping to gently tap one student. The student has to identify what kind of tooth he or she is and what function he or she performs. If the student answers correctly, he or she gets to select the next "tooth." If the student answers incorrectly, the tooth is lost and is removed from the row of teeth.

This game can also be played similarly to musical chairs. When the music stops playing, the one "tooth that is left without a socket" has to explain how he or she got "knocked out" (e.g., while playing baseball the ball hit him or her in the mouth). If the student can also describe a precaution that could have helped prevent the accident, he or she gets to remove a chair from the game and start and stop the next round of music.

○ □ ☆
Teethingo

If there are twenty-five students in your class, prepare twenty-five Teethingo cards by dividing an 8-by-5-inch index card into sixteen equal boxes (see Figure 11B-1). Print one word or term in each box. If possible, a piece of clear contact paper should be placed over the index card to prolong its use. (Remember, as with bingo, the cards will *not* be identical to each other.)

Prepare forty or more question cards using 8-by-5-inch index cards. Include the correct answer on each card. Possible question cards might be:

What are the front teeth that bite off large pieces of food (incisors)?

If a person must have all his or her teeth pulled, what do we call the manufactured replacements (false teeth)?

Should aspirin be placed next to an aching tooth (no)?

Each student will need sixteen markers. They can be small squares of poster board, buttons, bottle caps, etc.

After reading a question card, give the students time to think of the answer and place a marker on their cards if the correct answer appears.

Before each game is started, stipulate what will qualify as a Teethingo, for example, four in a row, four corners, everything covered.

When a student feels he or she has met the qualifications, check the answers. (The game could also be used by individual students in a learning center as review.)

FIGURE 11B-1 Sample bingo card

Incisors	Yes	Molar	Cutting Food
Appearance	Dentist	Grind Food	Space Retainer
Tearing Food	False Teeth	No	Bicuspid
Gum Injury	Speech	Antibiotic	Mixed Dentition

LIFESTYLE VALUE

○ □ ☆

Have each student list at least three reasons why teeth are important and rank the reasons according to what is most important to them. Compare the lists.

UNIT II: DIETARY HABITS AND ORAL HEALTH

The purpose of this unit is to help the student understand that it takes many different kinds of foods for optimum growth and healthy teeth. A lifestyle that encourages food and snacks consisting of meat, fish, and poultry; milk and cheese; fruits and vegetables; and bread and cereals is essential for proper development and maintenance of teeth, gums, bones, and tissues. Snacks that are selected just for their taste and without concern for the nutritional value are often high in sucrose and low in nutrients. These snacks are associated with cavity formation and obesity.

OBJECTIVES

1. The student will demonstrate her or his understanding of orally safe foods (without sugar) and orally hazardous foods (containing sugar) by placing pictures of various foods in the correct bulletin board bag.

2. Given a handout of orally safe and hazardous snacks, the student will draw pictures of orally safe foods that she or he enjoys that are juicy, crunchy, thirst quenching, and hunger satisfying.

3. The student will develop an awareness of his or her snacking behavior by keeping a personal snack food diary for three days.

MATERIALS

1. Atlas Figure 87, Orally Safe and Hazardous Snacks.

2. Orally safe foods, paper plates, utensils, napkins.

3. Food models or magazine pictures of food.

4. Poster board (28 x 22 inches), metal paper fasteners, sugar cubes, two medium-size brown paper bags, construction paper, scissors, glue, crayons, and felt-tip markers.

Methods

○

Favorite Foods

Have the students bring in pictures of their favorite foods from magazines and mount them on construction paper. During the week they are to place their foods in the bag in which they believe it belongs—Timothy Toothache (orally hazardous) or Charlie Chew (orally safe). See Figure 11B–2. At the end of the week,

FIGURE 11B-2 Dirty Dan and Shiny Sam bulletin board (Developed by Mary Ungarvsky)

Shiny Sam

Dirty Dan

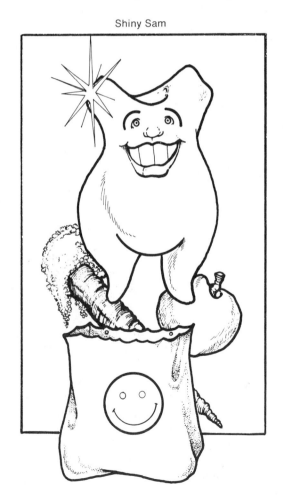
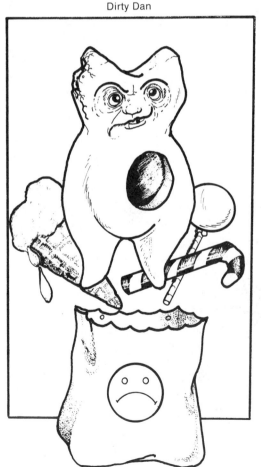

remove all of the food models from the bags and discuss with the class if each food is in the correct bag, what kind of food it is, who likes it, and what food appeared most often.

To construct the bulletin board, paper one side of the bulletin board with one color of construction paper and the other side with another color. Draw Charlie Chew and Timothy Toothache. Add two paper bags with a happy face or a sad face for the children to place their food pictures in.

○ □

Tasting Party

Have a tasting party featuring foods that make orally safe snacks, or display models and photographs of safe snacks and have the students select foods from the food groups that are nutritious and safe for the teeth.

□ ☆

Food Diary

Have the students keep a personal snack food diary for three days and list each snack they eat on a sheet of paper with two columns labeled "Safe" and "Hazardous." Ask them to classify each snack as either orally safe or orally hazardous by checking the appropriate column.

○ □ ☆

Continuum

Have the students identify their positions on a snack continuum.

Sugar Sweet	Nancy Nutrition
Sherry eats only	eats only orally
candy and foods	safe foods from
that are sweet.	the four food
	groups.

○ □ ☆

Sugar Cube Chart

Several students may wish to help you make a sugar cube chart, designed to visually demonstrate the amount of sugar in common snack foods. Glue pictures of common snacks to the left of a piece of poster board, and write the number of teaspoons of sugar in the various foods (see Table 11B–1 for suggestions). Graphically illustrate this quantity by gluing sugar cubes to the poster board (one sugar cube represents one teaspoon of sugar).

Evaluation

LIFESTYLE CONTENT

○ □ ☆

Snack Spin

The object of the snack spin game (courtesy of the American Dairy Council) is to choose orally safe foods. The player or team with the most points wins. Directions for the game are as follows:

1. Number of participants (one or two players, or two class teams).
2. Equipment
    a. 1 poster board (28 x 22 inches)
    b. 1 spinner
    c. 16–20 Dairy Council food models or magazine food pictures
    d. 16–20 flip-up answer tabs
    e. 16–20 metal paper fasteners
3. Construction directions
    a. Gameboard (draw and cut a 21–3/4-inch circle from poster board).
    b. Spinner
        Cut arrow from poster board (see pattern in Figure 11B–3).
        Punch small hole in center of arrow.
        Punch small hole in center of gameboard.

TABLE 11B-1 TOO MUCH SUGAR IS A TOOTH WRECKER

Picture of Food or Snack	Amount of Snack	Amount of Sugar in Teaspoons (shown in sugar cubes)
Chewing gum	1 stick	½
Average cookie	1	1–3
Jams and jellies	1 tablespoon	2½–3
Soft drink	8 ounces	5
Cocoa	6 ounces	4
Ice cream	⅛ quart	5–6
Apple pie	⅙ of 9″ pie	12
Devil's food cake	1/12 of 9″ cake	15
Gelatin dessert	½ cup	4½
Raisins	4½ tablespoons	4
Chocolate pudding	½ cup	4
Orange juice	½ cup	2
Grapefruit	½ medium	3½
Milk chocolate bar	1 ounce	8
Chocolate syrup	2 tablespoons	4
Cake type of doughnut	1	6

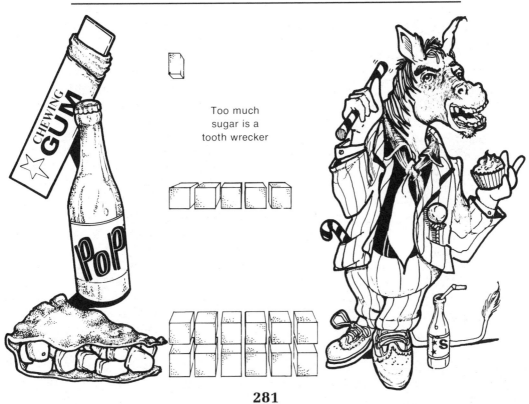

Too much sugar is a tooth wrecker

FIGURE 11B-3 Patterns for snack spin game

Arrow spinner pattern

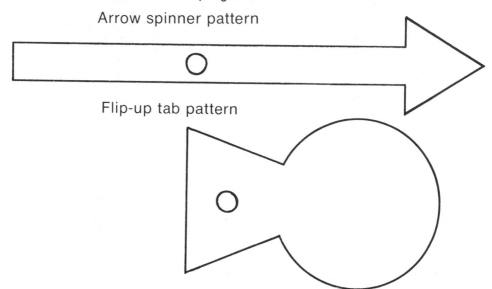

Flip-up tab pattern

Attach arrow with metal paper fastener in center of gameboard. (Arrow should spin freely.)

c. Select orally safe foods and orally hazardous foods to use on gameboard from the following:

Dairy Council food models—attach to gameboard around outside circumference with tape so that they can be removed and used in other teaching activities.

Magazine food pictures—permanently attached to gameboard.

Orally safe foods might include cheese, celery, carrots, potato chips (not nutritious), milk, apple, orange, banana, cottage cheese, hard-boiled egg, popcorn, pizza.

Orally hazardous foods might include soft drinks, cake, cookies, pie, candy bar, jelly, raisins, sugar-coated cereal.

d. Answer tab

Draw and cut flip-up tab from poster board (see pattern in Figure

11B–3). Make a flip-up tab for each food placed on gameboard. Draw either a smiling face or frowning face on each tab to correspond with orally safe or orally hazardous foods.

Punch a small hole 3/4 of an inch from edge of gameboard.

Punch a small hole 3/4 of an inch from edge of flip-up tab.

Attach tab to back of gameboard with metal paper fasteners. (Tabs should move freely.)

4. To play game (all tabs should be behind the gameboard).

Player spins spinner and decides if the food is orally safe or orally hazardous.

The flip-up tab is used to see if the student answered correctly.

If the answer is correct, the student or team receives a point.

The student or team with the most points wins the game.

Game may also be used for self-evaluation.

LIFESTYLE VALUE

○ □ ☆
Rank-Order Game

To construct, horizontally divide a piece of poster board in half. Divide the top half into three sections and number them. If the game is to be held up in front of a class rather than played on a table, attach three small pieces of hook and loop tape on the bottom half of the poster board. Mount pictures of snacks on construction paper and attach a small piece of hook and loop tape to the back of each one (or use Dairy Council food models).

Object of the game is to have the student rank the three food models from most cariogenic (cavity causing), to least cariogenic.

UNIT III: TOOTH DECAY AND DISEASE PREVENTION

Tooth decay is a prevalent disease that strikes almost all children but could be greatly reduced with regular and thorough cleansing of the teeth, a balanced diet low in sweets, and regular trips to the dentist. It is the teacher's responsibility to assist parents in teaching the child proper oral hygiene techniques and the value of good dental health.

OBJECTIVES

1. The students will identify bacteria in dental plaque as a causative factor in tooth decay.

2. After participation in classroom activities, the students will demonstrate their understanding of bacteria by writing a short paragraph describing how they feel about bacteria in the mouth.

3. The students will identify parts of the tooth affected as decay progresses and correctly explain the process that leads to tooth decay.

MATERIALS

1. Atlas Figures 20 and 21, Parts of a Tooth and Process of Tooth Decay.

2. Nitrazine paper, sterile cotton swabs, and color comparison chart if the student is to test his or her saliva for acidity/alkalinity (see science experiments in Unit V, Interdisciplinary Activities).

FIGURE 11B-4 Rank-order game

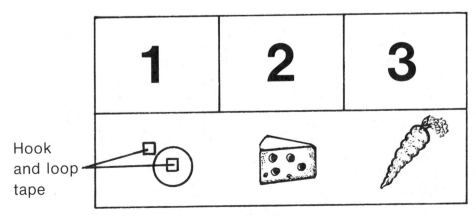

Hook
and loop
tape

3. The science experiments also show the presence of bacteria in the mouth and ways in which acid will weaken substances containing calcium. These experiments involve two eggs, two teeth, a jar of vinegar or 10 percent hydrochloric acid or soft drink containing sugar and phosphoric acid, gelatin, sugar, two shallow dishes, a pressure cooker or oven, and toothpicks.

Methods

○

Tooth Story

Young children are often motivated to learn through stories. Make up a story which relates to the students in your classes. It could be similar to the following story found in *Guidelines for a Dental Health Curriculum for Public Schools* (2, pp. 60–62).

Susan's Beautiful Tooth

Once upon a time there was a tooth which lived in the mouth of a little girl named Susan. Susan was five years old. Susan's tooth was beautiful.

In a little box in a drawer, Susan's mother had a string of pearls that were the same color. It was important that the tooth was beautiful because every time Susan smiled, everyone could see the tooth. The tooth was very proud to be so white and shiny. Susan's tooth had a job to do every day, and it worked hard at this job. It had to cut up Susan's food at every meal and it also had to help Susan whenever she talked to someone. The tooth was very busy all day long.

One day when she was working, Susan's tooth saw a very mean-looking germ go past her. He had a gang of his

friends with him. They were very nasty, ugly germs. They sat down on the beautiful tooth and they looked all around. They saw a place on Susan's tooth that Susan did not keep very clean. It was a sticky fuzzy place—just the kind of place germs like.

"Let's spend the night here," said one of them. "What if that little girl brushes us off here with her toothbrush?" asked another. "Look around you," said someone else, "she hasn't brushed this spot in days. Let's stay awhile and see if it's safe."

For two days they stayed and they watched and they waited. Many times Susan came very close to them with her toothbrush, but she never quite reached them. When the toothbrush came near them they held their breath and waited in great fear, but after a week the gang of big ugly germs decided that this was a safe ·hideout. They sent for all of their friends. They came by the thousands and built a large strong city. They waited and they watched.

One day Susan ate a piece of cake. The germ city was flooded with sugar—and germs love sugar. It makes them grow big and strong. They make acid out of sugar and you know acid is very strong and eats holes in anything it touches. On Susan's tooth there were so many germs making acid out of all that sugar that soon there was a hole in the tooth. Now the tooth was no longer new and shiny and beautiful. The tooth was very unhappy. How it hoped Susan would clean off the hideout of the germs. The next day Susan ate a piece of candy. Again the germs had an enormous meal and they made more acid. The hole in the beautiful tooth became bigger. Now the tooth was getting sick. It was in great pain. "Mother, my tooth hurts," Susan said.

Susan's mother looked and saw the city the germs had built. She took Susan's toothbrush and helped her destroy the city and brushed it away until the beautiful tooth was once again clean and shiny. But alas, the hole would never go away and Susan's beautiful tooth was ashamed because it had an ugly spot on it. Susan's mother said, "We will go to the dentist and he will make your tooth well again. He will put a shiny silver filling in it. It will never again be as beautiful as a pearl, but if we take care of it, it will last forever."

Susan looked in her mouth and saw all of the other beautiful teeth that were hers to take care of and she said, "Never again will I be careless about a single tooth. I will clean every one of you every day and I will be very careful not to miss a single place."

Susan's beautiful tooth smiled and once again was happy.

The important things to keep in mind when telling the story are those facts you want the students to retain.

1. The need for thorough cleaning.
2. The consequences if people neglect to clean.
3. An explanation of what causes teeth to decay.

○ □

Filmstrip

Older students will enjoy watching the filmstrips contained in *Toothtown, USA* * and creating their own stories.

□ ☆

Parts of a Tooth

Use Atlas Figure 20, Parts of a tooth, to

*Available from the local branch of the National Dairy Council.

review the structure of a tooth, and offer the following corresponding definitions:

A—Enamel: covers the crown and is the hardest substance in the body.

B—Dentin: an ivorylike tissue that makes up the main portion of the tooth.

C—Pulp: the pulp cavity contains blood vessels, nerves, and connective tissue. It is the heart of the tooth.

D—Cementum: a bonelike substance covering the root.

E—Periodontal membrane: lines the tooth socket and covers the root. This membrane helps hold the tooth in its place and serves as a cushion to lessen the force as the teeth come together in the process of chewing.

F—Jawbone.

Explain that the tooth is the most highly specialized organ of the body. It is made up of hard and soft tissue. The following points should be kept in mind during classroom discussion:

1. There is no single cause of cavities.
2. There is no total method of prevention.
3. There is a possibility that one may inherit a tendency to dental decay.

○ □ ☆

Process of Tooth Decay

Use Atlas Figure 21, Process of Tooth Decay, to supplement your explanation of tooth decay. Explain that plaque is a translucent film of threadlike bacteria that adheres to teeth and surrounding membranes. It can be removed temporarily by cleaning the teeth. This plaque provides a protective medium for the bacteria, which work on the trapped food (substrate) and produce acid that destroys the enamel of the tooth.

○ □ ☆
Experiments

(Perform science experiments Nos. 3, 4, and 5 found in Unit V.) Explain that if the bacteria are not removed in brushing and more sugar is consumed, more acid will be created, which leads to destruction of the dentin. If not treated, the pulp will become infected. An abscess (a collection of pus along with swelling) develops at the root end, and the bacteria can be carried by the bloodstream to distant parts of the body.

□ ☆
Bulletin Board

Encourage the students to develop a bulletin board illustrating the far-reaching effects of tooth decay. Pictures can include the following:

Soft foods (if teeth are decayed or the gums are sore, the act of chewing becomes a problem, which will lead to the selection of soft foods and increase one's chances of receiving an inadequate diet).

A person in a hospital bed, or a tombstone (tooth decay resulting in an abscess is dangerous and has been known to result in serious illness and death).

A person all alone (poor teeth can influence a person's personality and mental health).

□ ☆
Poster

Another bulletin board or poster can illustrate several factors in tooth decay:

1. Strength of the destructive acids.
2. Power of saliva in the mouth to neutralize the acid.
3. Length of time teeth are exposed to the destructive acids.
4. Frequency of exposure—sucking hard candy for twenty to thirty minutes or eating fermentable foods—sugars and starches—at bedtime without brushing the teeth afterward can be highly damaging to the tooth enamel.

DISCUSSION

Discuss with the class what can be done to reduce the risk of tooth decay from the factors illustrated on the bulletin board.

Evaluation

LIFESTYLE CONTENT

□ ☆
Beat Tooth Decay Game

The object of the Tooth Decay game is to correctly answer questions relating to dental health.* The player with the fewest number of decayed teeth wins. The game is especially useful for self-evaluation.

Equipment consists of one Dairy Council poster, Have a Happy Healthy Smile, one empty hosiery box, thirty-two drawing cards made out of poster board and cut into rectangles, and thirty-two cavity tokens that are simply holes punched out of black construction paper with a hole punch.

Construct gameboard according to the following directions:

Option 1. Use the teeth jaw structures on the back of the poster, Have a Happy Healthy Smile, as the gameboard.

Option 2. Trace the teeth structure from the poster, Have a Happy Healthy Smile. Mount the upper teeth jaw structure on the lid of a flat empty box. Mount

*Courtesy of the American Dairy Council.

the lower jaw on the bottom of the box. The hosiery box method can hold all the parts and be used as an individualized learning activity.

For the drawing cards, on one side of the poster board write a dental question and on the other side write the dental answer.

Play the game by observing the following rules:

1. Back of poster will serve as gameboard. (Each player will use one teeth jaw structure for the hosiery box method).

2. First player takes top dental question card and tries to answer the question correctly. If the question is answered incorrectly, a cavity (black punched-out dot) is placed on one tooth in the teeth jaw structure. No action is taken when the question is answered correctly, resulting in a healthy tooth.

3. The second player follows the same procedure.

4. The game continues until all questions are answered.

5. The player with the "healthiest teeth" wins the game.

(*Note*: Make a copy of the game instructions for Beat Tooth Decay and place in game box.)

This game can be played by one child, two children, or, if more games are constructed, several pairs of children at the same time. Bonus points might be given if the student can name different parts of the tooth.

LIFESTYLE VALUE

□ ☆

Have the students write a short paragraph concerning how they feel about bacteria in their mouth.

UNIT IV: PERSONAL AND PROFESSIONAL DENTAL CARE

A student's decision to prevent dental disease involves information and personal responsibility. The purpose of this unit is to present important skills that can be employed daily (brushing, flossing, and use of a disclosing agent) by the individual and to help students develop an appreciation for professional dental care.

OBJECTIVES

1. The student will correctly describe the main function of a toothbrush, disclosing agent, and dental floss.

2. The student will demonstrate the correct method for disclosing plaque.

3. The student will demonstrate a correct method for brushing the teeth and will present a clean mouth when her or his oral hygiene is evaluated.

4. The student will demonstrate a correct method for flossing teeth (on a model, if the child has not yet developed the required coordination to floss his or her own teeth properly and safely).

MATERIALS

1. Pamphlets, posters, and films, particularly the pamphlet *Cleaning Your Teeth and Gums*, which contains valuable information on proper techniques for cleaning the teeth.*

2. Disclosing tablets, mirrors, water, paper cups, toothbrushes, fluoride toothpaste, unwaxed dental floss, paper towels, and tissues. (Plaque Control Kits containing thirty-five toothbrushes, seventy

*A complete catalog is available from the American Dental Association, Bureau of Dental Health Education, 211 Chicago Avenue, Chicago IL 60611.

disclosing tablets, fifty yards of dental floss, thirty-five Eat-Brush-Floss stickers, thirty-five copies of *Happiness Is a Healthy Mouth* [for parents], and one copy of *Cleaning Your Teeth and Gums*, are available from the Order Section, BD–80, American Dental Association, for approximately $5.00.)

3. Large model of teeth, string, and a variety of toothbrushes.

4. Atlas Figures 22 and 23, Special Tools for Cleaning Your Teeth and Flossing Demonstration.

5. Dental X-rays and instruments.

Methods

○ □ ☆

Skills Pretest

Introduce this unit with a pretest. Students should demonstrate on a model how they brush and floss their teeth. Find out if they know what plaque is and how it can be exposed. The following multiple-choice quiz may also be given. (The letter of the correct answer is in italics.)

1. Describe your toothbrush.
   a. It has medium-soft bristles and is in good condition.
   b. It has stiff bristles.
   c. It looks like I stood on it; the bristles are curved and bent down.
   d. I don't have or use a toothbrush.
2. How do you feel about dental floss?
   a. I only use dental floss to hang mobiles from the ceiling.
   b. Dental floss is used as a substitute for fishing line or to tie around packages.
   c. Dental floss helps me clean between my teeth.
   d. I think waxed dental floss is better than unwaxed dental floss.
3. Fluoride is the best known dental decay preventive we have. How can it be taken to help the teeth?
   a. Drinking water can have fluoride added to it.
   b. Fluoride is added to some toothpastes.
   c. Fluoride gels can be applied to the teeth by a dentist.
   d. Fluoride can be taken in all of these ways.
4. How do you feel about visiting a dentist?
   a. I only go to a dentist when I have a toothache or see a cavity.
   b. I visit a dentist once or twice a year even when I don't think there is anything wrong with my teeth.
   c. It is a waste of money.
   d. I never visit a dentist's office.
5. Which of the following people are members of the dental health team?
   a. Dental assistant
   b. Dental hygienist
   c. Dentist
   d. All of these people are on the dental health team.

○ □

Demonstrate and Practice

Review the methods described for cleaning the teeth found in Chapter 11A and assist the students in learning how to use a disclosing tablet and properly brush and floss their teeth.

○

Toothbrushing Techniques

Demonstrate why it is important to brush the teeth after eating. Using a large comb (or model of teeth if one is available), have the children smear it with jelly, peanut butter, or fudge and take turns brushing it clean. Show how food catches between the teeth and requires the use of dental floss for removal.

○ ☆

Flossing Techniques

Dental flossing is a skill that can be developed with a little practice and should be given special attention in the classroom. Describe the procedure in the following manner. Break off about 18 inches of floss and wind most of it around one of your middle fingers. Wind the rest around the same finger of the opposite hand. This finger can take up the floss as it becomes soiled. Use your thumb and forefingers with an inch of floss between them to guide the floss between your teeth. A gentle sawing motion should be used to insert the floss between the teeth. When the floss reaches the gum line, curve it into a C shape against one tooth and gently slide it into the space between the gum and the tooth until you feel resistance. While holding the floss tightly against the tooth, move the floss away from the gum by scraping the floss up and down against the side of the tooth. Repeat this method on the rest of the teeth and then rinse your mouth vigorously with water. (Use Atlas Figure 23, Flossing Demonstration.)

Some students may not yet have developed the coordination required to floss their own teeth properly, and attempts to do so may result in injured gums. Learning opportunities on models or between the fingers are suggested prior to initiating flossing in the mouth. For the latter method, have the students choose partners. While one student holds hands together with fingers straight and held tightly together, the other student flosses between the fingers with string. Emphasize the importance of getting all the way down, but at the same time being gentle so as not to hurt the soft tissue of either the hands or gums. Explain that string should not be used when flossing real teeth. Another flossing technique that works well with younger students is to tie dental floss in a loop before flossing is started.

☐ ☆

Creative Writing

Have the students write themes about being a tooth. A student might explain the helpful and harmful actions his "owner" takes each day, as illustrated in the following story (2, pp. 96–97).

A Germ's Eye View

Hello! My name is Herman. I live in Bacteriaville, in the country of Tooth. I earn my living by making cavities. "Not much of a job," you may be saying, but when you think of all the unemployed among germs like me, you'll realize how lucky I really am. Depending on the mouth, of course, the work is usually pretty steady.

Every morning I get up early and meet the boys at the shop where we are assigned our stations. Take yesterday for instance. I was assigned to Enamel Avenue along with the usual crew. Fortunately, we arrived as breakfast was served and it was my favorite, all sugar and syrup. Immediately, we buckled down to the job at hand. We were almost through the hard stuff, you know, the enamel, when the street cleaner came along. I will describe the appearance of this monstrosity for you.

The street cleaner is a peculiar long-handled device with many bristles on the end. Some idiot down at the sanitation department thinks this place needs cleaning four or five times a day. This is pretty rough on us cavity-makers, but we can usually find cover. This time the cleaner missed us so we finished there.

My brother George was not so lucky.

His job was on Deciduous Street, formerly known as Baby Tooth Lane. He and his crew had almost demolished this tooth when along came a big red wafer and colored all their camouflage. Well, when the street cleaner came along, there they were, completely exposed, so of course they were destroyed. Well, we germs will fight back, yes indeed! We'll rebuild our cities and store up our sugar. There's only one thing that has us really worried. That fellow running that street cleaner seems to be getting a whole lot smarter!

□ ☆

Dental Scrapbook

Have the students collect advertisements of dental care products, such as toothpastes, dental floss, mouthwashes, breath mints. Ask them to evaluate the validity of the claims made for each product. Mount advertisements and class evaluations in a dental health scrapbook that can be referred to throughout the year.

Reserve one section of the scrapbook for members of the dental health team. Reports describing the training and duties of dentists, dental hygienists, and dental assistants should be included.

□ ☆

Professional Services

Divide the class into small groups and encourage them to list as many major services of the dental health team as they can think of in ten minutes. Compare lists. Services include performing dental examinations and diagnosing dental problems, cleaning the teeth (dental prophylaxis), filling cavities (restoring teeth), giving fluoride treatments, treating injured teeth and gums, replacing missing or knocked-out teeth, treating gum diseases, straightening teeth, performing root canals, and teaching patients about the cause and prevention of dental diseases.

○ □ ☆

X-rays

Show the class real dental X-rays. Explain that dental radiographs (X-rays) are used to locate tooth decay and to detect abscesses, impacted teeth, and other abnormalities that cannot be seen with the unaided eye or felt with instruments.

○ □ ☆

Dental Instruments

Show the class real dental instruments if available, or use the Atlas figure, Special Tools for Cleaning Your Teeth. Explain that a dentist or dental hygienist uses special tools to remove stain, dental plaque, and heavy deposits of calculus from the teeth.

○

Field Trip

After discussing who the members of the dental health team are and what their functions are, you might take the class on a field trip for a visit to a dental office or dental clinic. If this cannot be arranged, ask a dentist or dental hygienist to speak to the class and describe the services they perform.

Evaluation

LIFESTYLE CONTENT

○ □

Evaluate the students on their success at demonstrating a correct method for disclosing plaque and brushing and flossing their teeth.

□

Puppet Script

Have each student write a script for a puppet show, "Going to the Dentist." Select several of the best scripts and have the students divide into groups and stage a puppet show for another class.

LIFESTYLE VALUE

○ □ ☆

Put the following open-ended sentences on the chalkboard and have the students complete them on a sheet of paper.

Going to the dentist is _____ .
I think dentists are _____ .
I think the dental hygienist _____ .

Discuss the following questions with the class:

Should you encourage your brother or sister to clean his or her teeth? Why?

Do you feel that brushing your teeth is necessary to prevent losing them?

Do you think your teeth feel clean right this minute?

UNIT V: INTERDISCIPLINARY ACTIVITIES

By occasionally correlating health education with other areas of study, the teacher can reinforce health concepts while broadening the student's outlook and experiences. While most health topics can be successfully presented in this manner, the authors have chosen dental health as an example of this technique.

OBJECTIVES

1. The students will improve their spelling and writing skills by working puzzles, presenting reports, and writing a play.
2. The students will compare and contrast the diets of other cultures and determine how this has affected people's teeth.

3. The students will learn investigative techniques by performing simple experiments in the classroom.

4. The students will develop manual dexterity and creative art skills through a variety of art projects.

MATERIALS

Materials will vary according to the activities chosen and are listed with each activity.

Methods

LANGUAGE ARTS

○ □

Spelling

Present a spelling lesson with words related to dental health. Depending upon the age of the students you might use words such as teeth, gums, cavities, roots, enamel, dentin, pulp, molar, caries, periodontal, gingiva, calculus, tartar, plaque, dentist, orthodontist, bacteria, nutrition, incisors, deciduous, cuspids, fluoride, sugar, saliva, lingual, dentrifice, abrasive, pyorrhea, and malocclusion.

○ □

Skit

Have the students write or perform a play or do both. Another version of this idea is a grab bag skit, during which students perform impromptu skits with props from the grab bag. Props might include toothpaste, toothbrush, dental floss, disclosing tablets, mirror, candy, fruits, dental instruments.

□

Writing Assignments

Have the students write dental rhymes, poetry, and creative stories.

□ ☆

Book Reports

Have students present book reports related to dental health to the class on such books as *I Want to Be a Dentist* by Carla Greene, *The Riddle of Teeth* by Winifred Hammond, *The Tooth Trip* by Thomas McGuire.

○

Telephone

Have the students pretend to call the dentist for a dental appointment (using a play telephone). Encourage the students to be courteous. Students should be told that changing appointments must be done at least twenty-four hours before the appointed time.

MATHEMATICS

○

Using the sugar cube chart explained in the Dietary Habits and Oral Health lesson (Unit II), have the students count the number of sugar cubes in a snack and determine how many teaspoons are in a tablespoon, a stick of butter, an ounce, ½ cup.

□

Ask the students to determine if they were to eat three meals a day plus one snack for seventy-two years, how many meals and snacks would they have eaten.

□ ☆

Have students visit grocery stores and write down the name of the store and the cost of three different brands of toothpaste or mouthwash. Have them compare costs and graph the results.

□ ☆

The students may also wish to compare costs of toothpaste, toothbrushes, and dental floss. Have them figure the cost per use of toothpaste and dental floss.

□ ☆

Have the students compare the cost per serving of an orally safe food to the cost per serving of an orally hazardous food.

SOCIAL STUDIES

□ ☆

Discuss with the class the diets of other cultures. Ask the questions What kinds of food used to be eaten by the Eskimos? What kind of foods do they eat now? Has a different diet affected their teeth?

□ ☆

Have the students research information discussing dentistry during Colonial times, including diet and toothbrushing methods.

□ ☆

Find out how astronauts take care of their teeth. See "How Would an Astronaut Take Care of a Toothache?" (1, p. 100).

SCIENCE

○

Experiment #1: Dentifrice

Have the students make a simple dentifrice in class by combining one teaspoon salt with two teaspoons of baking soda. For flavoring, they may want to add a drop or two of oil of peppermint, wintergreen, or cinnamon. Let the students take home some of the mixture to use when brushing their teeth.

□ ☆

Experiment #2: Mouth Acidity

Have the pupils learn the acidity or alkalinity of their mouths by using a strip of nitrazine paper. Have them soak sterile cotton swabs with saliva and apply to the paper. The degree of acidity or alkalinity can be determined by comparing the resulting color of the paper strips with the color chart provided by the manufacturer. A pH of 7 indicates a neutral mouth, less than 7 indicates an acid mouth, and greater than 7 shows an alkaline mouth (3). Litmus paper may also be used to indicate the presence of acid in the mouth.

○

Experiment #3: Acid Power

To show that acid will weaken substances containing calcium (such as eggshell and tooth enamel), place a whole egg in a bowl of white vinegar (acetic acid) for about twenty-four hours. The eggshell should become soft as the vinegar decalcifies the shell. You might also want to soak an egg in stannous fluoride or another fluoride substance that a dentist can help you obtain before exposing it to the vinegar. Observe if the shell has become stronger. A variation of this experiment is to drop a tooth in a glass of white vinegar or soft drink containing sugar and phosphoric acid and leave it for about a week. See if the class can see a difference when it is compared with another tooth. A tooth may also be placed in water and another tooth in 10 percent HCL acid. In one week, a softening of the enamel from the acid should be evident.

□ ☆

Experiment #4: Bacterial Growth

To show the presence of bacteria in the mouth, sterilize some gelatin (sweetened with sugar) in a pressure cooker for fifteen minutes (or heat in oven at 100° to 120°F. for one hour). Prepare two shallow dishes of the gelatin. Carefully scrape between the teeth and near the gum line to remove food debris (may use a tooth-

pick). Place this material in one dish and cover both dishes, label, and place in a warm section of the room. The students should be able to see fungus growth in the dish exposed to mouth bacteria after several days have passed. The uncontaminated dish should show little or no growth.

○

Experiment #5: Tooth Models

Either an apple or an egg can be used as models to compare with the parts of a tooth:

Enamel: skin of apple or eggshell
Dentin: white of apple or egg white
Pulp: core of apple or egg yolk

By breaking the skin of an apple and leaving it for several days, the students can observe the progress of decay.

ART

○ □ ☆

Borrow or buy the book *Construction and Utilization of Visual Aids in Dental Health Education* by Florean Dearth.

○ □

Have the students design posters for Children's Dental Health Week in February.

□

Have the class create a bulletin board around the theme Until Death Do Us Part, showing the marriage of two teeth, decay of one of them, and one tooth left alone.

○ □ ☆

Have the students make dental collages for a bulletin board: have different groups of students working on smile collages, nutritious and orally safe snacks, toothpaste and other oral products, cartoons, etc.

○ □

Have the students make models of teeth and foods. Clay may be molded, baked, and colored. Combine 1 cup salt and 4 cups flour with food coloring to make a simple clay. Add water until mixture is doughlike. Teeth can be made from papier-mâché, paraffin, and wood, or carved out of white soap.

□

Have the students make tooth mosaics using seeds, pieces of eggshell, or floor tile.

○ □ ☆

Have the class draw dental cartoons on typing paper with a soft lead pencil. Select the best drawings and convert them into overhead transparencies.

○ □

Have the students cut out shapes of teeth, a beaker of acid, their interpretation of bacteria and tooth decay, candy, fruits, and vegetables from felt to be used with the felt board for story telling.

○ □

Have the class make puppets out of paper sacks or from papier-mâché and put on a puppet show for another class. Background scenery and other props can also be constructed.

○

Have the students draw (or supply them with) an outline of a tooth. Ask them to draw in the features they think their teeth would have if teeth had faces. Ask them, for instance, if they think their teeth are happy, sad, dirty.

Evaluation

LIFESTYLE CONTENT

○ □ ☆

Have the students complete Atlas Figure 88, the Mystery Mouth Worksheet. (Answers: Since the person has 28 teeth, but is missing the third molars or wisdom teeth, he or she is probably a teenager—assuming the wisdom teeth have not been pulled. Most people do not develop wisdom teeth until they are in their twenties. The teeth are too large for the person to be a child; 1. Central *incisor*; 2. First *bicuspid*; 3. Second *bicuspid*; 4. *Cuspid*; 5. *Cuspid*; 6. First *molar*; 7. First *molar*; 8. Central *incisor*.)

LIFESTYLE VALUE

○ □ ☆

Show Atlas Figure 24, What Is Your Dental I.Q.? The top row of teeth describe various dental health topics for possible classroom discussion. Ask the students to study the boy's lower row of teeth and write down those things that they do for their teeth. Ask them which three things they think are the most important to do every day.

REFERENCES

1. Julius B. Richmond, Elenore T. Pounds, Irma B. Fricke, and Dieter H. Sussdorf, *Health and Growth*, Grade 4, Teacher's Edition (Glenview, Ill.: Scott, Foresman, 1971).

2. Nancy Jane Reynolds, *Guidelines for a Dental Health Curriculum for Public Schools* (Columbus, Ohio: The Ohio State University, 1974).

3. Ruth Rich, "Tests for Acidity of the Mouth in Relation to Susceptibility to Dental Caries," *Journal of School Health* 33 (February 1963): 61.

CHAPTER 12

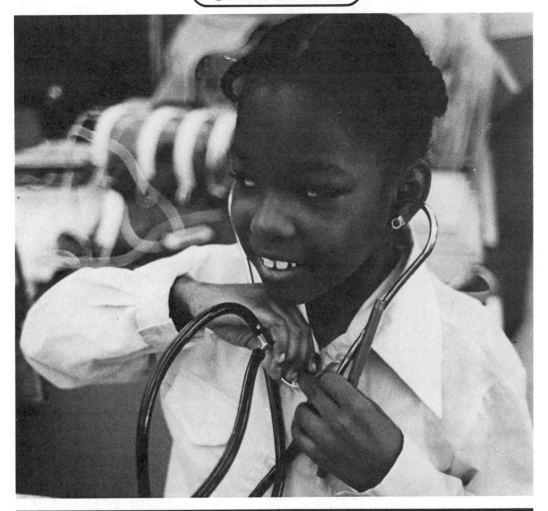

PART A: DISEASE CONTROL AND PREVENTION

Chapter 4, School Health Services, emphasized the importance of recognizing the existence of various medical problems in the classroom and facilitating delivery of medical services to those students who require such specialized attention. The authors observed that teachers come into contact with children on a sustained basis more often than any other professional group in society and consequently are able to make a significant contribution to preventive medicine.

Through early identification and diagnosis of medical conditions, many disorders can be remedied before they cause severe physical damage or interfere with a child's learning and development.

Such medical conditions may include orthopedic problems, mental retardation, nutritional deficiencies, psychiatric disorders, and impairment of sensory functioning resulting in student underachievement. The focus of this chapter, however, will be upon the management and prevention of acute and chronic diseases.

THEORIES OF THE CAUSE OF DISEASE

From the time of birth, until the time our bodies eventually decompose after death, our lives are spent in contact with microorganisms. Our health and well-being are influenced by the presence or absence of various microorganisms in the environment. Mounting information indicates, however, that people are not born with equal chances of catching diseases. There appears to be a complex interplay between one's genes and the environment that ultimately determines a person's susceptibility to a particular disease organism.

MICROORGANISMS—GOOD GUYS OR BAD GUYS?

Uncountable numbers of microorganisms surround everyone daily. Some of these organisms assist in the utilization of vitamins by breaking down organic matter and by destroying harmful microorganisms in the intestinal tract. Other microorganisms, however, are pathogenic and capable of killing. Some microorganisms have the ability to produce poisonous substances (toxins). When toxins are excreted into the body tissue or the surrounding medium, they are called exotoxins. A poison that is retained within the organism until the organism dies is called an endotoxin. The action of endotoxins has not been clearly established, but exotoxins can cause degeneration of host cells, block essential enzymes, and prevent enzyme synthesis.

Exotoxins lose their toxicity when heated or treated with acids. When the toxicity is lost, the resulting substance is a toxoid that has the ability to stimulate production of antitoxins. Since antitoxins can neutralize toxins in the body of the host, medical science has a powerful tool in protecting susceptible individuals from diseases caused by bacterial toxins.

FACTORS INFLUENCING INFECTION

Some microorganisms have a particular preference for certain cells and tissues which they may injure or destroy. For example, the poliomyelitis virus likes nerve cells, and the typhoid bacillus chooses the cells of the lymphoid tissue of the intestinal wall. To be destructive, these organisms must find a portal of entry and be of a significant number. If the host is hypersensitive to certain microorganisms, the result may be a chronic disease. The host species is another factor in determining virulency. The number of organisms capable of causing disease in a given host (infective dose) may be ineffective in another animal because of different defense mechanisms.

Although it usually takes only a small number of extremely virulent microorganisms to establish an infection, less virulent strains must enter the host in numbers inversely proportional to their virulence. Furthermore, many microorganisms lose their virulence for a given species after repeated transfers, for example, on laboratory culture media or after repeated transfers through laboratory animals.

Pathogens are also dependent upon their ability to find susceptible hosts to infect and an escape route before they are ultimately destroyed. Since pathogens bring on their own destruction, either by destroying the host or by stimulating the production of antibodies that will destroy them or prevent further spread, epidemics are self-limited. Unfortunately, much suffering and death may occur before the limits of an epidemic are reached. One's personal habits and lifestyle can do much to aid or restrict the possibility of infection by many pathogenic organisms (see Table 12A-1).

RESISTANCE

When external preventive and control measures fail to eliminate disease-causing organisms, the host's body takes over. Resistance comes in two forms: natural and acquired.

Natural Resistance

Natural resistance provides defense against infection by a number of mechanical and chemical barriers, but only a few of the more important factors will be mentioned here.

FIRST LINE OF DEFENSE

Unbroken skin and mucous membranes form an effective barrier to infectious agents, although it is possible for some microorganisms to enter through openings of the sweat glands and hair follicles. Sticky mucous membranes line natural body openings, and mucous secretions serve to trap microorganisms until they can be disposed of or lose their strength. Once inside the body, organisms encounter still more mucus and the sweeping action of cilia, which helps the body remove bacteria from susceptible areas.

Coughing, sneezing, shedding tears, and perspiring are other cleansing methods the body has at its disposal. Some of these secretions contain substances such as the enzyme lysozyme, which has the ability to destroy microorganisms. Other enzymes and hormones aid in the reduction of susceptibility to infection.

SECOND LINE OF DEFENSE

If pathogenic microorganisms manage to enter the body through breaks in the skin or irritated membranes, they find a comfortable, warm, moist haven in which to start an infection. At this point, the body mobilizes a cellular defense where specific cells called phagocytes gather to seek out and destroy the invading organisms. Phagocytes (eating cells) can be either leucocytes (white blood cells) or wandering macrophages (large phagocytes) and fixed phagocytes—cells of the reticuloendothelial system (RES). Macrophages are sometimes called scavenger cells, because they can move around to the site of an infection.

When a body tissue is damaged or poisoned by microorganisms, the infected area becomes tender and sore. The swelling, heat, tenderness, pain, and red appearance associated with inflammation are an indication that the body is attempting to localize and destroy harmful organisms. During the battle, phagocytes engulf and destroy invading microor-

TABLE 12A-1 TRANSMISSION AND PREVENTIVE MEASURES FOR INFECTIOUS DISEASES

Method of Transmission	Common Portal of Entry	Diseases Spread	Available Immunization	Prevention and Control
Airborne Direct (coughs and sneezes) Indirect (drinking glasses, eating utensils, soiled handkerchiefs)	Mouth or nose; then the respiratory tract (diseases often localize in throat or lungs)	Colds Diphtheria Scarlet fever Tuberculosis Pneumonia Whooping cough Smallpox Chicken pox Rubella (German measles) Measles Mumps Polio Influenza (flu)	No Yes No Yes Not practical Yes Yes No Yes Yes Yes Yes Yes	Avoid crowds when possible; exclude from school; disinfect contaminated articles; use tissues when sneezing; build resistance by getting enough sleep and eating properly; use individual towels; encourage immunization
Food borne Through contaminated food; improper food handling	Mouth (diseases often localize in the digestive tract)	Botulism and other kinds of food poisoning Typhoid fever Dysentery Cholera Infectious hepatitis	No Yes No Yes Short-term	Treat human carriers; practice proper disposal of human wastes; use sanitary food production and handling (wash hands); properly cook and store foods

Mode of entry/transmission	Disease	Immunization available	Prevention
Waterborne Through contaminated water Mouth (diseases often localize in the digestive tract)	Typhoid fever Dysentery Ear, eye, nose, and throat infections	Yes No No	Swim in chemically treated water; improve sanitation measures; dig deep wells
Direct Contact Through breaks in the skin or mucous membranes from (1) infected human Direct contact with lesions; mucous membranes; urogenital tract	Venereal diseases such as syphilis and gonorrhea Yaws Impetigo Boils Athlete's foot Conjunctivitis Head and body lice Ringworm of skin or scalp Scabies	No No No No No No No No No	Avoid intimate contact with infected people; have premarital blood tests; get medical treatment following possible exposure; improve sanitation and personal hygiene habits; do not share grooming articles; wear sandals in areas used by other people (showers at school); shampoo hair frequently; wear clean clothing
(2) wound or injury Opening in the skin—(circulatory system)	Tetanus Cutaneous anthrax	Yes No	Avoid wounds; when wounded, clean area thoroughly and bandage; consider need for tetanus shot; wear protective gloves when working

TABLE 12A-1 (cont.)

Method of Transmission	Common Portal of Entry	Diseases Spread	Available Immunization	Prevention and Control
(3) animals (when bitten or scratched); more than 100 diseases can be transferred from vertebrate animals to humans	Through a break in the skin (involvement of the circulatory system)	Rabies (bite from dog, bat, skunk, etc.)	Short-term (after bite)	Immunize dogs; be wary of wild animals; avoid contact with rodents; immunize farm animals; keep farm animals well nourished; control insects; quarantine infected animals, cremate carcasses of infected birds; pasteurize milk; completely cook meats
		Cat-scratch fever (bite or scratch from cat, bird, or other animal)	No	
		Ringworm (from dogs, cats, etc.)	No	
		Undulant fever (from cattle, hogs, goats, and sheep)	Cattle may be immunized	
		Leptospirosis (from cattle, dogs, horses, pigs, and sheep)	Domestic animals can be vaccinated	
		Q fever	No	
		Bovine tuberculosis	Not practical	
		Tularemia (rabbit fever)	Rather ineffective	
(4) insects (when bitten)	Through a break in the skin (involvement of the circulatory system)	Bubonic plague (rat fleas)	Yes (short-term)	Get rid of rats; when walking through woods, wear long socks and the appropriate boots; keep clothes clean; get rid of stagnant water; put up screens; use insecticides
		Rocky Mountain spotted fever (ticks)	Yes (short-term)	
		Typhus fever (human louse)	Yes	
		Malaria (anopheles mosquito)	No	
		Typhoid fever (house fly)	Yes	
		Encephalitis (mosquito)	No	
		Yellow fever (mosquito)	Yes	

ganisms; but in the process, many leucocytes and macrophages are killed. The material that accumulates is called pus and may be different colors depending upon the type of bacteria involved in the infection. Pus is transported to lymph nodes, where surviving invaders can be filtered out and destroyed.

Successful phagocytosis depends upon several factors:

1. Adequate blood circulation.
2. Successful passing of the leucocytes through the distended capillaries and into the damaged tissue.
3. An attraction of the leucocytes to the invading microorganisms caused by a chemical stimulus.
4. The presence of an antibodylike substance known as opsonin, which makes bacteria more susceptible to being engulfed.
5. Complete digestion of the pathogens.

Fever, or an increase in body temperature, is a result of phagocytosis and another means of defense, since many microorganisms are unable to reproduce at temperatures much above 98.6° F.

ACQUIRED RESISTANCE

THIRD LINE OF DEFENSE

In addition to phagocytes, the blood also contains antibodies, which are substances formed by the body in response to stimulation by each new toxin or species of microorganism. Antibodies may remain in the blood and provide immunity or protection from new attacks by the same toxins. This is called acquired immunity. Some acquired immunities are only temporary, as in the case of immunity to the common cold; other acquired immunities may provide lifelong protection against such diseases as measles and chicken pox.

Acquired resistance differs from natural resistance in that it is not inherent in the body but is acquired during life and is specific for a single type of microorganism. It may be active or passive.

IMMUNITY

As mentioned earlier, active immunity develops when antibodies are produced in the host as a result of contact with microorganisms or their products. Active immunity may be acquired by natural means (while recovering from an infectious disease) or artificially (by injection of an antigen, such as smallpox vaccination). A healthy lifestyle includes immunizations against polio, diphtheria/tetanus/pertussis, measles, mumps, and rubella before the first grade.

Passive immunity occurs when antibodies produced by another person or animal are injected into a person without the specific antibodies. Since no antigen is introduced, there is no stimulus for producing antibodies and the immunity is of short duration. This method is useful in preventing or modifying the disease in a person who has not been actively immunized before exposure to the disease.

As with active immunity, passive immunity may be conferred through artificial or natural means. Artificial immunity requires an injection of serum from an immune animal or human; natural immunity may occur if material antibodies are transferred to a newborn baby in colostrum (the first milk secreted after childbirth) or to an infant in utero by placental transfer of antibodies from the mother's blood.

VACCINES

Not all vaccines are alike. We have seen that active immunization induces the body to create the needed antibodies itself. The word "vaccine," incidentally, comes from the Latin word *vacca*, meaning cow. In 1796, a British physician named Edward Jenner took fluid from a girl suffering with cowpox (a mild disease) and used it as a vaccine to immunize a child from the more deadly disease of smallpox. Although Jenner did not understand how the inoculation caused the body to immunize itself against smallpox, he learned that it worked.

Vaccines used in active immunization contain antigens, or substances that stimulate the production of antibodies. They may be made from killed microorganisms (as in typhoid fever and Salk polio vaccines); attenuated or weakened organisms (as in the oral Sabin polio vaccine and rabies vaccine); or a live microorganism, which is not highly infectious in humans but is still capable of producing antibodies that afford protection (as in the smallpox example). Antigens may also be made from toxoids (toxins that have been treated to render them harmless without interfering with their ability to stimulate antibody production). Toxoids are used for protecting individuals against diphtheria, tetanus, and other diseases caused by toxins or toxin-producing microorganisms.

TREATMENT OF INFECTIOUS DISEASE

It was not until the early 1900s that a specific drug capable of curing disease without great danger to the patient was synthesized. Paul Ehrlich's contribution was significant, because his systematic search yielded a drug that was potent but low in toxicity for humans yet chemically stable.

A useful chemotherapeutic agent must also be able to penetrate the cells and tissues of the host in effective concentrations and not interfere with such natural defense mechanisms as phagocytosis and the production of antibodies. Chemotherapeutic agents are chemical substances used for the treatment of infectious diseases and may be obtained naturally (from microorganisms, plants, and animals) or made synthetically in the laboratory. Antibiotics and sulfonamides are perhaps the two most well known groups of chemotherapeutic agents.

Sulfonamides

The sulfonamides are a group of compounds that are effective against a wide variety of diseases ranging from urinary infections caused by gram-negative organisms to respiratory infections caused by *Streptococci* and *Staphylococci*. They are especially useful in the treatment of infections caused by meningococci and aid in the prevention of rheumatic fever as well.

Antibiotics

Antibiotics differ from most other chemotherapeutic agents in that they are usually obtained from living organisms (bacteria or fungi) but like other successful drugs are able to destroy many kinds of pathogens without being toxic to humans. It is sometimes possible to combine two or more antibiotics to eliminate organisms that are not completely susceptible to the action of a single antibiotic.

Penicillin

Several thousand antibiotic substances have been isolated and identified since penicillin was first discovered in 1929 by Sir Alexander Fleming, a British bacteriologist. Penicillin was found to be effective against certain types of pneumonia, as well as gonorrhea, strep throat, and other bacterial infections. Although it is the least toxic antibiotic presently known, some people suffer allergic reactions to it, ranging from a mild skin reaction to death. Some strains of bacteria have developed resistance to penicillin, thus reinforcing the need for continued research.

Streptomycin

Another important antibiotic is streptomycin, a drug which inactivates bacteriophages and helps treat tuberculosis and other bacterial infections. It is particularly important because it inhibits many organisms that are resistant to penicillin and sulfonamides.

WARNING SIGNS

When a pathogenic organism invades the body, there are warning signs or symptoms which require a quick response in order to aid in diagnosis and treatment of a disease. Warning signs of infection include fever, pain, loss of weight, shortness of breath, chronic fatigue, and bleeding. When pain persists or seems unusual, one should consult a physician. A doctor should be called when a cough lasts more than two weeks, when there is pain upon urination or a definite change in the color or volume of urine, or when excessive fatigue persists despite adequate rest. Refer to Table 12A-2 for help in identifying possible communicable diseases.

TABLE 12A-2 COMMUNICABLE DISEASE SYMPTOMS AND CONTROL MEASURES

Communicable Disease	Incubation Period	Common Symptoms	Control Measures
Rubeola (measles)	Usually 10 days; about 14 days before rash appears	Cough, watery eyes, runny nose, fever followed by red blotchy rash; possibly red spots on cheeks inside mouth	Exclude from school for at least 7 days following appearance of rash; encourage immunization
Rubella (3-day measles)	14 to 21 days; usually 18 days	Skin rash and mild fever; glands at back of head behind ears may be swollen	Exclude from school at least four days from onset of symptoms or appearance of rash; encourage immunization

303

TABLE 12A-2 (cont.)

Communicable Disease	Incubation Period	Common Symptoms	Control Measures
Chicken pox	2 to 3 weeks, usually 13 to 17 days	Skin rash with small blisters which leave a scab; eruption comes in crops	Exclude from school for at least 7 days from appearance of first crop of blisters; may return if only dry scales remain
Common cold	12 to 72 hours, usually 24 hours	Irritated throat, watery discharge from eyes and nose, sneezing, chills, general body discomfort	Exclude from school; symptoms may precede other communicable diseases
Impetigo	4 to 10 days, occasionally longer	Blisterlike lesions which later develop into crusted puslike sores	Exclude from school until adequately treated and sores no longer drain; infected persons should use separate towels and wash cloths
Conjunctivitis (pinkeye)	24 to 72 hours	Redness and swelling of membranes of the eye with burning or itching; thick, yellow discharge; sensitivity to light	Exclude from school until discharge from eyes has ceased; use separate towels
Infectious hepatitis	10 to 50 days; commonly 30 to 35 days	Loss of appetite, fever, nausea, fatigue; jaundice may appear	Exclude from school during first 14 days of illness and at least 7 days after onset of jaundice or longer if physician recommends (resuming activities too soon may cause a relapse)
Mumps	12 to 26 days; usually 18 days	Fever, painful swelling under jaw or in front of ear	Exclude from school at least 9 days from onset of swelling or until swelling is gone; encourage immunization

Communicable Disease	Incubation Period	Common Symptoms	Control Measures
Scabies (itch)	Several days to weeks before itching is noticed	Small raised areas of skin containing fluid; tiny burrow lines frequently in finger webs; itching is intense, especially at night	Exclude from school until adequately treated; use individual towels; observe for signs in other family members
Head lice (pediculosis)	Eggs (nits) of lice hatch in one week; reach sexual maturity in two weeks	Irritation and itching of the scalp; presence of small, light gray insects or eggs attached to hairs, especially behind ears and at nape of neck	Exclude from school until disinfestation is completed; all family members should be inspected; treat all headgear of infected persons
Ringworm of the scalp	10 to 14 days	Patchy baldness, lusterless hair; inflamed areas of scalp; brittle hair	Exclude from school until under medical control; hang hats and coats separate from others; avoid use of common towels, combs, and brushes
Ringworm of the skin	10 to 14 days	Ringlike lesions with slightly raised edges, gradually enlarged in size; itching and burning possible	Exclude from school until under medical control; exclude from gym and swimming pools; avoid common use of towels; examine family members and pets
Ringworm of the foot (athlete's foot)	Unknown	Scaling, cracking of skin, especially between toes; blisters containing thin fluid	Exclusion not feasible since organism is widely distributed; however, severe cases should not be permitted in school showers; wear socks with shoes

TABLE 12A-2 (cont.)

Communicable Disease	Incubation Period	Common Symptoms	Control Measures
Streptococcal sore throat/ scarlet fever	2 to 5 days	Scarlet fever: sudden onset, fever, head-ache, sore throat, vomiting and rash, followed by peeling of the skin; strep sore throat same as scarlet fever without rash or peeling	Exclude from school for duration of illness and until discharged from isolation requirements by physician; early diagnosis and treat-ment essential to prevent serious com-plications
Sore throats and fevers	Sudden onset	Headache; eyes may burn; general body discomfort	Exclude from school until recovery is complete (suggested that stu-dents be fever free for 24 hours before returning to school)
Whooping cough	7 to 21 days, usually 10 days	Cold, cough; whoop develops in about 2 weeks; cough may end in vomiting	Exclude from school for at least 10 days from onset or until recovery is complete; immunize

PART B: TEACHING ABOUT DISEASE CONTROL AND PREVENTION

The study of disease in the elementary school years is extremely important for several reasons. For one thing, students in this age group are highly susceptible to infectious diseases. In addition, students need to understand how their lifestyles, habits, and other personal factors influence their susceptibility. And finally, students need to learn to cover their coughs and sneezes, to get plenty of rest, and to take it easy when symptoms of disease appear.

In the elementary school years, students are often exposed to chronic health conditions and diseases for the first time. Coping with a personal condition or accepting a condition in another child fosters good mental health. Misconceptions about one's personal condition or that of another child may lead to fear or ridicule. Educating students about conditions such as epilepsy, diabetes, and rheumatic heart helps to dispel stigma.

A further task of the elementary teacher is to provide the framework of healthy habits and commitment to those habits which will reduce the student's risk of disease from a poor lifestyle. Although poor-lifestyle diseases may be without symptoms until a person reaches his or her forties, their beginnings can be traced to the habits which a person develops at an early age.

The elementary school curriculum should recognize the following needs of students in a teaching plan on disease control and prevention:

1. The student needs to learn about health conditions commonly experienced, such as diabetes, epilepsy, rheumatic heart, cross-eye.

2. The student needs to be comfortable with the changes that a health condition may cause (seizure, fainting spell) in himself or herself as well as in others.

3. The student needs to recognize the symptoms of childhood infections.

4. The student needs to desire to demonstrate habits which reduce the spread of infectious disease.

5. The student needs to learn about diseases that are aggravated by a poor lifestyle.

6. The student needs to commit herself or himself to a lifestyle that will reduce the risk of disease.

UNIT I: DISEASES FROM SMOKING

Research findings of the United States Public Health Service indicate that too many children now living in the United States will die prematurely and unnecessarily from lung cancer. Who are these children? They are those who most likely will begin to smoke at an early age. Of those people who smoke, 25 percent or more begin in the elementary school. They begin smoking to imitate adults and impress others. The greatest influence on their decision to smoke is attributed to peer pressure.

If educators are going to have an impact on smoking behavior, education regarding the effects of smoking needs to begin at a very early age. Children need to learn the health hazards of smoking as well as the value of making their own decisions. The lesson Diseases from Smoking covers many of the health hazards of smoking. It also gives the child a chance to join an I'll Never Start Club. Perhaps club membership can become the peer substitute for smoking.

OBJECTIVES

1. The student will draw a picture to illustrate one of the harmful effects of smoking depicted in one of the four smoking stories.

2. The student will be able to identify vocabulary words from this unit on a matching or fill-in exam.

3. The student will complete five unfinished sentences to express his or her attitudes toward smoking.

MATERIALS

1. Copies of the smoking word search.

2. Copies of *What's Your I.Q. on Smoking.**

*Available from the American Heart Association.

Appropriate grade levels are suggested for each teaching strategy and appear as ○, □, ☆ in the left-hand column.

○ = most suited for the primary grades;

□ = most suited for the intermediate grades;

☆ = most suited for the upper elementary grades.

3. Thank You for Not Smoking posters.*

4. I'll Never Start pledges, cards, and badges.

5. Bookmark (Best Tip Yet) from the American Cancer Society.

Methods

The four stories included in this unit were written to communicate the hazards of smoking to elementary children. In upper elementary school, the stories may be read to the children or the children may read them themselves. In the lower grades, it is best for the teacher to explain each story to the students. (The material is best suited for upper elementary.)

The main approach is to develop certain concepts by examining the stories. The material to be emphasized and the analogies used in the lesson are outlined below for the teacher.

THE SICK ENGINEER

The first story is "The Sick Engineer." Read the story, emphasizing the following:

1. One of the main points made in this story is the control of the cell by DNA, which does the following:
   a. is the boss of the cell
   b. tells the cell what to do
   c. controls cell growth
   d. stops cell growth
   e. replaces old cells
   f. makes new cells
   g. makes DNA for new cells
2. Another point made is that the cells help each other by:
   a. sharing food
   b. fighting disease

*Available from the American Heart Association.

UNFRIENDLY PASSENGER ON A CELL TRUCK

Read the second story emphasizing the following points. The information needed to understand this story is based upon the cell's construction and distribution of energy.

1. The cell combines ATP with oxygen to make energy.
2. The waste material made is carbon dioxide.
3. Oxygen is transported in the following manner:
   a. The red blood cells are made in the bones and are replaced every four months.
   b. The red blood cells are carriers.
   c. The special part of the red blood cell that does the carrying is called hemoglobin.
   d. The red blood cells go to the lungs to pick up oxygen.
   e. Hemoglobin and oxygen are attracted to each other (like magnets).
   f. Oxygen is carried to the body cells and used.
   g. Carbon dioxide is carried to the lungs to be exhaled (breathed out).
4. Smoking affects oxygen usage in the following way:
   a. When a person smokes, he or she breathes in carbon monoxide.
   b. The lungs will have both oxygen and carbon monoxide in them.
   c. The red blood cell (hemoglobin) goes to the lung to get a fresh supply of oxygen.
   d. The hemoglobin sees both carbon monoxide and oxygen.
   e. Hemoglobin likes carbon monoxide better than oxygen and fills up with carbon monoxide first.
   f. The red blood cell carries carbon

monoxide around the body, but the carbon monoxide cannot be used.

g. To get enough oxygen when there is also carbon monoxide, a person must breathe more and has a higher heart rate.

A FALSE ALARM

"A False Alarm" is intended to explain one of the theories linking smoking to atherosclerosis. The story begins by explaining the role of the circulatory system.

1. The blood vessels carry fuel to the cell.
2. To keep the fuel in the blood vessels moving, the heart beats from 50 to 100 times each minute.
3. When food is needed, more blood is sent to the stomach to pick it up.
4. When nicotine gets into the body, it sends a false alarm out.
5. Although the muscles do not need the food, it is still dumped into the blood.
6. Fats and sugars travel around the body's blood vessels but are never deposited in a cell for use.
7. These fats and sugars eventually stick to the wall of the blood vessel, resulting in atherosclerosis.

The story continues with an explanation of the role of atherosclerosis in the development of coronary heart idsease.

1. The fats and sugars can deposit in any blood vessel—leg, brain, or heart.
2. This is especially dangerous when the vessel is completely closed off, because no blood can get to that area.
3. If this happens in the brain, it leads to a stroke.
4. If it happens in the blood vessels leading to the heart itself (the coronary arteries), it results in a heart attack.

5. This is why people who smoke have seven times more heart attacks than those who do not smoke.

AN ARMY WITH NO GAS MASK

The final story explains why persons who smoke suffer more respiratory ailments and also why they cough a great deal.

1. The inside of the throat is a double passageway.
   a. The esophagus leads to the stomach.
   b. The trachea leads to the lungs.
   c. Sometimes food goes down the wrong barrel.
   d. Sometimes the particles people breathe get into the lungs.
2. In the trachea are cilia to protect the lungs.
   a. Small hairlike projections beat constantly in the trachea to keep foreign particles from getting into the lungs.
   b. Some of these particles go down the food barrel and chemicals in the stomach destroy them.
3. Some things will destroy the cilia.
   a. Tar and nicotine paralyze the cilia. After a person quits smoking, the cilia will work again.
   b. Tar and nicotine will eventually kill the cilia. A person will then cough continually to clean the trachea.

The Sick Engineer

The human body is made up of many small parts called cells. The cells are like the bricks on a house: it takes many bricks to make a house, and it takes many cells to make a boy or girl. Some of your cells make it possible for you to move; these are called muscles or muscle cells.

309

The cells that allow you to think are called brain cells. Other cells produce tears to wash your eyes out. Some cells help you to fight disease or get well after you have been sick. And the food that you eat is taken from your stomach to your muscles through a tunnel that is made of cells.

A car, like a person, is made of many parts. It has tires, an engine, windows, seats, and other parts. But a car needs a driver to make it go. The driver decides how fast it will go and in what direction it will move.

Likewise, a train has many boxcars, but it needs an engineer to make it go. The engineer determines how fast and in what direction the train will go.

Each of the cells in your body has its own driver or engineer. His name is Mr. DNA. He is not a real man, but he is the boss of the cell. Scientists refer to the boss of the cell as Mr. DNA. And Mr. DNA is a real bossy boss, because he tells the rest of the cell just what it can and cannot do.

Mr. DNA is a very wise boss, because he was passed on to you by your parents. Half of the Mr. DNA in each of your cells came from your mother and half came from your father. And the Mr. DNAs in the cells of your mother and father came from your grandmother and grandfather. So you see, Mr. DNA has been around for a long time and has a great deal of wisdom. There are a lot of Mr. DNAs in your body: one in every cell. They know just how to boss the rest of the cells. They know when you need to grow and when you should stop growing. They know when to make new cells to replace old worn-out ones and just how many new ones to make. And when new cells are made, the old Mr. DNA makes a new Mr. DNA for the new cell.

Your body is made up of many different kinds of cells, but each cell has its own engineer. Some cells are large and some are small. Some are long and some are short. Some move quickly and some do their work without moving. Some reproduce (make new cells) frequently and some never reproduce at all.

The best thing about human cells is that although they are different in size, shape, and color, all of the Mr. DNAs get along very well with each other. They share the food. They take turns. They help each other out of trouble. The reason that the cell bosses get along so well is that they have learned by hundreds of years of experience that the only way that they can continue to live is to work together. If one becomes greedy and eats more than his share of the food, it would mean that some of the other cells would have to go hungry or even die.

When a person smokes cigarettes, the brown tar in the smoke (previously demonstrated with smoking machine kit) gets on the cells in the lungs. When this happens, other cells rush to the lungs to help out. They try to eat up and destroy this poisonous brown tar. These special fighter plane cells are called white cells. And Mr. DNA in the white cell is a very good fighter pilot. If only small amounts of tar get into the lungs, the white cells will break it down into harmless substances. However, if the person continues to smoke, the white cells can only fight a losing battle, because there is too much brown tar.

If too much tar collects in the lungs, the poison makes Mr. DNA sick. Without killing him, it destroys a part of his brain. Now he cannot think properly. In this condition, he is no longer able to get along with the other cells. Because he is sick, Mr. DNA becomes greedy. The wisdom of the years is lost because of his sickness. In this greedy state, the sick cells eat up the food that properly belongs to other cells. The healthy cells then starve to death. Finally, because of the greed of these cells the whole body dies. The final blame probably should be placed on the brain cells because people who really think first would never start to smoke.

QUESTIONS

1. Who is the boss of the cell?
2. What are some of the things that he does?
3. What made the engineer sick?
4. How were the sick cells different from the normal cells?

VOCABULARY

cell, DNA, tar, white cells, reproduce

An Unfriendly Passenger on a Cell Truck

Mr. Muscle DNA is one of the hardest workers in your body. He works twenty-four hours every day to be sure that your muscles are well fed and ready to go to work when you want to get somewhere in a hurry. And whether you want to run, walk, climb, or swim, your muscles are always ready to go.

Mr. Muscle DNA has to do a lot of bookkeeping to keep his muscle cell working. He has to put in an order for so many truckloads of food and another order for so many truckloads of oxygen. And when the muscles are working, more and more orders must be sent out. Also, Mr. Muscle DNA has to send out for garbage trucks to take away all of the leftover material. You see, the muscle cell has to make its own fuel to burn while it is working. To do this, Mr. Muscle DNA combines the food you eat with the oxygen you breathe to make a high-test fuel. Mr. DNA calls his high-test fuel ATP. And so long as the ATP is available, your muscles can do many hours of work and play. But, if the ATP fuel gives out, the muscle cell dies.

You will remember that your family car also burns fuel. This fuel makes the engine run and the engine makes the wheels turn to move the car. When your car engine is running, it gives off some waste material that goes out the exhaust pipe. Your muscle cells also give off some waste materials when they burn ATP. This waste material is called carbon dioxide. Garbage truck cells come by your muscles every second of the day to pick up this waste material. The truck cells take this carbon dioxide to the lungs where you blow it out. And then while they are up at the lungs, they pick up a load of oxygen.

Mr. Muscle DNA has one very big worry: that something will happen to the trucks that bring him oxygen and take away carbon dioxide. He knows that if something happens to those trucks he is in real trouble. Fortunately, there is a factory inside your bones that makes new truck cells. The old truck cells break into small parts which are destroyed. Mr. Muscle DNA is very pleased about the fact that the old trucks are replaced by new truck cells every four months. Yet, he cannot help but worry that something might happen to his fleet of trucks.

There is one thing that you can do to relieve some of Mr. Muscle DNA's worries: never smoke cigarettes. When a cigarette burns, it gives off waste materials like the exhaust of your car. If this waste material from cigarettes gets in your lungs, it makes a big problem for Mr. Muscle DNA. You see, this cigarette waste gets into your truck cells and partly fills them up. And the bad thing is that this cigarette waste holds very tightly to the truck cells and just keeps riding around and around. This means that the truck cells can now only take part of a load of oxygen. Mr. Muscle DNA really starts to worry now. He knows that if the muscles have to do some hard work, he will be in trouble because his fleet of trucks can only bring him part of a load of oxygen; and without a full load of oxygen, Mr. DNA cannot make all the fuel he needs. He knows that if you enter a race, you will not be able to run as fast or as far as you would be able to if he could get full loads of oxygen. That, of course, is why good athletes do not smoke.

The material found in cigarette smoke that sticks in the back of the truck is called carbon monoxide. And by the way, this same material is found in the waste that comes out your exhaust pipe on the family car. Do not ever breathe this or stay in a closed garage in which a car is running. The exhaust of a car contains much more of this carbon monoxide than cigarettes. And if you breathe it even for a few minutes, your truck cells will become so filled that they cannot carry any oxygen. In this case, you will quickly die.

QUESTIONS

1. What is Mr. Muscle DNA's job?
2. What was the unfriendly passenger?
3. Where is the unfriendly passenger found other than in cigarette smoke?
4. How does smoke affect an athlete?

VOCABULARY

oxygen, ATP, carbon dioxide, carbon monoxide

A False Alarm

When Mr. Muscle DNA sends out an order for food or oxygen, he knows that he will get a delivery at once. He is thankful to the highway department of the body for this.

Inside your body, the highways are made up of many tunnels. These tunnels are necessary because the highways must pass under or through many of the different parts of the body. The tunnel highways are called blood vessels.

The delivery trucks that pass through the blood vessels do not have motors. Therefore, they must be pushed. It is your heart that does the pushing. It pushes all day and all night without stopping. And it pushes 72 to 100 times every minute. But it does slow down a little at night. This happens because you do not use your muscles while you are sleeping, and Mr. Muscle DNA can get along without so many trucks of oxygen and food.

Your heart is a very strong muscle which squeezes blood through the blood vessels just like you would squeeze water out of a balloon with the muscles of your hand. The human heart is about the size of your fist. It is small compared with a mouse's heart, which is about the size of a raspberry. But a giraffe needs a heart larger than yours because his heart must pump blood through many more tunnels. Thus, a giraffe heart is about the size of a basketball.

You have already learned that when Mr. Muscle DNA needs more food, he sends out an order to the heart. The heart then pushes more cars through the stomach area to pick up more food. However, if Mr. Nicotine gets in your body, he also sends out an order for food. But Mr. Nicotine sends out a false alarm, because the muscles do not really need more food.

The heart, unfortunately, does not know that this is a false alarm, and many trucks are loaded with fats and sugar and sent to the muscles. The trucks find out that it is a false alarm when they get to the muscle. The muscles do not have any room to unload the fats and sugar, and these foods have to ride around and around in the blood vessels.

If a lot of nicotine gets in the body, the trucks become overloaded. As these overloaded trucks pass through the highway tunnels, some of the fats and sugars spill onto the tunnel wall and start to block up part of the tunnel. This is very dangerous if it happens in the small tunnels that take food and oxygen to the heart muscle. If these tunnels become blocked, the person has a heart attack and may die. People who smoke have more heart attacks than people who do not smoke.

QUESTIONS

1. What are the highway tunnels?
2. What is Mr. Nicotine?
3. What was the false alarm?
4. Which highway tunnels are blocked during a heart attack?

VOCABULARY

nicotine, blood vessels, heart attack

An Army with No Gas Masks

Did you know that the inside of your throat is like a double-barreled shotgun? One barrel takes food to your stomach and the other barrel takes air to your lungs.

Put your finger on your Adam's apple. This is the beginning of your air barrel. Now, keeping your finger on the Adam's apple, swallow. What happened? The Adam's apple moved up. Each time you swallow the air barrel moves upward and partly closes so that food or drink will go the other way—down the food barrel to the stomach. But sometimes food goes down the wrong barrel and you are choked.

Your air barrel is made up of many cells and each cell has its own DNA boss. The DNA bosses in these cells work together on one big job—cleaning. Sloppy housekeeping by this group of cells would be very dangerous. The air barrel must always be kept open and clean.

The inside of the air barrel has many very tiny fingers. You have only five fingers on each hand, but the air barrel has thousands of tiny fingers that are always moving. These fingers catch small bits of dust or germs that enter the body when you breathe.

Hold your hands in front of you. Now move your fingers up and down quickly. The fingers in your air barrel move like this all of the time, even when you are sleeping. These fingers push anything that gets inside right out again. When these materials are pushed out, they fall down the food barrel and chemicals in the stomach destroy them. These fingers do such a fine job that if you were to put black ink down a chicken's air barrel, not a spot would be left after a short period of time.

The fingers in your air barrel are called cilia. These cilia do a wonderful job of keeping the air barrel clean. Coughing also helps to keep the barrel clean. But, if the cilia fingers were to stop working, you would have to do a lot of coughing to make up the difference.

Your lungs are very happy that the cilia fingers are there to protect them. These fingers are the lung's army. They are well trained and always ready to fight. What they lack in size, they make up for with courage. This fine army has only one weakness, poison gas. They are too tiny to carry gas masks. Therefore, they are in great trouble when the enemy uses gas.

The poison gas in cigarette smoke immediately paralyzes the cilia fingers. And if the person continues to smoke, the poison gas kills the cilia. That is why a person who smokes a lot also coughs a lot. The cilia fingers have been killed and coughing is the only way to keep the air barrel clean.

QUESTIONS

1. Can you think of another name for your air barrel?
2. What is the main job of the cilia fingers?
3. What is the main weakness of the cilia army?
4. Why do cigarette smokers cough a lot?

VOCABULARY

Adam's apple, chemicals, cilia, paralyzes

○ □

Pictures

Each student can draw a picture to illustrate his or her favorite part of one of the four stories that were examined.

○ □

Smoking Word Search

Several vocabulary words appear at the end of each story on smoking. To review the vocabulary, give the students the following word search and have them work it together. As each word is discovered, one of the students will explain the meaning of the word. The words which

can be found in the search are cell, DNA, tar, oxygen, carbon monoxide, nicotine, vessel, attack, cilia, air, poison, smoke, army, sick, alarm, heart, food, breathe, cough, germ, muscle, and brain.

D	N	A	R	M	Y	C
A	C	I	L	I	A	A
L	E	R	X	Y	T	R
A	L	T	A	R	T	B
R	L	N	O	U	A	O
M	G	E	R	M	C	N
P	B	S	I	C	K	M
O	X	Y	G	E	N	O
I	L	F	J	H	I	N
S	M	O	K	E	C	O
O	G	O	T	A	O	X
N	A	D	J	R	T	I
I	Y	D	C	T	I	D
C	O	U	G	H	N	E
K	V	E	S	S	E	L
B	R	E	A	T	H	E
J	B	R	A	I	N	Z
U	M	U	S	C	L	E

○ □ ☆

Thank You for Not Smoking Posters

Each student can make a Thank You for Not Smoking poster, which can be displayed throughout the school for a Thank You for Not Smoking week.

○ □

I.N.S. Club

As a culminating activity for a unit on smoking and diseases, the Franklin County Unit, Ohio Division of the American Cancer Society has developed the idea of forming an I.N.S. (I'll Never Start) Club. The student is given a pledge card to sign, a membership card to carry, and a badge to wear. The I.N.S. Clubs in Franklin County have been rechecked to see if the students have stuck to their pledges. The program has been successful thus far.

FIGURE 12B-1 Pledge card

"I.N.S." CLUB

I hereby promise that "I'll Never Start" SMOKING.

I realize that smoking is injurious to my health and can possibly cause cancer and other diseases.

Date _____ Signed _____

School _____

Grade _____

Teacher _____

FIGURE 12B-2 Membership card

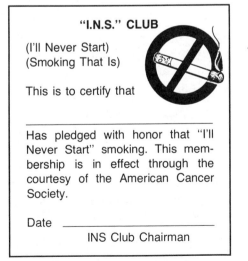

"I.N.S." CLUB

(I'll Never Start)
(Smoking That Is)

This is to certify that

_____

Has pledged with honor that "I'll Never Start" smoking. This membership is in effect through the courtesy of the American Cancer Society.

Date _____
　　　　　INS Club Chairman

FIGURE 12B-3 Badge

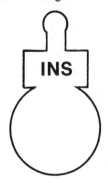

Evaluation

☐ ☆

LIFESTYLE CONTENT

The teacher can design a fill-in or matching test using the following words.

(cells) _____ 1. Small parts that make up the human body.

(DNA) _____ 2. The boss of the cell.

(white cells) _____ 3. Special cells that destroy the enemy in the body.

(tar) _____ Found in cigarette smoke. Makes the cell in the lungs dirty.

(ATP) _____ 5. A high test fuel for energy.

(carbon dioxide) _____ 6. The waste material that the body gives off.

(carbon monoxide) _____ 7. A gas that comes from cigarettes and the exhaust pipe of the family car.

(oxygen) _____ The body needs this gas to do work. People breathe it in through their lungs.

(heart) _____ A strong muscle that squeezes blood through the blood vessels.

(blood vessels) _____ Tunnels which carry blood to the cells.

(nicotine) _____ A false alarm in cigarettes that calls for sugar.

(cilia) _____ Small fingers that clean out the air barrel.

(cough) _____ Smokers need to do this to keep their air barrels clean.

LIFESTYLE VALUE

☐ ☆

The students can complete the following unfinished sentences:

Smoking is _____ .
When someone smokes _____ .
My parents _____ .
If someone asked me to smoke _____
_____
I think smoking _____ .

UNIT II: COMMUNICABLE DISEASES

Every preschooler should be immunized against the Big Seven: polio, measles, rubella, diphtheria, pertussis, tetanus, and mumps. Immunizations against these diseases greatly reduces the risk of illness to children and leaves a child susceptible to only the communicable diseases for which no immunity is afforded, such as chicken pox, the common cold, and pink-eye.

The lesson on Communicable Disease includes activities to learn about the Big Seven plus other communicable diseases. The students learn the symptoms of these illnesses and ways to reduce the risk of their becoming afflicted.

OBJECTiVES

1. After the potato experiment, the student will describe the growth of microorganisms.
2. The student will identify ten ways to prevent communicable diseases using the bowling game activity.
3. The student will use a health dictionary to locate one word associated with disease for each letter of the alphabet.
4. The student will give five correct clues about a disease in the germ mystery activity.
5. The student will complete "Happiness is" statements which reflect a desire to prevent the spread of communicable disease.

MATERIALS

1. Potatoes, three small saucers, and plastic bags.
2. Copies of the bowling sheets.
3. Copies of *Shots for Tots*.
4. Several health dictionaries.
5. Felt, wood board, glue, scissors.

Methods

○ ☐

Introductory Experiment

Are there microbes on your fingers? Are there microbes in your coughs? Are there microbes in your sneezes? The students will be able to answer these questions through performing the following experiment:

1. Put three pieces of sliced, cooked potato on three small, clean saucers.
2. Have someone rub a finger over the potato on the first saucer. Label the saucer.
3. Have someone cough on the potato on the second saucer. Label the saucer.
4. Have someone sneeze on the potato on the third saucer. Label the saucer.
5. Put each saucer in a clear plastic bag and seal it with tape. Look at the potato slices every day. Discuss how you will be able to see the microbes if they appear. (They will be in large clumps containing millions of microbes.) Do not

uncover the dishes at any time. Ask the students why and discuss the reasons.

□ ☆
Communicable Disease Bowling Game

Give each student a bowling sheet similar to the accompanying illustration:

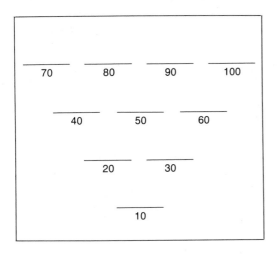

In this activity, a perfect score is 100. To knock down a pin, the student must write down a means of preventing disease. Answers may include cover your sneeze, avoid crowds, do not become overtired, avoid chilling, get immunized, do not use dirty handkerchiefs, wash hands after using toilet, wash hands before eating, use separate towels and wash cloths, properly cook and store foods, swim in chemically treated water, get premarital blood tests. See who can knock all the pins down first.

□
Drawing

Give each student a copy of *Shots for Tots*.* After they have read the booklet,

*A scriptographic booklet by Channing L. Bete Company, Inc., Greenfield, Massachusetts, 1975.

let the students draw pictures of a person who is ill. The picture may be of a person with a rash or runny nose or of someone who is coughing or sneezing. A headache, loss of appetite, and chills could be illustrated. Ask each student to show his or her drawing to the rest of the class and describe the symptoms of the ill person. If the correct illness has not been diagnosed after three guesses, the student should provide the class with additional facts, such as the methods by which it can spread, incubation period, and so on.

□ ☆
Disease Alphabet

In disease alphabet, the students think of words related to diseases that begin with different letters of the alphabet. The game can be played two ways. One way is to have the winner be the first student to find a word for each letter. The second way would be to give a certain time limit and the winner would be the student with the most words. This activity might be combined with a lesson on how to use a medical dictionary.

A—antibody, agent, antibiotic, antigen
B—bacteria, BCG
C—conjunctivitis, cell, cancer, chicken pox, communicable, chancre, cold
D—disease, diphtheria
E—earache, eye infection
F—fungi, fever
G—germ, gonorrhea
H—hepatitis, herpes, handkerchief, habit, harmful
I—immunity, illness, impetigo, influenza, immunization, infectious, incubation
J—jaundice, jungle fever
K—kissing, kidney
L—lungs, lice
M—microorganism, morbidity, mor-

tality, mumps, measles, medicine, malaria, malaise

N—nausea, nicrosis

O—organism, ointment, observation

P—pinkeye, pneumonia, pediculosis, polio, protozoa, parasite, plague

Q—quarantine

R—ringworm, rickettsiae, rabies

S—Sabin, Salk, scabies, strep throat, symptoms, syphilis, smallpox, swine flu

T—tuberculosis, treatment, trachoma, tetanus, typhus

U—ulcer, urethritis

V—vaccine, virus, vaccination, venereal disease, vomit

W—whooping cough

X—X-ray

Y—yaws, yellow fever

Z—zoonosis, zoosis, zinc ointment

Evaluation

LIFESTYLE CONTENT

☐

Germ Mystery Felt Board

The students can use a felt board activity to demonstrate their knowledge of communicable diseases. Each student makes a germ out of felt to put on the board. To make the felt germs, the students can use scrap pieces of felt, scissors, and glue. Have them draw the faces on the germ and cut out different pieces and glue them together. The germs should be dried for several hours before being used with the felt board. The students take turns putting their germs on the felt board. Ask the class to guess the disease caused by each student's germ. The student gives the class up to five clues. If the class guesses the disease before all five clues are given, the student must still

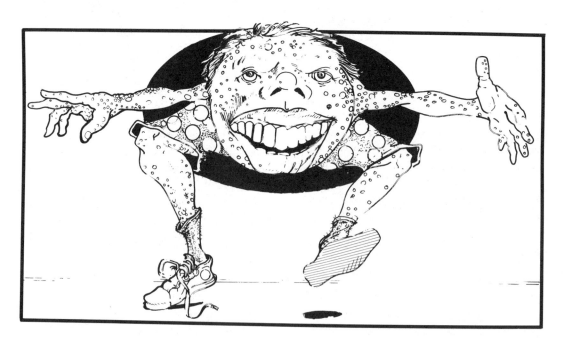

identify at least five facts. The teacher uses these five statements for evaluation.

The germ in the accompanying illustration represents rubeola or measles. The student might say the following:

1. I am caused by a virus.
2. I am spread by direct contact with infected people.
3. My incubation period from exposure to symptoms is ten to twelve days.
4. I will make you very tired, you will cough, and your eyes will be sensitive to light.
5. I am usually around in the spring.

LIFESTYLE VALUE

○ □

Ask the students to complete "Happiness is" statements about disease. Examples:

Happiness is getting a DPT shot.
Happiness is covering coughs and sneezes.
Happiness is using disposable tissues.
Happiness is not being chilled.
Happiness is being free of disease.

UNIT III: DIABETES

There are about 10 million diabetics in the United States, although the exact number is not known, since the condition may go undetected for many years. It usually occurs in people between the ages of thirty-five and sixty who are overweight. When insulin production is limited but not stopped, pills, proper diet, or a weight loss (or any combination) can often bring the condition under control.

Juvenile diabetes usually has its onset before age fifteen and accounts for about

5 percent of the diabetic population. This form is much more severe, since the ability to manufacture insulin deteriorates rapidly and daily injections of insulin are needed to live.

Both heredity and environment appear to affect the incidence of diabetes. Medical authorities believe that a predisposition to diabetes is inherited—possibly as the result of not one but several genetic abnormalities. The disease is then triggered by environmental factors, including obesity, exposure to certain viruses, and stress associated with surgery and pregnancy.

The child with diabetes in the teacher's classroom is special—just as is every other child. The child does not want to be singled out as being different from his or her schoolmates, yet his or her anxieties and those of the children in the classroom can be alleviated through education and understanding. The lesson on diabetes helps explain the condition and presents ways that students can help a friend who has diabetes.

OBJECTiVES

1. After viewing a series of transparencies and discussing them in class, the student will recognize at least ten words associated with diabetes and will be able to unscramble them.
2. After viewing the film *My Friend EDI*, the student will be able to write one paragraph describing the importance of exercise, diet, and insulin in the life of a diabetic.
3. Using a fact board, the student will demonstrate his or her ability to distinguish between signs of impending diabetic coma and insulin shock by placing the correct fact cards under the appropriate heading.

MATERIALS

1. Atlas Figures 25 through 33, Diabetes Series.

2. Board, nails, paper punch, index cards.

3 Film, *My Friend EDI* (15 minutes, color.).*

4. Copies of pre/post test.

Methods

□ ☆

Begin your discussion of diabetes by asking the class Can You Guess the Illness?

Clue No. 1: Two thousand years ago a Greek physician called it a disease in which the flesh melts away and is syphoned off in the urine.

Clue No. 2: It is a condition in which the victims' bodies cannot turn sugar into energy.

Clue No. 3: It is a condition in which, before treatment, the skin may itch, the vision may blur, and the victim may drink several gallons of water a day and always be hungry.

Clue No. 4: Before 1922, severely stricken victims had the choice of dying quickly or slowly starving to death.

Clue No. 5: In 1923, Fred Banting and Charles Best were awarded the Nobel Prize for their discovery of insulin, a substance normally found in the human body but missing (or present only in small amounts) in the body of a person with this condition.

(The answer is diabetes.)

□ ☆

Pretest

Determine how much the class knows

*Available through many local diabetes associations or from Eli Lilly Company, Indianapolis, Indiana.

about diabetes. Ask if the following statements are true or false.

(false) 1. Insulin is the sugar that the body uses for fuel.

(true) 2. Fat can be used for fuel or energy.

(true) 3. People who develop diabetes when they are an adult continue to make some insulin.

(false) 4. Insulin raises the blood sugar.

(true) 5. Insulin is formed in the pancreas.

(false) 6. Insulin is a cure for diabetes.

(false) 7. If you get diabetes as a child, you outgrow it by the time you are an adult

(true) 8. Key symptoms of diabetes are frequent urination, excessive thirst, and unusual weight loss.

(false) 9. Diabetes is contagious.

(true) 10. People with diabetes can participate in sports and even become champions.

□ ☆

Transparencies

Make nine transparencies from the illustrations provided in the Atlas and use them as the basis for a lecture/class discussion. You may wish to include the following supplementary information.

Diabetes mellitus is an inherited condition which prevents the body from using sugar properly. A hormone known as insulin is usually produced in the pancreas, a gland behind the stomach. Insulin allows the body to take a sugar called glucose from food; insulin lowers the blood sugar. The pancreas also produces digestive juices and another hormone called glucagon, which raises the blood sugar. We need these hormones to keep the level of blood sugar (glucose) at an even level.

Why do we even need this blood sugar (glucose)? Our bodies are made up of many, many cells. Glucose is the fuel needed by our cells so they can work. The bloodstream carries glucose to all of the cells in the body, but the glucose cannot enter the cells unless insulin is present. If the glucose cannot be used, it increases in the blood and some of it is lost in the urine, along with minerals and water.

Fat can also be used for energy. Fat does not require the presence of insulin. When fat is used as the main source of energy, some of it is changed to ketones. One of the ketones is acetone. As the level of ketones increases in the blood, some of them spill over into the urine.

As sugar is lost in the urine, the amount of urine increases, and the person becomes very thirsty. The person loses weight because she or he is losing urine water and the body is using fat for energy. If the body continues without insulin, ketones and acids build up in the blood and make the person very sick.

Diabetes is not contagious. You cannot catch it from your friend.

There is not yet a cure for diabetes, but much research is being done. Meanwhile, diabetes can be controlled by (a) regulating the amount of sugar eaten in foods, (b) regulating the amount of sugar used up through exercise and other activities, and (c) by taking the insulin that is prescribed by a doctor.

□ ☆
Films

Show the film *My Friend EDI.* EDI (Exercise-Diet-Insulin) is an elflike creature seen only by Davy to help him get his parents and friends and himself adjusted to life as a diabetic. The film is designed to assist in the explanation and treatment of diabetes.

(The 20-minute film *Low Blood Sugar Emergencies in the Diabetic Child* is recommended for in-service training of teachers, nurses, and other school personnel who may come in contact with a diabetic child.)*

□
Puppet Show

Puppets can be used to explain why people with diabetes need to carefully control the amount of foods and sweets they eat. Meals should be eaten at regular times, since a delay may result in insulin reaction. The puppets can give a party showing foods that could be permitted, such as artificially sweetened beverages, gelatin, or ice creams.

In another situation, the puppet with diabetes can be shown skipping lunch to save some money for a present. Unfortunately, this results in a blood sugar level that is too low, thus causing an insulin reaction. An insulin reaction may also be caused by too much insulin, nervous or emotional tension, or strenuous exercise not covered by extra food.

(See Chapter 14A for symptoms of diabetic coma and insulin shock and appropriate treatment.)

☆

Read to the class the article "Victory over the Sugar Sickness" by Charles H. Best.†

Evaluation

LIFESTYLE CONTENT

Facts surrounding diabetes mellitus may be confusing to the class unless the topic

---

*Available on loan from the Juvenile Diabetes Foundation, Greater Washington Area Chapter, P.O. Box 48, Silver Springs, MD 20907, as well as from many local diabetes chapters.

†As told to J. D. Ratcliff and appearing in the March 1964 issue of *Today's Health.*

is covered slowly and adequately reviewed. Several different evaluations may be helpful as learning tools.

□ ☆

Unscramble the Word

1. *IATBDEES LLESUTMI* is an inherited condition which prevents the body from using *USARG* normally.

2. Eating a lot of *SETWES* does not cause diabetes.

3. The *APNCREAS* makes *NILUSIN* and NAGOCULG.

4. In the human body, the source of energy is a *LECL*.

5. The fuel for the cell is *GELSUOC*.

6. *INNISUL* is the key that allows glucose to enter the cells.

7. After meals, the blood glucose level *RSEIS*.

8. Without glucose, our body uses *TAF* for energy.

9. When fat is used as a major source of energy, the liver converts some of it to *EKSENOT*.

10. The amount of sugar in the *RUINE* reflects the amount of sugar in the blood.

(bonus) 11. When glucose is lost in the urine, it carries a lot of *REWTA, IMRELASN* and other substances with it.

□ ☆

Post test

Administer the test as given before the lecture about diabetes. Determine whether the students have improved in their understanding of diabetes.

□

Drawing Activity

After the students have seen the two transparencies What Happens When There Is Not Enough Insulin? and Weight Loss (Atlas Figures 28 and 29), have each child draw a picture of what may happen when a diabetic does not receive enough insulin. The picture could illustrate thirst, weight loss, or hospitalization.

TABLE 12B-1 SIGNS OF DIABETIC COMA AND INSULIN SHOCK

Diabetic Coma	Insulin Reaction
Slow onset (unconsciousness is slow in developing)	Rapid onset (fainting may develop without warning)
Too much sugar in the blood	Not enough sugar in the blood
Not enough insulin	Too much insulin
Intense thirst, dry mouth, and frequent urination	Hunger
Skin is dry and flushed	Skin is pale and sweaty
Loss of appetite, nausea, and vomiting	Gnawing sensation in stomach
Large amounts of sugar and ketones in urine	Headache, jittery feeling, trembling
Breath has a peculiar fruity odor	Impaired vision, dimness of vision
No adequate first-aid treatment	Personality change, irritability
Call the doctor at once	Requires food containing sugar (candy, soft drink, fruit juice)

□ ☆
Fact Board

Construct a fact board by pounding nails in rows onto a large board. Use a paper punch to make holes in index cards. Facts about diabetes can be written on the index cards and displayed or rank ordered. The signs of impending diabetic coma and insulin shock (as listed in Table 12B-1) may be written on individual cards, which are shuffled. The students can then be asked to draw a card and place it under the appropriate heading: Impending Diabetic Coma or Impending Insulin Shock.

LIFESTYLE VALUE

□ ☆

Ask the students to discuss or write a short paper answering the questions: How do you think Dr. Banting felt when he gave up his little medical practice and sold his office furniture, books, and almost everything he owned to stake his resources on a hunch that he could cure the sugar sickness? Do you think you would have done the same thing?

Tell the class that scientists soon hope to develop a test that will help physicians recognize at an early stage a person who is prone to diabetes. Ask the students whether, if this were to happen, they think everyone should be tested, and why.

Have the students rank order the following age groups by placing a 1 by the group they think should be tested first, a 2 by the next group, etc.

_____ 6 months to 6 years old
_____ 7 to 15 years old
_____ 15 to 34 years old
_____ 35 to 60 years old
_____ Over 60

UNIT IV: SEXUALLY TRANSMITTED DISEASES

Educators are aware that sexually transmitted or venereal diseases (VD) are rampantly on the increase. Among the infectious diseases reportable to public health authorities in the United States, gonorrhea currently ranks number one. This disease is more common than strep throat, mumps, and measles.

What can be done about the sexually transmitted disease epidemic? The increase in these diseases is most likely related to ignorance, apathy, and a lack of responsibility. Because medical scientists know the cause, transmission, and treatment for these diseases, the responsibility for the eradication of VD is on educators' shoulders. Some will argue that providing education about sexually transmitted diseases in the fifth, sixth, or seventh grade is too soon. Statistics indicate, however, that providing it later than these grades may be too late.

OBJECTIVES

1. The student will demonstrate an increase in cognitive knowledge by taking tests.

2. After playing To Tell the Truth and participating in other class activities, the student will be able to list five misconceptions surrounding syphilis and gonorrhea and give correct information concerning them.

3. The students will demonstrate their knowledge of syphilis and gonorrhea by playing the VD game.

4. The students will anonymously respond to statements concerning personal responsibility for their own health and that of others by checking the appropriate columns of a VD values quiz.

5. The student will place himself or

herself on a continuum with regard to contracting sexually transmitted diseases and be able to discuss his or her position.

MATERIALS

1. 3-by-5-inch index cards.
2. Pretest, which will also be used as a post test.
3. Films, *VD—Attack Plan and VD—A New Focus.* *
4. VD gameboards and game cards, Atlas Figures 89 and 90. One die per four students and individual markers.
5. Construction materials, such as paper, scissors, paints.

Methods

☐ ☆

To get an idea of each student's level of VD knowledge, give a pretest without prior notice.

Pass out 3-by-5-inch index cards and have each student write down questions about VD she or he would like answered.

☐ ☆

Movie

Select a movie from your local health department to introduce the topic of sexually transmitted diseases. After viewing the film, divide the class into groups of three or four and have them complete the sentences based on the film. (The stem sentences may also be completed individually.)

☐ ☆

Stem Sentences

I thought the most shocking fact presented in the movie was _____.

*Information on how to obtain appears at the end of the unit.

The biggest problem for females who get VD is _____.

The first signs of gonorrhea in the male are _____.

When a male goes to the doctor and learns that he really does have gonorrhea (or another sexually transmitted disease) he has a responsibility to _____.

Gonorrhea can be cured if _____.

Have the students write their own stem sentences.

☆

Guest Speakers

Invite a physician or nurse from your local health department to talk about the VD program in your community. Guest speakers may also come from a hot line or a community VD clinic.

☆

Original Play

Have the students plan, write, and produce a play about sexually transmitted diseases. The characters may include Willy Wise, a knowledgeable student; Irma Ignorant, a student full of myths and misinformation about venereal disease; Carl Clapp, the gonococcus germ (gonorrhea); Suzie Syph, the spirochete (syphilis); and possibly Harry Herpes II, a virus germ. By researching information to be included in the play, the students will be provided with added facts and materials about sexually transmitted diseases.

☆

Math Related Activities

Have the class prepare charts showing the VD case rates for the 13 to 19 age group—nationally, statewide, and locally. The students can also prepare a graph that compares the amount of money spent on controlling VD with that spent on controlling other diseases, such as cancer and heart disease.

□ ☆
To Tell the Truth

Conduct a panel discussion based on the format of the TV show "To Tell the Truth."

A simple modification of the game is to have the teacher act as the moderator and direct questions to three students identified as VD Expert No. 1, No. 2, and No. 3. Only one of the contestants will answer all of his or her questions correctly. After all the questions have been asked, the class will then be polled as to who really is the VD expert. The following script may be used.

VD Expert No. 1

1. What do the terms clap and morning drip refer to? Answer: syphilis

2. Describe the chancre of syphilis. Answer: soft, very painful, usually large, and easily identified

3. Can a person be vaccinated against syphilis and gonorrhea? Answer: yes, just like smallpox, polio, and other diseases

VD Expert No. 2

1. What is the best known treatment for syphilis and gonorrhea? Answer: penicillin

2. Can I get these diseases if I am a virgin? Answer: yes, if you come into contact with an infected person and are sexually intimate

3. Can syphilis and gonorrhea be gotten at the same time? Answer: yes, as a matter of fact, they frequently are

VD Expert No. 3

1. What is one of the most common methods of contracting syphilis and gonorrhea? Answer: from public fixtures such as doorknobs, toilet seats, and drinking fountains

2. Is a person immune from these diseases if he or she has had one or the other? Answer: no, a person can get them over and over even after being treated and cured of them

3. If the sores and rashes of syphilis disappear, is the person cured of the disease? Answer: yes, if they go away you have nothing to worry about

Correct Answers

Expert No. 1—1. gonorrhea
2. hard, painless, often goes unnoticed
3. yes

Expert No. 2—1. penicillin
2. yes, if you come into intimate contact with an infected person
3. yes, they frequently are

Expert No. 3—1. Any intimate sexual contact,
2. no, you can get the diseases over and over
3. no, you are simply progressing to a different stage of the disease

(The real VD expert is No. 2.)

VENEREAL DISEASE GAMES

To review the many facts about venereal disease, you may want to use one of the following games.

☆
Game No. 1

Make the gameboard from a large square or rectangular shaped sheet of ⅜-inch plywood (see pattern in Atlas*). Paint

*Gameboard and directions developed by Mary Anne Mead, School of Health, Physical Education and Recreation, Ohio State University.

different spaces on the board. VD can be painted in the middle of the board with six spaces for piles of cards. The six spaces should be painted orange, blue, green, yellow, red, and purple. A die can be made from balsa wood. The six sides of the die should be painted to correspond to the spaces painted on the gameboard. The cards are placed in these six spaces. The cards are made of colored construction paper or colored index cards. Print the question and its numerical value (1, 2, or 3) on the card. Divide the cards equally, making them the six different colors. It would be a good idea to have each student or team make a marker to use with the game.

The teacher should decide which player or team will go first. The player rolls the die to see what color comes up. He or she takes a question from the pile of cards that corresponds to that color. The question will also have a number on it (1, 2, or 3). If the player answers the question correctly, he or she moves ahead the indicated number of spaces. If the student answers incorrectly, he or she must move back the indicated number of spaces. The first player or team to circle the board is declared the winner.

Sample Questions and Answers

(Numerical value for each correct answer is given in parentheses.)

(1) What is the cause of gonorrhea? (bacteria called gonococcus)

(1) How is gonorrhea transmitted? (spread almost exclusively by sexual intercourse)

(1) How is gonorrhea transmitted to the newborn child? (through an eye infection that may occur in a baby who passes through the birth canal of an infected mother)

(2) What is the incubation period for gonorrhea? (three to seven days)

(1) What are the symptoms of gonorrhea in the male? (1 point for each correct symptom with a maximum of 3) (painful, burning urination; yellowish discharge from penis; swelling of urethral tissue)

(1) What are the symptoms of gonorrhea in the female? (usually none [90%]; lower abdominal pain in advanced stages)

(2) What is the treatment for gonorrhea? (a single dose of oral medication [combination of ampicillin and probenecid] or injected penicillin)

(2) What happens if gonorrhea goes untreated? (may result in sterility, arthritis, or heart disease)

(1) Can gonorrhea be prevented? (yes, by using a condom which prevents contamination of the urethra)

(1) What is the cause of syphilis? (caused by a spirochete)

(2) What conditions will kill the spirochete? (a spirochete is susceptible to drying, to temperatures higher than that of the body, and to soap and water)

(1) What are the best conditions for the spirochete? (moisture, such as in sexual intercourse and intimate kissing)

(1) How is syphilis transmitted? (the spirochete from the lesion of an infected person passes through the intact mucous membranes or open skin of a second person)

(1) Name a misconception about the transmission of syphilis. (mistakenly believed by some that syphilis can be transmitted by doorknobs, drinking fountains, or toilet seats)

(2) What is the incubation period for syphilis? (ranges from 10 to 60 days, with an average of three weeks)

(1) What is the primary stage of syphilis? (the appearance of a chancre)

(1) Describe a chancre. (usually hard, does not itch or hurt; is not tender to touch; usually does not fill with pus)

(1) How long does the chancre appear? (for about two weeks)

(1) How is primary syphilis diagnosed? (absolute diagnosis can be made only from finding the spirochete in the chancre)

(3) How is primary syphilis treated? (with penicillin; for those sensitive to penicillin, erythromycin and tetracycline may be used)

(2) What symptoms appear in secondary syphilis? (skin lesions which appear as a flattened, slightly raised red rash; white patches which may occur in the mouth and anus; lymph nodes may enlarge)

(3) How long does secondary syphilis last? (from three months to several years; average is two years)

(2) How is secondary syphilis diagnosed? (the body develops antibodies during secondary syphilis; syphilis can be diagnosed from a blood test)

(2) What happens during late syphilis? (also called symptomatic syphilis; organs of the body—heart, blood vessels, brain, eyes, spinal cord—may be damaged)

(2) How is secondary syphilis treated? (with penicillin)

(1) How is late syphilis treated? (with antibiotics; however, damage cannot be reversed)

(2) What is congenital syphilis? (a condition in which the syphilis organism has passed from the infected mother to the unborn baby through the placenta)

(1) What is nongonococcal urethritis? (urethritis, or inflammation of the urethra, that is not caused by gonorrhea)

(2) What is herpes genitalis? (an acute inflammatory dermatosis)

(1) What is the cause of herpes genitalis? (a virus)

(2) What are the symptoms of herpes genitalis? (lesions that appear in the genital area, possibly accompanied by fever, headache, loss of appetite, and tender and swollen lymph nodes)

(2) How is herpes genitalis treated? (with isoprinosine, an antiviral drug; compresses of silver nitrate and boric acid; better treatments are currently being evaluated)

(1) What is Operation Venus? (the toll free telephone number, 800-523-1885, which anyone who needs more information about VD can call)

□ ☆

Game No. 2

Use the gameboard found in the Atlas or make a larger and more permanent board using poster board or a rectangular sheet of ⅜-inch plywood. Each student will need six syphilis and six gonorrhea cards (pattern for cards is included in Atlas). One die is required for every four students.

Each player receives twelve cards, six syphilis and six gonorrhea. Roll die to determine first player; students move clockwise in turn after that. The player throws the die to find out the number of boxes to move. Each box represents a situation involving VD. The players must decide which kind of VD. When a player lands on a box, he or she must lay down the correct kind of VD card (syphilis or gonorrhea). If the player lands on a box already covered by a card, better luck next turn! Next player moves. If the player lands on a box requiring a kind of VD card he or she has run out of, better luck next turn! Next player moves. Challenges: if a player thinks another player has laid down an incorrect card, the player may challenge. If correct, he or she gets to lay down the right card. Player challenged removes his or her card. If incorrect, original player may put the correct card on top of the first. The winner is the player who uses up all of his or her cards first or has the fewest cards left at the end of the game.

Evaluation

LIFESTYLE CONTENT

☐ ☆

Give the students the following multiple-choice test.

_(b)_ 1. Venereal diseases are caused by
   a. body strain
   b. germs
   c. injury
   d. toilet seats

_(a)_ 2. Which of the following applies to both syphilis and gonorrhea?
   a. two different diseases
   b. two names for the same disease
   c. two stages of the same disease
   d. two noncommunicable diseases

_(c)_ 3. What is the most common venereal disease?
   a. herpes genitalis
   b. common cold
   c. gonorrhea
   d. syphilis

_(b)_ 4. Gonorrhea is transmitted to the newborn child
   a. through the placenta
   b. through the birth canal
   c. through the bloodstream
   d. all of the above are correct

_(d)_ 5. Untreated gonorrhea may result in
   a. arthritis
   b. heart disease
   c. sterility
   d. all of the above are correct

_(b)_ 6. Gonorrhea can often be prevented by
   a. using a spermicide
   b. using a condom
   c. having a vasectomy
   d. having intercourse only during menstruation

_(c)_ 7. A chancre is
   a. painful but disappears in two weeks
   b. filled with pus and contains spirochetes
   c. painless and disappears in two weeks
   d. red, itches, and filled with bacteria

_(b)_ 8. Secondary syphilis is diagnosed by
   a. examining the chancre for spirochetes
   b. a blood test
   c. examining the urine for pus
   d. a Pap smear

_(d)_ 9. Against which of these diseases may a person be vaccinated?
   a. gonorrhea
   b. syphilis
   c. both gonorrhea and syphilis
   d. neither gonorrhea nor syphilis

_(c)_ 10. If the seminal duct of a man is blocked by scar tissue from a

gonorrheal infection, which of the following would result?
a. arthritis
b. blindness
c. sterility
d. heart attack

LIFESTYLE VALUE

☆

The student will anonymously respond to statements concerning personal responsibility for her or his own health and that of others by checking the appropriate column.*

S/A = Strongly Agree
U/D = Undecided
S/D = Strongly Disagree

	S/A	U/D	S/D
I would report all my sexual contacts.	___	___	___
I would tell my contacts myself if I had VD.	___	___	___
I would refer my steady to his or her doctor to get checked for VD.	___	___	___
VD is nobody's business but my own.	___	___	___
If I thought I had VD, I'd be ashamed and embarrassed to do anything about it.	___	___	___
Knowing I had VD, I'd no longer indulge in sexual activity until I was cured.	___	___	___

*Adapted from *VD: Getting the Right Answers* by Lenore Zarate, American School Health Association, 260 Sheridan Avenue, Palo Alto, CA 94306, pp. 42–43.

I would follow the doctor's instructions to the letter.	___	___	___
I recognize the relationship between VD and danger to unborn children.	___	___	___
If I heard my sexual partner had VD, I would be very upset and disappointed.	___	___	___
I see no need to take any type of precaution against VD.	___	___	___

☐ ☆

Continuum

The student will place herself or himself on the following continua with regard to contracting sexually transmitted diseases and be able to discuss her or his position.

How do you feel about VD in general?

Not worth discussing because it won't happen to me	Extremely serious and can cause death

What would you do if the person you are dating says, "Prove to me you love me."

Do anything, including taking risks	Forget him or her

What would you do if you thought you had syphilis?

Wait and see if the symptoms go away	Get help immediately from doctor or clinic

□ ☆

Thought Question

Have the students discuss or write their thoughts about the question How do you think sexually transmitted diseases can be stopped?

FURTHER READINGS

What Everyone Should Know About VD—Facts About Venereal Disease, scriptographic booklet by Channing L. Bete Company, Inc., Greenfield, Massachusetts.

What You Should Know About VD, Alton Blakeslee and Brian Sullivan, The Benjamin Company, Inc., 485 Madison Avenue, New York, NY 10022.

FILMS

VD—Attack Plan (1973) 16 minutes; Walt Disney Educational Materials Company, 800 Sonora Avenue, Glendale, CA 91201.

VD—A New Focus (1972) 15 minutes; American Educational Films, 331 North Maple Drive, Beverly Hills, CA 90210.

ADDITIONAL DISEASE CONTROL REFERENCES

Pamphlets: Contact the local branch of the following organizations before writing to the national headquarters: American Cancer Society, American Heart Association, American Lung Association, American Medical Association, American Optometric Association, Arthritis Foundation, Muscular Dystrophy Association, National Association of Hearing and Speech Agencies, National Foundation, National Multiple Sclerosis Society, National Society for the Prevention of Blindness, National Society for Crippled Children and Adults, and United Cerebral Palsy Association, Inc.

Allergy Foundation of America, 801 Second Avenue, New York, NY 10017. (The following pamphlets are available: *Hay Fever; Handbook for the Asthmatic; Allergy in Children; The Skin and Its Allergies; Insect Stings Can Be Dangerous; Mold Allergy; Food Allergy; Drug Allergy; Cosmetic Allergy; Asthma, Climate and Weather; Tips for Teachers;* and *Answers to Some Questions About Allergy.*)

"Childhood Diseases," Prudential Insurance Company of America, Public Relations and Advertising, Newark, NJ 07102.

"The Common Cold" (a scriptographic booklet) (Greenfield, Mass.: Channing L. Bete).

Current Health magazine features a new disease each month, ranging from appendicitis to zoonoses. (Curriculum Innovations, Inc., 501 Lake Forest Avenue, Highwood, IL 60040). One issue of special interest appeared September 1977: "The Ten Least Wanted" (heart disease, cancer, stroke, accidents, influenza and pneumonia, diabetes mellitus, cirrhosis of the liver, arteriosclerosis, infant death, suicide). (The featured condition in this issue is lice. The issue also discusses antibiotics.)

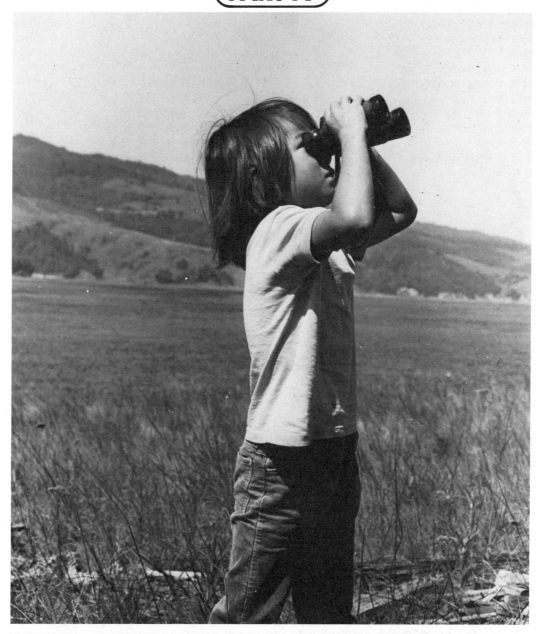

PART IV

TOWARD A HEALTHY ENVIRONMENT

CHAPTER 13

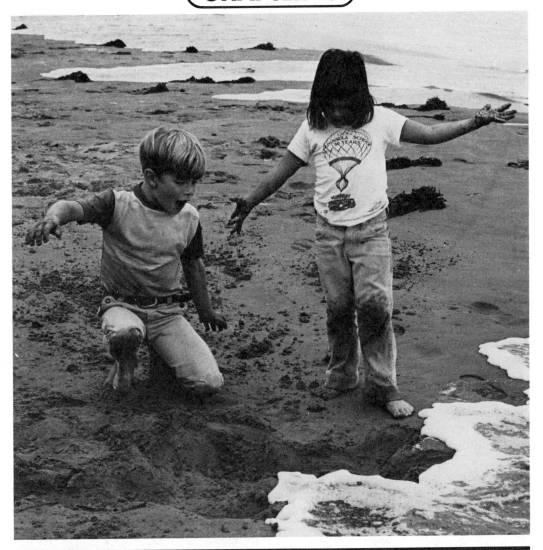

PART A: THE ENVIRONMENT

Until now, Americans have met environmental stresses by gradually adapting the environment to meet lifestyle expectations. However, it appears that these external controls, pressures, and changes have not been totally successful in meeting the environmental needs of persons desiring optimal health. Not long ago, Americans witnessed the closing of schools because of shortages of oil and gas, and many young children shivered in chilly homes while learning by television. A blackout in New York resulted in large economic losses from theft and crime. Sore throats and itchy eyes plague persons residing in Manhattan, Los Angeles, and Denver.

The consequences of an environment contaminated and abused by Americans' lifestyle selections are apparent. Americans are now faced with the task of reversing these selections so that they can ensure an environment fit for quality living.

As with most types of behavior, the best time to positively influence attitudes and habits is at an early age. The intelligent selection of alternatives in lifestyle regarding the environment should therefore be a focus of concern for the elementary schoolteacher.

A HEALTHY ENVIRONMENT

The environment is the surroundings in which people live and it includes homes, schools, places of business, recreation areas, and neighborhoods. On a larger scale, the environment includes cities and wilderness areas, air, water, the continents, and the oceans.

A healthy environment is one that allows people to grow and develop in order to become physically, mentally, and socially healthy individuals. It provides a variety of beautiful scenery, neat and clean neighborhoods, and quiet surroundings.

POLLUTION

As population has increased, people's activities have produced substances that are hazardous to the environment. These substances are called pollutants and may be chemical, physical, or electromagnetic in nature. Pollutants are found in the air

that people breathe, the water that they drink, and the soil in which they grow their food. While it appears doubtful that people will ever do away with pollutants entirely, they can and must find ways to limit their daily exposure to these substances in order to ensure a quality lifestyle.

Air Pollution

The human body utilizes about five quarts of air each minute. In order to meet this demand for air, it is necessary to take fourteen to eighteen shallow or eight deep breaths a minute.

ATMOSPHERIC LAYERS

The air that people breathe is the atmosphere, a covering of gases held close to the earth by gravity. The innermost layer is known as the troposphere and extends about six miles above the earth's surface; the next layer is the stratosphere, which extends to about thirty miles above the earth's surface; the third layer is the mesosphere, extending fifty miles above the earth's surface; the last layer is the ionosphere, which extends about 180 miles above the earth's surface.

The atmosphere becomes less dense (thinner and thinner) with increases in altitude, since gravity holds most of the air close to the earth's surface. Because of this, 99 percent of the molecules of gases that make up the atmosphere are found within the first twenty miles of the earth's surface.

GASES

Only the lower portions of the atmosphere are thus capable of supporting life. This thin area of the atmosphere consists primarily of nitrogen (78 percent); oxygen, the gas which supports animal and plant life (21 percent); argon, an inert gas (0.9 percent); and carbon dioxide, the gas needed by plants for photosynthesis (0.03 percent).

In addition to these gases, which account for the bulk of the dry atmosphere, the atmosphere contains water vapor, which varies in volume from 0 percent to 5 percent, depending upon local conditions. To these naturally occurring constituents the activities of humans have added a variety of pollutants.

SOURCES OF POLLUTANTS

Pollutants in the air come from many sources, some of which are the exhaust from automobiles, buses, and jets; smoke from oil refineries, power-generating plants, and steel mills and from residential heating; and natural causes such as volcanic eruptions, dust storms, and forest fires.

In general, pollutants in the air arise through the processes of combustion, vaporization, or attrition. Combustion is the process of burning. When fuel is burned, the oxygen in the air combines with the carbon in the fuel to produce carbon dioxide and water vapor. When burning is not complete, another gas, carbon monoxide, is produced.

Carbon monoxide is produced when cigarettes are smoked, resulting in one hazardous and frequent form of air pollution adversely affecting an otherwise quality lifestyle. Since carbon monoxide is also produced when cars and buses consume fuel, heavy traffic will guarantee frequent breathing of this noxious gas.

When fuel that contains sulfur, such as coal and oil, is burned, a poisonous compound called sulfur dioxide is produced. When this is combined with water vapor, the result is sulfuric acid.

Automobile engines produce another gas known as nitrogen dioxide. This pollutant irritates the eyes and throat and is harmful to plant life.

Air pollutants are sometimes the result of vaporization. This is the process by which a liquid is changed into a gas. Many chemical plants release such vapors into the air.

Attrition is the process of wearing away. Through this process, many small particles are released into the atmosphere. These small particles or particulates come from grinding, blasting, and drilling processes.

Particulates, also known as aerosols, may come from natural sources such as land dust, volcanic eruptions, pollen, and forest fires. About 90 percent of the particulate matter in the atmosphere comes from natural sources. Particulate matter affects the lungs of animals, contributes to smog, and reduces the amount of light penetrating the atmosphere.

SMOG

Smog (the word is formed by combining smoke and fog) is common to many large cities. Natural air movements usually carry smog away from the cities where it is produced and disperse it through the atmosphere. However, under special atmospheric conditions, an inversion (a layer of warm air covering a layer of much cooler air) may develop. This layer of warm air acts as a lid or cover, trapping pollutants and preventing their dispersion into the rest of the atmosphere.

Such conditions are common in many parts of the country and may exist for long periods of time, causing smog and pollutants to accumulate in the atmosphere. Smog that builds up in cities during inversions may be of two types: sulfurous and photochemical smog.

Sulfurous Smog

Sulfurous smog is caused by the sulfur dioxide formed by the burning of fuels that contain sulfur. Most sulfur smog comes from the burning of coal, but fuel oil is also an important source of this kind of smog. As pointed out previously, when sulfur dioxide combines with water vapor in the atmosphere, it produces sulfuric acid, a very strong acid. In vapor form, sulfuric acid sticks to small particulates and becomes a severe eye and lung irritant. As a person breathes, the acid attacks and destroys the lining of the upper airway and penetrates the air sacs at the ends of the lungs causing irreversible lung damage.

In high concentrations, sulfurous smog can cause death. Over 1,000 deaths were attributed to one episode of sulfurous smog in London in December 1952. The Thanksgiving Episode smog of New York in 1966 was held responsible for over 168 deaths in seven days.

Sulfuric acid also attacks plants and in high concentration is destructive to several forms of plant life. It damages marble, limestone, and mortar, thus wearing away buildings, statues, and many priceless art relics that are exposed to it.

Photochemical Smog

A second form of smog, photochemical, is produced from the internal combustion engine of the automobile. This engine produces exhaust which contains nitrogen dioxide and hydrocarbons (unburned gasoline).

Nitrogen dioxide is a brownish gas. As it absorbs energy from sunlight, it breaks down into nitrogen monoxide and oxygen—a highly active form of oxygen. This active form of oxygen combines with ordinary oxygen to form ozone. The ozone and the nitrogen dioxide combine with hydrocarbons from automobile exhaust to form a substance called PAN (peroxyacetyle nitrate).

PAN is the main constituent of photochemical smog. It is brownish in color and reduces visibility. In small amounts, it is irritating to the eyes, which causes them to smart and water. In larger doses, PAN causes throat irritation and difficulty in breathing, which is especially harmful to those already suffering with emphysema or bronchitis. PAN is also damaging to green plants, as evidenced in Southern California, where thousands of acres of forest land are being damaged by photochemical smog.

OTHER AIR POLLUTANTS

Aside from smog, other pollutants affect the atmosphere, including lead, carbon monoxide, carbon dioxide, and asbestos.

Lead

Lead in the atmosphere comes primarily from automobile exhaust. It is added to gasoline to raise its octane rating. When gasoline is burned, the lead is released into the atmosphere and can travel great distances. Lead was discovered in the polar ice caps at about the same time it was introduced into gasoline, and its level has increased yearly with each new layer of ice.

As much as 50 percent of the lead that a person breathes is retained in the body. As lead accumulates in the body, it may cause irreversible damage to the nervous system. Fortunately, many people are now using lead free gasoline in their cars, which will do much to solve the problem.

Carbon Monoxide

Carbon monoxide, another pollutant, is a colorless and odorless gas that is produced when combustion is not complete.

It is found in automobile exhaust and is a by-product of cigarette smoking. Exposure to even small amounts produces headaches, dizziness, confusion, and fatigue while large amounts of carbon monoxide can be fatal.

Exposure to 10 to 15 parts per million (ppm) of carbon monoxide for eight hours impairs time judgment, while 30 ppm for the same period of time affects vision and physical response. Tests show that people driving in traffic may be exposed to 50 ppm of carbon monoxide, while heavy expressway driving in Los Angeles or New York may result in carbon monoxide levels of 140 ppm.

Carbon Dioxide

Carbon dioxide, another gas produced by burning, is not normally considered a pollutant because it is a necessary part of the life processes of green plants. While the amounts of carbon dioxide produced by automobile exhaust, home heating, and industrial combustion do not have a direct harmful effect on humans, the indirect effects appear to be damaging to the environment. The carbon dioxide in the air will combine with water vapor to form carbonic acid. This weak acid erodes stone monuments and works of art in addition to corroding magnesium and other metals.

Asbestos

Asbestos is a fibrous mineral compound that is used in brake linings, roofing, insulation, ceiling tiles (for its insulating and sound-deadening qualities), and talcum powder. It is also found in the crushed stone used to pave rural roads and parking lots.

When small fibers of asbestos are inhaled, they lodge in the lungs of the victim and produce fibrous tissue which reduces the ability of the victim to breathe properly. Recently it has been discovered that asbestos may have a carcinogenic (cancer-producing) effect on the lungs. For this reason, asbestos ceiling tiles are being replaced in many schools and office buildings with less hazardous materials, and roads are no longer being paved with crushed rock containing asbestos.

Noise Pollution

Noise as a pollutant is difficult to define. What may be an agreeable sound to one person is noise to another. In general, however, noise can be defined as unwanted sound.

Noise is measured in units called decibels. One decibel (db) is the faintest sound that a person can hear. Some familiar sounds with their ratings in decibels follow:

rustling leaves, 20 db
window air conditioner, 55 db
ordinary speech, 60 db
heavy traffic, 90 db
power mower, 100 db
motorcycle, 110 db
rock band, 120 db
jackhammer, 130 db
jet liner at takeoff, 140 db

HARMFUL EFFECTS

Noise produces a number of harmful effects in humans. Hearing losses result from noise levels of 80 db over a period of time. Usually, this loss is temporary, but with prolonged exposure to noise, hearing can be permanently impaired. It has been generally accepted that a loss of hearing accompanies the aging process. However, studies have found that persons who live in quiet, rural environments maintain their hearing into old age much better than do people who live in noisy environments.

Noise pollution has a variety of other irritating effects: it can increase blood pressure and heart rate, cause headaches or restless sleep, and produce pain as the result of the stress and tension experienced with noise. Noise pollution also appears to hinder communication and concentration. Elementary schoolchildren who live in quiet environments tend to get better grades in school than children who live in noisier environments.

Radiation

Radiation or radioactivity is high-level energy released from the decay of radioactive elements such as uranium, radium, thorium, and radon. Natural background radiation has always been present in the ground, water, and air and is usually not harmful.

However, radiation from manufactured sources is cause for concern. They include radiation therapy (X-rays), radioactive isotopes, industrial X-rays (such as were used to check welding joints on the Alaskan pipeline), radioactive wastes produced from the processing of radioactive materials, and radioactive fallout from atomic weapons testing.

Radioactive fallout (or the return of radioactive particles to the earth from the atmosphere) following the explosion of an atomic or nuclear bomb poses the greatest threat. Rain carries these particles back to earth sometimes thousands of miles from the explosion site, contaminating water supplies, vegetation, and animal life. These particles can appear even in the milk of cows and humans.

DANGERS

Exposure to high levels of radiation produces nausea, radiation burns, changes in blood cells, disorders of the digestive and central nervous systems, and death. Even exposure to low levels of radiation over a prolonged period of time can produce birth defects, cataracts, a variety of cancers, and a shortened life span. It is therefore imperative to a healthy lifestyle to minimize one's exposure to radiation.

Water Pollution

Next to the air that is breathed, water is the most vital substance for continued life. Unfortunately, most American lifestyle selections have abused the water supply as badly as they have the atmosphere. In many areas of the United States, lakes and rivers have been heavily polluted by industrial and sewage wastes. The pollution in the Cuyahoga River flowing through Cleveland, Ohio, became so bad several years ago that it caught fire and burned.

Many sources contribute to water pollution. When raindrops form, they often form around air pollutant particles. Thus, by the time the rain splashes to the earth, it carries pollutants from the air. Radioactive particles, metal pollutants (such as lead), and gaseous pollutants (such as sulfur dioxide and oxides of nitrogen) find their way into the water supply in this manner. In addition to the pollutants added to the water supply by rain, there are the pollutants added directly by humans. One of the main pollutants is untreated or poorly treated sewage.

PHOSPHATE

Untreated sewage is high in phosphate, a chemical necessary for plant growth.

High levels of this chemical in the water of streams, lakes, and rivers promotes a fantastic growth of single-celled plants called algae, or algae bloom.

Algae blooms turn the water dark green and sometimes create an obnoxious odor. When this happens, the aging process of a lake is speeded up hundreds of times, causing an increased amount of sediment to build up in the bottom of the lake, filling it in, and making the lake shallower and shallower. This process is known as eutrophication. After the algae blooms use up all the phosphates, they begin to die in great numbers. When the algae die, they sink to the bottom of the lake and decompose. During decomposition of the algae, great amounts of oxygen dissolved in the lake are used up. When there is not enough oxygen in the lake, the fish and other aquatic animals die, eliminating a vital source of food and recreation.

BACTERIAL CONTAMINATION

Untreated sewage dumped into lakes and streams carries a more deadly menace. Bacteria and viruses from untreated or poorly treated sewage bring dysentery, hepatitis, and other diseases to persons who bathe in or drink the polluted water. In the hot summer months, many public beaches are closed because of bacterial contamination from sewage pollution.

THERMAL POLLUTION

Another form of water pollution is known as thermal pollution. Many industries use water from lakes and rivers for cooling purposes. When the water is used for cooling, it picks up heat from the substance that it has cooled. When the industries discharge this heated water back into the river or lake, over a period of time the water in the lake or river becomes warmer. As it becomes warmer, it is not able to hold as much dissolved oxygen. Many forms of sport fish, such as trout and bass, that require large amounts of dissolved oxygen in cold water die or disappear from the lake or stream. In addition, the heated water stimulates the growth of algae blooms, which cause eutrophication processes to increase.

PESTICIDES

Water running off agricultural lands and industrial wastes from pesticide processing plants add pesticides to water sources. Some of these pesticides, such as DDT and kepone, are long-lasting poisons with the ability to be stored in the cells of plants and animals. When this happens, pesticide levels tend to build up in the bodies of animals that eat plants and build up higher in the bodies of the animals that eat plant eaters until the levels become toxic. Since people eat a variety of both plants and animals, they are especially vulnerable to DDT effects.

Pesticide Dangers

In humans, pesticides are capable of causing cancer, nerve damage, sterility, and leukemia. Pesticide pollution has also upset ecological balances between insect populations and their predators. Many animals, fish, and birds feed on the poisoned insects and then become ill and die. Several predator birds, such as the peregrine falcon and the bald eagle, are approaching extinction from sickness induced by pesticide use.

Even the vast oceans have not been spared from the pollution of humans. Many coastal areas which formerly produced large numbers of fish and shellfish for human consumption are now off limits for fishermen as a result of sewage, industrial waste, and pesticide pollution. For instance, recently the James River in Virginia and portions of the Chesapeake

Bay were declared off limits because of high levels of kepone, a deadly pesticide, which was dumped into the river by a manufacturing plant.

Oil spills caused by accidents involving oil tankers and mishaps in offshore oil-drilling rigs have been another source of pollution in recent years. The oil slicks produced by these spills spread across the ocean's surface and sink to the ocean floor, killing many forms of plant and animal marine life.

Perhaps the seriousness of ocean pollution will be more apparent when one recalls that tiny green plants called plankton exist in the upper waters of the oceans. Plankton produce 60 percent of the world's supply of oxygen. Thus, destruction of the plankton will cut off the major supply of oxygen.

Land Pollution

Land pollution is any practice or the addition of any substance which degrades the earth's surface or soil. It appears that a lifestyle filled with trash has health as well as aesthetic consequences. In recent years, the development of an economy geared toward disposable and single-use products has created a very real problem of land pollution. The problem has reached such a magnitude that the amount of throwaway trash from 10,000 people in one year would cover one acre to the depth of seven feet. With the United States population at about 220 million, this means that each year Americans could pile up trash seven feet high on 22,000 acres.

How can people get rid of their garbage? An old method of dealing with trash was the open dump, an area in which trash was unloaded. Open dumps are subject to water runoff, are plagued by rodents and insects, and are generally sources of disease and pollution.

Another method of disposing of the trash is the use of a sanitary landfill. In landfill, trash is dumped into specific areas, where it is covered with dirt and compacted by heavy equipment. Landfills that are properly managed are sanitary areas that upon completion can be used as recreational areas.

Of all the methods of dealing with trash, however, recycling appears to be the best. In this process, glass and metal are separated from the trash to be recycled. The remainder of the materials may be burned to generate power or may be treated by composting to produce a type of soil conditioner.

ADAPTING TO THE ENVIRONMENT

This chapter has discussed various kinds of pollution and their effects on the human and natural environments in which people live. Rene Dubos, a prominent biologist, has pointed out that human beings have an enormous capability to adapt to the changing environment. While this has enabled humans to survive a variety of environmental insults and thus seems to be a positive attribute, it also has allowed people to survive low levels of pollutants and ignore them as not being important. The danger in this type of response is that people will tolerate conditions that are of low quality rather than make selections that promote a high level of health.

PART B: TEACHING ABOUT THE ENVIRONMENT

Health is a quality of life. It is abstract in nature and reflects the well-being of the individual. This quality represents the dynamic relationship of the individual's *total* nature, that is, the physical, mental, and social dimensions, and can best be represented graphically by an equilateral triangle, each side of which is represented by one of these dimensions. To explain further, if one were to construct a pinwheel using this triangle, he or she could literally see the spinning triangle becoming a circle even when knowing the structure is a triangle. Further, if all sides of the triangle are equal with regard to a person's functioning at his or her best, the triangle will form a more perfect circle. However, if only one of the sides is too long or too short, the spinning structure would not represent so fine a circle. It can be seen, then, from the above explanation that an individual's health is not represented by just one factor, for example, freedom of disease, but by all factors at all times. Therefore, in order for a person to live most and serve best, it is imperative that she or he function at all levels as efficiently as possible.

The sphere in which this entire process occurs is termed one's environment and includes all the living and nonliving factors which directly or indirectly affect the well-being of that person. Some of the living factors are one's friends, peers, family, and social relationships. Nonliving factors include the land, air, water, and industry.

It is easy to see that these factors can and do affect how a person functions. However, it must also be remembered that individuals have an effect on their surroundings. The study of the reciprocal relationship between an individual's effect on the abiotic environment and the effects of the abiotic environment on the individual is called human ecology. It is essential that students in the elementary grades examine the principles of ecology in order to help them realize the importance of the environment in their own lives.*

UNIT I: OUR EARTH

In the lesson Our Earth, the students learn that the planet earth is made up of many different ecosystems. This concept builds the foundation for other concepts and principles of environment in the elementary grades.

OBJECTIVES

1. The student will define the term "ecosystem."

*Chapter written in consultation with Elaine M. Vitello, Environmental Methods and Materials Specialist, Southern Illinois University.

Appropriate grade levels are suggested for each teaching strategy and appear as ○, □, ☆ in the left-hand column.
○ = most suited for the primary grades;
□ = most suited for the intermediate grades;
☆ = most suited for the upper elementary grades.

2. The student will be able to identify the function of each part of the six parts of the ecosystem.

3. The student will be able to match pictures with the six different parts of the ecosystem.

4. The student will make a collage of an ecosystem including:

    a. sun
    b. nonliving matter
    c. primary producers
    d. primary consumers
    e. secondary consumers
    f. decomposers

MATERIALS

1. Atlas Figure 34, An Ecosystem.
2. Magazines, poster board, scissors, glue.

Methods

○ □

The planet earth is composed of many different ecosystems. Show the class a picture of an ecosystem (in Atlas) and identify the following six parts:

1. sun
2. nonliving matter: air, rock, soil
3. primary producers: green plants
4. primary consumers: mice, rabbits
5. secondary consumers: animals (including humans) which eat little animals
6. decomposers: fungus, molds

Ask the students if they can now define an ecosystem and identify the function of each part (e.g. plants make food).

○

Make six large cards, one for each of the six parts of an ecosystem. For example, on one card put Nonliving Things. Col-lect a number of pictures and place them around the room. Have the students match each picture with the correct part of the ecosystem (e.g., they would match the Nonliving Things card with a picture of a rock).

○ □

Divide the students into groups of three or four. Give them a large poster board, several magazines, scissors, and glue. Have them make a collage of an ecosystem. Each group can explain its ecosystem to the class.

○ □

Take the students on a brief trip around the school yard and have them identify the different parts of an ecosystem.

□

Relate the term "ecosystem" to other classes. Students could develop an ecosystem for a foreign country. In other words, they could determine what kinds of things would make up an ecosystem in another part of the world, why the whole world needs sun, why the world needs green plants, and whether some parts of the world have better ecosystems than other parts.

Evaluation

LIFESTYLE CONTENT

○ □

The teacher will utilize the following checklist to evaluate the group explanations of the collages.

Checklist

____ Is able to define the word ecosystem.
____ Contains the sun.

____ Contains nonliving matter.
____ Contains primary producers.
____ Contains primary consumers.
____ Contains secondary consumers.
____ Contains decomposers.

LIFESTYLE VALUE

○ □

Following are some statements regarding some of the items or conditions, living and nonliving, found in an ecosystem. The students can give their opinions as to whether or not they would like to have these items or conditions in their ecosystem. The spaces provided allow a range of feelings between yes and no.

I would like to have mice in my ecosystem.
Yes _____ No

I would like to have air pollution in my ecosystem.
Yes _____ No

I would like to have air in my ecosystem.
Yes _____ No

I would like to have fungi in my ecosystem.
Yes _____ No

I would like to have mold in my ecosystem.
Yes _____ No

I would like to have mud in my ecosystem.
Yes _____ No

I would like to have rain in my ecosystem.
Yes _____ No

I would like to have dogs in my ecosystem.
Yes _____ No

I would like to have rocks in my ecosystem.
Yes _____ No

I would like to have bees in my ecosystem.
Yes _____ No

UNIT II: WHERE I LIVE: MY ENVIRONMENT

In a text designed with a lifestyle philosophy in mind, special focus should be placed on factors that are central in influencing lifestyle alternatives. The lesson Where I Live should be included at the lower (primary) grades to allow the students to appreciate and explore what is tangible to them before examining the environment at large.

OBJECTIVES

1. The students will be able to describe their environment in detail.

2. Through use of an almanac activity, the student will be able to describe the number of people living in local urban and suburban areas.

3. By use of a map activity, the students will be able to contrast their environment with other environments in which children may live.

4. Through community exploration, the students will become aware of how they can keep their environment nice and will express this desire during the picture puzzle activity.

MATERIALS

1. Floor covering (cardboard, canvas, etc.) and arts and crafts materials.

2. Copies of Atlas Figure 91, Environment Puzzle.

Methods

○

My Community

Plan a walk (or bus ride) for the class to explore the community in which the students live. Before the walk, have the students discuss the many things they may

343

observe. When the students return, they may want to make a model of their community. This activity can be combined with the area map described in Chapter 14B, units II and III.

○ □

In addition to having the students make the model, have them draw pictures of their homes and the streets on which they live. The pictures should be drawn in detail, showing trees, flower gardens, street signs, etc. Have each student share his or her poster and tell a story about his or her special environment.

○

Discuss with the students how to keep their special environment a nice place in which to live. Utilize the Environment Puzzle activity in the Atlas.*

MY CITY

After the students have completed the discussion of My Community, expand the concept of their environment to My City. The following activities can be used.†

○ □

Have the students use an almanac to gather data about the cities in their own state. After first finding the population figure which determines whether a community is considered a city, the students can list all of the cities in their state and add the populations of each city. In a parallel column, they can list the area for each city. After totaling the two columns, they will know the number of people in their state who live in cities and the

amount of land on which these people live. The figures can be related to the total population and size of the state in any of several ways by:

1. Determining the percentage of urban people and the percentage of land on which they live.

2. Constructing two pie graphs, one showing the percentage of urban land and the other showing the percentage of urban people.

3. Constructing two bar graphs, one showing the number of the total population who live in the city and the other showing the part of the total area of the state which is city land.

The method used to present the student's findings can be determined by the level of mathematical maturity they have achieved.

○

Have the students prepare a graph showing that out of 100 children, three-quarters of them live in the city. Have them use a tree to represent ten country children and a skyscraper to represent ten city children. The resulting graph will have 7-1/2 skyscrapers and 2-1/2 trees.

○

Have a contest to see who can collect, that is, list and identify, the largest number of street covers. Explain that there are many more covers than most people are usually aware of on both the streets and the sidewalks, and they are by no means all manhole covers.

○ □

Using a simple legend, have the students show on a map some of the different biomes, that is, environments, that are

*From *A Place to Live,* pp. 42–43. Reprinted with permission from the Environmental Information and Education Division, National Audubon Society, 950 Third Avenue, New York, NY 10022.

†From *A Place to Live,* pp. 12, 13.

found in the United States, such as desert, prairie, and tundra.

○ □

Have students who used to live elsewhere compare their present neighborhood with the one they left.

○

Have the students make a bar graph to show the populations of the ten largest cities in the country.

○

Ask the students to think about their community, their homes, and themselves as individuals and then list what they share with many people, few people, no people.

Evaluation

LIFESTYLE CONTENT

○ □

After the lesson, have the students gather around the community model and divide them into teams. The team members will take turns describing something in the model. As they describe some aspect of their community, the other team can ask them questions to guess what the team is describing.

LIFESTYLE VALUE

○

Have the students look at the Environment Puzzle that they completed during the lesson and discuss the differences in the two pictures. Ask them to complete the following statements.

I love my neighborhood because _____
_____.

To make my neighborhood a nice place to live, I could _____
_____.

The thing I like best about my city is
_____.

UNIT III: WE DEPEND ON EACH OTHER

In the lesson We Depend on Each Other, students design their own terrarium and learn that all living things depend on each other in one way or another to live.

OBJECTIVES

By putting together a terrarium, the student will be able to describe how soil, plants, and animals thriving within the confines of a container depend upon the life and death of each other.

MATERIALS

1. Items for a terrarium.
   a. a container that light rays can penetrate
   b. gravel or sand
   c. charcoal
   d. soil with some humus (decayed plant material)
   e. small plants and tree seedlings (dig soil up with the roots); moss, fern, violets (keep in plastic bag until ready for use)
   f. small saucer of water
   g. a pretty rock or two
   h. plastic wrap or glass to cover the terrarium
   i. a few grass seeds
   j. a small thermometer to keep in the corner of the terrarium
   k. animals (a snail or slug, bugs, beetles, frog, toad, ant, grasshopper, snake, or caterpillars)

2. Copies of Atlas Figure 92, What's in the Terrarium?

3. Copies of Atlas Figure 93, Terrarium Jigsaw Puzzle.

Methods

○ □

The Terrarium

To show the students the interdependence of all living things, have them make a terrarium for the classroom. A terrarium can be made in anything from a baby-food jar to an aquarium (even a leaky one). The principles of constructing a terrarium are as follows:*

1. Put in a 1- to 2-inch layer of gravel for the excess water to drain into.

2. Add some pieces of charcoal to the soil. (Charcoal is burned wood with lots of air spaces, and its addition will keep the soil well aerated and will absorb gases.) To use commercial charcoal briquets effectively, break them into small pieces to increase aeration. Better yet, if the briquets are burned, the alkalinity or sweetness of the soil increases. For greater effectiveness, add burned wood ashes to improve both the physical and chemical structure of the soil. (An alkaline or sweet soil contains more elements of calcium, potassium, and compounds such as lime. Some plants thrive better in sweet rather than in sour soil.)

3. Add 2 to 3 inches of topsoil. Do not use playground clay but soil from under

bushes, along fences, or from other areas where some humus has accumulated.

4. Add a small water dish to serve as a pond from which the animals can drink and to supply a good, humid environment.

5. Add the plants. Space the plants to allow room for growth. (The children may also want to plant a few seeds or nuts.)

6. Add the animals (no large animals or mammals; a snake or toad needs more room; snails, worms, and ants need less room).

7. Place the terrarium near a window, but do not let the sun shine directly on the terrarium or it will be an oven rather than a terrarium. Do not set the terrarium on a radiator or other heat source.

The purpose of the terrarium is to demonstrate how soil, plants, and animals thriving within the confines of the container depend upon the life and death of each other. The terrarium plants and animals may exist totally independent of any outside forces. This is representative of a closed system. The miniworld in a terrarium is self-supporting.

○ □

In learning about the interdependence of all living things, the students can do individual projects. They can learn about one part of the terrarium and report back as an "expert" to the class. You can aid this additional learning by having an Interest Center. The following are books you might include:

Be Nice to Spiders by Margaret Bloy Graham
A Fly Went By by Mike McClintock
The True Book of Insects by Illa Podendort
Let's Get Turtles by Millicent E. Selsam

---

* Ideas from *Environmental Learning Experiences,* prepared by The Center for the Development of Environmental Curriculum, Willoughby-Eastlake City Schools, Willoughby, Ohio; and Ohio Department of Education, Columbus, Ohio, 1973, p. 12.

Evaluation

LIFESTYLE CONTENT

○

Two activities to accompany the terrarium project are the Terrarium Jigsaw Puzzle and the puzzle What's in the Terrarium? (provided in Atlas).

LIFESTYLE VALUE

○ □

Have each student complete the following open-ended statement with a written paragraph.

When humans change the balance of nature, I feel that _____ .

UNIT IV: KEEPING THE BALANCE

By observing two experiments, the students can see how smog, dust, exhaust gases, and other pollutants affect plants and animals. The concept derived from the lesson Keeping the Balance is that certain things when added to an ecosystem can upset or even destroy the system.

OBJECTIVES

1. Following the experiments, the student will be able to describe the effect of smog, dust, exhaust gases, and other pollutants on plants and animals.

2. The students will express their feelings about a healthy environment by making a collage using magazine pictures which show the way they would like their city to look.

MATERIALS

1. Materials listed with experiments.
2. Rolls of white paper, scotch tape, crayons.

3. Magazines, scissors, glue, poster paper.

Methods

○ □

Give each student two pictures, one of an environment free of pollution and one showing some type(s) of pollution. Ask the students to explain the difference between the pictures to the class and tell which picture is preferred and why. From the pictures with pollution, compile a list of different types of pollution.

EXPERIMENTS

○ □

Disinfectants

To allow the students to examine pollution, have them conduct the following experiment to show how disinfectants work:*

1. Equipment (alcohol, Lysol, iodine, dried beans, four test tubes, sterile absorbent cotton).

2. Process
   a. Soak the beans in cold water.
   b. Number the test tubes.
   c. Put several beans in each test tube and cover the beans with water.
   d. Do not add anything to test tube 1.
   e. Add a little iodine to test tube 2.
   f. Add a little Lysol to test tube 3.
   g. Add a little alcohol to test tube 4.
   h. Stopper all the test tubes with cotton and put them in a warm place for two days.

*This experiment and the following smog experiment are taken from *Strand IV Environmental and Community Health, Environmental and Public Health*, University of the State of New York, State Education Department, Bureau of Elementary Curriculum Development, Albany, NY 12224 (1970).

3. Follow-up

a. Remove the cotton and smell the contents of the test tubes.

b. Discuss whether any of the test tubes have an odor.

c. Discuss what the presence of an odor indicates.

d. Determine how to make certain that microorganisms caused the odor.

Smog

Have the class perform the following experiment to produce smog. (Smog can be produced by the condensation of water vapor or other vapors on solid particles such as smoke):

1. Insert a lighted match in a gallon jug to make a small amount of smoke.

2. Blow with your mouth pressing firmly on the mouth of the jug and release quickly the compressed air. A smog should form in the jug.

3. Try this blowing activity without the smoke from the match.

The students can observe the effect of smog, dust, and exhaust gases on plants. Have them select two or three leaves of a healthy geranium plant and coat them with petroleum jelly, making sure that all surfaces are covered. Have the class observe the condition of the leaves on the same plant over a period of time.

An interesting variation of this experiment would involve coating one leaf on the bottom surface only and one leaf on both sides. Discuss the conclusions that can be drawn from this experiment.

○ □

Our City

Cover all the bulletin boards and the chalkboard with white paper. Place several crayons around the room. Allow each student to draw a part of their city. When the mural is finished, have the students discuss their city by answering such questions as How do people travel? Where do people live? What kinds of work do people do? How many parks and bodies of water are there? Is there an airport?

Ask the students to identify as many kinds of pollution in their city as they can and discuss how these different pollutants affect their environment.

LIFESTYLE CONTENT

Evaluation

Ask the students, after completing the two experiments, to describe the effects of smog, dust, exhaust gases, and other pollutants on plants and animals.

LIFESTYLE VALUE

○ □ ☆

Bring magazines, scissors, and glue to the classroom. Give the students sheets of poster paper and ask them to make collages from magazine pictures showing a healthy environment.

UNIT V: SAVING THE ENVIRONMENT

It has been said by many that people return to nature for serenity and peace and to collect their thoughts. The role of nature in tranquility and mental health is attested to by many poems and pictures. In the lesson Saving the Environment, the students will recognize their roles in maintaining our precious land, trees, and waters.

OBJECTIVES

1. The student will be active in saving the environment by launching a

classroom campaign to do one of the following: collect newspapers, collect returnable bottles, collect litter.

2. The student will demonstrate a knowledge of the environment by completing a crossword puzzle and a word search.

3. The students will express their feelings about this country's natural resources by participating in a bulletin board assignment. Each day, a student will put a new saying on the board: Smokey says _____ .

4. The student will demonstrate an interest in saving the environment by selecting an individual project for one month and evaluating it by checking a calendar.

MATERIALS

1. Pictures of people utilizing their natural resources and polluting their natural resources.

2. Balance scale, newspapers.

3. Large sheets of bulletin board paper.

4. Wire, papier mâché.

5. Contact paper.

6. Speaker (the custodian).

7. Atlas Figures 94 and 95, Environment Word Search and Environment Crossword Puzzles.

Methods

○ □

Begin the lesson by showing the class pictures of people utilizing their natural resources and polluting them. Examples of such pictures may be a lamp left on; someone driving an automobile; wood burning in a fire; a washing machine; and factory smoke.

Have the students discuss the saying,

"You can't get something for nothing." Follow the discussion with an explanation of how the earth has only so many raw materials, and if we use them all up, we cannot get any more.

SAVING THE ENVIRONMENT CAMPAIGN

Launch a classroom campaign to save the environment. Several activities can be engaged in to make the unit meaningful, involve the students, and keep it fun to do.

○

Recycling

Obtain a balance scale and have the students collect newspapers for one week. Have the class figure the following problems:

1. Find the smallest newspaper and suspend it on the hook beneath the scale. How much does it weigh?

2. Suppose the newspaper weighs the same amount every day except Sunday. What would the total weight be for six days?

3. Now weigh the largest newspaper (the Sunday paper). How much does it weigh?

4. How much would the largest newspaper weigh for an entire week?

5. If there are twenty-five students in the classroom, and if each student brought in newspapers for one full week, how much would all of the newspapers weigh together?

6. How much would the newspapers weigh for one month?

7. There are several local companies in town that recycle newspapers. They pay $2.00 for 100 pounds of newspapers. How much money could the class earn by saving their newspapers for one month?

○

Litterbug

Use a large sheet of bulletin board paper or newspaper to make a litterbug. Staple around the edges and stuff with the litter found around the classroom at the end of the day.

○

Litter Tree

Use some litter to make collages for a tree. Decoration will be put on a tree made from a wood post and wire branches. Interrelate paper and trees in a discussion.

○

Mural

Use paper scraps, material, pictures, etc., to make a Litter States of America mural.

○

Litter Walk

Give each student his or her own litterbag to collect trash found in and around the school building.

○

Trash Can Litter Heads

Have preformed wire heads unless you have enough time to let students help. Use litter paper, cover with papier mâché, then paint. Give names such as Litter Monster, Trash Eater.

○ □

Litter Stickers

Use precut contact paper to make stickers. Examples: Save a Tree, Don't Be a Litterbug. (Have students use original phrases.)

○

Custodian

Invite the school's custodian to explain the job and suggest ways the students can help keep their school clean and nice.

○

Pin a large drawing of Smokey the Bear on the bulletin board and let students take turns putting a new saying on the board, Smokey says _____ .

○ □

Some students may wish to memorize the Conservation pledge of the U.S. Department of Agriculture, Forest Service:

I give my pledge as an American to save and faithfully defend from waste the natural resources of my country—its soil and minerals, its forests and waters and wildlife.

Evaluation

LIFESTYLE CONTENT

○ □

To evaluate the students' knowledge of their environment, use the Environment Crossword Puzzle and Word Search found in the Atlas.

Answers

ACROSS: 1. waste 2. sanitarian 3. car 4. environment 5. ecology 6. pesticides 7. conserve 8. noise 9. Pasteur 10. healthy DOWN: 1. water 2. recycle 3. everyone 4. pollution 5. smog 6. natural resources 7. disease 8. ecosystem 9. litterbug 10. lungs

LIFESTYLE VALUE

○ □ ☆

Have each student select an individual project related to saving the environment that they would like to work on for a month. It might be a home project for the whole family.

Ditto off one-month calendars, leaving about 6 inches at the top for the students to draw a picture depicting their projects. Ask the students to make a check (√) in the calendar spaces for each day that they work on saving the environment through their projects.

FURTHER READINGS

In addition to using the lessons in this chapter on teaching about the environment, the teacher will want to obtain two excellent teacher's guides. The "Ecology Action Pack" developed by McDonald's Corporation, 1974, contains excellent lessons and overlays for each instruction. Write to McDonald's Corporation, 1 McDonald Plaza, Oakbrook, IL 60521. Another good resource is available from Metropolitan Life Insurance Company, a teacher's packet, "Exploring Your Environmental Choices: An Inquiry and Decision-Making Approach," which also contains teaching ideas for the elementary classroom.

ADDITIONAL ENVIRONMENTAL RESOURCES

Current Health Magazine, Curriculum Innovations, Inc. 501 Lake Forest Avenue, Highwood, IL 60040, explores a different environmental issue during each month of the school year. Recent issues have dealt with the following concerns:

October 1978, "Health Hazards of PCBs."

September 1978, "Asbestos: Environmental Time Bomb?"

May 1978, "Pesty Pesticides."

April 1978, "How Does a Nuclear Reactor Work?"

March 1978, "Urban Ecology."

February 1978, "Impact of Airports."

January 1978, "Alternatives to a Dump."

December 1977, "Solar Energy Update."

November 1977, "Water Purification."

October 1977, "Mercury at Minamata."

September 1977, "What Really Killed Smokey the Bear?" (vanishing wildlife).

CHAPTER 14

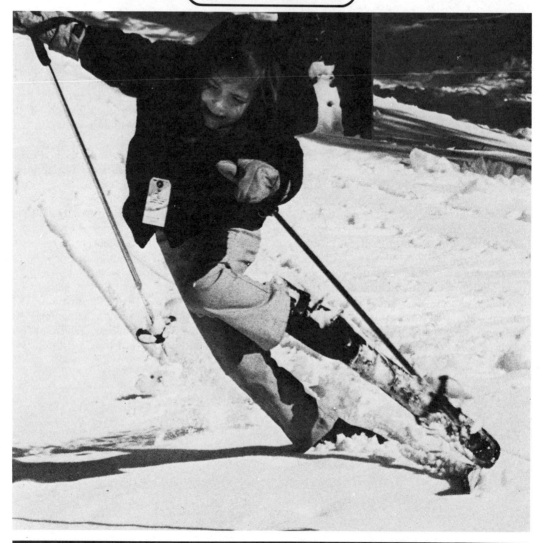

PART A: SAFETY AND FIRST AID

Accidents are the most common health problem of elementary schoolchildren; they account for more deaths among children between the ages of five and ten than do all diseases combined. However, most of these disabling injuries and deaths can be avoided. "Like other events, accidents are caused and, therefore, can be controlled when their causes are identified and understood" (4, p. 5).

Accidents often occur through carelessness—people making mistakes. They result through ignorance—what we don't know *can* harm us. However, it would be a mistake to oversimplify the causes of accidents. In fact, several authorities suggest that the term "accident" be discarded.

They believe it more reasonable to classify the resultant injuries as electrical, chemical, mechanical, and the like. The misconceptions that accompany the term *accident* can also be avoided by this classification. In science, if the cause of an event is known, that event is not an accident; most accident causes are known, but we still persist in calling them accidents (4, p. 6).

John J. Brownfain makes a discerning observation about defining accidents:

If we label all of life's unpleasant surprises as accidents, then we come to perceive ourselves as the playthings of fate and we cultivate a philosophy of carelessness and irresponsibility. On the other hand, if we look for causes and hold ourselves accountable for the mishaps in our lives, we become people of resource and confidence, increasingly able to control the direction of events (4, p. 6).*

The purposes of the two chapters on safety are to increase awareness of the main accident problems, provide factual knowledge, and suggest ways for students to use the safety knowledge they acquire.

Quoting accident statistics, using scare techniques, and stressing safety rules are not so effective as taking the conceptual approach to teaching safety. Full understanding of a concept enables the student to make good decisions in a variety of situations without relying on rote recall of specific safety rules.

*Original article, "When Is an Accident Not an Accident?" by John J. Brownfain, *Journal of the American Society of Safety Engineers* (September 1962): 20.

The teacher should remember that safety is not an end in itself; it is a means to a more productive life. Thygerson (4) believes that life is at its best when taking risks for things worthwhile and that safety education reduces the risks in living. Similarly, Robert Russell reminds us that "many real pleasures, exciting experiences, and true accomplishments result only from taking risks. Consistently cautious behavior can stunt a person's functioning—and stunted functioning is not healthy. What this boils down to is that healthy people take certain risks and certain precautions. They balance their risks" (3, p. 103). This chapter is therefore devoted to specific risks and precautions associated with home, traffic, community, recreation, and medical problems.

SAFETY IN AND AROUND THE HOME

Although people think of their home as a shelter and retreat, it actually represents the site of two out of five accidents. The National Safety Council estimates that there is a home accident every eight seconds and a death resulting from such an accident every twenty minutes.

Fire

Fire is the leading cause of death resulting from accidents in the home. It takes the lives of 7,000 to 9,000 Americans each year and hospitalizes 70,000 more.

Most home fires start in the kitchen or basement, but many start in bedrooms. More than half of the burn cases studied at the Shriners Burn Institute in Galveston between 1966 and 1970 were found to have been caused by space heaters (usually gas), matches, outdoor fires, gas hot-water heaters, and kitchen stoves. Fifty-four percent of the children burned had been wearing combustible clothing, primarily cotton dresses and nightgowns, although shirts, skirts, and trousers were also involved. A survey of forty-one adult burn patients over age sixty at the University of Texas medical branch in Galveston revealed similar results; but cigarettes were added as an important cause of burns, and bedding as well as clothing was involved.

CLOTHING FLAMMABILITY

Since clothing materials vary considerably as to their flammability, federal law now requires that all clothing be labeled to show the exact fiber content. These labels are especially important to read when clothing is being bought for children or elderly people. Although federal standards prohibit flammable materials in children's sleepwear up to size 6X, it is still wise to be wary.

People need to keep in mind that cotton is highly flammable unless it has been treated with flame-retardant; this is also true of linen and cellulose synthetics such as rayon and acetate. Fabrics with a loose weave, fluffy pile, or soft nap also catch fire easily. Long, loose sleeves pose another threat to safety when working in the kitchen.

KITCHEN HAZARDS

Besides presenting the danger of fire, kitchen hazards include falls (slipping on spilled liquids, grease, or food or unsafe climbing practices), unclean kitchen tools (such as meat grinders, blenders, can openers, and wooden chopping blocks that often do not receive the special cleaning they should), kitchen knives that are not stored out of the reach of children, and food that becomes contaminated through unsanitary handling or improper refrigeration.

Refrigerators should be set at the coldest point before freezing. This is especially important during the summer months. Salmonella organisms can survive up to three months in the refrigerator, but they flourish best at the 60- to 140-degree temperature range. Although no refrigerated food should be held at room temperature very long, it is important to be especially cautious about foods containing eggs, such as custards, sauces, or mayonnaise. If an egg is cracked, it is best to throw it out or use it in a cake or recipe requiring cooking at a high temperature. Frozen foods should be kept thoroughly frozen and meat and poultry should be thawed in the refrigerator. One should buy only government-inspected meats and poultry.

Food Poisoning

Food poisoning is caused by toxins and bacteria. Although toxins do occur naturally in seafood, seafood poisoning is quite rare as a result of constant surveillance of offshore fishing areas. Some mushrooms are toxic, but those purchased at a grocery store are safe. The vast majority of food poisonings are caused by bacteria. Several of the most common types of food poisoning are outlined in Table 14A-1.

Botulism is a deadly food poison so potent that merely one half pound of the toxin could eliminate the entire population of the world. The name botulism, derived from the Latin *botulus* meaning sausage, was assigned after the first botulism incident was traced to contaminated sausage. Fortunately, trouble rarely

TABLE 14A-1 FOOD POISONING

	Botulism	Salmonella	Common Ubiquitous Bacteria
Disease-producing organism	Caused by a toxin produced by the bacterium clostridium botulinum (anaerobic —grows only in absence of air).	Caused by rod-shaped bacteria (almost 1,300 varieties, but only about a dozen are harmful to humans).	A variety of bacteria including staphylo-coccus aureus, clostridium perfrin-gens, escherichia coli, bacillus subtilis.
Action in the body	Absorbed from the in-testinal tract into the bloodstream; a neurotoxin—affects the nervous system.	May infect victims in three ways: multiply in the intestinal tract (salmonella gastroenteritis), multiply in the blood, localize and produce abscesses else-where in the body (rare).	Staph attacks the intes-tinal tract.
Symptoms	Fatigue, muscular weakness, double vision, drooping eye-lids, dilated pupils, dryness of mouth, swelling of tongue, difficulty in swallow-ing and speaking. In fatal cases (about 65%) respiratory fail-ure occurs. (Onset of symptoms will depend on amount ingested—varies from a few hours to a few days.)	Severe stomachache or cramps, vomiting, and diarrhea; may be followed with fever and a headache. Usually subsides after a few hours or days but has been fatal to infants, the elderly, and the infirm. Serious com-plications are possible.	Symptoms are often similar to those of intestinal flu, ranging from mild to fairly severe. Usually symptoms last only a day or two.
Prevention	Use pressure canner correctly; throw out cans that bulge or have split seams. (Usually occurs in underprocessed home-canned foods.)	Keep work surfaces clean. Scrub knives, cutting board, blender, meat grinder, and can opener. Wash hands before eating; keep refrigerator cold. Cook meat properly.	Cook and store food properly; wash hands before eating; throw out food that tastes, looks, or smells odd. Keep all kitchen uten-sils scrupulously clean.

occurs with sausage in the United States. Either cooked meat is used in the manufacture of sausage and other specialty meats or cooking instructions are clearly stated on the label of those products that require cooking before consumption. Although antitoxins for botulism have been developed, they are effective only when small amounts of the toxin have been ingested and when treatment is initiated promptly.

Exposure to salmonella poisoning is increasing as the lifestyle of most Americans now includes more eating out. The resulting centralization of food preparation in the hands of relatively few food processors and cooks increases the risk of a single source infecting many people at once. Experts estimate that about 2 million Americans (about 1 percent of the population) suffer with salmonella poisoning annually. In terms of lost school days and working days and the cost of medical treatment, the National Academy of Sciences brands salmonellosis "one of the most important communicable disease problems in the United States today."

Food tainted with salmonella looks and smells like any other food. Despite its name, salmonella has nothing to do with salmon. The bacterium is named after a nineteenth-century American veterinarian, Daniel E. Salmon, who discovered the microbe in pigs in 1885.

A person who becomes ill with what seems like salmonella poisoning should call a doctor, who will probably prescribe fluids, a bland diet, and perhaps an antidiarrheal drug. People should remember that because the infection can spread to others, they should observe basic rules of cleanliness.

Two other food-related items that may be dangerous are microwave ovens and pottery, earthenware, and dinnerware that contain lead or other toxic metal compounds. Microwave ovens made prior to October 1971 should be tested for radiation leakage. When buying a microwave oven, one should make sure that it contains a label certifying compliance with federal standards. It is advised that one follow the manufacturer's instructions for safe operation, stay at least an arm's length away from the front of the oven while it is operating, and have the oven checked periodically by a qualified person.

Toxic metals in some glazes applied to dinnerware or cookware may be dissolved when they come into contact with acidic foods such as fruit juices, cider, vinegar, and tomato products. The danger is increased if the food or beverage is warm or stored in the container overnight. The hazard is not high in American-made, commercially available pottery and dinnerware, however.

Although the authors have emphasized the kitchen as a major source of potential hazards, a careful inspection of the entire house is recommended. The home is the site of 75 percent of all accidents that befall children under age five. Several factors combine to threaten the young child:

1. Children are active, curious, and fast moving and are fascinated by the world around them.

2. Young children lack the knowledge and experience that often serve to protect adults; they lack the ability to read warning labels as well.

3. Size, strength, and muscular coordination are not sufficiently developed to protect the young child.

Accidental poisonings (aspirin and

vitamin tablets are most frequently involved), fire, and drowning are the main causes of death among children under five years. Injuries from falls, sharp objects, electric cords and outlets, and stoves and suffocation from plastic bags have also proven to be prevalent.

Many precautions could be listed; for example, toxic substances should be stored out of reach of small children, and a child's toys and playground equipment should be inspected for rust, sharp edges, and splinters. But the most effective rule is to let common sense prevail.

TRAFFIC SAFETY

Motor-vehicle accidents are a leading cause of death for all people under forty-four years of age. The risk of serious injury or death, however, can be reduced in several ways.

Automobile Safety

Children should understand that they are not to interfere with the driver. They should be required to wear a seatbelt or other restraint and reminded not to stick their arms, legs, or head out the window. During a long trip, it is important to provide games and activities that will keep youngsters from becoming bored. Finally, children should not be permitted to operate the controls of a car. Cars are not toys. Proper instruction and a license should always precede a first driving attempt.

Much has been said about the use of safety belts and various other restraints. Despite reluctance on the part of some people to wear them, safety belts unquestionably minimize injury in head-on ac-

cidents. Although most children are big enough to use regular lap belts by the time they are four or five years of age, a shoulder belt should not be used until the child is at least four and one-half feet tall. Younger children need the protection of a sturdily constructed car bed or infant carrier specifically designed for use in automobiles. All children need the example of adult use of safety belts.

Bicycle Safety

Every year, according to Department of Health, Education, and Welfare estimates, one in every fifty bike owners is injured—a total of one million riders. More than half of the injured are between the ages of five and fourteen, and most of them are boys. Therefore, in the interest of a healthy lifestyle, certain bike safety rules should be reviewed.

The bicycle should fit the rider and be in good condition. Children should be made aware of the fact that they are operating a vehicle and must follow all traffic rules. They should not race down a road or steer their bicycles in a reckless manner any more than a responsible automobile driver would. The practice of riding double or carrying a friend on the handlebars should be discouraged.

When riding in heavy traffic in the city, it is a good idea to dismount and walk the bicycle across busy intersections, using the pedestrian crossing lanes. Additional care must be taken when one is riding a bicycle at night. The bike should have a light that is visible for 500 feet and a reflector that is visible for 300 feet. Riders should wear light-colored clothing. It is also recommended that the bicycle frame be outlined with reflective tape so that motorists can readily spot the cyclist.

The three types of signals should be reviewed with children:

1. Light signals
   a. red (stop)
   b. yellow (caution)
   c. green (go)
2. Arm signals
   a. right turn
   b. left turn
   c. slowing and stopping
3. Basic traffic signs and shapes
   a. stop (octagon)
   b. danger or caution (diamond)
   c. yield (triangle)

Motorcycle Safety

Anyone who rides a motorcycle should realize that the motorcycle is a hazardous machine which offers far less protection than even a small car. Consequently, a helmet with triangles of retroreflective taping; goggles with impact-resistant protective lenses; and retroreflective tape on the wheel rims, fenders, and entire frame should at least be utilized. Like an automobile or bicycle, a motorcycle should be in good repair, and the driver should be skilled in its operation before driving it on the highway.

Minibikes

Many states prohibit the use of minibikes on public streets and sidewalks, thereby limiting their use to private property. Most states also have laws governing the minimum age for minibike riders. The local police department can be contacted for more specific information. As with other motor vehicles, safe operation depends upon the skill of the driver and the condition of the machine. A helmet should be worn for added protection.

COMMUNITY SAFETY

Although the city dweller must contend with heavy traffic, air pollution, and crime, there are actually fewer risks associated with urban life than with rural life. The nonurban dweller has a lifestyle that often includes faster driving, greater yard and garden hazards, and a larger number of animals. According to the National Safety Council, more people are killed each year in farmwork accidents (3,000 to 4,000) than in any other major industry. Tens of thousands more are injured. Those who are injured are frequently the inexperienced, and many of the accidents are preventable.

The chances of having a fire are multiplied when living on a farm because many of the buildings are made of wood. An abundance of combustibles (dry crops, grain, weeds) and fuels and ignition sources (lightning, gasoline, kerosene, and matches) are often found in farm areas. The farm also is usually quite a distance from fire-fighting equipment and adequate water sources.

Tractors and farm machinery pose another hazard and are extremely dangerous when mishandled. The Department of Agriculture states that children must never be permitted to operate such machines. It is common sense never to wear loose, flowing clothing or hair when around farm machinery, to make repairs on machinery that is in motion, or to refuel or oil a machine while the engine is still running.

Animals, like machinery, should be treated with respect. They should be approached cautiously and tended with care. It is important that fences and gates enclosing animals be kept in good condition. Animals need to receive vaccinations against diseases just as humans do. If an animal appears ill, a veterinarian should be called.

Any substance that is capable of killing unwanted plants and pests is capable of killing livestock and people as well. Such substances should be stored safely out of the reach of children and pets. The Department of Agriculture recommends the following safeguards when using pesticides:

• Wear head-to-toe protective clothing (including natural rubber gloves) for mixing as well as spraying.
• Wear a special respirator that has been tested and approved for this purpose.
• Spray on a day when there is very little wind.
• Wash yourself and your clothes thoroughly after using pesticides.

Plants can present several problems. Some look edible but are not. The National Safety Council and outdoor-safety experts warn that humans cannot rely on observation of animals and birds to determine what is edible. Other plants secrete oils that can cause a blistery rash and intense itching. About three out of four persons in the United States are allergic to the chemcial urushiol, contained in the oils secreted by the species *Rhus toxicodendron*—commonly known as poison ivy (widely prevalent), poison oak (West Coast), and poison sumac (Southwest).

Urushiol is found in every part of the plant—leaves, flowers, berries, twigs, stems, and roots. Burning these plants will disperse the chemical into the air. A rash will develop from several hours to forty-eight hours after exposure to urushiol by susceptible individuals.

Treatment involves removing the contaminated clothing, immediately washing the exposed area with soap and water, and applying rubbing alcohol. (Any clothing that may also be carrying the oil must be washed thoroughly.) In an effort to relieve itching, calamine lotion or other soothing skin lotions may be applied if the rash is mild. If a severe reaction occurs (or if the face or genitals are involved), one should seek medical advice. People can prevent allergic reactions from occurring by learning how to recognize poisonous plants common to their area and avoiding contact with them.

OUTDOOR RECREATIONAL AND SEASONAL SAFETY

Vacations away from home provide an opportunity for recreation, relaxation, and a change in lifestyle, but the very strangeness of a new place or activity can make the vacation hazardous as well as exhilarating. The following precautions should be observed when participating in outdoor activities.

1. *Hiking*
   a. When doing a lot of walking be sure you are in good physical condition.
   b. Wear sturdy, comfortable boots.
   c. When hiking in cool climates, wear wool or cotton socks and long pants and carry some heavy sweaters.
2. *Water Activities* (Drowning ranks second only to motor vehicles as a cause of fatal accidents among young people; most of these deaths can be prevented.)
   a. Always swim with some other individual that can come to your aid in an emergency.
   b. Do not become overtired.
   c. Swim in areas free of fishermen, boats, and skiers.

d. Do not swim when there is lightning.

e. Children should swim only when there is adult supervision.

f. Learn how to give artificial respiration.

g. Get instruction from an expert before going water skiing or scuba diving. (Swimming experience and good physical conditioning are important.)

h. Wear a life belt when water skiing.

i. Double-check scuba equipment before diving.

3. *Boating*

a. Wear a life jacket when in a small rowboat or canoe.

b. Learn how to right a canoe that has capsized.

c. Learn how to properly fuel and operate a motorboat before leaving shore.

4. *Skiing* (Downhill skiing injures 200,000 Americans annually. Poor conditioning is often responsible for many of the bruises, strains, sprains, dislocations, and broken legs that occur.)

a. Get in shape before skiing through active exercise such as swimming, cycling, jumping rope, and jogging.

b. Make sure equipment is in good order.

c. Consider the need for expert instruction.

d. Do not overestimate your ability. To protect the eyes, one should also consider the use of goggles or dark glasses.

Bites and Stings

Bites and stings are a hazard of outdoor living that should be discussed. When a person is bitten by an animal and the skin is broken, he or she should have someone try to capture and confine the animal. The animal should be kept alive if possible, or, if killing is necessary, precautions should be taken not to damage the animal's head. The wound and surrounding area should be cleansed with soap and water, the bitten area flushed, and a sterile gauze or clean handkerchief applied before a victim is taken to the hospital. Movement of the affected part should be avoided until a physician can be reached.

Most of the approximately 45,000 snakebite incidents that occur in the United States each year are not inflicted by poisonous snakes; fatal cases do occur, however. Figure 14A-1 reproduces an American Red Cross Poster of 1978 describing first aid for snakebite.

INSECT BITES

Spiders in the United States are generally harmless, except for the black widow spider and the brown recluse. The following are symptoms of bites from these two spiders (1, pp. 110–111).

1. *Black widow*
   a. slight local reaction
   b. severe pain produced by nerve toxin
   c. profuse sweating
   d. nausea
   e. painful abdominal cramps
   f. difficulty breathing and speaking
2. *Brown Recluse*
   a. severe local reaction produced by the venom which forms an open ulcer within one to two weeks
   b. destruction of red blood cells
   c. chills
   d. fever
   e. joint pains
   f. nausea and vomiting

FIGURE 14A-1 First aid for snakebite

POISONOUS OR NONPOISONOUS

Poisonous or nonpoisonous, a snakebite should have medical attention. A snakebite victim should be taken to a hospital *as quickly as possible*, even in cases when snakebite is only suspected.

FIRST AID

1. As stated above, *get the victim to a hospital fast*. Meanwhile, take the following general first aid measures:

- Keep the victim from moving around.
- Keep the victim as calm as possible, preferably lying down
- Immobilize the bitten extremity and keep it at or below heart level.

If a hospital can be reached within 4 to 5 hours and no symptoms develop, this is all that is necessary.

2. *If mild to moderate symptoms develop, apply a constricting band* from 2 to 4 inches above the bite but NOT around a joint (i.e., elbow, knee, wrist, or ankle) and NOT around the head, neck, or trunk. The band should be from ¾ to 1½ inches wide. NOT thin like a rubber band. The band should be snug, but loose enough to slip one finger underneath. Be alert to swelling: loosen the band if it becomes too tight, but do not remove it. To ensure that blood flow has not been stopped, periodically check the pulse in the extremity beyond the bite.

3. *If severe symptoms develop, incisions and suction should be performed immediately.* Apply a constricting band, if not already done, and make a cut in the skin with a sharp sterilized blade through the fang mark(s). Cuts should be no deeper than just through the skin and should be ½ inch long, extending over the suspected venom deposit point (because a snake strikes downward, the deposit point is usually lower than the fang mark). Cuts should be made along the long axis of the limb. DO NOT make cross-cut incisions; DO NOT make cuts on the head, neck, or trunk. Suction should be applied with a suction cup for 30 minutes. If a suction cup is not available, use the mouth. There is little risk to the rescuer who uses his mouth, but it is recommended that the venom not be swallowed and that the mouth be rinsed.

IF THE HOSPITAL IS NOT CLOSE (cannot be reached within from 4 to 5 hours)

1. Continue to try to obtain professional care by transportation of the victim or by communication with a rescue service.

2. *If no symptoms develop*, continue trying to reach the hospital and give the general first aid described above.

3. *If ANY symptoms develop*, apply a constricting band and perform incisions and suction immediately, as described above.

OTHER CONSIDERATIONS

1. *Shock:* Keep the victim lying down and comfortable and maintain body temperature.

2. *Breathing and heartbeat:* If breathing stops, give mouth-to-mouth resuscitation. If breathing stops and there is no pulse, cardio-pulmonary resuscitation (CPR) should be performed by those trained to do so.

3. *Identifying the snake:* If the snake can be killed without risk or delay, it should be brought, *with care,* to the hospital for identification.

4. *Cleansing the bitten area:* The bitten area may be washed with soap and water and blotted dry with sterile gauze. Dressings and bandages can be applied, but only for a short period of time.

5. *Cold therapy:* Cold compresses, ice, dry ice, chemical ice packs, spray refrigerants, and other methods of cold therapy are NOT recommended in the first aid treatment of snakebite.

6. *Medicine to relieve pain:* A medicine *not containing aspirin* can be given to the victim for relief of pain. DO NOT give alcohol, sedatives, aspirin, or other medications.

7. *Snakebite kits:* Keep a kit accessible for all outings in snake-infested or primitive areas.

SYMPTOMS

1. *Mild to moderate* symptoms include mild swelling or discoloration and mild to moderate pain at the wound site with tingling sensations, rapid pulse, weakness, dimness of vision, nausea, vomiting, and shortness of breath.

2. *Severe* symptoms include rapid swelling and numbness, followed by severe pain at the wound site. Other effects include pinpoint pupils, twitching, slurred speech, shock, convulsions, paralysis, unconsciousness, and no breathing or pulse.

The information on this poster is based on a report prepared for the American Red Cross by the National Academy of Sciences—National Research Council.

American Red Cross

Snakebite prevention practices that can eliminate needless illness and worry may be learned in a Red Cross first aid course. Call your chapter to enroll.

One should perform the following in the case of a bite from a black widow or brown recluse spider (1, p. 113).

1. Give artificial respiration if indicated and apply a constricting band above the injection site (as described previously).

2. Keep the affected part below the level of the victim's heart.

3. Get medical help immediately.

4. If medical care is delayed, remove the band after thirty minutes and apply ice contained in a towel or cold cloths to the site of the bite.

"Bites or stings from fleas, mosquitoes, lice, gnats, chiggers, and other common insects produce local pain and irritation, but are not likely to cause severe reactions. Some of these insects may transmit disease to man, but are not harmful in themselves. . . . Minor bites and stings may be treated with cold applications and soothing lotions, such as calamine" (1, pp. 110, 112).

Ticks adhere to the skin or scalp and can transmit germs of several diseases, including Rocky Mountain spotted fever. The following steps should be taken to remove ticks.

1. Do not forceably remove a tick if its head has penetrated the skin.

2. Cover the tick with heavy oil (mineral, salad, or machine) to close its breathing pores. The tick may disengage at once; if not, allow the oil to remain in place for a half hour before carefully removing the tick with tweezers. (Be sure all parts are removed.)

3. Gently scrub the bitten area with soap and water to help remove germs that may be present.

4. See a medical doctor if symptoms of illness appear.

Stings from ants, bees, wasps, and hornets and yellow jackets have been known to cause death, usually from acute allergic reaction. If there is no reaction suggesting allergy, one should apply cold compresses and perhaps a soothing lotion. In the case of a bee sting, one should remove and discard the stinging apparatus and venom sac. Acute allergic reactions require immediate medical attention.

Team Sports

Team sports pose different problems. Although skinned knees, bumps, and bruises are probably unavoidable, care should be taken to prevent more critical injuries.

Statistically, basketball is America's most dangerous team sport. Players should take care to strengthen muscles and tendons in the legs, since this game often results in sprains and dislocations. Glasses should be secured with a band around the head and the lenses should be impact resistant.

Although football injuries may not number as many as in basketball, they are apt to be more serious. In fact, in 1971 there were twenty deaths attributable to nonprofessional football injuries. To avoid severe injury, a football player should be in good physical condition and participate in preseason conditioning. Proper protective outfitting and rigid enforcement of the rules should be insisted upon. The use of amphetamines should definitely be avoided.

Baseball is also responsible for hundreds of thousands of accidents. Precautions include never flinging the bat away after hitting the ball, avoiding trick pitches, remembering to slide into base feet first, and always keeping one's attention on the ball.

There are any number of fine sports that provide both enjoyment and risks, but it is really up to individuals to learn all they can about the activities that fit their particular lifestyles as well as how they can participate in them with minimum harm.

CHRONIC CONDITIONS AND PREDICTABLE EMERGENCIES

Almost every family has at least one member with a special medical problem that could require emergency treatment under certain conditions. Since awareness of the problem can prevent a crisis from becoming a catastrophe, victims of chronic conditions and wearers of contact lenses, pacemakers, etc., should consider wearing a necklace or bracelet bearing the *Medic Alert* emblem. Medic Alert is a foundation that exists to protect victims from the risk of wrong treatment or nonrecognition of a problem by providing data vital in an emergency situation. Such data include the condition (e.g., allergic to penicillin), an identifying serial number, and a telephone number that can be called collect at any hour of the day or night by medical personnel, police, or anyone else in a position to help. The telephone number is that of a central file that contains all relevant information that a person may wish to have available. For further information one can write to the Medic Alert Foundation, Turlock, CA 95380.

The authors have also included basic information about seven chronic conditions and hope that readers will become better informed about their family's particular chronic conditions and the procedures to follow in case of an emergency.

Allergies

Allergies are defined as "hypersensitivity to certain irritating substances with which one comes in contact" (2, p. 13). Most allergies are not serious, although they can cause great discomfort. Asthma (see the section on chronic respiratory disorders) can be serious if it precipitates a respiratory crisis. Poison ivy, drugs, certain marine life, and a few insects can also be responsible for a life-threatening condition.

Immediate treatment is needed if symptoms of shock begin to develop. Artificial respiration and cardiac massage may also be necessary. People who are allergic to insect stings should discuss the advisability of hyposensitization with their doctors; such treatment (using specific insect extracts) can decrease future susceptibility to severe reactions. They should also consider a lifestyle that includes wearing clothing of such light colors as white, light green, tan, and khaki. The American Medical Association suggests that persons with a proven allergy to insect stings avoid dark clothing; bright flowery patterns; scented lotions, soaps, shampoos, hairsprays, and perfumes; and bright jewelry and belt buckles. Wearing long pants, long-sleeve shirts, and shoes outdoors from April to October will also afford more protection.

Diabetes

People with chronic diabetes are susceptible to two types of crisis: impending diabetic coma and impending diabetic shock. Family members should be familiar with the signs and symptoms of each condition and know what to do. Table 14A-2 provides key symptoms; but if the situation is not clear, one should assume that an insulin reaction is occurring. If the ingestion of sugar brings no response within a few minutes, treatment for impending diabetic coma should begin. The diabetic should consider the use of Medic Alert tags.

Epilepsy

In order to prevent panic on the part of other students, teachers should be fully informed about students with epilepsy or other neurological disorders that can involve disorientation. (People with epilepsy, muscular dystrophy, cerebral palsy, Parkinson's disease, and myasthenia gravis should always wear a Medic Alert necklace or bracelet to prevent inappropriate action on the part of strangers.)

A major epileptic seizure is often dramatic and frightening but usually lasts only a few minutes. It does not require expert care and seldom is anything gained by transporting the person to a hospital emergency room. The Epilepsy Association of Franklin County recommends these simple procedures to be followed by the classroom teacher or concerned bystander:*

*Adapted from information sheet distributed by the Epilepsy Association of Franklin County, 144 East State Street, Columbus, OH 43215.

1. Keep calm. You cannot stop a seizure once it has started; the seizure will run its course. Reassure other students that their friend is not in pain, will not die, and will be all right very soon and that they cannot catch it.

2. If you can, ease the person to the floor; try to prevent him or her from striking the head or body against any hard, sharp, or hot objects, but do not interfere with the person's movements.

3. Do not force a blunt object between the victim's teeth. There may be violent teeth clenching as part of the seizure, and teeth or gums could be injured in attempting to introduce objects into the mouth.

4. When jerking is over, loosen clothing around the neck. Turn the person on the side, face pointed downward so that saliva or vomitus can drain out and is less likely to be inhaled. Maintain an open airway.

5. Do not be frightened if the person having the seizure seems to stop breathing momentarily; breathing usually resumes spontaneously. If this does not happen, check the airway and give artificial respiration.

6. During a seizure, there is increased salivation and the saliva may appear frothy and bloody. Do not be alarmed. A small amount of blood (from injured tongue or other mouth parts) mixed with a large amount of saliva looks much worse than is really the case.

7. After the movements stop and the person is relaxed, allow sleep or rest if it is desired.

8. If jerking of the body does not stop within five minutes (time the seizure) or keeps recurring, medical assistance should be obtained.

9. If the person is a child, the parents

TABLE 14A-2 DIABETES EMERGENCIES

	Impending Diabetic Coma	*Impending Insulin Shock*
Cause	Hyperglycemia (too much sugar in the blood, not enough insulin)	Too much insulin or too little food with usual doses of insulin; children are prone to it because of their higher level of activity and lower sugar reserves
Onset	Unconsciousness usually fairly slow in developing	Sudden; fainting may develop without warning
Hunger and thirst	Intense thirst, dry mouth, frequent urination	Hunger
Skin	Dry, flushed	Cold sweat, pale
Breathing	Deep and rapid	Shallow or normal
Gastrointestinal symptoms	Nausea and vomiting sometimes occur	Gnawing sensation in stomach
Other symptoms	Drowsiness, confusion, breath has a peculiar fruity odor	Weakness, dizziness, jittery feeling, tremor of the hands, dimness of vision, change in personality
First aid	No adequate first-aid treatment; immediate hospital treatment necessary, including an injection of insulin	If person is conscious, raise blood sugar concentration as quickly as possible (candy, soft drinks, sugar, fruit juice, or anything sweet); hypoglycemia with unconsciousness is an extremely urgent medical emergency—rush person to hospital for an immediate intravenous injection of dextrose or glucagon

(Refer to Chapter 12B for additional information concerning diabetes.)

or guardians should be notified that a seizure has occurred.

10. After a seizure, many people can carry on as before. If after resting, the person seems groggy, confused, or weak, see that he or she is accompanied home.

A minor seizure with or without motor activity can also be a confusing experience for the observer. During such seizures, confusion or nonresponsiveness may occur and may be accompanied by a display of some simple nonpurposeful movements such as smacking the lips, fingering the clothing, chewing, or rhythmically moving the eyes.

Heart Conditions

Children do not generally have heart attacks, but sudden chest pain is a symptom that calls for attention by a doctor. Children should be taught the name of their family doctor and where to locate his or her telephone number. All members of the family should be alert to the symptoms that could signal an emergency situation, know where prescribed emergency medications are located, and know how to administer artificial respiration.

Hemophilia

Hemophilia is usually an inherited disease occurring in males, in which the blood clots improperly. There is danger from any wound that involves bleeding as well as from episodes of internal bleeding triggered by a bump or bruise. If there is the remotest suspicion of bleeding in a hemophiliac, the person must be rushed to the hospital. Every member of the family should be familiar with symptoms of internal bleeding and know what action to take. A hemophiliac should also wear a Medic Alert tag.

Chronic Respiratory Disorders

Teachers should be aware that asthma is a chronic allergic condition that may occur in people of any age. During an attack, shortness of breath may appear without warning. The victim feels as if he or she is suffocating and will sit up or stand up to devote all of his or her energy to breathing. A slight, dry cough will eventually become worse and produce considerable white sputum. Exhalation is especially strained, and there is a loud wheezing sound which is prolonged. Many drugs are used to counter the violent spasms and relieve distress. Fluid intake should be increased to combat dehydration. Tests should be run to detect the causative agent so that specific treatment can begin. It is essential to remove the cause of emotional stress when there is a psychological factor apparent, which is often the case with asthmatic children.

Chronic bronchitis (not common in children and young adults), chronic pulmonary tuberculosis (often associated with poverty), and chronic cystic fibrosis (a hereditary abnormality of the secretion of various exocrine glands) are associated with many life-threatening complications that demand medical treatment.

Sickle-Cell Anemia

Sickle-cell *disease* is a condition in which abnormal genes have been inherited from both parents. A change in one of the amino acids that make up the hemoglobin molecule causes the red blood cell to assume a sickle or crescent shape. These abnormally shaped red cells are more easily destroyed than normal cells, thus causing the *anemia* part of the disease. They also have greater difficulty passing through small blood vessels and may become stuck, resulting in a sickle-cell crisis.

Crisis may occur unpredictably and cause severe abdominal pain, shortness of breath, joint pain which may mimic arthritis, or obstruction of the blood supply to the brain or heart. Obviously, such a crisis requires medical attention. This disease affects almost one percent of Blacks living in the United States.

Sickle-cell *trait* results when only one abnormal gene from one parent is inherited. These people have much less abnormal hemoglobin in their red blood cells and will develop sickle-shaped cells only under extreme conditions of low oxygen. People with the sickle-cell trait are known as carriers; they have the trait, but usually do not know it without appropriate testing. The trait is found in about nine percent of Blacks in this country. By taking a simple blood test, couples can learn whether they are carriers of an abnormal gene and what the chances are that their children would get sickle-cell disease or trait.

Although there is no cure for sickle-cell disease, many things can be done to help alleviate the symptoms. Treatment includes administering blood transfusions, medications for pain, and oxygen. Unfortunately, most people with the disease have a shortened life span.

Other Chronic Conditions

If other conditions have been diagnosed by a physician, such as hypertension (high blood pressure), peptic ulcer, or kidney stones, children should be informed of the condition and what to do in the event of a crisis. They should also be aware of the medications prescribed for someone in the household and whether the medication poses certain risks, such as toxic overdose or allergic reaction, or is dangerous when combined with alcohol or other drugs.

MAJOR MEDICAL EMERGENCIES

All individuals should know how to cope with emergency situations involving severe bleeding, stoppage of breathing, and poisoning by mouth, even though they may not have had the advantage of first-aid instruction.

Severe Bleeding

Wounds with severe bleeding require immediate action, since shock and loss of consciousness can occur rapidly. The American Red Cross lists four important objectives when bleeding is involved:

1. Immediately attempt to stop the bleeding.

2. Protect the wound from contamination and infection.
3. Provide treatment for shock.
4. Obtain medical attention.

When the bleeding is severe, one should apply direct pressure over the wound, using a clean cloth or sterile gauze pad if one is available. It is possible to bleed to death in a matter of minutes if a large artery has been severed, but in most cases the natural clotting process will soon diminish the flow of blood. After the bleeding has been controlled, one should apply additional layers of cloth without removing the original dressing and disturbing the blood clots, and bandage firmly.

The injured part of the body should be elevated above the level of the victim's heart, unless there is evidence of a fracture. Gravity will help reduce blood pressure in the injured area, but direct pressure on a thick pad over the wound is still necessary.

If bleeding continues, one should exert pressure with the fingers or hand over the nearest arterial pressure point to temporarily compress the artery supplying blood to the affected limb. One should not use a pressure point in conjunction with direct pressure and elevation any longer than is necessary to stop the bleeding. The brachial artery should be used for the control of severe bleeding from an arm wound. Pressure should be applied at the point located "on the inside of the arm in the groove between the biceps and the triceps, about midway between the armpit and the elbow" (1, p. 27). The femoral artery should be used for the control of severe bleeding from a leg wound. The pressure point is located "on the front, center part of the diagonally slanted 'hinge' of the leg, in the crease of the groin area, where the artery crosses the pelvic bone on its way to the leg" (1, p. 28). Pressure points are illustrated in Figures 14A-2 and 14A-3.

A tourniquet is an extremely tight bandage applied around an arm or leg to stop hemorrhaging. It is a dangerous device that is rarely justified except in critical emergencies that are life threatening. According to the American Red Cross, "The decision to apply a tourniquet is in reality a decision to risk sacrifice of a limb in order to save life" (1, p. 28). Once the serious decision to apply a tourniquet has been made, the tourniquet should not be loosened except on the advice of a physician. One should make a written note of the location of the tourniquet and the time it was applied and attach the note to the victim's clothing.

One should not attempt to cleanse serious wounds but should immobilize the injured area and adjust the victim's lying position so that the affected limb can be elevated if possible.

FIGURE 14A-3 Pressure points (Arm)

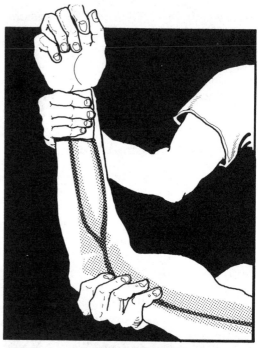

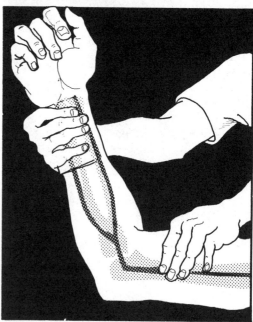

FIGURE 14A-2 Pressure points (Leg)

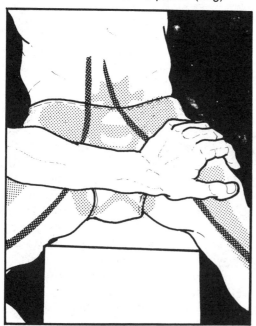

(Adapted with permission from *Standard First Aid and Personal Safety*, copyright 1973 by the American National Red Cross, pp. 27, 28.)

Stoppage of Breathing

"Artificial respiration is a procedure for causing air to flow into and out of a person's lungs when his natural breathing is inadequate or ceases" (1, p. 66). Artificial respiration can be life saving when breathing has stopped because of electric shock; drowning; gas poisoning; drugs such as morphine, opium, barbiturates, and alcohol; compression of the chest; choking and strangling; and partial obstruction of the breathing passages. Many studies have proven mouth-to-mouth resuscitation to be the easiest, most direct, and most effective way of forcing air into the victim's lungs. See Figure 14A-4, "When Breathing Stops," which duplicates the American Red Cross poster, for appropriate first-aid procedures.

Artificial respiration should be continued until:

1. The victim begins to breathe for herself or himself.
2. The victim is pronounced dead by a doctor.
3. The victim is dead beyond any doubt.

In the case of a person who has been eating or may have a foreign body in the mouth and is suddenly unable to speak, cough, or breathe, the possibility of complete airway obstruction should be recognized. The victim may clutch at the throat, appear dusky blue in color, and proceed to collapse. Prompt action is urgent. By using the Heimlich Maneuver, one can exert pressure that forces the diaphragm upward, compressing air in the lungs, and thus expelling the object that is blocking the breathing passage. The procedure is as follows:*

*Ohio Department of Health, *First Aid for Food Choking,* 1977.

When the victim is standing, stand behind the victim and wrap your arms around victim's waist (when victim is in sitting position, rescuer should kneel behind to apply the maneuver).

Place a fist thumb-side in against victim's abdomen below rib cage, slightly above navel.

Grasp your fist with other hand.

Press the fist forcefully, with a quick upward thrust into the victim's abdomen.

Repeat several times if necessary.

When the victim is lying face up, kneel astride the victim, face to face.

With one hand on top of the other, place heel of bottom hand on victim's abdomen below the rib cage, slightly above the navel.

With a quick upward thrust, press forcefully into the victim's abdomen and repeat several times if necessary.

The American Red Cross recommends delivering four sharp blows with the heel of the hand over the victim's spine between the shoulder blades before administering abdominal thrusts as described in the Heimlich Maneuver.

Poisoning

Poisoning is often a cause of death in young children, chiefly because they cannot distinguish between what should and should not be eaten. If poisoning occurs, the American National Red Cross recommends the updated information found in Figure 14A-5 (used with permission).

Unfortunately, the authors cannot give teachers all the first-aid information that is necessary to meet every crisis situation. They do highly recommend that teachers enroll in a first-aid course every few years and encourage students to value safety and first aid in their own lives.

FIGURE 14A-4

WHEN BREATHING STOPS

AMERICAN RED CROSS ARTIFICIAL RESPIRATION

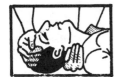

IF A VICTIM APPEARS TO BE UNCONSCIOUS — TAP VICTIM ON THE SHOULDER AND SHOUT, "ARE YOU OKAY?"

IF THERE IS NO RESPONSE — TILT THE VICTIM'S HEAD, CHIN POINTING UP. Place one hand under the victim's neck and gently lift. At the same time, push with the other hand on the victim's forehead. This will move the tongue away from the back of the throat to open the airway.

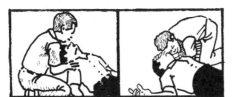

IMMEDIATELY LOOK, LISTEN, AND FEEL FOR AIR.
While maintaining the backward head-tilt position, place your cheek and ear close to the victim's mouth and nose. Look for the chest to rise and fall while you listen and feel for the return of air. Check for about 5 seconds.

IF THE VICTIM IS NOT BREATHING — GIVE FOUR QUICK BREATHS.
Maintain the backward head tilt, pinch the victim's nose with the hand that is on the victim's forehead to prevent leakage of air, open your mouth wide, take a deep breath, seal your mouth around the victim's mouth, and blow into the victim's mouth with four quick but full breaths just as fast as you can. When blowing, use only enough time between breaths to lift your head slightly for better inhalation. **For an infant,** give gentle puffs and blow through the mouth *and* nose and do not tilt the head back as far as for an adult.

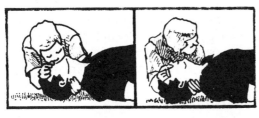

IF THERE IS STILL NO BREATHING — If you do not get an air exchange when you blow, it may help to reposition the head and try again.

AGAIN, LOOK, LISTEN, AND FEEL FOR AIR EXCHANGE.

CHANGE RATE TO ONE BREATH EVERY 5 SECONDS **FOR AN ADULT.**

FOR AN INFANT, GIVE ONE GENTLE PUFF EVERY 3 SECONDS.

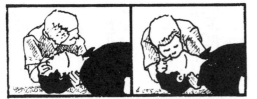

MOUTH-TO-NOSE METHOD — The mouth-to-nose method can be used with the sequence described above instead of the mouth-to-mouth method. Maintain the backward head-tilt position with the hand on the victim's forehead. Remove the hand from under the neck and close the victim's mouth. Blow into the victim's nose. Open the victim's mouth for the look, listen, and feel step.

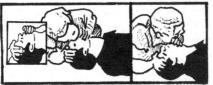

For more information about these and other life-saving techniques, contact your Red Cross chapter for training.

FIGURE 14A-5 The American Red Cross Attacks Poisons

IS IT POISON?

Symptoms vary greatly. Base your suspicion that a person has swallowed poison on—

- Information from the victim or an observer
- Presence of a poison container
- Sudden onset of pain or illness
- Burns around the lips or mouth
- Chemical odor on the breath
- Pupils contracted or dilated

FIRST AID FOR POISON BY MOUTH

Conscious victim:

- *Dilute* the poison *with a glass of water or milk* if the victim is not having convulsions.
- *Call the poison control center* or your doctor or dial 0 or 911; call the emergency rescue squad.
- Save the label or container for identification; save vomited material for analysis.
- *Do not* neutralize with counteragents. *Do not* give oils.
- If the victim becomes unconscious, keep his airway open.

Unconscious victim:

- Maintain an open airway.
- Call the emergency rescue squad.
- Give mouth-to-mouth resuscitation or cardiopulmonary resuscitation (CPR) if necessary.
- *Do not* give fluids; *do not* induce vomiting; if the victim is vomiting, position his head so that vomit drains from his mouth.
- Save the label or the container for identification; save vomited material for analysis.

Convulsions:

- Call the emergency squad as soon as possible.
- *Do not* attempt to restrain the victim; try to position him so that he will not injure himself.
- Loosen tight clothing.
- Watch for obstruction of the airway and correct it by tilting the head; give mouth-to-mouth resuscitation or CPR if necessary.
- *Do not* force a hard object or finger between the teeth.
- *Do not* give any fluids.
- *Do not* induce vomiting.

- After a convulsion, turn the victim on his side or in the prone position, with his head turned to allow fluid to drain from his mouth.

Instructions on product labels for specific treatment of poisoning *may* be wrong; contact your doctor or a poison control center for instructions.

Have on hand

These products should be used *only* on the advice of your doctor or the poison control center.

1. *Syrup of ipecac* (to induce vomiting)
2. *Activated charcoal* (to bind, or deactivate, poison)
3. *Epsom salts* (a laxative)

If poisoning occurs where medical help is unavailable (e.g., camping), you may induce vomiting if the victim has taken an overdose of drugs or medication, but *not* if a strong acid, alkali, or petroleum product has been swallowed. Then get the victim to a hospital as quickly as possible.

Emergency telephone numbers

DOCTOR _____

RESCUE SQUAD _____

POISON CONTROL

CENTER _____

Write in these numbers now! Have the family memorize them. Also place them on your telephone.

The information on this poster is based on a report prepared by the National Academy of Sciences—National Research Council, Committee on Emergency Medical Services.

REFERENCES

1. The American National Red Cross, *Standard First Aid and Personal Safety* (Garden City, N.Y.: Doubleday, 1973).

2. Robert E. Rothenberg, *Medical Dictionary and Health Manual*, rev. ed. (New York: New American Library, 1975).

3. Robert D. Russell, *Health Education* (Washington, D.C.: National Education Association, 1975).

4. Alton L. Thygerson, *Safety: Concepts and Instruction* (Englewood Cliffs, N.J.: Prentice-Hall, 1976).

PART B: TEACHING ABOUT SAFETY AND FIRST AID

A rather long chapter is being devoted to safety, partly because accidents are the number one killer of young people today. New lifestyles demand ever increasing human adaptability. Americans must adapt to physical strains, psychological stresses, and hazardous conditions if they are going to survive in this society.

In industry, in school, at home, and on the highway, the accident-prone individual is a potential threat to everyone. Teachers can teach students to value safety as a worthy lifestyle component by dealing with some basic needs of students:

1. Students need to recognize safe and unsafe patterns of behavior.
2. Students need to recognize that their safety depends upon adjusting to various environments.
3. Students need to realize that everyone has an obligation to help prevent accidents from occurring.
4. Students need to appreciate the value and quality of their lives.
5. Students need to know how to react in an emergency situation.

The safety lessons in this chapter involve students practicing safety at home, at school, on the playground, and on sidewalks and streets. Through constructing a mock community, taking a home survey, role playing, and participating in games, the students are helped to make decisions and consider possible outcomes. The students learn to take responsibility for their actions and how to respond in emergency situations.

UNIT I: HOME SAFETY

The purpose of this lesson is to remind students that every member of the family has a responsibility to recognize possible dangers around the home and to help safeguard against accidents.

OBJECTIVES

1. The students will decide how safe their homes are by conducting a survey in their home using standards discussed in class. With the assistance of their par-

Appropriate grade levels are suggested for each teaching strategy and appear as ○, □, ☆ in the left-hand column.

○ = most suited for the primary grades;

□ = most suited for the intermediate grades:

☆ = most suited for the upper elementary grades.

ents, they will try to eliminate any hazards discovered.

2. The students will decide from their surveys what are the most common causes of accidents in the home.

3. The students will participate in role-playing activities that demonstrate what to do in the event of fire.

MATERIALS

1. Atlas Figure 96, Potential Home Hazards Checklist.

2. Paper, pencil, poster board, construction paper, felt-tip markers, cardboard box, scissors, and paste.

3. Atlas Figure 35, Policeman Fred Says: Never Open the Door for Strangers.

Methods

○ □ ☆

Home Survey Checklist

Discuss potential hazards around the home and help the class prepare a checklist to be used as a home survey, or use the checklist included in the Atlas.

○ □

Safety Detective

Let each student make a badge to wear and give the students the assignment of being safety detectives over the weekend after informing their parents that they will be doing so.

The students should report to their parents any hazards they find and ask their parents to help them eliminate the hazard. For example, a child can clean up rubbish in the basement but should not move power tools; if a child finds poisons and medicines within the reach of children, the parents should move them to a safe place.

○ □

Tabulate Research Findings

As a follow-up activity, the class should tabulate their findings to discover which were the most common hazards around their homes. The students may also each draw a picture of one hazard they discovered and a second picture showing how it was eliminated.

○

Stevie Safety

To introduce this unit to primary-age children, construct a puppet, Stevie Safety, who tells the students about simple safety rules. While Stevie tells his story from a stage constructed from a cardboard box and cloth or paper, the students should be thinking of possible safety hazards in their homes and how they can be corrected.

○ □

Three Little Pigs Bulletin Board

A bulletin board about safety can be based on the story "Three Little Pigs." Each of the pigs should have a house on the bulletin board. These houses can be made in booklet form, using construction paper or poster board as the outside and regular white paper inside to represent different rooms in the house. If each house has six pages or rooms in it, eighteen children could be responsible for drawing a room. Other children may construct house coverings, draw additional scenery, and draw the wolf lurking nearby who is going to check for possible home hazards.

The cover of the first little pig's house should be colored to look like straw, or, better yet, have real straw glued to it. The straw house is not sturdy and invites many accidents.

The pages in this house could picture a kitchen with a burner left on and food boiling over, cleaning fluids close to heat, liquids spilled on the floor, meat and vegetables left unrefrigerated, dirty dishes in the sink, cupboards left open, many flies, and a child trying to climb out of her or his high chair.

The second page might represent the living room. Toys could be shown strewed over the floor, a fire burning in a fireplace with no screen, a burning cigarette that somebody has forgotten, an extension cord in bad condition, and marbles left in a walking area.

The third page could be a bedroom showing a girl leaning out an open window, a bottle of pills on the nightstand along with a package of cigarettes, and a fan blowing close to some curtains.

The fourth page might be the bathroom showing too many appliances plugged into an outlet, a radio plugged in next to the tub, only one drinking glass for the family, shampoo spilled on the floor, and razor blades left out with the razor.

The fifth and sixth pages could show the basement and garage with similar hazards. For instance, mousetraps and rat poison could be shown on the basement floor, and gasoline and matches stored close together in the garage.

The second little pig's house should be made to appear it is made out of wood and represent hazards that are not so obvious as in the first house. The inside walls could have old paint chipping off, a gas stove leaking gas, a lamp with a defective plug, unclean water, flies on the food, poor lighting, sagging beds, and matches within reach of a child.

The third little pig's house should be a hazard-free house demonstrating good overall safety habits. It should appear to have a firm foundation and to be built with bricks. Each room is clean, orderly, and not overcrowded.

After the bulletin board is completed, ask the students to discuss the hazards depicted in each room.

The following activities acquaint students with the most common fire hazards and means of removing or compensating for them. Urge students to cooperate in building a strong fire-safety program; help them develop safe habits in handling fire and flammable materials.

○

Drawing

To get the class thinking about fire safety, have them draw a picture of a good use of fire (to provide warmth from a fireplace, to cook food, to provide light).

□

Match Demonstration

Demonstrate how to use matches safely, reminding students to:

1. Use only safety matches.
2. Close the cover before striking.
3. Make sure they are not wearing long, loose sleeves that could easily catch on fire.
4. Dispose of used matches by running water over the end or breaking them and placing them in a glass or tin container.
5. Take care not to let a match burn too long and burn their fingers.

○ □

Role-Playing Situations

Role play how a child and adult should react in the following situations:

1. Your oven catches on fire. (Call an adult to turn off the source of heat and close the oven door if it is open. Smother small fires with ordinary table salt.)

2. Grease in a frying pan catches on fire. (Cover pan with lid or throw lots of baking soda on the flame to smother the fire. *Water should not be poured on flaming grease*, since it will cause it to spread.)

3. Your clothing catches on fire. (Wrap yourself in a heavy rug, blanket, bedspread, or coat and roll slowly on the floor or grass. *Do not run*, since running will fan the flames.)

4. You are caught in a room filled with smoke. (Keep close to the floor where the air is purest. Crawl on your hands and knees. If possible, cover your nose and mouth with a damp piece of cloth.)

○

Fire Drills

Help students recognize the importance of fire drills. Before a school fire drill, go through all the steps involved and make sure every student knows what to do. You may want to make an eye-catching poster concerning proper behavior (keep in line, remain quiet, lock windows).

○ □

Teach students how to identify and use a water/chemical fire extinguisher and fire alarm box. (To use a fire alarm, break the glass if necessary, open the door, pull down the lever.)

□

Home Fire Escape Plan

As homework, let each student make his or her own family nighttime fire escape floorplan with the help of his or her parents according to the following directions:

1. Outline the entire floor area.
2. Label bedrooms, windows, doors, and stairway. (Determine if any rooftops can be used as a fire escape.)

3. Select the best window in each bedroom for an emergency escape.
4. See if you can open the window.
5. Draw black arrows to show normal exit through hall or stairway and colored arrows to show emergency exit in case fire blocks hallway or stairs.

Evaluation

LIFESTYLE CONTENT

○

Flash Card Game Have the students each draw a picture of a potential home hazard (such as shoes left on stairsteps) and mount the picture on construction paper or poster board. On the other side of the card, have them draw a picture showing how the accident can be prevented (taking shoes off the steps).

You now have a set of safety flash cards that can be used for individual review or as a game. Divide the class into two teams and hold up a flash card. The students must identify what accident could occur and how it could be prevented.

LIFESTYLE VALUE

□

Have the students discuss the following questions:

Suppose your mother asked you to make the toast for breakfast and the toast got stuck in the toaster. What would you do?

What would you do if you were in a high-rise apartment and a fire broke out?

Do you think most accidents can be prevented? Why?

Why do accidents happen wherever there are people?

When the doorbell rings, do you open your door if no one else is in the house with you? (Distribute copies of Atlas Figure 35, Policeman Fred Says: Never Open the Door for Strangers, for the students to color and discuss.)

UNIT II: TRAFFIC SAFETY

Teachers cannot hope to change their students' lifestyles by having them only *talk* about the safest way to school. It is important that students are taught to visualize their paths, discriminate between the safe and unsafe routes, and discuss street safety with their parents, teachers, policemen, and peers. It is only then that teachers may hope to affect students' behavior in a positive manner.

OBJECTIVES

1. Each student will draw a map showing the safest way to school from home.
2. The student will demonstrate knowledge of safety rules for riding a bicycle (or tricycle) by making replicas of road signs and participating in class activities such as making a classroom safety town.
3. The students will be able to recite at least five rules that are necessary for riding the school bus safely.
4. The students will share their knowledge of traffic safety with other students informally and through a formal multimedia presentation.
5. The student will research a safety program (such as the school safety patrol, green pennant program, or safety town) and report her or his findings to the class.

MATERIALS

1. *A Teacher's Guide for the Safest Route to School Project.*
2. Bicycle.
3. Simple camera, slide film, tape recorder, slide projector.

4. Pencils, felt-tip markers, paper, construction paper, poster board, scissors, and glue.
5. Atlas Figures 36 through 41—Policeman Fred says: Obey Traffic Signals; Be Extra Careful on Rainy Days; Riding Double Leads to Trouble; Always Use Bike Hand Signals—Obey All Traffic Signs and Signals; Obey Your School Patrol; and Play It Safe—Keep the Green Pennant Flying.

Methods

The Traffic Engineering and Safety Department of the American Automobile Association in Falls Church, Virginia, has developed *A Teacher's Guide for the Safest Route to School Project*, which is available from your local AAA Club. The department has also recently revised the film *The Safest Way*, telling how a class of boys and girls discovered their safest routes to school. The students take a field trip, develop an area map, and then trace their own routes. They learn that the safest way applies not only to going to school but also going to the playground, to church, to the movies, or to any place. This film is available from your local AAA Motor Club or film rental library and is useful for launching a safest route to school project, which the authors highly recommend.

SIGNS FOR SAFETY

Teach young children the meanings of the colors of a traffic signal; help them recognize the basic shapes of signs and learn their meanings; review safety tips on crossing a street.

○

Workable Traffic Signal

Some communities have police officers that will bring a life-size workable traffic signal to the school. The police officer can demonstrate how a drum causes the lights to change colors and can explain safety related to traffic signals. Group discussion could take place on questions such as What are some of the things that can happen if a car does not stop at a red light? Why are there traffic signals? What might happen if there were no traffic signals?

○

Make and Obey Signs

Let the students make cardboard or poster board replicas of road signs in the appropriate colors. The signs could be hung in the classroom and obeyed for several days. For instance, place the stop sign at the children's eye level on the wall to the right of the exit door. A yield sign could be placed on a stick with a holder or taped to the floor where two schoolroom traffic patterns meet. A railroad sign could be placed near a picture or model of a train. A diamond-shaped

sign could indicate a possible danger in the classroom.

○

Role Playing

Have the students create their own little town by placing masking tape on the floor to mark streets and intersections. Have some of them role play various situations while other students tell what rule the actors performed and whether they demonstrated it correctly.

○□

Bulletin Board

On one side of a bulletin board, place various signs (with older children, you may only want to use various shapes for signs and not include any lettering). On the other side of the bulletin board write the meaning of the sign: railroad crossing ahead, curve to the right ahead, stop, traffic light, yield right of way, warning, or school nearby. Let the students match the sign with its meaning by connecting yarn

FIGURE 14B-1 Safety signals

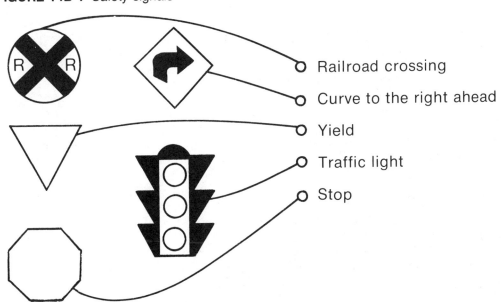

Railroad crossing

Curve to the right ahead

Yield

Traffic light

Stop

between the meaning and its sign. (See Figure 14B-1.) This may be an individual activity or a game.

FORMAL TRAFFIC SAFETY PROGRAM

○ □

Have the students share their knowledge of traffic safety with other students by preparing a safety program. Several students might learn a bicycle safety song to teach to another class. Students interested in photography could be taught how to operate an instamatic camera and take slides of safe and unsafe situations. (Stress the importance of being careful with a camera because it is fragile.) Let the students practice using the camera without film, and have them draw or describe situations they wish to photograph before the camera is loaded. Show the students how a slide projector works and let each student practice running it.

BICYCLE SAFETY

In teaching a unit on bicycle safety, it is important to find out how many students have a bike and how many know all of the hand signals. You might want to begin a discussion by asking the students whether they think riding a bicycle is healthy and if a bicycle is a toy or means of transportation or both.

○ □

Have the class make up a list of rules for safe bicycling.

○

Bicycle Demonstration

Consider bringing a bicycle to school and asking the students to correctly demonstrate getting on and off a bicycle, applying foot or hand brakes or both, stopping and parking the bicycle.

□

Field Trip

Arrange a visit to a bicycle shop. Let the students see various kinds of bicycles and learn how to take care of the bicycles. If possible, have a worker in the shop show the students how to make some minor bicycle repairs.

□

Bicycle Club

Determine whether the students would like to form a bicycle club at school or participate in a bicycle safety day at which they demonstrate their ability and skill to ride a bicycle safely. Activities might include a bicycle mechanical test and a bicycle skill test.

○ □ ☆

Bicycle Institute of America

Write to the Bicycle Manufacturers Association of America, 1101 15th St. N.W., Washington, D.C. 20005, for pamphlets, a bicycle safety checklist, and other related information.

○

Record

Play the record *Songs of Safety* by Frank Luther and let the students choose their favorite safety song.

○ □

For many more class activities regarding traffic safety, call or write your local American Automobile Association. Especially helpful booklets include *10 Otto the Auto Stories* for teachers of primary grades, and *10 Traffic Safety Guides* for grades K–3 or 4–6.

○ □

Bus Safety

Have the students make a bus out of construction paper and list at least five rules

FIGURE 14B-2 Bicycle Safety Check (Courtesy the Bicycle Manufacturers Association of America, Washington, D.C.)

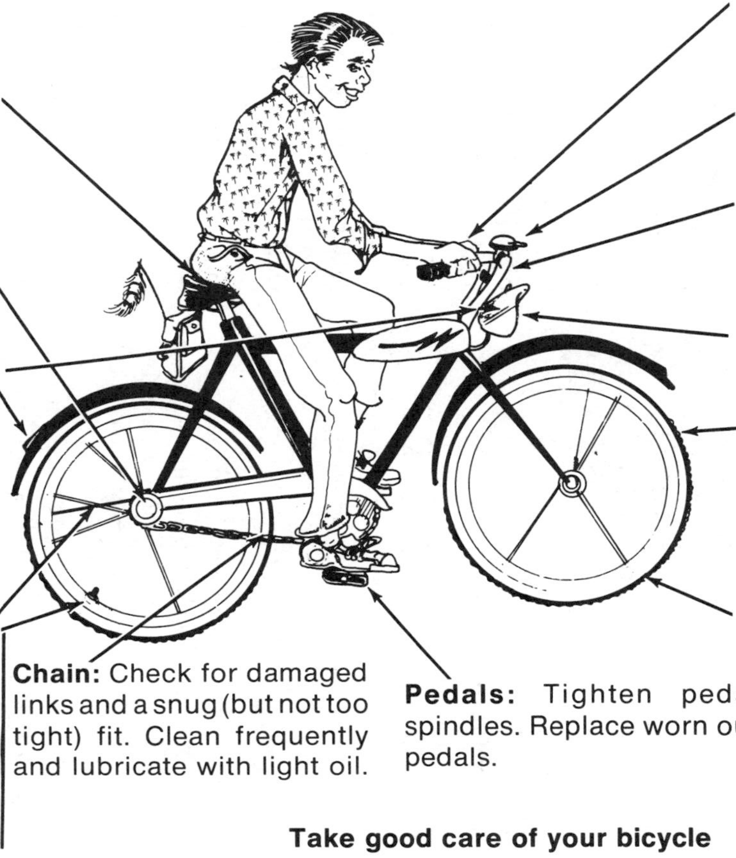

Have your bicycle checked twice a year by a reliable serviceman

Handle grips: Replace worn grips. Make sure they fit snugly.

Bell or horn: Be sure it works properly.

Handle bars: Adjust for your comfort. Keep stem well down in fork. Tighten securely.

Light: Must be visible for 500 feet.

Tires: Inflate to correct pressure. Check tires frequently. Remove imbedded glass, cinders, etc. Don't ride on worn out tires.

Wheels: Tighten wheel nuts.

Pedals: Tighten pedal spindles. Replace worn out pedals.

Saddle: Adjust height so leg bends only slightly with ball of foot on pedal at bottom of stroke. Tighten securely.

Coaster brake, hand brakes: Must brake evenly everytime. No slippage. Have it adjusted by a trained serviceman.

Lights and reflectors: Should be visible at dusk and at night for 500 feet. Federal law requires that bicycles be equipped with reflective devices, including front, rear and pedal reflectors. If damaged, replace immediately for your own safety.

Spokes: Replace broken ones promptly. Keep them tight.

Tire valve: Inspect for leaks and straightness.

Chain: Check for damaged links and a snug (but not too tight) fit. Clean frequently and lubricate with light oil.

Take good care of your bicycle   Always ride with caution

on it that are necessary for riding the bus safely. A variation of this activity is to have the students cut out a large bus and attach it to the bulletin board. In each window of the bus, they can insert a small cardboard tab that can be pulled out to reveal a safety rule.

○

Have a bus driver speak with the students.

○

Dramatize getting on and off a bus and observing other safety rules by placing classroom chairs in rows representing seats in a bus.

□ ☆

Safety Programs

Help the students investigate various safety programs that exist in their community. Have each student report to the class any information gathered.

○

Safety Town

Some communities have developed elaborate preschool safety programs similar to Safety Town in Upper Arlington, Ohio. To build their safety town, citizens marked the paved area at Wickliffe School to resemble miniature streets with crossings. They built small homes, churches, schools, and shops to simulate a village; and they installed small road signs and signals.

The summer program includes safety songs and rules. Children dance the Hokey Pokey to help learn right and left. They color pictures of their friends the policeman, the fire engine, and the traffic light. On special days, the children might even climb aboard a school bus or fire engine or marvel at a helicopter. They learn to use a telephone for emergency help, and they ride tricycles and pedal

cars through the streets of Safety Town, always stopping for the red light and practicing other safety habits. Following their two weeks of safety lessons for three hours each day, the children are presented certificates of achievement.

THE GREEN PENNANT SAFETY PROGRAM

The Green Pennant Safety Program sponsored nationally by General Motors has also helped reduce the number of young people involved in traffic accidents and increase their awareness of safety. Contact your local Chamber of Commerce for more information regarding this fine program.

SCHOOL SAFETY PATROL

The School Safety Patrol was started in 1920; today more than a million members are on duty each day of the school year helping schoolmates at hazardous crossings near schools.

A patrol member never stops cars. Only police officers and adult guards have the right to stop vehicles. A patrol member holds back only schoolmates and sets an example by knowing and practicing safe walking. Call the local division of the American Automobile Association for information about the pamphlets *School Bus Patrols*, *School Safety Patrols Information Test*, *School Safety Patrol Member's Handbook*, and *Policies and Practices for School Safety Patrols*.

Evaluation

LIFESTYLE CONTENT

○

Have the class play Sign-O, a safety game played like bingo.* Make nine squares on

---

*Courtesy of the American Automobile Association, *Traffic Safety Guide for Teachers*, K–3, 1974–1975.

an 8-by-11-inch plain piece of paper or poster board. Draw in various road and pedestrian signs (see illustration in Figure 14B-3 for guidance) in place of the numbers and letters that would be used on a bingo card. Make several different variations of the sign-o sheet, and produce enough copies for the entire class.

Play the game by calling out the different signs to the class or giving a description of where the signs would be located. Provide chips or pieces of paper for the children to mark their answers. Whoever fills a row first—up and down, sideways, or diagonally—has sign-o. (Call the local AAA Club for the pamphlet *New Road Signs Coming Your Way*, Stock #3556.)

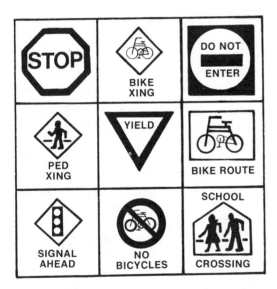

FIGURE 14B-3 Sign-O game

LIFESTYLE VALUE

☐
Have the students complete the following open-ended statements:

Being alert means ＿＿＿＿＿＿ .
By crossing at a corner, the children are ＿＿＿＿＿＿＿＿＿＿ .
The traffic light ＿＿＿＿＿＿ .

Hitching or holding on to moving vehicles is ＿＿＿＿＿＿＿＿＿ .
Using streets or sidewalks rather than shortcuts is ＿＿＿＿＿＿＿ .

Play-area safety hunt is described in *Traffic Safety Guide for Teachers.** Make a composite list obtained from the entire class of areas in which each student has played in the past week. Write down these places on the chalkboard and, using a scale of 0 to 5, have the class rank the play areas by accident potential or danger. 0 would indicate little or no danger; 5, much danger.

Tabulate and rank these areas yourself from least to most dangerous, based on the students' evaluations. Ask the students to identify the possible hazard in each area. Record their evaluations on the chalkboard, and ask the students if they see any prominent or common dangers. Ask the students to suggest ways in which particular hazards can be avoided in each play area.

UNIT III: COMMUNITY SAFETY

The purpose of this unit is to assist students in developing coping and decision-making skills that will enable them to grow safely with the community.

OBJECTIVES

1. The student will be able to identify hazards that exist in the school and on the playground upon completion of a large bulletin board and playground activity.
2. The student will learn about specific problems of community safety, such as dealing with strangers, construction

*For grades 4–6, available from the American Automobile Association.

sites, and parking lots, and about community helpers through the construction of a neighborhood model and informal discussion.

3. After completing the lesson which discusses strangers, the students will be able to distinguish between family friends, police officers, and strangers. They will be able to orally identify boundaries in which they are allowed to play and discuss why they should not take food, money, a ride, or anything else without their parents' permission.

4. The students will begin to understand the inner workings of city government by interviewing city personnel and trying to have a hazard in their community corrected.

MATERIALS

1. Construction paper, scissors, crayons, paste, gummed stars, colored yarn, index cards, cardboard, and masking tape.

2. Outside playground equipment.

3. Felt board, felt (including red and green), hand puppets, self-hardening clay, rolling pin, paper clips, table knife, small pieces of sponge, tempera paints (optional).

4. Camera and film.

5. Atlas Figures 42 through 44—Policeman Fred says: If You Are Lost or Go Astray; Taking Candy from a Stranger; A Trip Through Safetyland.

Methods

○ □

Introduction

Introduce the concept of community safety with the film *Primary Safety: In the School Building.** You may also want to

*A Coronet instructional film.

send for "Checklist of Safety and Safety Education in Your School."[†]

○ □

Thought Questions

Ask the class the following questions:

Why do we need safety in the school building?

Do you run in the halls?

Do you race up the stairs?

Do you carry such a large stack of books that you cannot see where you are going?

Do you use the handrail?

Do you always follow safety procedures when performing science experiments?

Do you push and shove at the water fountain?

○ □

Bulletin Board

Make a school safety bulletin board showing a floorplan of a school, complete with classrooms, stairs, fire escapes, cafeteria, water fountains, workshop, gym, etc. Leave room for a playground and playground equipment outside. Paste stars on the places where index cards containing safety information have been made and use colored yarn to connect the stars with the appropriate information cards that surround the bulletin board display.

This bulletin board idea can also be used as a game. Turn the index cards over so that the information does not show and see if the students can identify the various danger points on their own.

[†] Available from National Commission of Safety Education, National Education Association, 1201 Sixteenth Street, N.W., Washington, DC 20036.

○

Playground Safety

Take the students out to the playground swings. Ask them why there are often boundaries around the swing area. Have three students swing as high as they can on the swings. The rest of the students can decide how close they can be to the swing without being hit (front, back, and sides). They may even want to mark boundaries on the ground if none already exist.

Have two students get on a teeter-totter and get off it. Lead into a discussion about the safe way to get on and off such equipment.

Discuss safety rules for using other available playground equipment, such as climbing on a jungle gym and playing tetherball.

Ask the students what is important to keep in mind when walking or running across the playground.

○ □

Neighborhood Model

Expand the area map described in the *Safest Route to School Project* guide in Unit II. In addition to adding model houses and a school, add other buildings including stores, a hospital, fire and police stations, a church. You might even add a quarry, construction site, farm, public park with woods and a lake.

If you do not have time to construct models, simply divide paper or a window shade into city blocks. Color the pond with a blue felt-tip marker or use foil paper to represent the pond. Label squares representing houses and build-ings. Write the telephone numbers of the police and fire departments in the appro-priate squares. The students may also want to include the telephone numbers for a nearby hospital and poison control center on their neighborhood model. Let the students make a *Community Safety Telephone Numbers* pamphlet to take home and give their parents.

○ □ ☆

Safety Directory

Have the students use a telephone direc-tory to learn where to get help for public problems. Have them research the tele-phone numbers and addresses of the agen-cies that would deal with the following:

Fires

Police matters

Abandoned vehicles on private or pub-lic property (check division of police)

Air pollution (check state environmen-tal protection agency)

Animal bites (check division of envi-ronmental health, city health depart-ment)

Animals dead in the street (check divi-sion of sanitation)

Animals running loose (check animal control center)

Building conditions (check division of housing, city health department)

Electricity off (check the electric com-pany)

Ice on residential street (check street cleaning)

Insect infestation (check environmen-tal health, city health department)

Playground complaints (check recre-ation and parks)

Sewer complaints (check sewage and drainage or sanitation department)

Snow removal and street cleaning (check division of engineering)

Traffic signals damaged or removed (check traffic engineering)

Trash collection (check division of sanitation)

Unresolved complaints (check to see if you have an ombudsman)

Water leaks (check with division of water)

○

Decision Making

Make sure you have included streets, intersections, traffic signs, and railroad tracks in the neighborhood model. Let the students bring toy trucks and cars from home and respond to various situations involving vehicles.

Strangers

Recent studies have shown that child molesters are not usually the strangers whom parents fear but often someone known to the child. The child molester may not be known to the parents, however. Teaching in this area must be positive to avoid frightening the child or giving him or her a feeling of distrust.

○

One way of approaching this subject is to discuss how people meet friends and the need for an introduction. Emphasize that children should not talk with strangers. Explain that children need to have freedom of movement, yet for their own protection they need to have definite boundaries for their play areas. To go beyond these boundaries should require parental permission.

○ □

Have the students discuss why they should not take food, money, a ride, or anything else from strangers.

Discuss the duties of a police officer. Point out that a security guard is not a police officer, even though he or she may be carrying a gun and wearing a uniform.

○

Speaker

Invite a police officer to speak to the class about the danger of talking to strangers. Let the students see that the police officer is their friend. Let them examine the police uniform.

○

Transparency

Use Atlas Figure 42, Policeman Fred says: If You Are Lost or Go Astray.

○ □

Movies

Show the movie The Riddle of the Friendly Stranger.* The movie tells why strangers can be a terrible danger and shows examples of what to do and what not to do when approached by someone unfamiliar.

You may also want to use the pamphlet, Gabby's Coloring and Game Book —The Riddle of the Unfriendly Stranger.* It includes games, coloring pages, and poems. A filmstrip package from SVE Films on child molesting, Patch the Pony, is excellent for the primary grades.

○

Use Atlas Figure 43, Policeman Fred says: Taking Candy from a Stranger. Ask questions such as Do you think the little girl is going to take the candy the man wants to give her? Would you take the candy? Should the girl talk to the man? Should she get into his car?

○

Hand Puppets

Afer discussing safety rules concerning strangers, use hand puppets for review.

*Available from Marathon Oil Company, Guidance Films, Inc., 1964, 20 min. color.

The hand puppets may also be used in discussing ways that people meet new friends and ways to make introductions. (Figures on a felt board may be substituted for puppets.)

○
Hello Plaques

Let the students make a plaque of their hello (right) hand. Give each child a square of cardboard and a lump of clay. (Self-hardening clay can be made with equal parts of salt and flour and enough cool water to make it fairly stiff but workable.) The clay should be placed on the cardboard and molded into an attractive shape. Instruct students to roll the clay until it is reasonably flat and then press their right hand firmly in the center with fingers spread. A piece of moistened sponge can be rubbed lightly around the edges of the plaque to give it a smooth appearance. Students may press a paper clip into the top of the clay on the back as a hanger. After the clay has thoroughly dried, it can be painted. Have the students compose a verse about friendship to accompany their plaques. Teach them a song about friends.

□ ☆
Social Studies

A social studies unit on city government can be correlated with community safety. The social studies unit would probably include a discussion of city personnel and their functions. Have various speakers (police officer, fire fighter, councilperson, sanitation worker) speak to the class and be interviewed about their contributions to community safety.

○ □
Community Safety

Take a walk with the class in search of hazards in the community (overgrown bushes on a corner, buildings obstructing a view, unclear crosswalk lines). Have the students photograph or draw pictures of these hazards. All of the pictures should be put on a big bulletin board under the heading "Before." Discuss how the hazards can be corrected: trash can lids can be put on the containers; litter can be picked up; agencies listed in the community safety telephone numbers project can be contacted.

□ ☆
Petition

If the class feels strongly about correcting a problem and nothing is being done about it, consider their circulating a petition or campaigning in the neighborhood. If some of the hazards are corrected or eliminated, ask the students to draw new pictures or take new photographs and display them on the bulletin board under the heading "After." Since this project benefits the community, of which the school is a part, the pictures could be put in a front showcase.

Evaluation

LIFESTYLE CONTENT

○ □

Have the class illustrate Things That Harm Us and Things That Help Us. Make a felt board using two pieces of cardboard that are attached on both sides with a masking-tape hinge. Cover one piece of cardboard with red felt and label it "Harmful." Cover the other piece with green felt and label it "Helpful." Have the students display pictures of such things as aspirin, guns, lawn mower, appliances, scissors, a police officer, a stranger with candy, hospital, and have each student select an item and decide

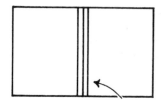

Make hinge by putting
masking tape on both
sides of the cardboard.

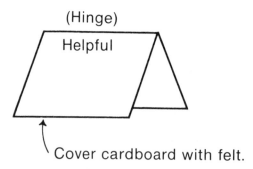

Cover cardboard with felt.

which side of the board she or he thinks it belongs on. Discuss when the object may be helpful and what could make it harmful. Promote a discussion about whether an object or situation can be both.

LIFESTYLE VALUE

○

Using Atlas Figure 44, A Trip Through Safetyland, have the students list all the possible hazards they see and rank them from most dangerous to least dangerous.

○ □

Have the students decide which response they think is best in the following situations and place a 1 by it. Have them rank the other three responses, with 4 being the worst response. The students may write in another best response if they would do something other than what is suggested.

1. If a stranger asks you to get in his or her car, what would you do?
____ a. Go with the stranger.
____ b. Tell the stranger you are not allowed to go for rides with people you do not know.
____ c. Tell the stranger you have to ask your mother first.
____ d. Find a police officer and tell him or her about it.

2. You and your friends are playing in a vacant lot. They see an old refrigerator and want to play in it. What would you do?
____ a. Help them get in it and then shut the door.
____ b. Tell them they should not play in there.
____ c. Play with them.
____ d. Go tell your parents that your friends are playing in an old refrigerator.

3. You are playing in your backyard when a stray dog that is acting strangely comes into the yard. What would you do?
____ a. Go inside immediately and tell your parents.
____ b. Continue playing.
____ c. Go over to the dog and try to pet it.
____ d. Chase the dog out of the yard.

4. You went for a walk and cannot remember your way back home. What would you do?
____ a. Keep walking until you see something familiar.
____ b. Find a police officer and tell him or her that you are lost.
____ c. Sit down on the sidewalk and cry.
____ d. Find a public telephone and call your parents.

UNIT IV: OUTDOOR RECREATIONAL AND SEASONAL SAFETY

Personal safety depends upon a person's ability to adjust to new environments by increasing his or her safety knowledge and skills. The purpose of this unit is to provide knowledge for recreation and seasonal safety. It includes a detailed calendar of safety rules. Like most other health topics, safety should be a year-round habit instead of a two-week lesson. The calendar at the end of the unit is one way of helping the teacher provide continuing emphasis upon safety.

OBJECTIVES

1. Each student will participate in at least one classroom activity for all five of the following areas: sports safety, camping and hiking safety, water safety, winter safety, and farm safety.

2. The students will assemble and display a survival kit that could help them survive if they became lost in the woods.

3. The students will participate in classroom activities and discussion designed to increase their awareness of the special precautions that should accompany special holidays.

4. The students will be able to cite possible safety hazards in activities they enjoy and suggest ways of reducing risks.

MATERIALS

1. Recreation and seasonal safety calendar.

2. Paper, pencil, brown paper sack, scissors, pictures of poisonous plants, snakes, insects, and farm equipment.

3. Metal tin can and lid, cardboard boxes, and glue.

4. Atlas Figure 97, Sport and Activity Word Search puzzle.

Methods

○ □

Sports Safety

Most of the accidents that happen to upper elementary school-age children occur during sports and activities on the playground or in the gym.

Have the students consider and discuss the following questions:

Do you think clothing can affect your safety in a game?

What kinds of words make you think of rough play (shoving, tripping, hitting)?

How should you go about finding a safe area to play in?

What are safety items that give protection in various sports (mouth protectors, padding, knee pads, masks)?

Do you play with children close to your own age and size when participating in active group games?

How can being tired make you more prone to accidents?

What does your school do to help prevent accidents on the playground or in the gym?

○

Display

Have the students create a display showing things that are safe and unsafe to throw.

□

Acrostic

Have the students make safety rule acrostics using the letters of various sports.

Examples are given for the words "soft-ball" and "football."

S—Slide into a base only if you have been taught the correct method of sliding.

O—Only a bat with tape on the handle should be used.

F—Fly balls should be called by the fielder.

T—Throwing the bat is dangerous.

B—Basemen should play near their bases and not in the baselines.

A—Always keep your eyes on the ball.

L—Look for bad pitches.

L—Look for a safe place to play softball.

F—Falling, rolling, and getting up should be practiced.

O—Only when you know you are in safe condition should you return to a game after an injury.

O—Organize a game of touch football away from busy streets.

T—Take time to rest.

B—Be sure you understand the rules of the game.

A—Always keep your head up to brace for the shock of a collision.

L—Look for rocks, broken glass, and other hazards before the game starts.

L—Learn to be alert to the opponent's probable action.

☐

Sport and Activity Search

Make copies of Atlas Figure 97, Sport and Activity Word Search, for each student in your class. See who can find the most sports and activities. Besides having the students circle the words, have them write the words on a piece of paper and compose a safety rule to correspond with each activity.

A perfect score would be to find the following forty-three words: basketball, tennis, baseball, football, sailing, archery, fishing, hockey, lacrosse, croquet, camping, gardening, picnic, skating, darts, hunting, canoeing, skiing, rowing, golf, sledding, hiking, swimming, boxing, jumping, racing, sing, carve, ball, roll, bowling, dance, judo, soccer, biking, slide, carry, climb, fencing, jog, flying, walk, and squash.

☐ ☆

Camping and Hiking Survival Kit

Ask the students if they were going to hike deep in the woods away from all other people and wanted to prepare a survival kit that had to fit in a tin can with a metal lid, what would they take? After listing the items on the chalkboard, have the students assemble such a kit and display it when they play A Day in the Life of a Camper. (Possible items include a single-edge razor blade, matches, soap, string, fishhooks, fishline, pocketknife, disinfectant, adhesive bandages.)

☐ ☆

A Day in the Life of a Camper

Set the room up to resemble a camp scene as much as possible and play A Day in the Life of a Camper. Invite other classes to learn about camping.

Have the students select one of the following groups in which to participate:

1. Camp gear (collect examples of proper clothing—comfortable, sturdy shoes or hiking boots, woolen socks, bright-colored jacket—flashlight, first-aid kit, compass, sleeping bag).

2. Food (demonstrate how to build a safe fire and the proper way to extinguish it; collect samples of typical foods that campers often carry; reconstitute some

dehydrated foods and let other students sample them).

3. Poisonous plants (draw or collect pictures of poisonous plants and demonstrate first aid for accidental contact with poison ivy, poison oak, and poison sumac; research the type and parts of plants that are edible in case a camper becomes lost).*

4. Snake and insect bites (display plastic spiders and other artificial insects in a natural setting to get the attention of the students; live insects may be displayed in a jar with a tight lid; draw or collect pictures of poisonous snakes and insects with correct coloring shown and research the appropriate first aid for accidental bites).

○ □ ☆

Water Safety Survey

Have the students answer the following survey questions:

Do you know how to swim?

Did you ever take swimming lessons from a certified instructor?

Do you swim only in supervised areas?

Do you stay out of deep water if you cannot swim?

Do you always swim with someone you know?

Do you ever swim when you are tired?

---

*Two valuable resource paperback books for the teacher are *Edible Wild Plants—The Complete, Authoritative Guide to Identification and Preparation of North American Edible Wild Plants* by Oliver Perry Medsger (Collier Books, 1966) and *Green Medicine—One Woman's Dramatic Story of the Search for Plants That Heal!* by Margaret B. Kreig (Bantam Books, 1964). *Color Treasury of Herbs and Other Medicinal Plants* by Crescent Books has beautiful photographs by Mirella Bavestrelli and could be included on a browsing table for the students to look through.

Do you ever pretend that you are drowning and call for help?

Do you ever push or shove other children in the water?

Do you dive only in deep water?

Do you know how to give mouth-to-mouth artificial respiration?

○ □

Swimming Hazards

Have the students draw a picture or construct a model of an unsafe place to swim and label the hazards (e.g., deep quarry, no lifeguard, sharp rocks, no chlorine in the water).

□

Have the students pantomime the correct and incorrect ways to get in and out of boats using several cardboard boxes as play boats.

□

Speaker

Invite someone from the Red Cross to explain to the class what to do if one is in a small boat that overturns. The speaker will tell the students not to swim to shore but cling to the side of the boat if it is still floating. Have the speaker teach the right way to right an overturned boat.

□ ☆

Demonstrate how to rescue a person who falls overboard from a boat.

□ ☆

Winter Safety Decision Making

Ask students what they would do in the following situations.

1. After playing outside for a long time, Timmy discovers that his hands are very cold and his skin is grayish-yellow, a symptom of frostbite. (Cover the frost-

bitten area with your warm hand. Do not rub the frostbitten area, since this increases risk of injury to the tissues. Get Timmy indoors and soak his hands in lukewarm water. Wrap him in warm blankets and give him a cup of warm cocoa.)

2. As you are skating on a frozen pond you hear your friend Susan screaming for help and see that she has fallen through some thin ice. (Do not start running towards her. Get a ladder or board and attach a rope to it. Push the board along the ice to her. When she gets hold of the board use the rope to pull her out. If no board or rope is available, have several people lie on the ice, each holding the feet of the person in front of her or him. The first person has her or his hands free to pull Susan out. Wrap Susan in warm blankets and give her something warm to drink. If Susan has stopped breathing, administer mouth-to-mouth artificial respiration while waiting for help to arrive.)

Value Situations

Ask the students what they would do in the following situations.

1. A group of your friends decide to throw snowballs at passing cars.
2. Your friend asks you to go sledding down a steep backcountry road that hardly ever has a car pass on it.

□

Matching

Have the students match the protective equipment with the activity described. Remind the class that more than one answer may apply.*

*From the 1975–1976 Traffic Safety Guide for Teachers. Grades 4–6, courtesy of the American Automobile Association.

1) Snow shoes
2) Umbrella
3) Bright-colored clothing
4) Rough-heeled boots
5) Warm coat
6) Raincoat
7) Rubber boots
8) Gloves
9) Water-repellant clothing

____ Walking to school in the snow
____ Riding a bicycle in rain
____ Winter hiking in northern woods
____ Sledding
____ Ice-skating
____ Playing in the snow
____ Walking in the fog
____ Skiing

Initiate a class discussion of reasons why the proper equipment is needed for each activity.

○ □

Farm Safety Mural

Have the students make a large mural of a farm and include representations of possible hazards such as tools, machinery, poisonous sprays and other chemicals, irrigation ditches, silos, and farm animals.

○ □

Have a class discussion after constructing the mural, and invite a farmer to speak to the class about special precautions that must be taken when living on a farm. If possible, arrange a field trip to a nearby farm.

HOLIDAY PRECAUTIONS

Special safety precautions are needed for holidays. The following information appeared in the 1974–1975 Traffic Safety Guide for Teachers.*

○ □

"Discuss the origin of Halloween with your students. Explain to them that the word Hal-

*For grades K–3, courtesy of the American Automobile Association.

loween means 'Hallow' or Holy Evening. This was a celebration where people became more aware of each other's needs. Rather than threatening people with 'Trick or Treat,' they kept a good spirit by saying 'Help the poor.' The object of the Halloween costume is that many people wanted to go unnoticed, so they dressed in 'costumes' different from their everyday clothes and distributed food, clothes, and money to the poor."

○

"To illustrate the fact that masks over the face cut off needed vision, you will need a brown paper bag large enough to cover the head and a pair of scissors. Take the bag and cut holes in it for the eyes. Select a student to stand at the front of the room and place the bag over his head. Now have him/her close one eye and count how many of his classmates he sees through the slit in the bag. Repeat the procedure with several students. If you cut off vision, you will not see all the problems of traffic. By not wearing a mask, you will be more aware by seeing everything going on around you, including approaching traffic. You can still be in costume by wearing face make-up."

CHRISTMAS SAFETY

It was the night before Christmas,
And all through the house,
There were dangers lurking,
And a fire to douse . . .

Ask the students to identify at least five possible causes of fires that occur during the Christmas season.

□ ☆

Dramatic Play

Have the students create an original play designed to make them aware of some of the possible dangers (physical, as well as psychological) associated with various types of toys.

○ □

Analyze Toys

Have the students bring various toys to school and see if they can discover any defects and hazards in them.

□ ☆

Analyze Advertising

Help the students tape record advertisements and analyze the claims made by toy manufacturers about their products. Also have them review claims in magazine advertising or on the product itself. Ask students if they think safety is already built into most toys or if they would be willing to pay extra for exceptional safety in a toy.

○ □

Bulletin Board

Create bulletin boards around recreation and seasonal safety. (Refer to the Recreation and Seasonal Safety Calendar, Figure 14B-4, for ideas.)

Evaluation

LIFESTYLE CONTENT

○ □ ☆

Recreational Safety Worksheet

Ask the students to make three columns on a sheet of paper. The first column should be headed "My Favorite Sports and Activities," the second column should be headed "Possible Danger," the third column should be headed "How I Can Help Protect Myself." After the sheet has been filled in by each student, discuss their answers with the class.

LIFESTYLE VALUE

○

Have students rank-order the following statements, giving the most important a 1.

FIGURE 14B-4 Recreation and seasonal safety calendar

September	October	November	December	January

1. *Pedestrian Safety*
  a. Safest way to school
  b. Traffic signs
  c. Safety patrol
2. *Bus Safety*
  a. Safety rules
  b. Bus operation
  c. Bus patrol
3. *Bicycle Safety*
  a. Bicycle rules
  b. Bicycle maintenance
  c. Bicycle skills
	1. *Fire Safety*
	  a. Extinguishing small fires
	  b. Fire escape plan
	  c. Reporting a fire
	2. *Halloween Safety*
	  a. Safe costumes
	  b. Stay with friends
	  c. Make-up instead of masks
	3. *Community Safety*
	  a. Dangerous areas
	  b. Beware of strangers
	  c. Community help
		1. *Home Safety*
		  a. Household medicines
		  b. Electrical tools and appliances
		  c. Falls
		2. *Frostbite*
		  a. Prevention
		  b. Symptoms
		  c. First-aid
		3. *Hunting*
		  a. Bright clothing
		  b. Safe gun handling
		  c. Gun and ammunition storage
			1. *Christmas Safety*
			  a. Christmas tree
			  b. Inspect lights
			  c. Clean up wrappings
			2. *Safe Toys*
			  a. Safe construction
			  b. Lead paint/toxic chemicals
			  c. Safety features
			3. *Winter Games*
			  a. Proper clothing
			  b. Snowball throwing
			  c. Skating
				1. *Safety Resolutions*
				  a. Know and practice safety
				  b. Decision making
				  c. Attitude and self-control
				2. *Basketball*
				  a. Proper warm-up
				  b. Avoid elbowing and rough play
				  c. Proper shoes
				3. *School Safety*
				  a. Halls and stairs
				  b. Gymnasium and playground
				  c. Classrooms

February	March	April	May	June

1. *First-Aid*
  a. Emergency care
  b. Home treatment
  c. Obtaining help
2. *Sledding*
  a. Good sportsmanship
  b. Watch for obstacles
  c. Stay off roads
3. *Hockey*
  a. Safe ice
  b. Good sportsmanship
  c. Proper equipment
	1. *Dress for Irregular Weather*
	  a. Proper clothing
	  b. Umbrella safety
	  c. Remove wet clothing
	2. *Dangerous Ice*
	  a. Safe walking
	  b. Prevention—ice removal
	  c. Safe rescue
	3. *Kite Flying*
	  a. Location
	  b. Weather
	  c. Power lines
		1. *Eye Safety*
		  a. Sharp objects
		  b. Chemicals
		  c. Eye protection
		2. *Yard Safety*
		  a. Insecticides
		  b. Outdoor grill
		  c. Outdoor power tools
		3. *Weather Safety*
		  a. Electrical storms
		  b. Tornadoes
		  c. Hurricanes
			1. *Swimming*
			  a. Learn how to swim
			  b. Swim with a friend
			  c. Supervised area
			2. *Water Safety*
			  a. Boating
			  b. Wear life preserver
			  c. Polluted water
			3. *Water Accidents*
			  a. Overturned boat
			  b. Person drowning
			  c. Artificial respiration
				1. *Sun Safety*
				  a. Prevention
				  b. Over-exposure
				  c. First-aid
				2. *Camping/Hiking*
				  a. Poison plants
				  b. Insect and snake bites
				  c. Proper clothing and equipment
				3. *Animal Danger*
				  a. Domestic animals
				  b. Farm animals
				  c. Wild animals

What do you feel is most important when choosing a place to play?

____ Playing away from traffic.

____ Not playing in driveways or alleys.

____ Playing at home.

____ Having a neighborhood park to play in.

How would you most like to spend Halloween?

____ Have a Halloween party at school.

____ Have a Halloween parade with prizes for the best costume.

____ Go Trick or Treating for candy in the neighborhood.

____ Help collect money for UNICEF.

UNIT V: FIRST AID

Encourage students to value first-aid training for how it can help themselves, their families, and other people. Through first-aid training and the following activities, students will increase their safety consciousness as well.

OBJECTIVES

1. The students will discuss various situations where first aid is needed and learn how to respond through use of the Jack and the Beanstalk bulletin board, To Tell the Truth in First Aid game, and acrostics.

2. After seeing the puppet show and posters, the students will demonstrate first aid for minor injuries on each other.

3. The student will be able to identify the four emergency situations in which first aid is urgently needed. The younger student will tell how to get help. The older student will demonstrate proper first aid for stoppage of breathing, severe bleeding, poisoning, and shock.

4. With the help of an adult, the student will conduct a medicine chest sur-vey in her or his own home using the list of basic essentials and nonessentials that has been handed out in class.

MATERIALS

1. Construction paper, scissors, paste, index cards, first-aid books or pamphlets.

2. Puppets, poster board, cardboard box (for puppet theater), washcloth, soap and water, antiseptic, and adhesive bandages.

3. Atlas Figure 98, Medicine Cabinet Checklist.

Methods

☐

Bulletin Board

Construct a bulletin board around the theme of Jack and the Beanstalk. Using construction paper, cut out a brown beanstalk and leaves of different colors (yellow, red, green, orange, blue, and purple). On the front of the yellow leaves print situations leading to burns. On the back of the leaf print the appropriate first aid that should be given. Do the same for red leaves (wounds), green leaves (shock), orange leaves (poisoning), blue leaves (stoppage of breathing), and purple leaves (other situations).

A situation on the yellow leaf might read, "Jack was chopping wood and lost track of the time that he spent under the hot sun. The next day he had blisters on his arms and a headache. What should he do?"

There should also be cutouts of a house, Jack chopping wood, a cow in a fenced pasture, the giant's castle, and clouds that serve as stepping stones connecting the top of the beanstalk with the castle. Jack's house could also represent a hospital, and the students would have to decide if the injury were serious enough to require treatment in a hospital.

Each day, pluck a leaf from the beanstalk and read the description of the accident to the students. Let them suggest what should be done for the injury. After giving them time for discussion, turn the leaf over and discuss the correct treatment. Conclude each mini-lesson with a short story in which Jack, a member of his family, or the giant is the main character. Describe an accident and let the students finish telling or writing the story. (Who came to the rescue? What kind of first aid was given? Why?)

Possible story ideas could include the giant's falling off the beanstalk and breaking his leg or cutting himself on sharp rocks when he landed.

☐ ☆

To Tell the Truth

By adapting the television program "To Tell the Truth," older elementary students can develop their research and speaking skills. For a class of thirty students you will need thirty index cards. Make fifteen word or phrase cards by writing one word or phrase per card. Decide on five situations that you want the students to research and write each one situation on three cards. For example, you may want to make up three sets of cards about epileptic seizure, insulin reaction, poisoning, wounds, and burns. Make fifteen letter cards by writing each letter (A, B, C, D, E) on three cards.

Let each student draw a card. Have the class form groups, with students with the same situation in one group and students with the same letter in another group. The students with situation cards should research their topic by looking through their class notes, health book, health

pamphlets, etc. They will be the contestants who will be questioned by the class. As in the television program, only one student will tell the truth. The other students will try to fool the class. Let the students in each group decide who will tell the truth. The students with letters on their cards will be told which group they will be questioning so that they can also research the topic. Each of the three members in the group will be permitted to ask two questions in an attempt to discover which person is telling the truth.

When the first group is called (e.g., epileptic seizure), the students should file into the classroom and be numbered Contestant No. 1, Contestant No. 2, and Contestant No. 3. Before sitting down, each person should say, "I have epileptic seizures."

The first panel will take turns asking the questions they have prepared. When they are finished, ask them to mark their ballots for Contestant No. 1, 2, or 3. Before their answers are shown, encourage the rest of the class to vote just from listening to the questions and answers given by others in the class. Follow the class vote with the panel vote and have the "real" person stand up.

If this game is played again with other words, switch panelists and contestants and see that the students work with different people each time.

☐ ☆

Acrostics

Students enjoy learning through acrostics. Use the following examples during class discussion or have the students make up some of their own.

Types of Wounds

P—Puncture (produced by a pointed

object that pierces the skin)

A—Abrasion (caused by rubbing or scraping the skin—floor burn)

I—Incision (a sharp cut, such as from knife or broken glass)

L—Laceration (jagged or irregular wound—often much tissue damage)

(PAIL—to carry soap and water in to cleanse the wound. Avulsions are another type of wound. They result when tissue is forcibly separated or torn from the body and usually occur with incised or lacerated wounds. Wounds are subject to infection, which means that germs are multiplying and destroying the tissue about them. Because germs need time to grow and multiply, evidence of infection usually appears from two to seven days after the injury.)

Signs of Infection

H—Heat (area feels warm)

A—Absence of motion (because it hurts to move the affected area)

R—Redness (also red streaks which may extend from the wound up the arm or leg and indicate infection is spreading)

P—Pain (and sometimes pus, which is an accumulation of white blood cells, germs, and tissue debris)

S—Swelling

(HARPS may be what you hear if you do not take adequate care. Wash hands thoroughly with soap and water. Cleanse the injury thoroughly and dry with a sterile dressing. Apply a bandage. See a doctor promptly if evidence of infection appears.)

Ways to Remember the Four Medical Emergencies

A—Asphyxiation (lack of oxygen)

B—Bleeding (severe)

C—Chemical poisoning

S—Shock

(ABC'S of first aid.)

H—Hemorrhage (severe bleeding)

O—Oxygen (lack of)

P—Poisoning

S—Shock

(Illustrated with a rabbit called HOPS.)

Signs of Fractures or Broken Bones

H—hear the snap

O—out of place (evidence of deformity)

S—swelling (requires some time to develop)

P—pain on motion

I—inside grating

T—tenderness

A—absence of motion (because it hurts to move the affected part)

L—local discoloration (because of ruptured blood vessels)

(HOSPITAL—your destination if symptoms of fracture are present. Keep the broken ends quiet, as well as the adjacent joints. First aid for shock may be needed. Control hemorrhage by direct pressure. Do not push a protruding bone back. Place ice bag over painful area to reduce swelling and pain.)

○ □

Burns

Have the students collect pictures of things that can result in burns. Divide a bulletin board into three sections and mount the pictures under the type of burn that may result (thermal—caused by fire or high temperature, sunburn—

caused by ultraviolet rays, chemical—caused by an acid or alkali).

□ ☆

Poetry

Ask the students to compose a poem that includes some first-aid instructions, using a current first-aid manual as a reference. The following anonymous poem has been used in several first-aid courses.

> Get him free and lay him down,
> Look him over, from sole to crown.
> Check for bleeding, breathing quick,
> Keep him warm with covers thick.
> Call a doctor, tell him all,
> If unconscious, no drink at all.
> Refuse advice to let him up,
> Care for every bruise and cut.
> Get a ride—this is alright,
> Tell his people of his plight.

○

Puppet Show

Divide the students into small groups and have them each make a puppet and help create a short puppet show. Each puppet show should contain simple first-aid pointers. For example, using a boy puppet, Steve Scratch, and a girl puppet, Betsy Bandage, the proper first aid for treating a scratch could be performed.

□

Posters

Ask the students to draw posters that help explain proper first-aid techniques. The students should be prepared to answer questions from the rest of the class after their presentation has been completed.

○ □ ☆

Medicine Cabinet Checklist

Make copies of the Medicine Cabinet Checklist Atlas Figure 98 for the students to complete at home with the help of an adult.

Evaluation

LIFESTYLE CONTENT

□ ☆

The Jack and the Beanstalk bulletin board described earlier may be used for review and to evaluate the responses of individual students.

Students may study and quiz themselves independently with the set of four very inexpensive books, *Basic First Aid* by the American National Red Cross. The books are used in the ARC basic first aid program for students up to age thirteen and provide first aid instruction for stoppage of breathing, severe bleeding, poisoning, shock, and less serious conditions.

LIFESTYLE VALUE

□ ☆

Have the students write a short essay entitled, "What First Aid Means to Me."

REFERENCES FOR FIRST AID AND SAFETY

Write to Consumer Services, Johnson and Johnson, Health Care Division, 501 George Street, New Brunswick, NJ 08903, for their booklet, *First Aid for Little People*. More advanced first-aid literature is also available.

Contact your local chapter of the American Red Cross for additional information concerning the following programs:

Basic First Aid. No minimum age requirement. Resources include basic first aid textbooks (set of 4).

Safety and First-Aid Multimedia. Must be at least thirteen years old or have completed the seventh grade. Resources include multimedia workbooks and standard first aid and personal safety textbook. This course was originally developed at American Telephone and Telegraph Company as a means of effectively training people in first-aid skills in a short period of time. The program usually consists of one 8-hour session or two 4-hour sessions.

Standard First Aid and Personal Safety. Must be at least thirteen years old or have completed the seventh grade. Resources include the standard first aid and personal safety textbook.

Courses in CPR, Canoeing, Rowing, Outboard Boating, Sailing, Lifesaving, and Water Safety are also available.

Write the following organizations for their literature:

American Association of Poison Control Center, c/o Academy of Medicine of Cleveland, 10525 Carnegie Avenue, Cleveland, OH 44106.

National Recreation Association, 8 West 8th Street, New York, NY 10011.

National Safety Council, 444 North Michigan Avenue, Chicago, IL 60611.

National Society to Prevent Blindness, 79 Madison Avenue, New York, NY 10016.

Aetna Life Affiliated Companies, Education Department, 151 Farmington Avenue, Hartford, CT 06115.

American Automobile Association, Traffic Engineering and Safety Department, Falls Church, VA 22040 (pamphlets and films on traffic safety, safety project materials).

American Insurance Association, Safety Department, 85 John Street, New York, NY 10038.

Bicycle Manufacturers Association of America, 1101 15th Street N.W., Washington, D.C. 20005.

Ford Motor Company, Information Department, Dearborn, MI 48127 (traffic safety).

National Fire Protection Association, Public Relations Department, 60 Batterymarch Street, Boston, MA 02110 (posters, pamphlets, comics, charts, and quizzes).

CHAPTER 15

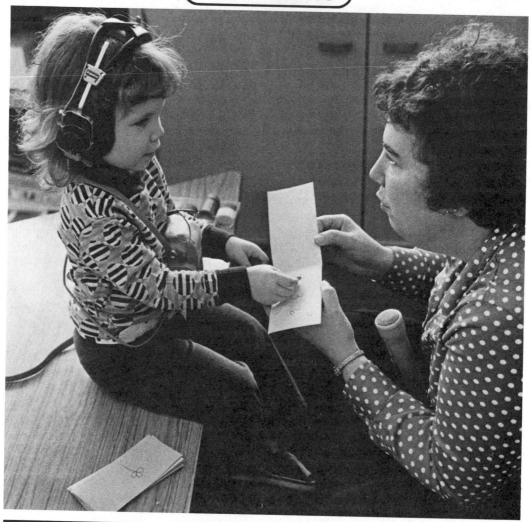

PART A: CONSUMER HEALTH

The importance of individual responsibility for human health is nowhere so evident as in the area of consumer health. Here people are faced with a large number of alternative products and services which may play a role in their future health. The food people eat needs to be safe and nutritious; the drinking water needs to be pure. People need to know how to select competent physicians, whether the drugs and cosmetics they are using are effective and safe, and whether the toys and games they select are safe. These needs are all relevant to the selection of a healthy, happy lifestyle.

Many people assume that all products on the market today are effective or at least safe; otherwise they would not be available. Unfortunately, this assumption is incorrect. As a result, everyone has the responsibility of selecting wisely. A number of government agencies on both the local and federal level help to protect the consumer, but these agencies are overworked and understaffed and thus are unable to monitor the thousands and thousands of new products that are coming out or are already available. Consequently, today's consumer needs to be informed and alert in order to sift through the volumes of information about the products she or he buys.

The chapter on consumer health is lengthy because of a long list of consumer products that require comment. It is intended as a resource chapter, and no attempt should be made to communicate all of the information to elementary students. However, when questions arise, this chapter can serve as an important source of information.*

FEDERAL LAWS

The Fair Packaging and Labeling Act, passed in 1966, requires the net contents of a package and the address of the manufacturer to appear on the product's label. While many products also require a listing of ingredients in order of decreasing weight, the consumer can still be misled. Some categories of foods, such as

*The authors are indebted to David Corbin for his help with this chapter.

soft drinks, ice cream, and many cheeses, are exempted from a listing of ingredients. They must, however, conform to certain standards.

Labels that require net weight may be misleading. Although two cans of the same product may weigh the same, one may contain a high percentage of water while the other contains a high percentage of the product. At the same price, one product is actually a better buy.

The consumer faces another difficulty when making comparisons to select the best alternative or product. Since most products come in several different size containers, it is difficult to approximate the unit price, especially when dealing with fractions of ounces.

Meats

In 1967, the Wholesome Meat Act was passed requiring all states to have their meat inspected by either state or federal officials from the U.S. Department of Agriculture and meet minimum standards in the sanitary condition of meat products. Although it has limitations, the law has been helpful. Standards have not as yet been established for honesty, refrigeration temperatures, or minimum grading procedures, however.

Currently, beef is graded U.S. Choice, U.S. Good, or U.S. Standard. In February 1976, the standards were lowered to the delight of the cattle raisers and the disdain of the consumer. Beef grading is based on the taste of the meat rather than on its nutritional value. The more expensive cuts and grades of beef generally have more fat or marbling and less protein per pound. Pork is usually not graded because all pork cuts are considered tender.

Milk Products

Grade A milk has a lower bacteria count than Grade B, but such voluntary grading is not related to milk's nutritional value. Pasteurization is a process which kills the bacteria in milk. Homogenization breaks up fat globules in milk in order to distribute them throughout.

Cheese may be labeled "Quality Approved" on a voluntary basis, but only American cheddar is graded by quality words and points—Extra Fancy (95+), Fancy (92–94), No. 1 (89–91), No. 2 (86–88), No. 3 (83–85) and culls (below 83). "U.S." must appear on the label if the cheese has been federally inspected.

Eggs

Eggs are graded by quality and size. Grades are AA, A, and B. Once again, the grading is not related to the nutritional value of the egg. Although the yolks of grade AA eggs may look better than those of grade A eggs, their nutritional value is the same. Eggs vary in size from jumbo (about 30 ounces per dozen) to small or pullet (at least 18 ounces per dozen). The color of the eggshell is not related to the nutritional value of the egg.

Pesticides

The USDA tests pesticides to decide what is safe for human consumption and has set the residue level at 100 times lower than the known minimum danger levels for humans. Nevertheless, many consumers believe that foods grown without the use of pesticides are more wholesome. As a result, they are willing to pay much more for them.

It is difficult to tell if a product has been grown without the use of pesticides, and no federal or state laws exist that set standards as to what constitutes organic or natural. The seller decides this.

Although there are biological programs to control insects and pests (e.g., sterilizing them), modern technology is still dependent upon the use of pesticides. Efforts have been made to control the use of hard pesticides such as DDT which do not break down into inert materials. Much research concerning the cumulative effects of DDT in the body is being conducted, and there appears to be a link between DDT buildup and cancer.

In February 1976, the Environmental Protection Agency (EPA) banned the production of most pesticides containing mercury because of its link to a nervous system disorder.

Since soft pesticides are biodegradable (capable of decaying and being absorbed by the environment) and do little harm to the environment, farmers are now encouraged to substitute soft pesticides for hard pesticides. Pesticides should be used very carefully and only when necessary. Certain pesticides have specific functions and need as careful consideration as that given by a doctor when prescribing a drug for a specific disease.

Sweeteners

The Delaney Clause is a law which prohibits the use of any cancer-causing additives. In 1969, the artificial sweetener cyclamate was banned because it caused cancer in rats. In 1976, after reviewing the evidence, the Food and Drug Administration (FDA) ruled to continue the ban, although existing products containing cyclamates were allowed to be sold over the following two years. Recently this ban was appealed, but the ruling was upheld.

In 1977, a proposal by the FDA to ban saccharin touched off great controversy in the United States that is a good example of the difficulty that surrounds the regulation of food products. The authors recommend "The Saccharin Ban" by Wayne L. Pines and Nancy Glick in the *FDA Consumer* (May 1977) for an important discussion of this topic.

DES and Red Dye No. 2

Another controversial substance banned by the FDA was diethylstilbestrol (DES), a substance used to fatten cattle just before slaughtering. DES is suspected to be a carcinogen. However, it is still used as the morning-after pill and, if taken under the supervision of a physician, is effective in preventing pregnancy.

Red Dye No. 2 is a food coloring additive that was banned in January 1976 by the FDA because of its relationship to cancer in laboratory rats. The purpose of food coloring in most instances is to make food look more attractive and appetizing.

Food Additives

The Food Additive Amendment requires that new chemical additives be tested and considered safe before they are put on the market. The FDA continually monitors additives on its Generally Recognized as Safe (GRAS) list. Since it is almost impossible to eliminate all undesirable substances from food products, the FDA has published, under consumer organization pressure, the legal limits of foreign substances allowable in specific foods. For instance, the maximum filth

allowance for chocolate is 150 insect fragments and four rat hairs per half pound. The filth allowance for peanut butter permits an average of 225 insect fragments or nine rodent hairs per pound. Consumers can find out the filth limits of other foods by contacting the FDA.

Some of the following additives in food today are being questioned as to their safety and their necessity.

Diethylpyro-carbonate (DEP) is used to preserve the freshness of soft drinks and inhibit fermentation in noncarbonated wines. DEP in combination with certain foods results in the formation of urethan, which is a carcinogen.

Sodium nitrite is used to preserve cured meats and give them a reddish color. When combined with some compounds in foods, it can develop into nitrosamine compound, which is cancer causing. Sodium nitrate is used for the same reasons as sodium nitrite, and the action of bacteria upon sodium nitrate is thought to convert it to sodium nitrite, affording it the same dangers.

Monosodium glutamate (MSG) is a flavor enhancer that is widely used in meat tenderizers and other foods. Since MSG has caused brain lesions and destroyed brain cells in infant laboratory animals, it has been voluntarily taken out of baby foods. Although some studies claim no side effects with the use of MSG, other studies claim the possibilities listed above as well as MSG headaches in adult human beings. These headaches often occur during or after one eats Chinese food, since this type of cuisine often contains large amounts of MSG.

In addition to the commercial addition of food additives, certain chemicals find their way into foods in the environment. Toxic levels of mercury, for example, have been found in some fish, especially swordfish. Metals such as mercury are not excreted from the body. Thus, small amounts eaten are accumulative and can cause crippling. In 1970, the FDA recalled from the market 12.5 million cans of tuna which were thought to contain too much mercury. In addition, fishing in or near industrial waterways where heavy metals may accumulate seems to be contraindicated.

GENERAL NUTRITION

Vitamins

Millions of Americans take vitamin pills every day. However, most nutritionists recommend a well-balanced diet in preference to vitamin supplements. Vitamin pills supply no dietary fiber and become ineffective with age. They can also be harmful if not taken as prescribed.

Many companies have added vitamins, minerals, and other nutrients to their foods to attract consumers. Fortified cereals, for example, are actually candy with vitamins and minerals added. It is not uncommon for a cereal to contain 30 to 50 percent sugar.

Companies argue that at least the consumer is getting some nutrition from the fortification that he or she probably would not otherwise get. Nutritionists argue that this practice only helps to foster bad eating habits and encourages obesity.

Michael G. Jacobson of the Center for Science in the Public Interest compared the prices of two equivalent cereals, one of which had been fortified. He found that the unfortified cereal cost 18 cents less per box. Further investigation revealed, however, that the fortification process cost only 0.6 cents per box. Thus, there was a 3,000 percent markup as-

sociated with the fortification process. While this practice is questionable, what nutritionists find even more disturbing is the excessive amounts of sugar and salt that are added to many of our foods.

Sugar and Salt

Sugar contains many calories and is not a source of nutrition. Some research indicates that it may contribute to cancer and play a role in cardiovascular disease. For these reasons, it is best to examine one's lifestyle and to cut down on sugar whenever possible. This means recognizing sugar in its different forms—dextrose, glucose, corn syrup, foods packed in heavy syrup. Sugar can be eliminated or reduced in most recipes; fruits and vegetables can be substituted for between-meal snacks which contain sugar; and fruit juice may be substituted for soft drinks.

Salt is added to almost all processed foods. Although salt is a necessary nutrient, the average American eats it in levels far above the necessary limits. Jean Mayer, the noted Harvard nutritionist, has stated that the average adult needs only a quarter teaspoon of salt per day. A bag of salted potato chips probably contains this amount.

Hypertensive patients are routinely asked to limit their salt intake, although it is still not clear whether salt restrictions on persons with normal blood pressure would yield beneficial results.

Salt tablets are generally of no value unless a person has been exercising vigorously for several hours; even then, the addition of salt to foods should be adequate for this purpose. It is probably best to cut down on highly salted foods such as pretzels, saltines, corn chips, and potato chips. Meat products contain enough salt without adding more.

The Role of the Consumer

By insisting on a label that contains a complete listing of ingredients, many people who are allergic to certain foodstuffs would be able to avoid foods which bother or harm them. It would be a great help to consumers if the percentages of each ingredient were also listed on the package. A customer seeing that a certain cereal is 55 percent sugar might think twice about buying it. A consumer with complaints about a certain food can write to the manufacturer and to a consumer organization or even to the FDA.

Many current standards regarding labels are confusing to the consumer. The wise consumer needs to learn present specifications. Many consumers think that fruit juice and fruit drink are synonymous. Yet specifications vary. Orange juice is 100 percent orange juice, orange drink blend has 70 to 95 percent orange juice; orange juice drink has from 35 to 70 percent orange juice, orange drink has from 10 to 35 percent orange juice; and orange-flavored drink has less than 10 percent orange juice.

Products which list the net dry weight would indicate to the consumer the cost of the product and not of the water packed with that product.

Junk food advertisements on children's TV programs and ads that misrepresent foods as being nutritious or packed with energy are of concern to many parents. Many consumers' groups are fighting for the removal of this type of advertising. It is especially important to remember that good eating habits begin at young ages and that children need to learn how to be good consumers.

Another practice helpful to the consumer is open dating. Some states require the manufacturer to supply easily readable dates on perishable items so that consumers know they are getting fresh products.

Tips on Shopping for Groceries

Before shopping, one should write a list of the things one needs. A consumer must not let bright displays and specials coax him or her into buying something that is really not necessary. In essence, one should not deviate from the shopping list.

Another tip is to be familiar with the layout of the store. Hundreds of thousands of dollars are spent by supermarkets to learn where and how to place items that attract customers. Specials should be checked to see if they are really a bargain. Higher priced items are usually placed at eye level, while the less expensive ones are placed on the bottom shelves.

Shopping less frequently saves gas and reduces chances for impulse buying. It is also best not to shop on an empty stomach, since consumers tend to buy more items when they are hungry.

Consumers tend to buy many unneeded items if they are sold on the value of coupons. It is best to look at the grocery list and see if any of the coupons can be used rather than to make a grocery list based on coupons.

Trading stamps are paid for by the consumer. Although gift items are received for the trading stamps, the consumer has been making installment payments on that gift by paying higher prices for products.

When buying a dated product, consumers should check to see that they are getting the freshest product possible by purchasing the one with the latest date.

In most cases, store brands are the best

buy for the money. Recent studies indicate that when consumers are asked to compare name brands with store brands they could not tell the difference. In addition to buying store brands, consumers should check the unit pricing listed on the shelf so that they can compare the price per unit of weight. In general, larger sizes are the most economical, and it is wise to purchase the larger quantity if the product will be used before it can spoil.

The label on an item can be helpful in making a wise purchase. The ingredients are listed in order of predominance in a package. If sugar is listed first, there is more sugar than anything else in the package.

The net weight should be checked to avoid purchasing a deceptively sized container. If fruits or vegetables are sold by the piece, it is best to weigh them and take the heaviest.

The nutritional value of foods is usually listed. A food with no nutritional value is an unwise buy. If no ingredients are listed, the food makes no claim for being nutritious.

It is much less expensive to buy protein foods such as fish, poultry, and cheeses. Beans, rice, and grains with cheese and eggs are also high quality sources of protein for less money. Meats such as hot dogs, bologna, bacon, and sausage have very little protein, are high in fat, and contain nitrates and nitrites.

There are other ways to cut food bills. Sugar is very expensive and, as indicated previously, has no nutritional value. By substituting yogurt for sour cream, consumers will save money and calories. Dry milk can be substituted for whole milk, especially in cooking where the difference in taste is not noticed. Margarine can be substituted for butter, frozen orange juice for orange drinks. Grade B

medium eggs are a good buy. Fruits and vegetables are priced lowest when in season; for example, apples taste best and cost less in the fall.

Except for canned fruits and vegetables, which cost more whole than cut up, it is best for consumers to do the cutting themselves. For example, grated cheese costs much more per pound than a wedge of cheese. One can save money by making his or her own bread crumbs and avoiding so-called convenience foods.

A consumer can conserve nutrients by salting meat only *after* it is cooked (early salting draws out the juices and nutrients) and not thawing poultry under running water, which washes away nutrients. Soaking and overcooking foods which contain water soluble vitamins causes a loss of these vitamins. Rinsing rice and pasta washes away many of the vitamins and minerals.

Proper knowledge of how to store and preserve foods will save money as well as help to prevent the foods from losing their nutrients. Exposure of eggs to air affects their protein (eggs should be stored in the carton), and exposure of milk to light reduces riboflavin. (See "A Storage Chart for Pantry Foods," Table 15A-1, reprinted from *Good Housekeeping*.)

Tips on Food Care

Frozen foods should be packaged in insulated bags.

Frozen foods stacked above the freeze line on the store's freezer are not a good purchase, since they may be spoiled.

Potato chips cost almost four times as much per pound as raw potatoes; products with boiling pouches cost more in general than equivalent products.

In summary, the wise consumer can select a shopping style at the grocery store than can save money as well as pro-

TABLE 15A-1 A STORAGE CHART FOR PANTRY FOODS

Suggestions: Store food in coldest cabinets, not over range or by refrigerator's exhaust. Use coolest spots (the cellar, etc.) for storing potatoes, onions, etc., and for long-term storage of canned foods. When buying, choose freshest looking packages. Do not buy cans with swollen ends. Dented cans may be purchased if there is no leakage, ends do not bulge. Most staples and canned foods will keep indefinitely, but flavors will fade and textures wilt; buy only what you expect to use in the recommended storage times, below. Date foods; use oldest items first.

Food	Time	Special Handling
STAPLES		
Baking powder, soda	18 months	Keep covered and dry.
Bouillon cubes, envelopes	1 year	Keep covered and dry.
Chocolate, semi-sweet	1 year	Keep cool.
unsweetened	1 year	Keep cool.
Coffee, cans (unopened)	1 year	Refrigerate after opening.
Coffee, instant (opened)	2 weeks	Keep lid tightly closed.
(unopened)	6 months	Keep lid tightly closed.
Coffee lighteners (dry) (opened)	6 months	Put in airtight container.
Flour (all types)	1 year	Keep in original packets.
Gelatin (all types)	18 months	
Honey, jams, syrups	1 year	Keep tightly covered.
Macaroni	1 year	Keep tightly closed.
Molasses	2 years+	Keep tightly covered.
Noodles	6 months	Keep tightly closed.
Rice, white	2 years+	Keep tightly closed.
Salad dressing (all types)	3 months	Refrigerate after opening.
Salad oils	1-3 months	

Food	Time	Special Handling
CANNED AND DRIED FOODS		
Fruits, canned	1 year	Keep in cool spot.
dried	6 months	Put in airtight container.
Gravies	1 year	
Meat, fish, poultry	1 year	Refrigerate after opening.
Milk, canned, sweetened, condensed and evaporated	1 year	
nonfat dry	6 months	Put in airtight container.
Pickles, olives	1 year	Refrigerate after opening.
Soups	1 year	Keep cool.
Vegetables	1 year	Keep cool.

TABLE 15A-1 *Continued*

Food	Time	Special Handling
Shortening, solid	8 months	Refrigeration not needed.
Spaghetti	1 year	Keep tightly closed.
Sugar, brown	4 months	Put in airtight container.
confectioners'	4 months	Put in airtight container.
granulated	2 years+	Keep tightly covered.
Tea, bags	6 months	Put in airtight container.
instant	1 year	Keep tightly covered.
loose	6 months	Put in airtight container.

MIXES AND PACKAGED FOODS

Food	Time	Special Handling
Bread crumbs, dried	6 months	Keep covered and dry.
Cake mixes	1 year	Keep cool and dry.
Cakes, prepared	1-2 days	If butter-cream, whipped-cream or custard frostings, fillings, refrigerate.
Casserole mixes	18 months	Keep cool and dry.
Cereals, ready-to-eat	check date on package	
ready-to-cook	6 months	Keep covered and dry.
Cookies, packaged	4 months	Keep box tightly closed.
Crackers	3 months	Keep box tightly closed.

HERBS, SPICES AND CONDIMENTS

Food	Time	Special Handling
Catchup, chili sauce (opened)	1 month	
Herbs and spices whole spices	1 year	Keep in airtight containers away from sunlight. At times listed, check aroma; when it fades, replace. Keep red spices in refrigerator.
ground spices	6 months	
herbs	6 months	
Hot pepper sauce, Worcestershire	1 year	
Steak and meat sauces	2 years+	
	2 years+	

Item	Time	Notes
Frosting, in cans or mixes	8 months	If opened, put in airtight container.
Hot roll mix	18 months	
Pancake mix	6 months	Put in airtight container.
Piecrust mix	8 months	
Pies and pastries	2-3 days	Refrigerate whipped cream, custard, chiffon fillings.
Potato mixes	18 months	Keep in original package.
Pudding mixes	1 year	Keep in original packets.
Rice mixes	6 months	
Sauce, gravy mixes	6 months	Keep in original packets.
Rice mixes	6 months	
Sauce, gravy mixes	6 months	Keep in original packets.
Soup mixes	6 months	Keep in original packets.
Toaster pop-ups	3 months	Keep in original package.

OTHERS

Item	Time	Notes
Coconut	1 year	Refrigerate after opening.
Hard-shelled squash	Few weeks	Keep cool.
Metered calorie products, instant breakfasts	6 months	Keep in cans, closed jars or original packets.
Nuts	9 months	Refrigerate after opening.
Onions, potatoes, rutabagas, sweet potatoes	1-2 weeks at room temperature	For longer storage, keep below 50°F, but not refrigerated. Keep dry, out of sun. Plan short storage in spring when sprouting is serious problem.
Parmesan cheese (grated) (opened)	1 month	Keep lid tightly closed. (Refrigerate shredded Parmesan cheese.)
Peanut butter (unopened)	6 months	Two months after opening. Refrigeration not needed.
Soft drinks	3 months	
Whipped topping mix	1 year	

vide better nutrition. It might be a good idea to briefly review these suggestions before a trip to the market.*

The Fast Food Chain

Millions of Americans eat one or more meals outside the home each day. Many of these consumers eat at one of the fast-food chains, where food can be purchased at a low price with quick service. The nutritional value of these types of meals has been analyzed and reported in *Consumer Reports*. That analysis is included in Figure 15A-1.

DRUGS

Americans spend billions of dollars on prescription drugs each year and have come to expect their doctors to prescribe drugs for every ailment. Surveys have shown that the most common means by which a doctor finds out about a new drug is through advertising in medical publications or from the drug salesperson.

If a doctor has been exposed only to the brand name of a certain drug, he or she will prescribe that drug. But after a new drug patent expires, other manufacturers will produce the drug under a generic name rather than the registered brand name. The generic drug may be up to 40 percent cheaper. For example, the brand name Librium is the same as the generic drug chlordiazepoxide.

Recently the U.S. Supreme Court upheld a decision to allow the advertising

*Adapted from *The Great American Food Hoax* by Sidney Margolius, copyright 1971 by Sidney Margolius, and used with permission of the publisher, Walker and Company; and *Consumer Survival Kit* from the television series by the Maryland Center for Public Broadcasting.

of drug prices so that the prices of brand-name drugs and generic drugs could be compared, as could prices between drug stores, thus enabling the consumer to do some comparison shopping and save money.

Regardless of whether a drug has been prescribed by a doctor or bought over the counter, it is important to realize that any drug can have adverse side effects, especially when combined with another drug. Anyone who is on medication should not use alcohol or any other drug unless under the strict supervision of a doctor.

In 1967, the National Academy of Sciences National Research Council reported that 1,700 brand-name drugs were ineffective. A more recent study by the National Academy showed that 14.7 percent of the 16,573 drugs they tested were ineffective. One of the purposes of the FDA is to get these ineffective drugs off the market.

Drugs that are effective for many people may cause dangerous allergic reactions in others. It is therefore imperative that each drug is tested carefully before it is put on the market so that all possible side effects are known and its actions in different situations are understood.

Thalidomide was a sleeping pill that was used in West Germany in the late fifties and the early sixties. Unfortunately, it was responsible for the malformation of more than 6,500 babies. Dr. Frances Kelsey, an alert FDA official, was instrumental in stopping the drug from being sold in the United States.

More than 10 million women in the United States use birth control pills despite the serious side effects that may occur in some women. Necessary warnings must now accompany all prescriptions for the pill.

The FDA is often "damned if they do

Which fast-food entrées are the most nutritious?

	Serving size	Calories	Fat	Carbohydrates	Total sugars	Sodium	Protein	Vitamin A	Thiamin	Riboflavin	Vitamin B₆	Vitamin B₁₂	Niacin	Calcium	Phosphorus	Iron
										Percentage RDA*						
Hamburgers																
BURGER KING WHOPPER	9 oz.	660	41 gm.	49 gm.	9 gm.	1083 mg.	57%	12%	51%	30%	19%	67%	55%	9%	29%	26%
JACK-IN-THE-BOX JUMBO JACK	8¼	538	28	44	7	1007	61	9	56	41	13	70	57	13	29	24
McDONALD'S BIG MAC	7½	591	33	46	6	963	59	5	52	33	13	63	55	23	44	23
WENDY'S OLD FASHIONED	6½	413	22	29	5	708	52	8	36	26	13	83	45	8	24	27
Sandwiches																
ROY ROGERS ROAST BEEF SANDWICH	5½	356	12	34	0	610	63	5	38	29	16	37	60	2	28	23
BURGER KING CHOPPED-BEEF STEAK SANDWICH	6¾	445	13	50	0.7	966	67	5	48	34	25	40	66	15	37	30
HARDEE'S ROAST BEEF SANDWICH	4½	351	17	32	3	765	41	4	36	22	10	47	42	8	29	17
ARBY'S ROAST BEEF SANDWICH	5¼	370	15	36	1	869	52	4	36	21	10	53	56	5	35	20
Fish																
LONG JOHN SILVER'S	7½	483	27	27	0.1	1333	72	5	17	12	16	133	24	3	46	3
ARTHUR TREACHER'S ORIGINAL	5¼	439	27	27	0.3	421	46	3	11	6	10	27	18	2	32	3
McDONALD'S FILET-O-FISH	4½	383	18	38	3	613	35	3	39	19	6	23	25	14	27	9
BURGER KING WHALER	7	584	34	50	5	968	48	3	38	20	7	60	31	8	50	12
Chicken																
KENTUCKY FRIED CHICKEN SNACK BOX	6¾	405	21	16	0	728	78	4	21	25	19	40	72	6	35	14
ARTHUR TREACHER'S ORIGINAL CHICKEN	5½	409	23	25	0	580	57	3	12	10	24	10	87	2	33	4
Specialty entrées																
WENDY'S CHILI	10	266	9	29	9	1190	50	54	20	169	18	47	8	9	27	27
PIZZA HUT PIZZA SUPREME	7¾**	506	15	64	6	1281	61	36	59	40	17	43	49	41	46	24
JACK-IN-THE-BOX TACO	5½***	429	26	34	3	926	35	25	16	13	15	27	18	20	33	12

* Recommended Daily Allowance for an adult woman, as set by the National Academy of Sciences/National Research Council.
** One-half of a 15½-oz., 10-in. Pizza Supreme Thin and Crispy.
*** Two 2¾-oz. tacos.

and damned if they don't" on the actions that they take on some drugs. Some people criticize the agency for its slow action in permitting certain drugs that have long been used in foreign countries. Others may rebut with the thalidomide example. Certainly the FDA is understaffed and overworked. When in doubt, perhaps the key word is "caution."

We have already commented upon the ineffectiveness of many drugs. It is common knowledge that nothing often works as well as anything. Countless tests and experiments have shown that placebos (inert pills with no active ingredients) often are effective in treating a wide variety of maladies. Many people claim great relief merely upon walking into a doctor's office. Since placebos often work, many people spend huge amounts of money on ineffective drugs that only work to reduce their pocketbook.

The Federal Trade Commission (FTC) reports that thirty-six cents of every consumer dollar paid for the ten leading headache medicines goes toward advertising. Just as people can get well by thinking positive thoughts, the opposite is also true. Advertising is considered by some to be a suggestion that maybe the person really is sick. Maybe people *are* constipated, maybe they *do* have bad breath or body odor. With the suggestion planted and the constant repetition of the commercials, the person may actually manifest some or all of the symptoms. For example, many people have been convinced that their bowel movements should be regular or on schedule, and if they are not they should take a laxative.

Millions of dollars are spent on laxatives in the United States each year despite studies that show that if a person eats a well-balanced diet (including dietary fiber) and if regular exercise is tak-

en, the need for laxatives should be negligible. Missing a bowel movement for one or two days is not unusual, nor is it a cause for concern. However, a change in bowel habits can be a sign of cancer, and a checkup is indicated if it persists.

It should be noted that if a person takes laxatives on a regular basis, a dependency may develop that necessitates the purchase of more and more laxatives and decreases the chances of ever being able to have a natural bowel movement again.

Antacids are another product that receives heavy advertising. These products supposedly neutralize stomach acids, although their effectiveness seems dubious for several reasons. Since the stomach is supposed to have a high acid content to aid in the proper digestion of food, the addition of an antacid would seem likely to inhibit the normal digestive processes. If increased stomach acid is due to nervousness or tension rather than the ingestion of food, the drinking of water or milk can effectively neutralize the acid. By reducing the amount of food consumed at one sitting, people could avoid many stomachaches.

COSMETIC AND PERSONAL PRODUCTS

Men and women, young and old, spend large sums of money on products to improve themselves or their looks. They rub, pour, spray, sprinkle, and soak all parts of the body in the hopes of becoming more attractive.

Since November 30, 1976, all cosmetic and toiletry products sold in the United States have listed their ingredients in descending order of predominance, meaning that the main ingredients of each product appear at the top of the list.

However, the FDA provides a loophole for protection of trade secrets by permitting fragrances and flavors to be labeled only as "fragrance" cr "flavor" and not by their actual chemical makeup. The listing of ingredients is especially important for people who are trying to avoid allergic reactions. In the past, they had to judge solely by the word "hypoallergenic" on the label, only to find that there were no legal requirements for using the word; thus the labeling was meaningless.

The Consumers' Union has concluded that aerosols are not good buys for many reasons—medical, environmental and financial. Medically, they can produce rashes, eye irritations, and lung problems (via inhalation). It is suggested that persons with known heart disease or lung conditions such as chronic bronchitis, emphysema, or asthma should avoid the use of aerosols.

Aerosol cans pose a safety hazard if exposed to temperatures of 120° F. or more, since they can explode and cause injury. Suntan aerosols left in closed automobiles in the hot sun fall into this category. While results are inconclusive, many scientists believe that the gases from aerosols end up in the atmosphere and reduce the ozone layer, thus permitting more ultraviolet rays to penetrate to the earth and increasing the incidence of skin cancer.

When buying aerosols, one is paying a great deal for the strong can and the propellants. Sometimes the propellant even outweighs the active ingredient. For these and other reasons, simple pump spray containers have become increasingly available. In fact, it is a goal of the FDA, EPA, and the Consumer Product Safety Commission to eliminate most fluorocarbon sprays from the market within the next few years. Over-the-counter drug sprays for asthma sufferers, contraceptive vaginal foams, and cytology fixatives used in diagnosing cancer are classified as essential and are not subject to the labeling requirements or the eventual ban.

Other Harmful Ingredients

Most cosmetic manufacturers have removed hexachlorophene from their products pending further studies on the effects it may have on infants; the decision was made after at least fifteen dogs died after eating half a bar or more of soap containing hexachlorophene.

The FDA recently banned the use of chlorophyll, which was used in some toothpastes and cough medicine to enhance taste. Its ingestion has been linked with cancer. The FDA also recommended against the use of the chemicals TBS, TCC, TFC, triclosan, and Vancide FP, because it appears that they can be absorbed through the skin from soaps that contain them and can produce damage to internal organs.

Some creams contain methyl mercury, which may be stored in the body. Although the immediate effects are not dangerous, continuous use can be detrimental. To make matters worse, many creams are excellent media for the growth of bacteria and may be the cause of staphylococcus and salmonella infections. The chemical 2.4TDA that is used in forty-three brands of hair dye was shown to be carcinogenic in 1966 when injected into laboratory animals. Its effect upon humans is unknown but is suspect.

What can the consumer do? Laws need to be passed that will require cosmetics manufacturers to list their ingredients, provide honest advertising, and subject their products to rigorous safety testing. Although the FDA requires that all eyeglass lenses be impact-resistant, there are no requirements for nonflammability of eyeglass frames; the buyer therefore should be careful to avoid open flames or extreme heat.

Contact lenses are much more expensive than glasses, but many people prefer them for esthetic reasons or because they are involved in athletics or some other endeavor that makes wearing regular glasses inconvenient.

Hard contact lenses are difficult to become accustomed to, although many people adjust very well and are very happy with them. Care should be taken to adjust slowly and have them fitted properly. Proper cleanliness is of the utmost importance. (A common bad habit is to clean the lens by placing them in the mouth. Since this could lead to bacterial infections, the practice should be avoided.)

Soft lenses are easier to adjust to than hard ones. Many people adjust to the soft lenses in a day or two and praise their effectiveness. However, they are usually more expensive. As with hard lenses, certain procedures should be followed to maintain soft contact lenses. They need to be sterilized in a special device that comes with the lenses. This is because they are porous and can absorb irritants and chemicals from the air. A person working around chemicals should not wear soft lenses. If not kept in solution, these lenses can dry up and become brittle and break.

HOME PERILS

Lead Poisoning

Estimates show that 200 children die from lead poisoning each year and another 6,000 are brain damaged or handicapped. The most frequent cause is eating the paint that has chipped off walls of older dwellings that have been painted with a lead-based paint. For a while, the U.S. Department of Housing and Urban Development (HUD) banned lead-based paints on government housing; they later rescinded the ban. By making phone calls and writing letters to the proper authorities, consumers can apply the pressure needed to help make homes safe and free of the perils of lead poisoning.

Detergents

Soap used to be the main cleansing agent, but now people are finding detergents with added enzymes and phosphates that are purported to get their clothes whiter than white or brighter than bright. Phosphates do help to get clothes cleaner, and they are biodegradable; but they also end up in lakes and streams and promote the growth of algae, which in turn chokes out the other life in the water and leads to the demise of the lake or stream (eutrophication).

People concerned about lakes and streams can use a low- or nonphosphate detergent, since most water treatment plants will not remove phosphates from the water. Care should also be taken when using detergents that contain enzymes. Although enzymes help break down stains, there is danger that they can also cause skin irritations and lung damage. A case of a child's dying from reportedly inhaling dust from an enzyme detergent has been cited in the medical literature. Contrary to popular belief, suds have nothing to do with cleaning power, and most detergent manufacturers recommend the use of far more detergent than is necessary to get clothes clean.

Toys

Toys represent another potential hazard to health. The National Commission on Product Safety estimates that 700,000 injuries including burns, cuts, deafness, strangulation, electrical shocks, bruises, broken bones, and sprains are caused by toys each year.

The FDA protects the consumer from flammable toys and is now authorized to protect children from unsafe toys. But as has been observed in other areas, the process of checking and removing unsafe products from the market is a long and tedious process. The best way to be safe is to be alert and observe the guidelines set up by the U.S. Department of Health, Education, and Welfare:*

1. Choose a toy appropriate for the child's age and development (many toys have age group labels on the package).

2. Remember that younger children may have access to toys bought for their older brothers and sisters.

3. Check fabric labels for nonflammable, flame-retardant or flame-resistant notices.

4. Check instructions; they should be easy to read and understand. Instruct the child in the proper use of any toy that might cause injury through misuse.

5. Avoid toys that produce excessive noise (even toy cap pistols fired too close to a child's ear can cause damage).

6. Avoid shooting games, especially those involving darts and arrows, unless the games are played under parental supervision.

7. When choosing a toy for small children, make sure it:

    a. is too large to be swallowed

*From *Playing Safe in Toyland,* U.S. Department of Health, Education, and Welfare, Rockville, MD 20852.

    b. does not have detachable parts that can lodge in the windpipe, ears, or nostrils

    c. is not apt to break easily into small pieces or leave jagged edges

    d. does not have sharp edges or points

    e. has not been put together with easily exposed straight pins, sharp wires, nails, etc.

    f. is not made of glass or brittle plastic

    g. is not poisonous or toxic

    h. does not have exposed flames or build up heat to dangerous levels

    i. does not have flimsy electrical wiring

    j. does not have parts which can pinch fingers or catch hair

    k. avoids long cords and thin plastic bag materials (for children under two)

8. Choose carefully. Any toy can be dangerous if misused. There is no substitute for parental judgment and supervision. Even after purchase, it remains the responsibility of the adult to examine the toy from time to time to assure that wear and tear has not uncovered a hazardous situation.

WARRANTIES

Some products are under warranty or guarantee. Whenever anyone has a faulty or dangerous product, he or she should return it for a new one or for a refund.

Good Housekeeping magazine offers a money-back guarantee for any product that advertises in the magazine. It even has its own institute that tests such products as toys. Consumers must remember that the guarantee only offers their money back and does not accept respon-

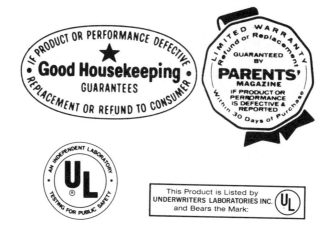

FIGURE 15A-2 Labels to look for

sibility for faulty installation. *Parents' Magazine* seals are for products advertised in the magazine. This guarantee offers money back if a product is proven defective. The magazine sometimes has private firms test products. Underwriters' Laboratories examines electrical appliances for safety. If and when an appliance passes the test, it receives a UL seal. Consumers should always check to see if both the product and the cord have the UL seal. (See Figure 15A-2.)

To find out about the safety of a food or other product, consumers can check the following consumers' magazines: *Consumer Reports, Consumers Digest, Consumers Research, Changing Times,* and *FDA Consumer.* Consumers who wish to know if one of the consumers' magazines has researched a product that they want can consult the latest *Consumer's Index—To Product Evaluations and Information Sources* edited by C. Edward Wall (Ann Arbor, Mi.: Pierian Press).

MEDICAL CARE

X-rays

The *FDA Consumer* states, "Although a single X-ray examination is not likely to cause damage, all exposure may involve some small risk. There is no known amount of ionizing radiation below which it can be said that no adverse health effect can occur. This does not mean that a needed X-ray should be shunned, for the potential benefits in diagnosing a serious disease or injury can far outweigh the possible damage from radiation exposure. But it does mean that all *unnecessary* X-ray examinations should be eliminated."

The FDA is currently inspecting X-raying equipment and facilities to determine their safety level. Because they have found that many people are receiving more radiation than is necessary, a continuing education program for X-ray technicians has been developed.

The FDA has also recommended a patient gonad shield to protect the testicles from unnecessary radiation during ab-

414

dominal or pelvic X-rays. Subjecting the testes to radiation might cause genetic mutations. Likewise, patients who are pregnant or who suspect that they might be pregnant should inform the doctor or technician before any X-rays are taken. Whenever possible, X-rays of a pregnant woman are avoided because of the danger to the fetus.

Chiropractors

Consumers' Union believes that "chiropractice is a significant hazard to many patients." Because the chiropractor's practice is limited to musculoskeletal complaints (specifically twenty-six nerves), CU thinks that chiropractic treatment should not involve the administration of X-rays or drugs for the treatment of disease and that chiropractors should be prohibited from treating children.

When selecting a physician, one should check with medical societies, local hospitals, nearby medical schools, and friends and not just pick a doctor out of the yellow pages of the phone book. Medical societies will be able to give a person the credentials of a doctor that he or she is interested in. Family practitioners or general practitioners can treat the majority of the maladies encountered by most families, and their services are cheaper. The family practitioner will refer a patient to a specialist if the occasion arises.

The following books will help inform people about various doctors and types of practices—group, osteopathy, laboratory, and X-ray facilities—as well as provide other useful information: *How to Be Your Own Doctor—Sometimes* by Dr. Keith W. Sehnert and Howard Eisenburg (Grosset and Dunlap), *Talk Back to Your Doctor* by Dr. Arthur Levin (Doubleday), and *Managing Your Doctor*, by Dr. Arthur S. Freese (Stein and Day).

PART B: TEACHING ABOUT CONSUMER HEALTH

Because proper maintenance of the human body should be important to everyone, a great deal of time has been spent in this book describing lifestyles conducive to personal well-being. The responsibility of maintaining optimum health does not rest just with the individual but with individuals working together to provide health services for everyone.

Although health services cover the entire world as well as the individual community, and their organization may be official, professional, or voluntary, this chapter will emphasize the voluntary health agency in the community.

An additional goal for the teaching plan is for the students to perceive the issues involved in their consumer choices and actions as important. For the students to do this, they must recognize consumer issues and value the results of being wise, concerned consumers. In other words, they must see that wise consumership can be healthy and actualizing and can promote happiness.

The following needs should be considered in a teaching plan for consumer health and medical care:

1. The students need to believe that their consumer selections and judgments can affect their well-being.

2. The students need to be aware of advertising aimed at their age groups and gimmicks used to appeal to them.

3. The students need to be encouraged to participate in consumer protection and should be committed to obtaining and reading reliable health sources regularly and reporting consumer abuse to authorities.

4. The students need to believe that regular health examinations are vital to their continued well-being.

5. The students need to know that their overall physical health will have a direct influence on their ability to learn in school.

6. The students need to recognize sources of good medical care and treatment and how to obtain them when threatened by a health problem.

7. The students need to become acquainted with the work of voluntary health agencies in the community and ways that these agencies are committed to preventing disease through programs of community service, public and professional education, and research.

Appropriate grade levels are suggested for each teaching strategy and appear as ○, □, ☆ in the left-hand column.

    ○ = most suited for the primary grades;
    □ = most suited for the intermediate grades;
    ☆ = most suited for the upper elementary grades.

UNIT I: THE WISE CONSUMER

The amount of money Americans spend on health aids and services increases by leaps and bounds each year. The 1970 consumer expenditures in this country totaled over $1 billion on nonprescription drugs, $28 billion on recreational drugs (alcohol and tobacco), and an estimated $2 billion on fake health aids (1). Much of the appeal of advertising these products is aimed at young persons. Students need to be acquainted with advertising techniques and given an opportunity to practice their skill in evaluating the advertising appeal of several products.

Students also need to establish the pattern of keeping abreast of current health information. In this lesson, students examine the evening news, weekly and monthly magazines, and national and local agencies to become cognizant health consumers. They learn to evaluate sources with the hope of establishing a desire to be informed consumers of health information.

OBJECTIVES

1. The student will hear a tape of ten commercials and will rate the commercials according to their appeal.

2. Using the information learned about advertising appeal, the student will design a mock product.

3. The student will express his or her values toward advertising when given play money to shop at a store.

4. The student will orally describe advertising appeal in a fishing game.

5. After the Friday ___ O'Clock News Report, the student will be able to answer five questions about the current health news of the week.

6. After the Friday ____ O'clock News Report, the students will rank the health topics reported from those of least concern to them to those of most concern and will give the rationale for their rankings.

7. The student will demonstrate that she or he can summarize news articles accurately by participating in the development of a health newspaper.

8. As part of a health science fair, the student will develop a booth on an organization or agency that provides health information.

9. The students will express their attitudes and values toward important health information by participating in a hidden treasure activity.

MATERIALS

1. Tape recorder.
2. Old cartons and packages, play money.
3. Magazine advertisements, glue, cardboard, string, and paper clips.
4. Metal box.

Methods

○ □ ☆

Open-Ended Sentences

As an introduction, have the students complete the following statements:

I use _____ toothpaste because _____ .

I use _____ soap because _____ .

I drink _____ soft drink because _____ .

I eat _____ cereal because _____ .

○ □ ☆

Commercials

Tape record ten different commercials for the class. Make certain that each commercial is identified by numbering them Commercial No. 1, Commercial No. 2, etc. The students will number from 1 to 10 on a sheet of paper. As they hear the tape, they will place a (✓) by the number of each commercial that appeals to them.

Play the tape again. Stop after each commercial and discuss why the commercial appealed to the students. Discuss factors that influence people to buy products:

cost and amount of money one has
availability of item
styles and customs
friends and what they have
family
emotional appeal
good advertising

○ □ ☆

Jingle Contest

Have the students divide into groups of five to participate in a jingle contest. The students will have twenty minutes to write down or tape record as many jingles as they can think of that are used to advertise products. (Jingle example: "Coke adds life.")

Sample Store

Have each student design a product package for a grocery store. To make the product, have the students use old food cartons and cover them with paper. The students should make their packages as appealing as possible, since the purpose will be to sell the product to the class.

After the packages are made, the

teacher can display them on shelves in a simulated store. The students can be involved in gimmicks to promote their products as follows:

1. The class may wish to make door-to-door handouts which include advertisements of each product.

2. The students can make coupons to attract customers.

3. The students can offer free prizes or games with their products.

4. The student can be a mock representative in the store trying to promote the product.

□ ☆
Television Show

Divide the class into groups of four or five students. Each group must collect written articles on health-related topics. (This lesson could be done throughout the year, and you could assign specific health topics to relate to the unit you are currently covering.) The group will select four or five articles which they want to report to the class.

Each week, one group is responsible for the Friday ___ O'Clock News Report. One student is the newscaster and coordinates the reporters. Other students are the reporters, who must summarize their chosen articles and present them to the class in reporter style.

After the news report, the students may ask for more information on any of the reports, comment, or criticize. The class discussion of the news report should include general comments, bias of articles, relevance to students.

After the discussion of the entire news report, the students may personally rank the health topics reported from those of least concern to them to those of most concern to them. The students must also give one rationale, describing why they ranked each topic as they did. Ask who (how many) ranked each topic first or second.

The students may also do value voting to describe their feelings as to whether the health topics presented in the news report were personal health problems, community health problems, or world health problems.

○ □ ☆
Health Newspaper

Determine whether the students would like to make a Health Newspaper to take home. The newspaper should be a collection of articles that the students feel are most important to them.

Have each student bring an article that he or she wants to include. Select one student to be the editor. The students may submit their news happening in one of two ways. They may write a summary of the article to give to the editor, or they may call the newspaper with the information.

Set up two telephones in the classroom. The student calling in the information must give an accurate summary. The student in the newspaper office will have to evaluate the call and determine if there was enough accurate information to warrant including the story in the paper.

○ □ ☆
Best Tip Yet

Each week you may give an award to the student who finds a health article that offers the "best tip yet." You may include the weekly winners in a booklet called Hints for a Healthy Lifestyle.

○ □ ☆

Health Library

Designate a display table of newspaper articles, magazines, bulletins, etc., as a research center. Articles should be grouped into categories. The students may add articles to each category and use them for reference. Reading at the research center can be a spare-time activity.

□ ☆

Health Science Fair

Divide students into groups to present reports on consumer groups which help people to be well informed. Booths could be set up to display the kinds of information or services available from an organization or agency, such as the Food and Drug Administration; Federal Trade Commission; Department of Health, Education, and Welfare; National Institute for Mental Health; Better Business Bureau; and American Medical Association. The parents or children from other rooms could be invited for Health Science Fair Day.

Evaluation

LIFESTYLE CONTENT

○

Fishing Game

Divide the class into two teams. Let each student cut out an advertisement from a magazine and glue it to a piece of heavy cardboard. Cut each cardboard advertisement into the form of a fish and punch a hole near the mouth. Construct a fishing pole out of a long rod and a piece of string. Use a paper clip at the end for a hook.

Put all of the cardboard fish into a tub behind a screen. The teams will take turns fishing. Let the students throw the string of their fishing poles over the screen. The teacher may attach a fish to one of the paper-clip hooks.

The lucky angler must describe the appeal of the advertisement in order to keep the fish. If he or she cannot describe the appeal, the fish must be thrown back. The team with the most fish wins.

□ ☆

The students should correctly answer at least five questions after the Friday ____ O'Clock News Report each week. The questions will be made up by the students doing the reports for that week.

○ □ ☆

Make up a quiz to accompany the Health Newspaper. The students will take the quiz and give the quiz to a parent when they take the Health Newspaper home to share.

□ ☆

Periodically have a quiz from the booklet *Hints for a Healthy Lifestyle*.

□ ☆

Design questions to be used at each booth at the health science fair.

LIFESTYLE VALUE

□ ☆

Each student will be given $15 in play money. (Use play money or have the students make play money.) The students will go to the store and spend their money. After shopping, the student should write down all of the products he or she was able to purchase with the $15 and explain why he or she chose each product.

Shopping List

Have the students write down all the things they bought, beginning with the one which cost the most and ending with the one that cost the least.

Product	Price	Why I Bought It
1. _____	_____	_____
2. _____	_____	_____
3. _____	_____	_____

☆
Hidden Treasure

Present this situation to the students: this civilization is dying out, and you want to leave behind some written information about the United States for the next civilization. The students can bring in important articles which deal with various aspects of the nation's health. The articles will be dropped into a small metal box. The students report to the class on why they think their article is valuable for the next civilization.

UNIT II: BEFORE YOU VISIT THE DOCTOR

The medical care a person receives is influenced by her or his knowledge and behavior. When one visits the doctor, it is helpful to have a basic understanding of how one's body works and be able to understand some of the technical terms the doctor seems to know so well. The purpose of this unit is to help students review their body organs and systems and appreciate the value of an accurate family medical record.

OBJECTIVES

1. After the students have studied all their body systems (as detailed in Chapter 8), they will be able to correctly match a description of nine body systems with the correct system.

2. The students will demonstrate a knowledge of basic anatomy by cutting out human body organs from the patterns provided and attaching them to a blank human form at their correct locations in the body.

3. The student will orally explain the importance of keeping an accurate family medical record and will encourage his or her family to fill out a family medical record if they do not already have a current record of their own.

MATERIALS

1. Felt board, different colors of felt, scissors.

2. Atlas Figures 100 and 101, Body Organs and Human Form Outline.

3. Atlas Figure 99, Body Organs Coloring Activity.

4. Atlas Figure 102, Family Medical Record.

Methods

Begin this unit by telling the students the following. When you go to the doctor he or she looks at you, asks you to say ah, and takes your blood pressure. The doctor carefully presses his or her fingers against your lymph glands and abdomen. In order to recognize an abnormality, the doctor must go to school for a long time and learn how the normal body looks and functions. You have been learning how the human body works too. Let's see how much you can remember.

□ ☆

Match Functions with Body Systems

See if the students can match each of the following nine body systems with its correct description. You may want to use individual handouts, the chalkboard, or a felt board. Pictures of organs in each system can be matched with the correct function instead of written body systems.

1. ___ Skeletal System
2. ___ Muscular System
3. ___ Circulatory System
4. ___ Respiratory System
5. ___ Digestive System
6. ___ Excretory System
7. ___ Endocrine System
8. ___ Nervous System
9. ___ Reproductive System

a. Holds bones in position and allows bones to move.
b. Filters watery wastes from the blood and sees that they are removed from the body.
c. Specialized tissues that deliver messages to the body and take messages to the brain.
d. Provides support for the body.
e. Takes food, oxygen, hormones, etc. to the body tissues and carries away waste products.
f. Breaks down food so that it can be absorbed into the bloodstream and eliminates unabsorbed materials.
g. Brings in oxygen through inhalation and disposes of waste carbon dioxide through exhalation.
h. Responsible for the development of sex cells and aids in sexual activity.
i. Produces chemical signals that begin the physical changes of puberty, maintains a certain carbohydrate level, tells muscles to work harder in situations of emotional stress.

(ANSWERS: 1. d 2. a 3. e 4. g 5. f 6. b 7. i 8. c 9. h)

□ ☆

Coloring Activity

To test whether the students understand the names of various body organs and in which system the organs belong, pass out copies of the Body Organs Coloring Activity (Atlas Figure 99), and ask the students to color the organs to match the following body systems:

Skeletal System: white (pelvis, clavicle, sternum, and humerus)
Muscular System: green (diaphragm—also a part of the respiratory system—bicep; heart is optional)
Circulatory System: red (heart)
Respiratory System: light blue (lungs; diaphragm may also be included)
Digestive System: pink (stomach, small and large intestines, gallbladder, pancreas; rectum may be included, but really belongs with the Excretory System)
Excretory System: brown (urinary bladder, kidneys, rectum)
Nervous System: orange (brain and spinal cord)
Endocrine System: yellow (pituitary, thyroid, adrenals, pancreas; also ovaries and testes, which may be included as a part of the reproductive system as well)
Reproductive System: dark blue (ovaries and testes, also included under Endocrine System; uterus and fallopian tubes; prostate)

The appendix may be colored pink, since it is attached to the lower end of the large intestine. The spleen may be colored red; it is actually a lymphatic organ which, during the life of the embryo, manufactures blood cells. After birth, one of its functions is related to disposal of old, worn-out red blood cells. Other functions are not yet completely determined.

□ ☆

Felt Board or Desk Activity

Students can also demonstrate their knowledge of anatomy by cutting out body organs (Atlas Figure 100) and placing them in the correct location on the human outline form (in Atlas Figure 101). For class use, the teacher may wish to glue the paper organs to cardboard backed with felt so that the organs can be used with a felt board.

□ ☆

Medical Terminology

Advanced students interested in being exposed to basic medical terminology will enjoy the activity "Itis-ectomy-ology: Speaking the Doctor's Language."* After the students have reviewed a list of medical prefixes, roots, and suffixes, two quizzes enable them to apply their new knowledge.

FAMILY MEDICAL RECORD

"Information about the health of your immediate family can prove helpful in early diagnosis and treatment of diseases that are known either to be genetic or to occur more commonly in some families." †

○ □ ☆

Ask the class why they think it is important for every family to keep an accurate

*Appears in *Go to Health* (New York: Dell, 1972.)
† Quote and accompanying Family Medical Record information reprinted by permission of the National Foundation—March of Dimes.

medical record. Following are some of the reasons that you can suggest:

Information is organized and readily available.

Helpful when filling out school and travel records.

Contains information needed to fill out insurance forms.

Helpful during routine medical consultations.

Can prove a valuable diagnostic tool for one's physician.

A family health history showing a genetic disorder can alert a doctor to early symptoms in time to avert advanced disease or disability in another.

A child's birth record that includes the Apgar score, which rates a newborn's respiration, muscle tone, reflexes, heart rate, and color on a scale of zero to two for a maximum of ten points one minute after birth, may also provide a clue to some difficulty the child may have later in life.

A record of individual problems, medications, or allergies can be crucial in an emergency and very important during a routine consultation, since it will help the doctor avoid prescribing a drug that might interact adversely with one that is already being taken.

○ □ ☆

Survey

Take a survey of your class and find out how many of their families have an up-to-date medical record.

○ □ ☆

Family Medical Record Booklet

Duplicate copies of the Family Medical Record (Atlas Figure 101) and let each student design a cover page. Staple all of the pages together and have the students give the books to their parents. The students should be able to explain the importance of keeping a current family medical record. Have them ask their parents to fill out the book for them. You may want to include a note to the parents explaining that their family health record, faithfully kept and passed along to their children as they mature, can become a valuable testament to your concern for the well-being of the generations still to be born.

Evaluation

LIFESTYLE CONTENT

☐ ☆

Using body organs cut from colored felt, ask different students to identify the organ and the system to which it belongs.

LIFESTYLE VALUE

○ ☐ ☆

Ask the students to write a brief paragraph in response to each of the following questions. What do you think is the most important reason for having an up-to-date family medical record? Before you visit your doctor, do you think of any questions that you want to ask him or her during your physical examination? What do you think would be good questions to ask your doctor?

UNIT III: A MEDICAL EXAMINATION

When did you have your last health checkup? You know the old saying, "An ounce of prevention is worth a pound of cure." That ounce of prevention is one of the main purposes for having a medical exam. A periodic physical examination is important for everyone, no matter what the age.

For children, a physical exam includes checking growth and development, as well as giving any necessary immunizations. For adult women, a physical exam will include a Pap smear (to check for cancer of the cervix) and a breast examination. Adult men should have a rectal examination to check for lumps in the prostate. All adults over age forty should be examined with a proctoscope that can illuminate the colon and rectum, thus aiding in the early detection of colon cancer.

Periodic examinations enable a doctor to know a patient better and be able to successfully discover and correct problems early.

OBJECTIVES

1. After participating in a classroom discussion utilizing transparencies of various instruments used during a physical examination, the student will be able to correctly name at least four instruments used by a physician or nurse and explain their function.

2. The student will tell what normal body temperature means, explain two ways the temperature may be taken, and explain three measures that are usually helpful in reducing a fever.

3. The student will correctly obtain an accurate temperature, pulse rate, respiration rate, and blood pressure reading and record his or her own vital-sign data on a graph.

MATERIALS

1. Atlas Figures 45, 46, 47, 48, 50, 51, 52, 54, 55, and 56–Scales, Thermometer, Sphygmomanometer, Otoscope, Tongue Depressor, Ophthalmoscope, Eye Chart,

Stethoscope, Hypodermic Syringe, and X-ray Machine.

2. Felt board and pictures of people in different age groups.

3. Thermometers, stethoscope, sphygmomanometer, stopwatch or watch with second hand, felt-tip markers, and graph paper.

Methods

□

Telephone Game

One way to begin a lesson concerning the importance of health checkups is to play the game of telephone. Have the class form a circle. The teacher whispers into the first student's ear, "It is important to visit your doctor at least twice a year in order to prevent disease, develop a friendly and trusting relationship with your doctor through health counseling, and establish an individual health history." Each child attempts to repeat what the last child whispered to her or him. The last student says the sentence out loud.

If the student is correct—fine. If not, repeat the statement to the class. Ask the class to discuss why each of the reasons for visiting a doctor is important.

○ □ ☆

Felt Board

Prepare a felt board with pictures of people in different age groups—infant, toddler, preschool, school age, and adult over forty-five. Ask the class to tell you how often each specific age group should see the doctor and why. Talk about how often one should usually visit the eye doctor, dentist, and other specialists.

Discuss what happens during a physical examination by utilizing the follow-

ing information, transparencies, and activities.

○ □ ☆

Urine Tests

When a healthy child visits the doctor for a physical exam, she or he will probably first meet the nurse, who will ask for a sample of urine. To prepare the student for this, invite a nurse to speak to the class about various kinds of urine tests, how they are done, and why they are necessary.

○ □ ☆

Scales

Show a transparency of the Scales (Atlas Figure 45) and explain that the nurse may want to weigh and measure the students. This is to check how they are growing and if they are the proper weight for their height. Explain that knowing their weight is important to the doctor when prescribing medicine for them.

○ □ ☆

Thermometer

Ask the students if they ever wondered why the nurse (or doctor) takes their temperature when they are not even sick (show transparency of Atlas Figure 46). An infection that they are not aware of may have started somewhere in their body. In that case, the doctor could decide to put off giving a booster shot that he or she had planned to give.

Ask the class if 98.6 degrees is normal body temperature. Explain that it is not always. Normal temperature differs slightly in various parts of the body. When a thermometer is placed under the tongue, 98.6 degrees is generally regarded as normal for most people, although physicians tend to consider a range between 97 and 99 degrees a normal zone. Temperature goes up and down normally all day. It is lowest from 2:00 to 5:00 A.M. for people who sleep at night and is usually at its highest point by late afternoon or early evening.

Oral Thermometer

Explain that an oral thermometer is used when taking an oral temperature. It is composed of two parts: a bulb and a stem. There is mercury in the bulb. The mercury, which is a metal, will expand when exposed to heat, causing it to rise in the stem. The long lines on the thermometer represent full degrees, but only the even numbers are written; the short lines represent two-tenths of a degree.

It is important that proper care be used in taking mouth temperatures. The reading can be raised or lowered by drinking hot or cold beverages just before the thermometer is inserted. If the patient is a mouth breather, the oral temperature is meaningless. Even smoking immediately before taking a mouth temperature can throw off the reading.

○ □ ☆

Demonstration

Explain to the class that to read a thermometer, one must rinse it in cool water and shake it down so that the mercury drops below 95 degrees. The thermometer should be held under the tongue with the mouth shut for a minimum of three minutes. Read and record the results. Body temperature may also be taken in the armpit or groin (normal temperature is about 98 degrees) and rectally (normally 99.6 degrees). The heat-regulating system in infants and young children is not fully developed, and they can run alarmingly high temperatures even if only a slight infection is present. A child who runs a temperature of 105 degrees may

have a bad cold; but if the child's mother or father registers 105 degrees, she or he is usually in serious trouble.

Ask what a person can do to reduce a fever. The following information can be presented:

1. Drink plenty of fluids. The body loses a great amount of water from sweating during a fever.

2. Since a high temperature very quickly burns up a lot of nutrients, increase your intake of solid foods that are easily digestible and get plenty of rest.

3. Aspirin will generally bring down a mild fever within thirty to sixty minutes. Drugs that lower body temperature usually do so by dilating the blood vessels of the skin.

4. Use light bed covers and keep the room comfortably cool and humid.

5. An ice pack may help when the fever is over 103 degrees.

6. If a low-grade fever persists for several days, despite all that you do, it may be a sign of chronic infection or some other condition. Let your physician examine you and diagnose what is wrong. The same is true for a raging fever that lasts more than one day.

Sphygmomanometer

Tell the class that during a physical examination, the nurse or doctor will use a sphygmomanometer to take the blood pressure (show transparency of Atlas Figure 47). Explain that blood pressure is the pressure exerted by the blood on the wall of any vessel. The highest point reached by the contraction of the heart is the systolic pressure. The lowest point to which it drops between beats is the diastolic pressure (when the heart is at rest). The normal range for systolic pressure is 110 to 146 and for diastolic pressure is 60 to 90. An average reading is 120/80, but this will vary depending on age and other factors. Blood pressure is best measured by the brachial artery, which runs from the shoulder to the elbow. A stethoscope and sphygmomanometer are needed.

○ □ ☆

Demonstration by School Nurse

Have a school nurse demonstrate the proper way to take a blood pressure reading as follows:

1. Wrap the blood pressure cuff around the arm (2 inches above elbow).
2. Place the stethoscope disc over the brachial artery.
3. Close valve on air pump and pump bulb.
4. Pump bulb to 180, then gradually relieve pressure valve.
5. Note the exact numerical line on the scale when the first beat is heard (this is the systolic reading). The last clear sound that is heard should be noted as the diastolic reading.
6. Record the results.

Explain that if the nurse has performed this test, she or he will give the results to the doctor, who will then want to check the ears, nose, throat, eyes, lymph glands, chest, abdomen, reflexes, and overall appearance.

○ □ ☆

Otoscope

Tell the class that to check the ears, the doctor uses an instrument that can light up the ear. It is called an otoscope (show transparency of Atlas Figure 48). The doctor can study the condition of the eardrum and look for changes and signs of disease. The doctor can also see accumulations of wax that may need removing.

○ □ ☆

Tongue Depressor

Explain to the class that when the doctor looks into the mouth, he or she is viewing the general condition of the tongue, teeth, tonsils, and mouth tissue (show transparency of Atlas Figure 50). The ahh itself may tell the doctor that one's voice is hoarse, and he or she will look at the vocal cords. Discolored teeth may be the result of one's mother receiving tetracycline during the pregnancy or of a child's receiving repeated doses while the second teeth were forming in the gums.

Have the students look at their tongues. Ask if they are moist, red, rough-coated, and still. See if they can stick their tongues out firmly and right in the middle of the mouth or if they pop out to one side.

○ □ ☆

Ophthalmoscope and Eye Chart

Tell the class that to study the condition of the eyes, the doctor will use an instrument called an ophthalmoscope (show transparency of Atlas Figure 51). It is used to light up the lining of the eye. The thin film of nerve cells that line the back of the eyeball is the retina. The retina is the only place in the body where nerve tissue and blood vessels can be clearly seen, because they are not covered by skin or muscles. By examining the retina, the doctor can often detect early signs of kidney disease, diabetes, and high blood pressure. To test visual acuity, the doctor uses an eye chart (show transparency of Atlas Figure 52).

Examination of Lymph Glands and Lungs

When the doctor presses his or her fingers against the throat, he or she is feeling the lymph glands. If they are swollen, the doctor will look for other signs of infection.

Next, the doctor will probably start tapping the chest. A drumlike sound will tell the doctor that he or she is tapping over air, a sign of normal lungs. A dull, flat sound tells the doctor that there may be an abnormal condition in one or both of the lungs.

○ □
Stethoscope

A stethoscope is used to study the heartbeat and passage of air into the lungs (show transparency of Atlas Figure 54). Have some students try holding an empty cardboard tube against another student's heart. Ask if they can hear the heartbeat any clearer.

Explain that the doctor will also press his or her hands against the abdomen to check for displaced or enlarged organs, including the spleen.

The doctor will often check the reflexes by tapping a small hammer on the knee or inside the arm.

Explain that during the time that the doctor is looking and listening and touching, he or she is learning more about the patient. The doctor will notice if the skin is pale or flushed, moist or dry, and will observe the posture.

○ □
Hypodermic Syringe

Explain that there are times when one should have an immunization (show transparency of Atlas Figure 55). Sometimes people must receive shots to protect them from getting diseases that could make them very ill.

○ □ ☆
X-ray Machine

Ask the students what they think the doctor would do if he or she thought a pa-tient had broken a bone or there was evidence of infection in the lungs. Explain that the doctor would want to take X-ray pictures (show transparency of Atlas Figure 56). Although an X-ray machine may look big and rather strange, it will not hurt a person. Ask the class if it hurts when they have their pictures taken. Show them what a real X-ray looks like.

Blood Test

Explain that if the doctor really wants to know what is going on inside someone, he or she may want to borrow a few drops of blood. A very small amount of blood may be taken from the finger and diluted. It is then spread out on a glass slide and looked at under a microscope. Red blood cells and white blood cells can be seen. If a person does not have enough red blood cells, she or he may have some form of anemia and need medicine or a change in diet. If someone has too many white blood cells, it can mean there is an infection in the body and more white blood cells have been made to fight the harmful germs.

People are fortunate that the doctor has so many instruments and has gone to school for such a long time so that he or she can help them stay well or make them better when they are ill.

○ □ ☆
Locating the Pulse

Ask the students if they can remember how to find their pulse. Remind them that every time their hearts beat, blood is sent through the arteries, and the pulse is the resultant throb of a heartbeat in the artery.

Tell the class that the American Heart Association accepts as normal for adults a pulse rate of between 50 and 100 beats per minute. However, the normal male pulse is usually between 60 and 65 beats per minute, and the normal female pulse is between 67 and 72 beats per minute. Explain that common places to measure the pulse are at the radial artery in the wrist and the carotid artery on the front side of the neck.

○ □ ☆

Describing the Pulse

List for the class the following ways to describe the pulse:

Strong and regular: even beats with good force.

Weak and regular: even beats with poor force.

Irregular: both strong and weak beats that occur within a minute.

Thready: weak force and irregular.

○ □ ☆

Timing the Pulse

Ask the students to each place three fingertips over the radial or carotid artery of another student (not using the thumb). Tell them to count the number of beats for one minute and record the results. Explain that the relationship between pulse and respiration is one respiration for every four heartbeats. To a degree, a person can control her or his own rate of respiration. When body temperature is elevated, the respiratory rate increases.

○ □ ☆

Describing Respiration

List for the class the following ways to describe respiration:

Rapid, shallow; very slow or very deep.

Regular, both in rate and depth.

Irregular, deeper than usual followed by a period of no breathing.

○ □ ☆

Recording Respiration

Explain to the class that to find the respiration rate, each student should continue to hold the other student's wrist after the pulse has been taken. The students should count the number of times the chest rises and falls during one minute (one rise and fall equals one respiration). Record the results.

Evaluation

LIFESTYLE CONTENT

□ ☆

Show your students the article "Peculiar Patients" by William Johnson.* Have the students each write similar creative stories about some famous fictional character (e.g., the giant in Jack and the Beanstalk, Tom Thumb, Snow White). The story should include correct medical terminology. Select the ten best stories and read them to the class for diagnosis, or display them on the bulletin board and let the students read and diagnose the "patients" in their free time.

○ □ ☆

Have the students correctly name at least four medical instruments used during a physical examination. You may want to show the transparencies, covering the names of the instruments. You can also have the students match a real instrument or picture of the instrument with its correct name.

□ ☆

Evaluation of a student's ability to take an accurate temperature, pulse, respira-

*From the April 1976 issue of *Family Health*.

tion, and blood pressure reading can be made through observation and completion of a graph that shows each student's vital sign data compared to normal readings.

LIFESTYLE VALUE

○ □ ☆

Discussion Questions

Ask the class the following questions: What do you think of the behavior of those who hesitate to visit the doctor for fear the doctor will find something wrong?

Why do doctors sometimes ask questions about the health of your parents or grandparents?

To maintain your very best health throughout your life, what do you think is most important (age, heredity, diet as a child, knowing how your body works and using that knowledge wisely, receiving the best medical care possible)?

Do you think that if you are born with good health, you will probably have good health all of your life?

UNIT IV: A VISIT TO THE HOSPITAL

Children often have many fears and misconceptions about hospitals. Some of these notions are acquired through conversations with friends, and some through watching television.

The purpose of this unit is to help students understand that hospitals exist to help people. Some hospitals not only treat people who are ill, but are associated with medical schools and provide clinical instruction during the various phases of undergraduate medical training.

OBJECTIVES

After participating in classroom discussion and activities, including the games Children's Hospital, Children's Hospital First-Floor Maze, and Health Specialists Concentration,

1. The student will be able to identify at least five specific sections in a hospital.

2. The student will be able to explain (either orally or in writing) at least three ways disease-causing microorganisms are accurately identified through the use of laboratory facilities.

3. The student will be able to name and correctly explain the function of at least three kinds of medical equipment found in hospitals.

4. The student will be able to correctly name at least five hospital occupations.

MATERIALS

1. Atlas Figure 104, Children's Hospital gameboard, colored poster board, scissors, felt-tip pen, game markers, one die.

2. Duplicates of Children's Hospital First-Floor Maze (Atlas Figure 105) and pencils.

3. Paper and crayons, other materials listed with supplementary activities.

Methods

Begin a discussion about hospitals by asking how many students watch "Medical Center" or whatever hospital-based program that happens to be on television at the time. Ask the students if they like the program and why and if they think real hospitals are like the ones they see on television. This kind of discussion will probably lead into a discussion about actual experiences in a hospital. Try to keep the discussion positive, and use the students' enthusiasm to teach them information they do not already know.

☆

Some students may be interested in researching the earliest hospitals, which date back to the ancient pre-Christian empires of India, Persia, Egypt, Greece, and Rome.

☆

Research Papers

The greatest stimulus to hospitals in modern times came from the discoveries concerning the nature of infection. Several of the students may want to research the success of English surgeon Joseph Lister in reducing postoperative infection through the use of the antiseptic phenol (carbolic acid), which opened the era of aseptic surgery.

Other students may want to research the development of the X-ray; uses of elaborate medical apparatus; and laboratory procedures for examining blood, urine, and spinal fluid for their important roles in today's modern hospital.

□ ☆

Pretest

To learn whether the students realize that a modern general hospital has many different sections which treat specific categories of illness, give a pretest, asking the students to each write down all the various medical and nonmedical sections in a hospital that they can think of. Compare their responses with the following information and supplement where necessary.

The Medical Section is subdivided into specialties including:

Hematology, which treats diseases of the blood.

Cardiovascular, which treats diseases of the heart and circulatory system.

Neurology, which treats diseases of the nervous system.

Endocrinology, which treats diseases of the endocrine glands, such as the thyroid and adrenal.

Metabolism, which treats diseases of body chemistry.

Gastrointestinal, which treats diseases of the digestive tract.

Pulmonary, which treats diseases of the lungs.

The Surgery Section includes subspecialties for:

General surgery.

Surgery for the brain and nervous system.

Heart surgery.

Eye, ear, nose, and throat surgery.

Other sections include Obstetrics, Psychiatry, and Dermatology.

The Medical Laboratory has various departments including:

Bacteriology, which identifies disease-producing microorganisms from specimens of sputum, pus, blood, and scrapings from various tissues.

Chemistry, which can detect abnormal concentrations of substances in urine and blood samples that may be clues to disease.

Pathology, which studies samples of tissues from tumors and distinguishes cancerous from noncancerous tissue.

The Radiography Unit takes X-rays to detect fractures and the presence of tumors. The Radiotherapy unit makes use of apparatus which generates radiation for treatment purposes, as in cases of cancer.

The Physical Therapy Section uses devices such as diathermy units which produce heat, whirlpool baths, ultraviolet lamps, and high-frequency (ultrasonic) sound generators.

The Occupational Therapy Unit exercises various parts of the patient's body through productive and creative handcrafts.

The Outpatient Department treats patients who have been released from the hospital and who require follow-up care or checkups and those who do not require hospitalization but who need special diagnostic or therapeutic services of the hospital.

Some hospitals specialize in the treatment of children's problems, tuberculosis, diseases of the eyes and ears, tumors, or joint diseases.

A hospital has patient rooms, a burn unit, a section for infant care, a section for food preparation, a section for research, and a pharmacy. There are emergency treatment rooms and offices for the medical staff and administration. Rooms must be devoted to medical records and patient services. There are also probably a gift shop, playroom, chapel, and volunteer services area, as well as a poison control center.

○ □

Hospital Models

After discussing what makes up a hospital, the students may want to create a model simulating a hospital. Cardboard boxes can be used, or some of the students may want to bring in dollhouses and turn them into various sections of a hospital.

○ □

Role Play

After making the hospital model, the students may want to role play various workers in a hospital. They can make hats and other props to add realism.

○ □

Map

Have each student draw a map from his or her home to the nearest hospital.

○

Name Bracelet

Have the students make name bracelets like those that must be worn by every patient in the hospital. Discuss with the class why these bracelets are necessary.

○ □

Hospital Rules

Ask the students to name some rules that a hospital must impose and discuss why young children cannot visit patient rooms. Have them find out what the visiting hours are at the hospitals in their community.

○ □

Puppet Show

Have the class write and produce a puppet show about a child who has to go to the hospital to have his or her tonsils taken out. The play should dramatize what happens and feature people the child meets while in the hospital.

□ ☆

Speaker

Ask the students if they know who candy stripers are. Have a high school student who is a hospital volunteer talk about what she or he does at the hospital. Explain how students may become volunteers when they are older.

○ □ ☆

Articles

Ask students to bring in articles about hospitals from the newspaper and magazines. Discuss with them the meaning of malpractice.

○ □ ☆

Malpractice Game

Have the class play the game Malpractice. You will need to make up a deck of fifty-three cards (old manila folders work well because they are sturdy and light colored). Print hospital occupations (see the accompanying suggestions) or hospital specialties on twenty-six cards, and make a duplicate card for each occupation or specialty. One card should be labeled "Malpractice."

This game can be played with four to eight children at one time. The object is to make the most pairs. Have one player deal the entire deck of cards. The first player draws a card from the person on the left. If the card matches one of his or her cards, the first player puts the pair down in front of him or her and receives another turn. The winner is the child who runs out of cards first and is not left holding the Malpractice card.

(Hospital occupations include Electrocardiograph Technician, Electroencephalograph Technician, Laboratory Assistant, Medical Assistant, X-ray Technician, Medical Illustrator, Medical Photographer, Music Therapist, Hospital Accountant, Hospital Purchasing Agent, Medical Record Librarian, Hospital Office Worker, Admitting Clerk, Hospital Librarian, Hospital Public Relations Director, Inhalation Therapist, Physical Therapist, Occupational Therapist, Prosthetist, Registered Nurse, Licensed Practical Nurse, Medical Doctor, Biomedical Engineer, Medical Technologist, Operating Room Technician, Cytotechnologist, Pharmacist, Medical Dietitian, Nurse Anesthetist, Medical Researcher, Circulation Technologist, Sanitarian, Ambulance Driver, Medical Secretary, Blood Bank Technologist, Geneticist, Histologist, and Pharmaceutical Sales Representative.)

○ □ ☆

Health Specialists Concentration

Another way to familiarize students with different kinds of health specialists and the kinds of general services they offer is through a Health Specialists Concentration game.* (A variation for use of this game with primary children would be to use pictures, for example, for an eye doctor, an eye; for a dentist, a tooth, etc.)

Game Materials   The materials for the game consist of a gameboard with twenty compartments. In ten random compartments, there are the names of various health specialists; and in the remaining ten, there are brief descriptions of the nature of the specialists' services. Each compartment has a numbered cover card which conceals the pertinent information. In addition, there is a judge's sheet with the correct combination of specialists and services identified.

Number of Players   For each gameboard, there are two players and one judge. (The game can be played with two teams and one judge; but this is a less desirable approach, because some members of a team could avoid involvement.)

Rules   The rules for the game are simple. Order of play can be determined by having the judge write a number between one and ten and allowing each player to choose a number. The one closest to the judge's is the first player. After order of play is determined, the first player chooses two numbers from the board.

The cover cards are removed, revealing two pieces of information. If there is no match, the cover cards are returned to

*Developed by Myrna A. Yeakle, Chairperson of Health and Safety Education Division, Eastern Michigan University, Ypsilanti, Michigan.

TABLE 15B-1 CONCENTRATION GAME SAMPLE KEY

Numbers	Description of Work	Specialist
5/20	Cardiologist	Heart Specialist
11/18	Dentist	General care of teeth
3/19	Dermatologist	Skin Specialist
1/16	General Practitioner	General Health care
4/7	Obstetrician	Cares for mother before baby is born
2/10	Ophtalmologist	Corrects vision problems/can perform eye surgery
6/13	Optometrist	Corrects vision problems
8/14	Oral Surgeon	Pulls teeth/performs mouth surgery
12/17	Orthodontist	Straightens teeth
9/15	Pediatrician	Children's doctor

their original positions on the gameboard and the second player takes a turn.

The game is terminated when all cover cards are removed from the board. The winner is the player who holds the most cover cards at the end of the game. In case of a tie, the player who received the last two cover cards loses.

Classroom Management of the Game Ideally, there would be sufficient gameboards for everyone in the class to be involved in a team of three. If you had thirty students in your class, you would need ten gameboards. Since there are so many different kinds of health specialists, each gameboard can be different, although there can be some repetition. In this way, the game can be used for sev-eral rounds before the students have a chance to learn all the health specialists.

Construction of the Game Construction of the gameboard is relatively simple and inexpensive. Use a large sheet of heavy display board to make the gameboard sturdy. Poster board can be used for the twenty health specialists and brief description cards, and construction paper can be used for the twenty cover cards. Use a small exacto knife to make slits in the display board to hold the game cards.

The key in Table 15B-1 (or another one of your choice) can be used by the judge.

□ ☆

Children's Hospital Game

The Children's Hospital gameboard can be made by taping together the four game sheets (Atlas Figure 104).* Fasten the entire game sheet to cardboard for more support. Cut sixteen small circles and thirty-eight larger circles (use pattern below) from colored poster board. *Label* the circles (e.g., "Infant Care Area") so that there are two matching circles for every circle on the gameboard except "Patient Services—Admitting," which will have

Pattern for cover circles

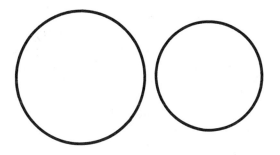

*Game developed by Sharon Pottebaum.

no cover. The four circles that remain should be labeled "Wild Card."

Markers can be two to four small squares of construction paper of different colors, colored wood tokens, etc. The only other material required is one die.

Rules for Playing   There are two to four players. The object of the game is to be the first player to match all his or her circles on the gameboard and land on the exit space after passing through the outpatient clinic.

Since there are two covers per medical area, it is likely that some of the areas will be covered by other players before a player can reach them. In that case, after a player has made all the matches open to him or her, he or she should head for the exit. The first player to land on the exit space may automatically dispose of one additional circle. The winner will be the player with the least number of circles (if any) remaining after one person has completed the game.

With two players, players draw (or deal) twelve circles (four small, eight large); with three players, eight circles (two small, six large); with four players, six circles (two small, four large).

Roll a die to see who goes first (largest number). To cover a circle on the gameboard with a matching circle, a player must move the number of spaces indicated after tossing the die and land exactly on the circle. Whenever a player makes a match, he or she may take another turn.

If a circle is already covered the player cannot land on it and must take another path or go backwards. A player may jump over a covered circle (counting it as one square) on the way to another circle. A player may also land on or pass over any other circle area on the gameboard that is not covered, counting the circle as one space, on the way. A wild card can be used to cover any circle.

○ □

Hospital Maze

The students can also learn the names of specific sections of a hospital by playing Children's Hospital First-Floor Maze (Atlas Figure 105). Duplicate enough copies of the pattern for all the students that want to complete the puzzle in their spare time.

Evaluation

LIFESTYLE CONTENT

○ □ ☆

Have the students identify at least five specific sections in a hospital. Were they able to list more than they did on their pretest?

□ ☆

After talking about laboratory tests can the students identify three ways disease-producing microorganisms are identified? (Through studying sputum, pus, blood, urine, tissue scrapings).

☆

Matching Quiz

Have the students match the instrument or test with the correct description:

_____ 1. Used to detect fractures and the presence of tumors.

_____ 2. These samples are sent to the chemistry lab to be searched for abnormal concentrations of substances which may be clues to disease.

_____ 3. Instrument that makes recordings of the electrical activity of the heart.

_____ 4. A special device used to produce heat in body tissues.

____ 5. An instrument that makes recordings of the electrical activity in the brain.
____ 6. A way for delivering oxygen to sick
persons at critical periods.
____ 7. A machine that can help people to
breathe.
  a. Diathermy
  b. Electroencephalograph
  c. X-rays
  d. Respirator
  e. Oxygen tent
  f. Electrocardiograph
  g. Blood and urine
  h. Samples of tissue

(ANSWERS: *1. c 2. g 3. f 4. a 5. b
6. e 7. d)*

LIFESTYLE VALUE

☆

Have the class debate whether the cost of
medical care is too high, covering the following subjects:

  doctors' salaries
  a day in a hospital
  the cost of new medical equipment

☆

Discuss with the class whether there
should be a limit on how much money is
spent to keep a person alive.

☆

Discuss with the class whether a hospital
should spend huge sums of money for a
new machine that could save the lives of
six people a year.

☆

Discuss with the class the following situation: a person cannot live without being
attached to a lot of machines in a hospital
and asks to have all the machines turned
off.
  Have the students consider whether

the people caring for the person should
turn the machines off when they are ded-
icated to keeping people alive.

UNIT V: SCHOOL AND COMMUNITY HEALTH HELPERS

Previous sections of this book have ex-
plored selecting good medical care, different kinds of medical specialists, and
hospital occupations. However, other
school and community health helpers
have not been discussed in much detail.

This unit is designed to give the students a general knowledge of the wide
variety of health services available in almost every community and to promote an
attitude of cooperation, respect, and appreciation for the health helpers they
meet.

OBJECTIVES

1. Each student will research the training and duties of a different health helper
and present an oral or written report of
his or her findings.

2. The students will be able to differentiate between different health helpers
by playing the What's My Line game, role
playing the duties of a health helper, or
both.

3. The students (in small groups) will
select a voluntary health organization,
write a letter requesting information
about the organization, and present their
findings to the class in the form of a skit,
puppet show, etc.

4. Given a drawing of twelve symbols,
the student will be able to correctly identify and match a minimum of six voluntary health agencies with their appropriate trademarks.

MATERIALS

1. Atlas Figure 60, Symbols of Voluntary Health Agencies.

2. Paper, pencils, crayons, small mirrors.

3. Various speakers from the school and community (optional).

Methods

○ □

Begin a discussion by asking the students to name people they think are health helpers. Remind them that parents and teachers are health helpers, because they look out for the well-being of children. The students will probably recall a doctor, dentist, dental hygienist, nurse, and eye doctor as well. Explain that a health helper is a person at school, home, or in the community who helps keep people healthy.

○ □

Bulletin Board

Cut pictures from magazines, or let the students draw pictures of health helpers in the community. The class may even decide to take photographs of health helpers they know and display the photos on the health helpers bulletin board.

○ □ ☆

Speakers

Invite the school nurse, school psychologist, and speech therapist to speak to the class.

○ □

Research

Make a set of cards, with each card containing the name of a health profession. Have each student draw a card and research the profession. The student should learn what kind of training is required for the profession and what some of the duties may include. Have each student present her or his findings to the class.

School Psychologist

Present the following introduction to the class. We all have some kinds of problems that we must cope with every day, don't we? I'm going to talk about some problems you might have at school or at home, and I want you to show me how you would solve these problems. (Allow the students to role play or discuss several different solutions.)

1. Imagine that you left your lunch money or your lunchbox at home this morning. How would you solve this problem? How long would this problem bother you?

2. What would you do if you had borrowed your brother's baseball bat, left it out on the playground, and couldn't find it when you went back to look for it? How long would this problem bother you?

3. You are sitting at the dinner table and accidentally spill your milk. How would you solve this problem? How long would this problem bother you?

4. You stayed up to watch the monster movie on TV and were very much frightened by the monster. You are afraid to go to bed, you don't go right to sleep, and when you do sleep you have nightmares that wake you up. What would you do to solve this problem? How long do you think it would take to solve this problem?

5. When you were younger you were bitten in the face by a big dog that knocked you down. Now whenever you see a large dog you get frightened and start to cry. Is there anything else you can

do to solve your problem? How long do you think it would take to solve this problem?

The students should begin to realize that some problems are easily solved, some must be worked out within the family, and some problems cannot be solved without outside help.

Explain that when someone has a problem that he or she cannot find an answer for or does not know how to solve, the person could go to the school psychologist, who helps with problems that people cannot solve by themselves— the ones that bother people for a long time.

○ □

Visit School Psychologist

Arrange to have the class visit the school psychologist's office. Have the psychologist show the class what he or she uses in his or her work and explain why the school district hires a school psychologist as a health helper.

○ □

Ask the students to tell a story about a problem they once had and the way they solved it.

SPEECH

Give the students the following directions:

Stand up.
Turn around three times.
Stamp your foot.
Sit down.

Ask the students how they knew what to do just now. They will probably say by the words that were said.

○ □

Mirror Activity

Tell the students that words are made up of different sounds. Ask if they want to see themselves making sounds. Let the students choose partners and share one mirror between the two of them. Tell them that you will write a list of words on the blackboard; ask them to say each word slowly three or four times, looking in the mirror as they say the word. Ask them to see if they can find out what parts of their mouths help them to form the words. Have them take turns saying the words and using the mirrors. (Have a list of eight to ten words prepared that you know the class can read.)

Ask the students what helps them make the sounds of the words they said (tongue, teeth, and roof of the mouth.) Ask what they think would happen if they could not say all of the sounds (they could not say all of the words they wished to say and might not be understood).

○ □

Speech Therapist

Introduce the speech therapist for the school. Explain that this person can help the students learn to say sounds that they have trouble with. Let the therapist explain what she or he does and describe some of the activities that are used during therapy.

○

Making Sounds

Have the students make the sounds of various animals, insects, or machines. Ask them to tell you what parts of their mouths they used in making each sound. Discuss how the animal, insect, or machine makes its sound.

○ □

Feeling the Throat and Lips

Have the students put their hands on their throat and lips to feel the movement that happens during speech. Call attention to sounds that they have difficulty with in words of songs, poems, or stories. Have the students try to say the following tongue twisters very fast three times:

The big black bug bled blue blood.
She sells seashells down by the seashore.

○ □

Veterinarian

Explain to the class that studies have shown that most families today have some kind of pet. Tell them that pets need medical assistance just as people do. Invite a veterinarian to your class or arrange a field trip to his or her office. Have the veterinarian discuss ways that he or she helps prevent illness and describe some of his or her other duties. Have the students write a short paper comparing the kind of work a veterinarian does with the work of a medical doctor.

○ □

School Custodian

Discuss with the class the kinds of things that are important in creating a healthy school environment (cleanliness, clean water supply, adequate lighting, good heating, proper ventilation).

Invite the school custodian to the classroom so that the students can get to know him or her. Have the custodian explain how he or she is a health helper and possibly suggest some simple ways the students can help keep the school clean and healthy.

○ □

School Walking Tour

Take the class on a walking tour through the school. Ask the students to examine the restrooms, lighting, vents, windows, heat registers, floors, walks, and emergency exits to see if they can discover any hazardous conditions. If they do find some, discuss what they think should be done about them. A class project may involve correcting or at least bettering the situation. Another project could be to make a bulletin board in the hall for others to see that stresses the necessity of healthy and safe school conditions.

○ □

Cafeteria Manager

Invite the cafeteria manager to speak to the class. Show the filmstrip *Safeguarding Our Food** or any other film that is appropriate and available. The film will probably raise some questions that the cafeteria manager can answer. She or he can discuss the importance of sanitary conditions (garbage and trash disposal, incinerators, kitchen grinders, clean restrooms, personal cleanliness of employees, ways to sanitize dishes, and the preparation and storage of food). The students could make a chart listing the most important sanitary conditions which should exist in the school cafeteria and check them throughout the year. Related activities could include planning well-balanced meals and improving sanitation in the home.

○ □

Sanitation Worker

Ask the students the following questions. Is the person who collects the garbage a

*By Young American Films.

health helper? What do you think would happen if this service were discontinued? Is there any way you can help with the problem of trash disposal? Do you know the names of any diseases that are connected with unsanitary conditions?

□ ☆
What's My Line?

After the students have learned about many of the health helpers, have them play the game What's My Line? Let each student select a health helper to portray or have her or him draw a name at random. You may want to give the students time to further research the persons they are supposed to represent. Divide the class into groups of four so that every student gets a chance to be on the panel. Each panelist may ask the contestant yes or no questions for so long as the answer is yes. If the answer is no, the next panelist takes a turn. Each no counts as one point. While taking a turn, a panelist who thinks he or she knows the occupation of the contestant may guess it. If the panelist is wrong, the game continues until the correct occupation is guessed or ten points have been collected.

Change panels and play a new game with another contestant. After all of the panels have had a chance to question a contestant, see which panel collected the fewest number of points. That panel is the winner. In the case of a tie, play two more games with one contestant for each panel.

□ ☆
Voluntary Health Organization

Give the students a list of the town's voluntary health organizations and their addresses. Divide the students into small groups and let them each select a differ-

ent voluntary health organization to research. The students should write a letter to their chosen organization and request information about it. After the information arrives, the students should be given time to prepare and present their findings to the rest of the class. The students may want to give a skit, compose a poem or song, produce a puppet show, etc.

□ ☆
Voluntary Health Agency Trademarks

Have the students draw the trademark that represents their chosen health organization if they can locate one. Make a bulletin board of various voluntary health agency trademarks. Show them a transparency of Atlas Figure 60.

□ ☆
What's My Organization?

A game called What's My Organization? can be played like What's My Line?, using voluntary health organizations rather than occupations. A list of voluntary health organizations follows.

Alcoholics Anonymous
American Cancer Society
American Diabetes Association
American Heart Association
American National Red Cross
Arthritis Foundation of America
Association for the Aid of Crippled Children
Epilepsy Association of America
Leukemia Society, Inc.
Muscular Dystrophy Association of America
The Myasthenia Gravis Foundation, Inc.
National Association for Mental Health, Inc.

National Association for Retarded Children, Inc.

National Council on Alcoholism

National Cystic Fibrosis Research Foundation

National Foundation—March of Dimes

National Hemophilia Foundation

National Kidney Foundation

National Multiple Sclerosis Society

National Parkinson Foundation, Inc.

National Society for the Prevention of Blindness

National Tuberculosis and Respiratory Disease Association

Parkinson's Disease Foundation, Inc.

Planned Parenthood Federation of America

United Cerebral Palsy Association

□ ☆

Perhaps the class would like to select a voluntary health organization to donate money to. Let the students decide ways that they could earn money, such as by washing cars, doing odd jobs around the house, mowing lawns or shoveling snow, babysitting, and having a bake sale.

Evaluation

LIFESTYLE CONTENT

□ ☆

After the students have completed the activities in this unit and played What's My Line?, they should be able to complete the following matching activities.

____ 1. Registered Nurse
____ 2. School Psychologist
____ 3. Speech Therapist
____ 4. Veterinarian
____ 5. School Custodian
____ 6. Cafeteria Manager
____ 7. Physician

____ 8. Sanitation Worker
____ 9. Dentist
____ 10. Health Agency Volunteer Worker

a. A person who tries to preserve health and prevent disease; may prescribe drugs and perform surgery.

b. A person who helps take care of sick people and assists the doctor.

c. A person who can help people with problems they do not know how to solve.

d. A person who helps prevent disease by removing the garbage.

e. A person who can help people say sounds that they have trouble with.

f. A person who tries to keep the school clean and healthy.

g. A person who tries to keep pets healthy and cares for them when they are sick.

h. A person who specializes in keeping people's teeth and gums healthy.

i. A person who helps educate the public about a special health problem and raise money for more research.

j. A person who is concerned with kitchen cleanliness and proper preparation and storage of foods.

(ANSWERS: *1. b 2. c 3. e 4. g 5. f 6. j 7. a 8. d 9. h 10. i*)

□ ☆

Again show the students the transparency Symbols of Voluntary Health Agencies (in Atlas). Have them number on paper from 1 to 12 and list as many of the organizations as they can that correspond with the symbols that are shown. For a variation, have the students match the symbols with the following organizations:

1. ____   a. National Society for the Prevention of Blindness

440

2. ____ b. Epilepsy Foundation of America

3. ____ c. The National Foundation—March of Dimes

4. ____ d. American National Red Cross

5. ____ e. National Multiple Sclerosis Society

6. ____ f. American Heart Association

7. ____ g. United Cerebral Palsy Association

8. ____ h. American Cancer Society

9. ____ i. National Tuberculosis and Respiratory Disease Association

10. ____ j. Muscular Dystrophy Association of America

11. ____ k. National Kidney Foundation

12. ____ l. Easter Seal–National Society for Crippled Children and Adults

(ANSWERS: *1. b 2. e 3. a 4. j 5. d 6. c 7. h 8. f 9. k 10. l 11. i 12. g*)

LIFESTYLE VALUE

○ □ ☆

To evaluate the feelings and values formed from the lesson School and Community Health Helpers, have the students answer the following questions.

I never thought of _____ as being a health helper until we had this unit on health helpers. Now I know that this person is important because _____
_____
_____ .

I think the three most important health helpers in my school are _____ , _____ , and _____ , because _____
_____
_____ .

I think the three most important health helpers in my community are _____ , _____ , and _____ ,

because _____
_____
_____ .

REFERENCES

1. "1970 Consumer Expenditures," *Supermarketing* 26 (1971): 39.

ADDITIONAL REFERENCES FOR CONSUMER HEALTH AND MEDICAL CARE

Consumer Health

American Medical Association. Many pamphlets are available, including *Chiropractic: The Unscientific Cult; Facts on Quacks; Health Quackery; Mail Fraud; The Merchants of Menace;* and *Your Money and Your Life,* to mention a few.

U.S. Food and Drug Administration. Pamphlets such as *Consumer Protection—Drugs and Cosmetics; Consumer Protection—Foods; Hot Tips on Food Protection; How Safe Is Our Food? Read the Label;* and *Safe New Drugs* are available.

American Dental Association. *Folklore and Fallacies in Dentistry.*

Pharmaceutical Manufacturers Association. Many pamphlets, including *Key Facts About the Drug Industry; The Medicines Your Doctor Prescribes.*

Money Management Institute. *Your Clothing Dollar; Your Food Dollar; Your Health and Recreation Dollar.*

Medical Care

American Academy of Pediatrics, P. O. Box 1034, Evanston, IL 60204.

American Chiropractic Association, 2200 Grand Avenue, Des Moines, IA 50312.

American Dental Association, 211 East Chicago Avenue, Chicago, IL 60611.

American Dietetic Association, 620 N. Michigan Avenue, Chicago, IL 60611.

American Hospital Association, 840 North Lake Shore Drive, Chicago, IL 60611.

American Medical Association, Department of Health Education, 535 North Dearborn Street, Chicago, IL 60610.

American Nurses Association, 2420 Pershing Road, Kansas City, MO 64180.

American Optometric Association, 243 N. Lindbergh Blvd., St. Louis, MO 63141.

American Podiatry Association, Council on Education, 20 Chevy Chase Circle, Washington, D.C. 20015.

National League for Nursing, 59th Street and Columbus Circle, New York, NY 10019.

Also contact Consumer Product Information, Pueblo, CO 81009, for information about health products and services.

TOWARD AN EXCITING CLASSROOM

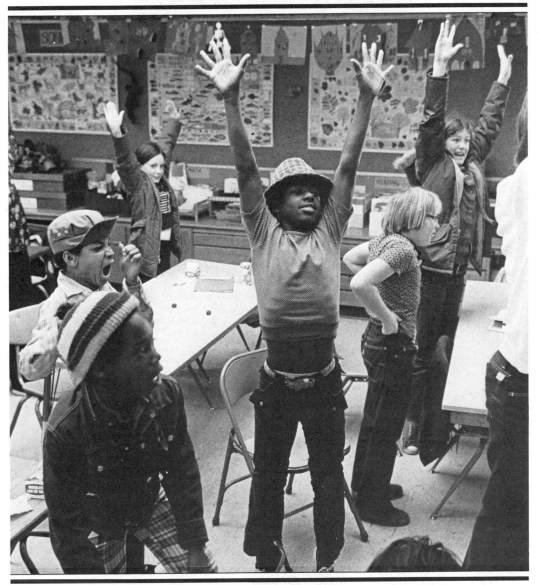

AN ATLAS OF
INSTRUCTIONAL MATERIALS

CHAPTER 16A
OVERHEAD PROJECTION
AND TRANSPARENCIES

The overhead projector is one of the simplest visual communication devices available. It is simple to maintain and can be used as easily for large group instruction as for conventional size classes and smaller groups. Since light is transmitted through translucent material to a nearby screen, the projected image can be viewed in a lighted room.

Many teachers are regular users of overhead projectors because they can completely control their presentation, encourage the participation of every student in the class, disclose ideas in sequence, and prepare their materials ahead of time. The teacher can hold student attention by writing, pointing, underlining with color, and using overlays as part of the presentation.

Commercially prepared transparencies range from simple printed materials on clear film to elaborate color presentations with multiple overlays. Transparency masters can be purchased in printed form in packages or in loose leaf binders or taken from this book. With the master sheets found in this section, transparencies can be prepared in a few seconds with the use of any thermographic (heat process) machine having an infrared light source to expose the film to original materials. Depending on the film selected, the image may be black on a clear background, black on any one of a number of colors, or clear on a black background.

Transparencies made with the heat process method require the original drawing to be done in india ink, soft lead pencil, or black printing ink, since these marks absorb heat. Drawings done with ballpoint pen or colored printing ink and spirit-duplicator copies will not reproduce.

Transparencies can be colored by using translucent inks, cellophanes and foils, and adhesive-backed films and translucent letters and lines purchased from an art supply house. Colored liquids can be mixed on glass trays to produce psychedelic effects. Movement can be suggested by employing patented Technamation materials to polarize light. When projected, the image from the transparency passes through a rotating spinner of polarized glass which makes wheels seem to turn and fluids to flow.

Some teachers move colored plastic cutout pieces around on the projector stage to tell a story rather than using a felt board or add additional acetate sheets (overlays) to a basic transparency. Progressive disclosure is a related technique in which the instructor covers a transparency with a piece of paper (temporary use) or hinged pieces of light cardboard (permanent use) and reveals information step by step.

Additional Hints When Teaching with Transparencies

The following ideas can be useful when using transparencies in the classroom:

1. Direct attention to details in a diagram by placing a pointer or sharpened pencil directly on the transparency.

2. Add details to transparencies with felt pen or wax-based pencil before or during projection, making sure the marks can be removed unless they are intended to be permanent.

3. Create your own overlays to add new material to commercial transparencies.

4. When you use prepared masters, such as the printed materials in this At-

las, consider adapting them to the needs of your class by changing vocabulary that is too advanced for your students; adding such indicators as underlines and arrows to the master with a soft lead pencil or carbon ink; and cutting up the master to eliminate certain parts, rearrange material, or make two transparencies from one master. If you do not wish to deface the original, use a copying machine to make a paper duplicate and do your editing on that.

Teaching Illustrations for Preparing Transparencies

The illustrations in this section can be used in any order, although they have been included under chapter headings to correlate with additional information in the textbook.

Chapter 7B Teaching About Drugs, Alcohol, and Tobacco

Figure 1, Mother Monkey Reads the Label and Follows the Directions

Figure 2, Physical and Emotional Effects of Alcohol

Figure 3, Smoking Cigarettes May Cause . . .

Figure 4, Maslow's Basic Needs Hierarchy

Figure 5, Decision-Making

Chapter 8B Teaching About the Human Body and Grooming

Figure 6, Your Body Is Made of Millions of Tiny Cells

Figure 7, Muscle Types

Figure 8, Animal Hearts

Figure 9, Front View of Urinary Organs

Figure 10, The Brain and Its Functions

Figure 11, Nerve Cell/Reflex Action

Figure 12, The Endocrine Glands

Figure 13, Male Secondary Sex Characteristics

Figure 14, Female Secondary Sex Characteristics

Figure 15, Inserting the Tampon

Chapter 9B Teaching About Exercise, Rest and Relaxation

Figure 16, Posture

Chapter 11B Teaching About Dental Health

Figure 17, Functions of Teeth

Figure 18, Primary and Permanent Teeth

Figure 19, How Does a Tooth Grow?

Figure 20, Parts of a Tooth

Figure 21, Process of Tooth Decay

Figure 22, Special Tools for Cleaning the Teeth

Figure 23, Flossing Demonstration

Figure 24, What Is Your Dental I.Q.?

Chapter 12B Teaching About Disease Control and Prevention

Diabetes Series (9 illustrations)

Figure 25, Location of Pancreas

Figure 26, Diabetes Symptoms and Risk Factors

Figure 27, Insulin-Producing Cells

Figure 28, What Happens When There Is Not Enough Insulin?

Figure 29, Weight Loss

Figure 30, Diabetic Acidosis Resulting in Hospitalization

Figure 31, Diabetes Roulette—Review the Facts

Figure 32, Tests and Treatments

Figure 33, Responsibilities of a Diabetic

Chapter 13B Teaching About the Environment

Figure 34, An Ecosystem

Chapter 14B   Teaching About Safety and First Aid

Policeman Fred Series (9 illustrations)

Figure 35, Never Open the Door for Strangers

Figure 36, Obey Traffic Signals

Figure 37, Be Extra Careful on Rainy Days

Figure 38, Riding Double Leads to Trouble

Figure 39, Always Use Bike Hand Signals—Obey All Traffic Signs and Signals

Figure 40, Obey Your School Patrol

Figure 41, Play It Safe—Keep the Green Pennant Flying

Figure 42, If You are Lost or Go Astray

Figure 43, Taking Candy from a Stranger . . .

Figure 44, A Trip Through Safetyland

Chapter 15B   Teaching About Consumer Health and Medical Care

Medical Instrument Cartoon Series (12 illustrations)

Figure 45, Scales (Reduce If Overweight)

Figure 46, Thermometer

Figure 47, Sphygmomanometer (Control High Blood Pressure)

Figure 48, Otoscope (Examining the Ear)

Figure 49, Audiometer (Ear Test)

Figure 50, Tongue Depressor

Figure 51, Ophthalmoscope (Examining the Eye)

Figure 52, Eye Chart

Figure 53, Refractor Machine Used for Prescribing Eyeglasses and Examining Eyes

Figure 54, Stethoscope

Figure 55, Hypodermic Syringe

Figure 56, X-ray Machine

Figure 57, Structure of the Human Ear

Figure 58, Function of the Lens and Brain

Figure 59, Structure of the Eye

Figure 60, Symbols of Voluntary Health Agencies

FIGURE 1
MOTHER MONKEY READS
THE LABEL AND FOLLOWS
THE DIRECTIONS

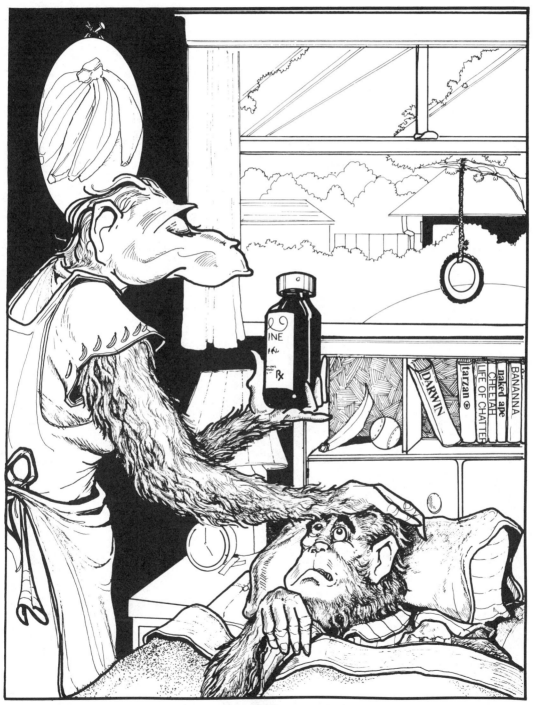

FIGURE 2
PHYSICAL AND EMOTIONAL EFFECTS OF ALCOHOL

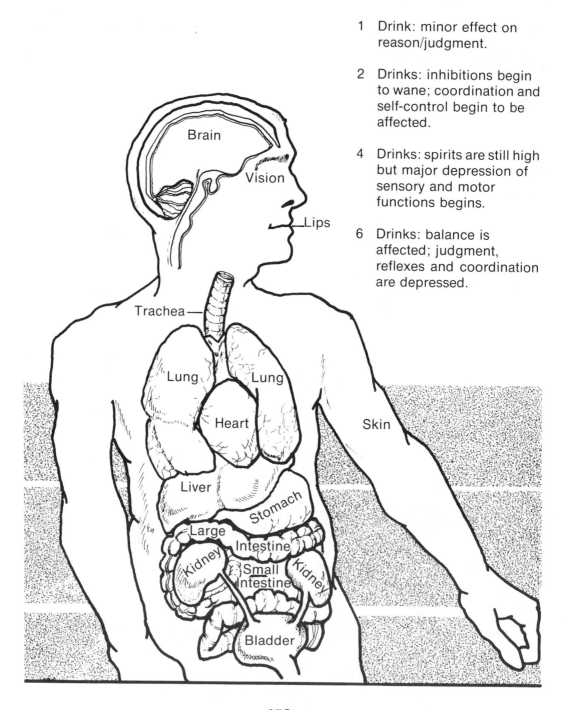

1 Drink: minor effect on reason/judgment.

2 Drinks: inhibitions begin to wane; coordination and self-control begin to be affected.

4 Drinks: spirits are still high but major depression of sensory and motor functions begins.

6 Drinks: balance is affected; judgment, reflexes and coordination are depressed.

FIGURE 3
SMOKING CIGARETTES MAY
CAUSE. . .

CHAPTER 7B, UNIT IV

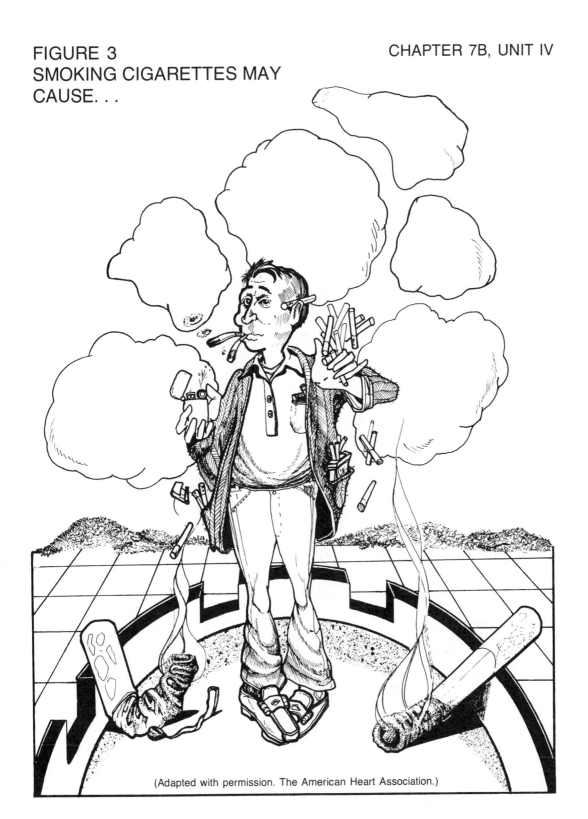

(Adapted with permission. The American Heart Association.)

FIGURE 4
MASLOW'S BASIC NEEDS
HIERARCHY

CHAPTER 7B, UNIT V

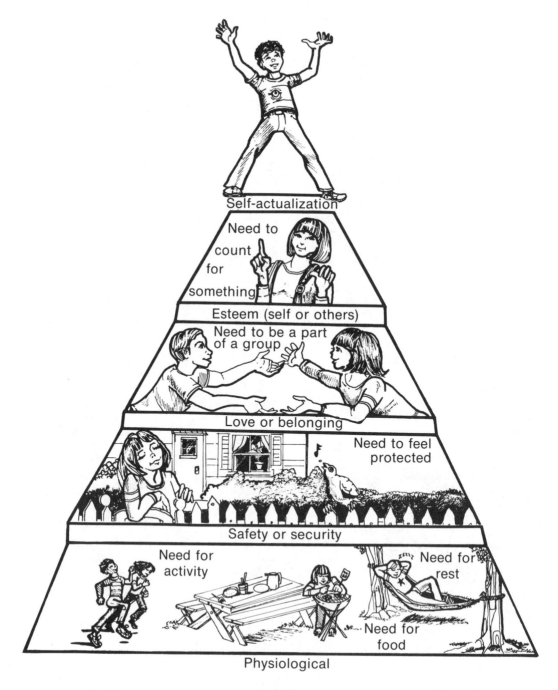

FIGURE 5   CHAPTER 7B, UNIT V

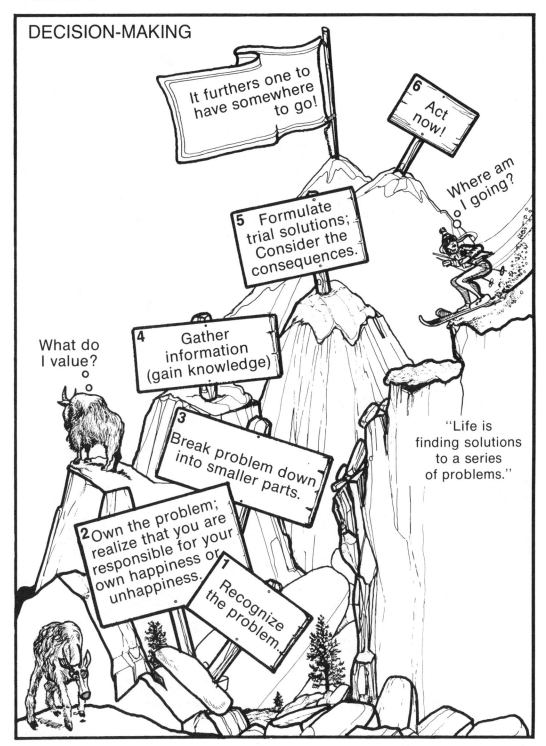

FIGURE 6
YOUR BODY IS MADE OF
MILLIONS OF TINY CELLS
JOINED TOGETHER TO
FORM BODY
TISSUE

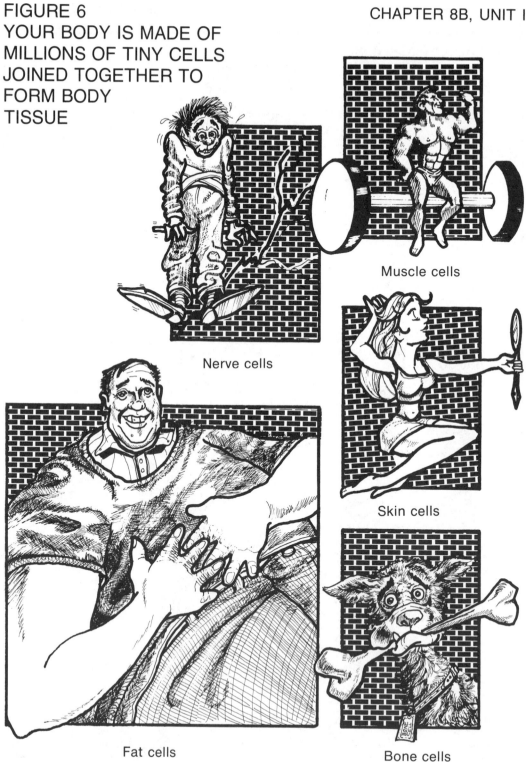

Nerve cells

Muscle cells

Skin cells

Fat cells

Bone cells

FIGURE 7
MUSCLE TYPES

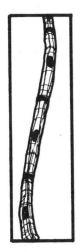

CARDIAC MUSCLE
(Imperfectly cross-striated, involuntary)
Single, centrally located nucleus.
Strong, rhythmical contractions.

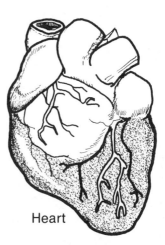

Heart

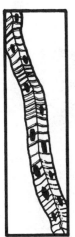

SKELETAL MUSCLE
(Striated, voluntary)
Fibers exhibit alternating light and dark
bands, called striations.
Multinucleated.
Quick, nonrhythmical contractions.

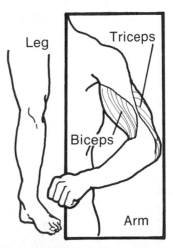

Leg

Triceps

Biceps

Arm

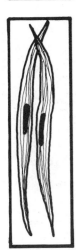

SMOOTH MUSCLE
(Visceral, involuntary)
No cross-striations.
Elongated oval nucleus.
Slow, rhythmical contractions.

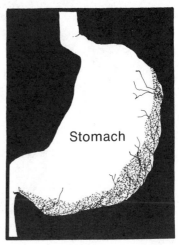

Stomach

FIGURE 8
ANIMAL HEARTS

CHAPTER 8B, UNIT III

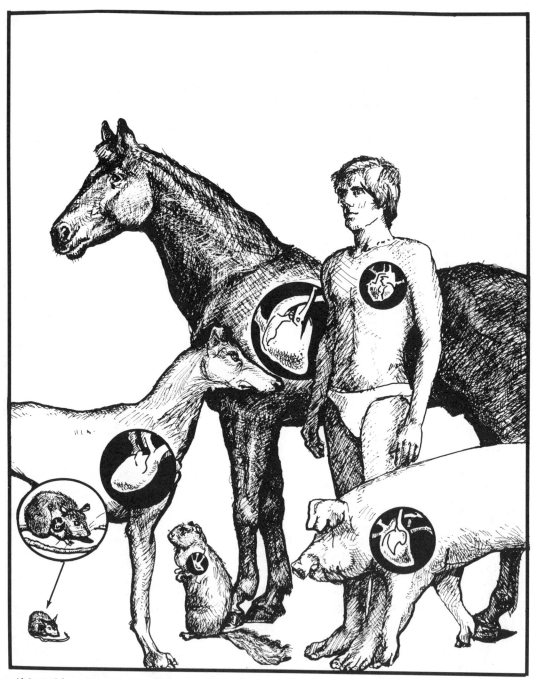

(Adapted from *Heart Project* with permission of The American Heart Association, Central Ohio Chapter, 200 East Rich St., Columbus, OH 43215. Format: New York State Education Department. Author: Donald Brown.)

FIGURE 9
FRONT VIEW OF URINARY
ORGANS

CHAPTER 8B, UNIT V

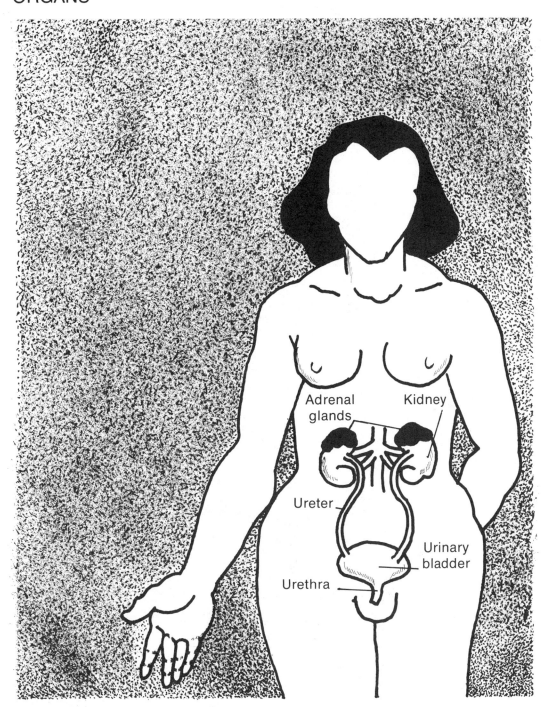

FIGURE 10
THE BRAIN AND
ITS FUNCTIONS

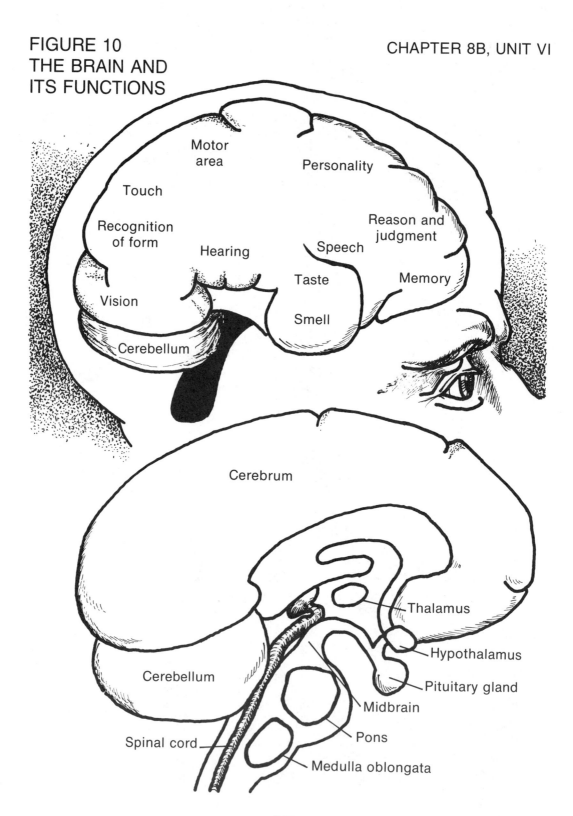

FIGURE 11
NERVE CELL/REFLEX
ACTION

CHAPTER 8B, UNIT VI

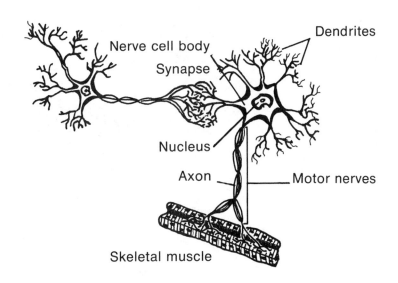

Nerve cell body

Synapse

Dendrites

Nucleus

Axon

Motor nerves

Skeletal muscle

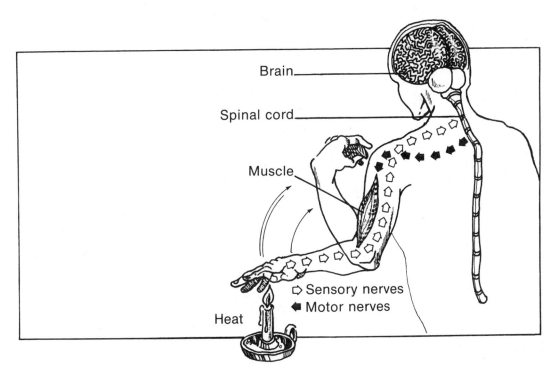

Brain

Spinal cord

Muscle

Heat

⇨ Sensory nerves
◄ Motor nerves

FIGURE 12
THE ENDOCRINE GLANDS

CHAPTER 8B, UNIT VIII

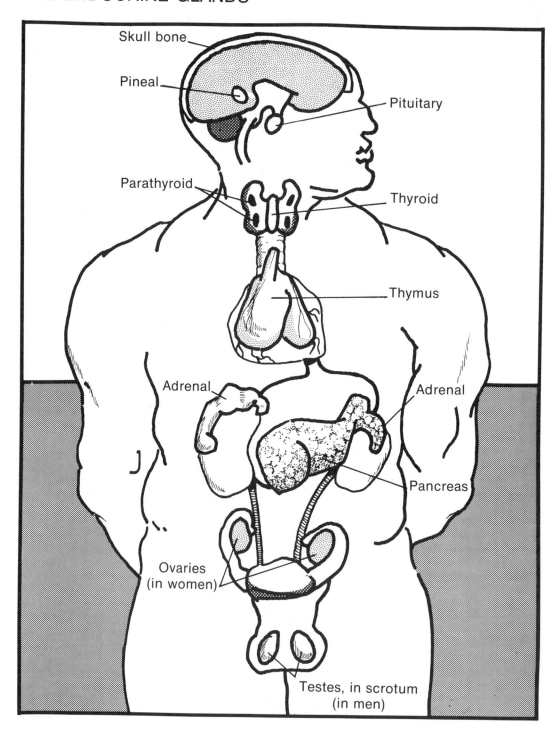

FIGURE 13
MALE SECONDARY SEX CHARACTERISTICS

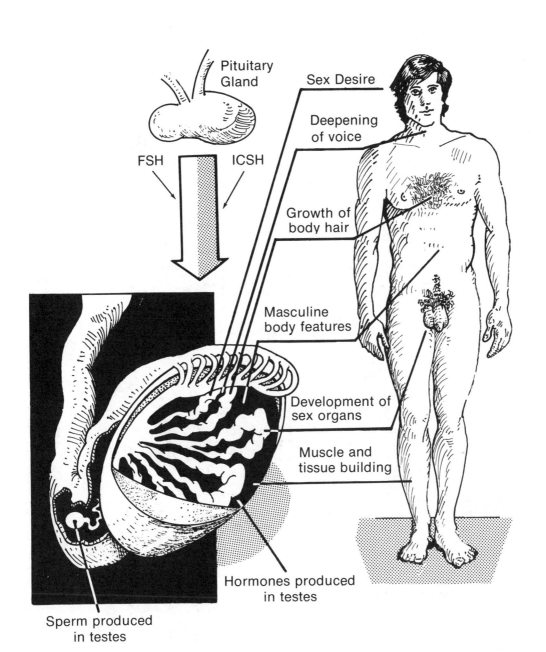

Pituitary Gland

Sex Desire

Deepening of voice

FSH   ICSH

Growth of body hair

Masculine body features

Development of sex organs

Muscle and tissue building

Hormones produced in testes

Sperm produced in testes

FIGURE 14
FEMALE SECONDARY SEX
CHARACTERISTICS

CHAPTER 8B, UNIT VIII

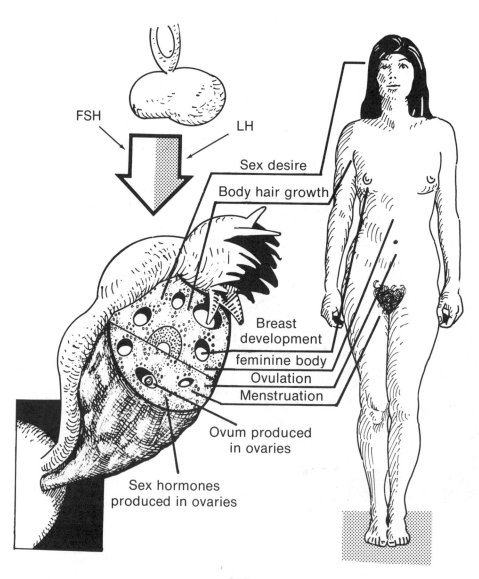

FSH

LH

Sex desire

Body hair growth

Breast
development

feminine body

Ovulation

Menstruation

Ovum produced
in ovaries

Sex hormones
produced in ovaries

FIGURE 15
INSERTING THE TAMPON

CHAPTER 8B, UNIT VIII

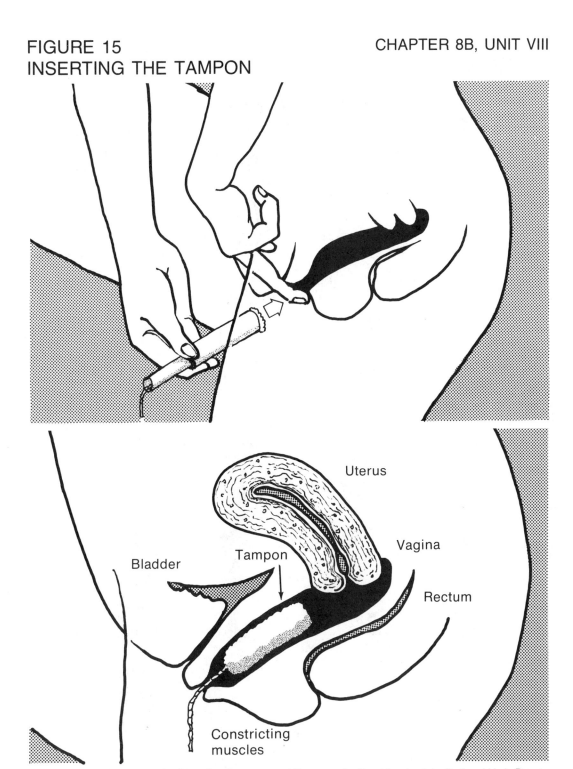

Uterus

Vagina

Bladder

Tampon

Rectum

Constricting
muscles

(Adapted from *Education for Sexuality: Concepts and Programs for Teaching,* by John Burt and Linda Brower Meeks, W. B. Saunders Co., 1970.)

FIGURE 16
POSTURE

CHAPTER 9B, UNIT III

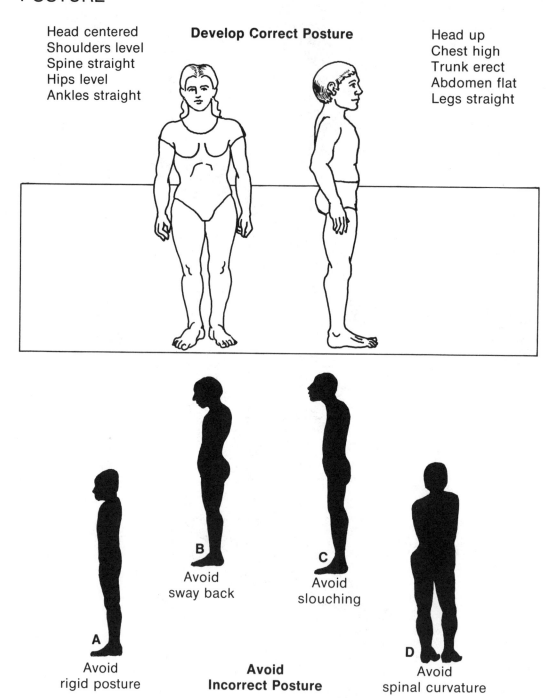

Head centered
Shoulders level
Spine straight
Hips level
Ankles straight

Develop Correct Posture

Head up
Chest high
Trunk erect
Abdomen flat
Legs straight

B
Avoid
sway back

C
Avoid
slouching

A
Avoid
rigid posture

**Avoid
Incorrect Posture**

D
Avoid
spinal curvature

(Adapted with permission of Reedco, Inc., 5 Easterly Ave., Auburn, NY 13021.)

FIGURE 17
FUNCTIONS OF TEETH

CHAPTER 11B, UNIT I

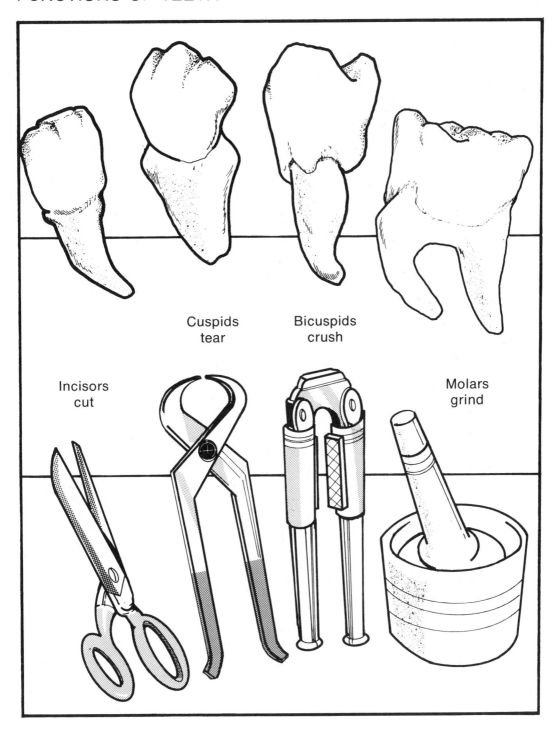

Cuspids
tear

Bicuspids
crush

Incisors
cut

Molars
grind

FIGURE 18
PRIMARY AND PERMANENT TEETH

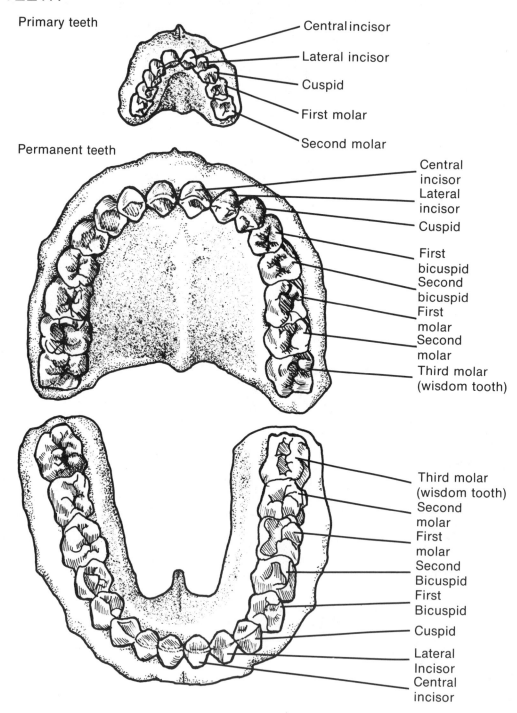

Primary teeth

Central incisor

Lateral incisor

Cuspid

First molar

Second molar

Permanent teeth

Central incisor

Lateral incisor

Cuspid

First bicuspid

Second bicuspid

First molar

Second molar

Third molar (wisdom tooth)

Third molar (wisdom tooth)

Second molar

First molar

Second Bicuspid

First Bicuspid

Cuspid

Lateral Incisor

Central incisor

FIGURE 19
HOW DOES A TOOTH GROW?

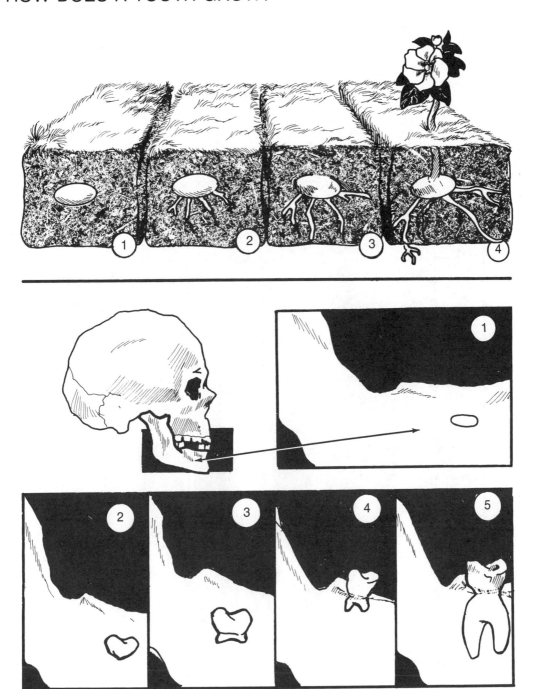

(Adapted from *Guidelines for a Dental Health Curriculum for Public Schools,* Columbus, Ohio. Courtesy Nancy J. Reynolds, D.D.S.)

FIGURE 20
PARTS OF A TOOTH

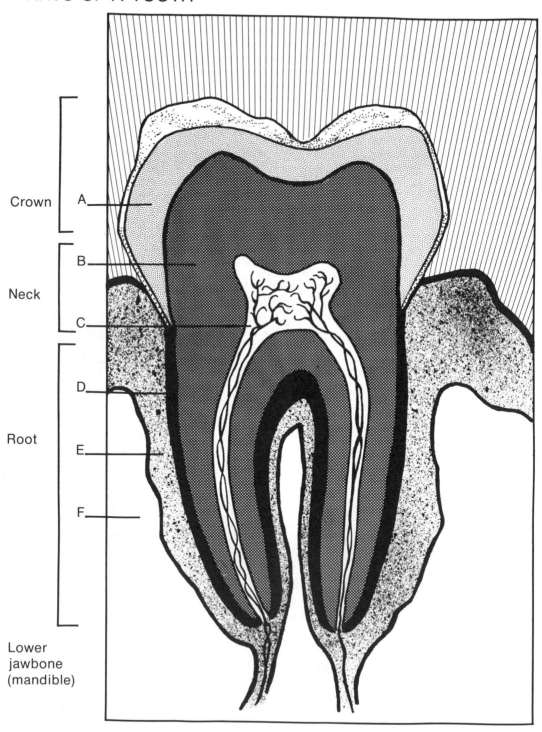

Crown

Neck

Root

Lower
jawbone
(mandible)

A

B

C

D

E

F

FIGURE 21
PROCESS OF TOOTH
DECAY

CHAPTER 11B, UNIT III

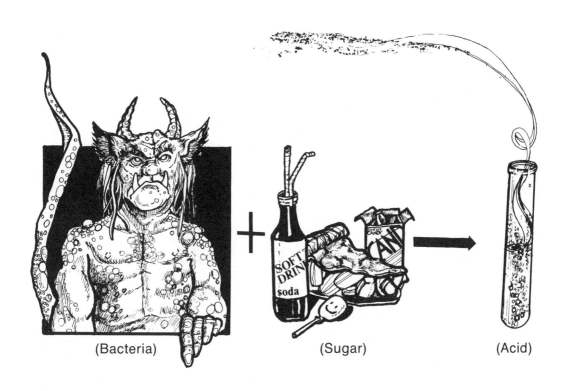

(Bacteria)   (Sugar)   (Acid)

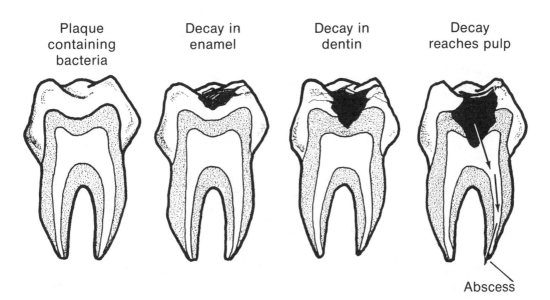

Plaque
containing
bacteria

Decay in
enamel

Decay in
dentin

Decay
reaches pulp

Abscess

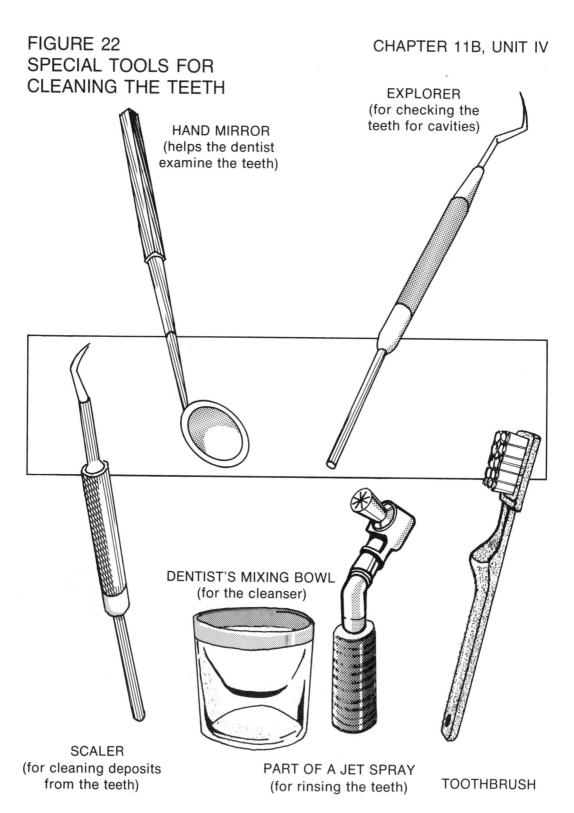

FIGURE 22
SPECIAL TOOLS FOR
CLEANING THE TEETH

CHAPTER 11B, UNIT IV

EXPLORER
(for checking the
teeth for cavities)

HAND MIRROR
(helps the dentist
examine the teeth)

DENTIST'S MIXING BOWL
(for the cleanser)

SCALER
(for cleaning deposits
from the teeth)

PART OF A JET SPRAY
(for rinsing the teeth)

TOOTHBRUSH

FIGURE 23
FLOSSING
DEMONSTRATION

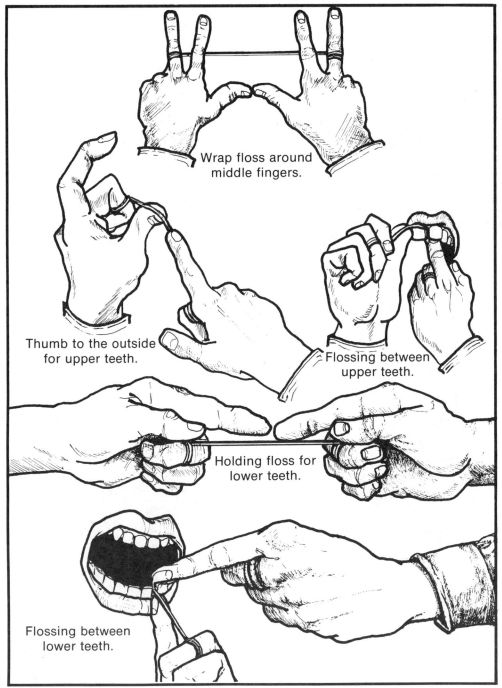

Wrap floss around middle fingers.

Thumb to the outside for upper teeth.

Flossing between upper teeth.

Holding floss for lower teeth.

Flossing between lower teeth.

(Adapted with permission, *The Ohio Program for Dental Health Education in Schools, Teachers Guide*, p. 48, and *Fifth Grade Manual*, p. 23, 1972, 1976. The Metropolitan Health Planning Corp., 908 Standard Building, Cleveland, OH 44113.)

FIGURE 24
WHAT IS YOUR DENTAL I.Q.?

CHAPTER 11B, UNIT V

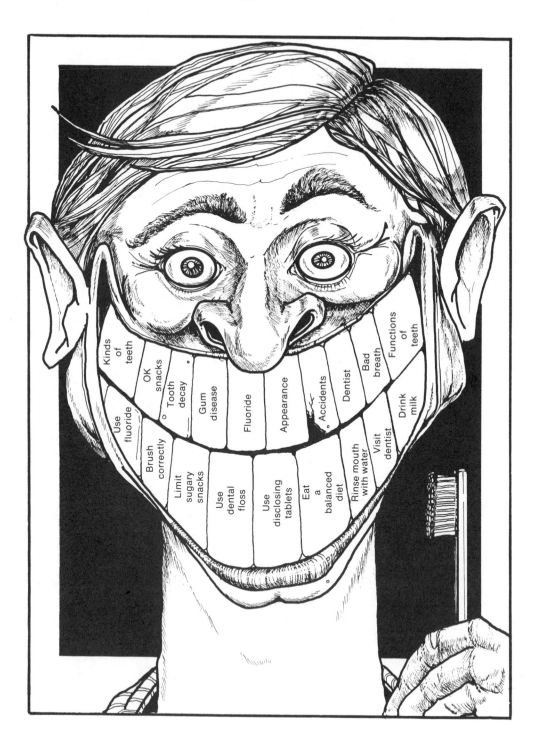

FIGURE 25
LOCATION OF PANCREAS

The pancrease is an organ in the body that makes insulin and glucagon.

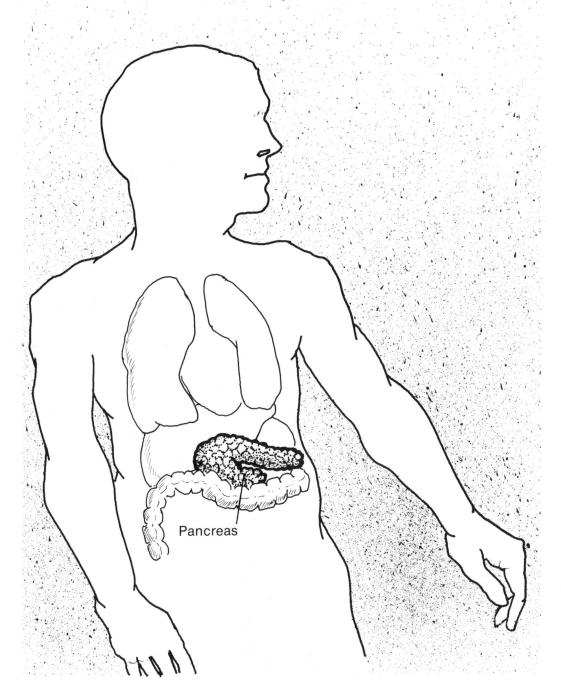

Pancreas

FIGURE 26
DIABETES SYMPTOMS AND
RISK FACTORS

CHAPTER 12B, UNIT III

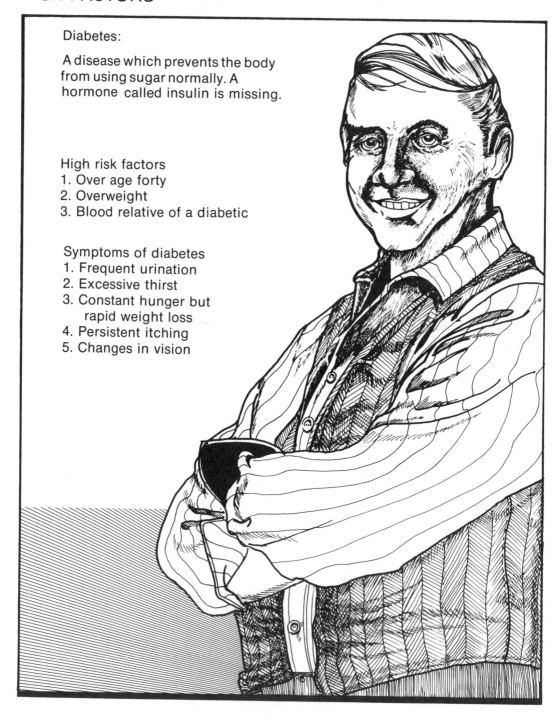

Diabetes:

A disease which prevents the body from using sugar normally. A hormone called insulin is missing.

High risk factors
1. Over age forty
2. Overweight
3. Blood relative of a diabetic

Symptoms of diabetes
1. Frequent urination
2. Excessive thirst
3. Constant hunger but rapid weight loss
4. Persistent itching
5. Changes in vision

FIGURE 27
INSULIN-PRODUCING CELLS

The normal pancreas produces several hormones including Insulin and Glucagon.

When an *adult* develops diabetes, *some* of the insulin-producing cells stop working.

When a *child* develops diabetes, *all* of the insulin-producing cells stop working.

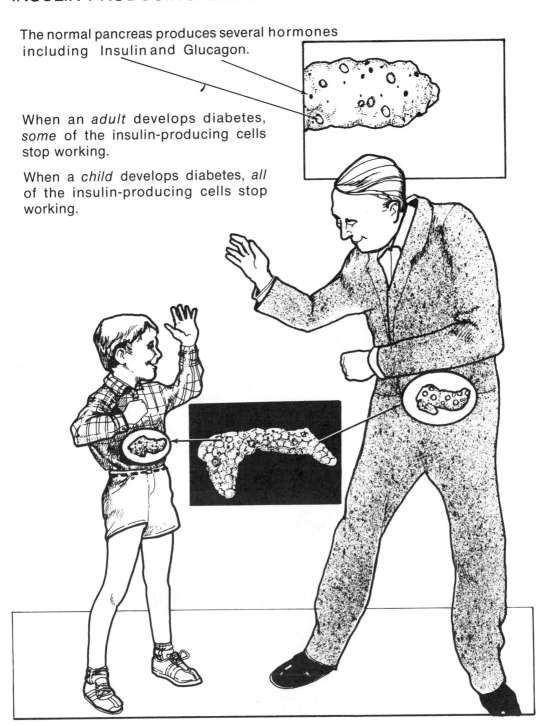

FIGURE 28
WHAT HAPPENS WHEN THERE IS NOT ENOUGH INSULIN?

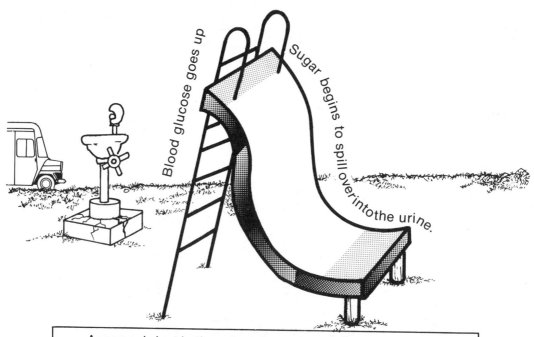

Blood glucose goes up

Sugar begins to spill over into the urine.

As sugar is lost in the urine, the amount of urine increases.

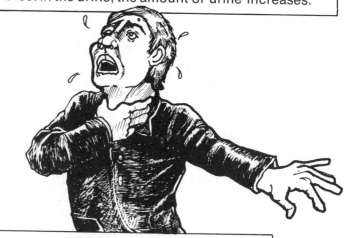

With the loss of urine water, the person develops an intense thirst.

FIGURE 29
WEIGHT LOSS

CHAPTER 12B, UNIT III

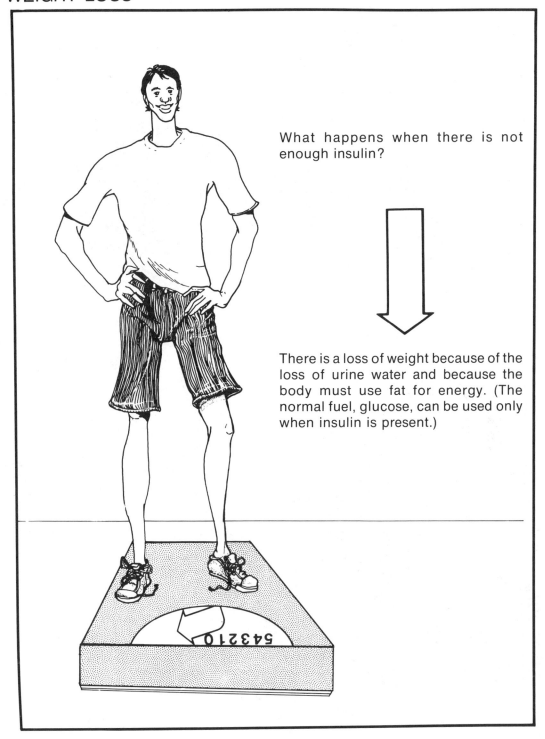

What happens when there is not enough insulin?

There is a loss of weight because of the loss of urine water and because the body must use fat for energy. (The normal fuel, glucose, can be used only when insulin is present.)

FIGURE 30
DIABETIC ACIDOSIS RESULTING IN HOSPITALIZATION

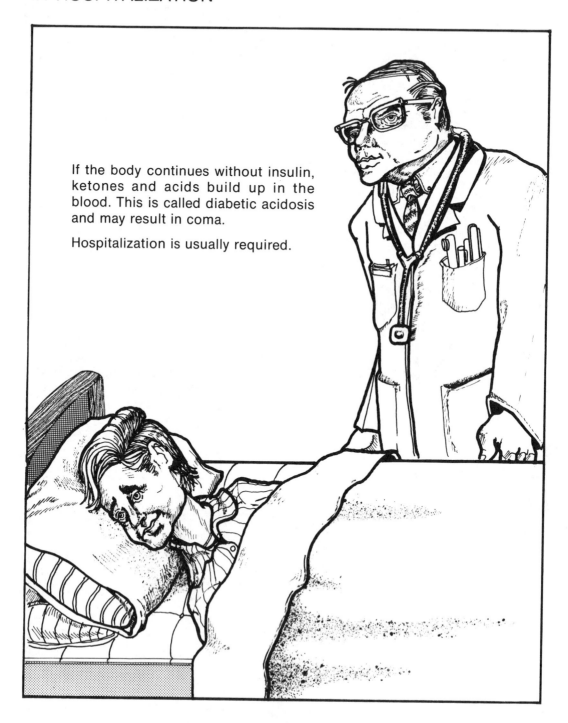

If the body continues without insulin, ketones and acids build up in the blood. This is called diabetic acidosis and may result in coma.

Hospitalization is usually required.

FIGURE 31
DIABETES ROULETTE—
REVIEW THE FACTS

CHAPTER 12B, UNIT III

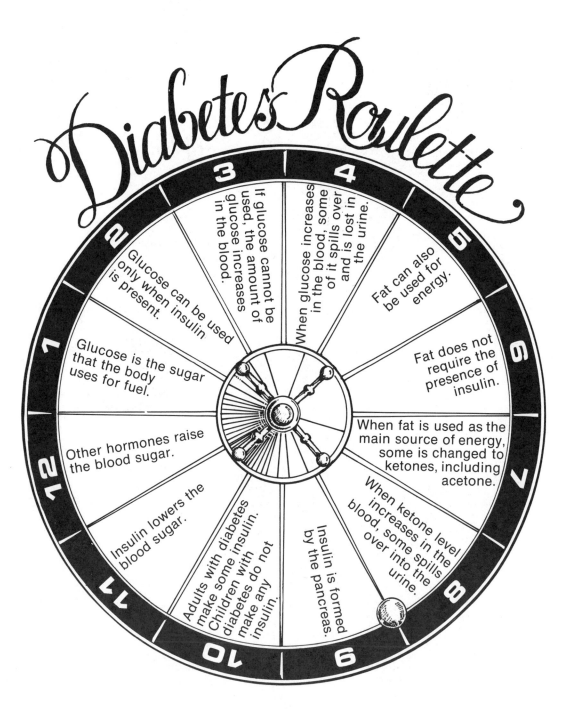

FIGURE 32
TESTS AND TREATMENT

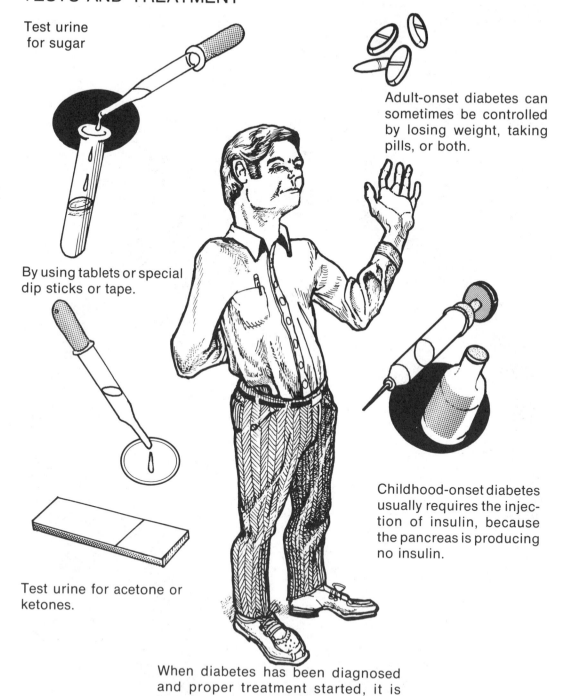

Test urine
for sugar

By using tablets or special
dip sticks or tape.

Test urine for acetone or
ketones.

Adult-onset diabetes can
sometimes be controlled
by losing weight, taking
pills, or both.

Childhood-onset diabetes
usually requires the injection of insulin, because
the pancreas is producing
no insulin.

When diabetes has been diagnosed
and proper treatment started, it is
important to learn what can be done
to stay healthy.

FIGURE 33
RESPONSIBILITIES OF A DIABETIC

The amount of insulin needed will vary from time to time.

The diabetic tries to balance insulin and food.

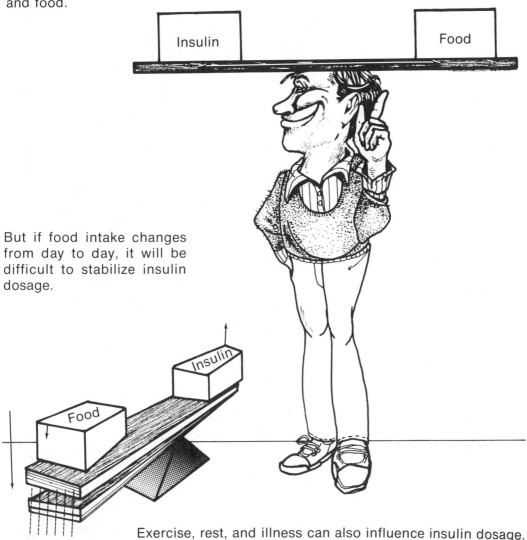

But if food intake changes from day to day, it will be difficult to stabilize insulin dosage.

Exercise, rest, and illness can also influence insulin dosage.

Responsibilities of a diabetic
1. Perform urine tests several times daily.
2. Follow diet prescribed by physician.
3. Regulate exercise.
4. Inject insulin or take oral medication.
5. Be alert to acute complications.

FIGURE 34
AN ECOSYSTEM

CHAPTER 13B, UNIT I

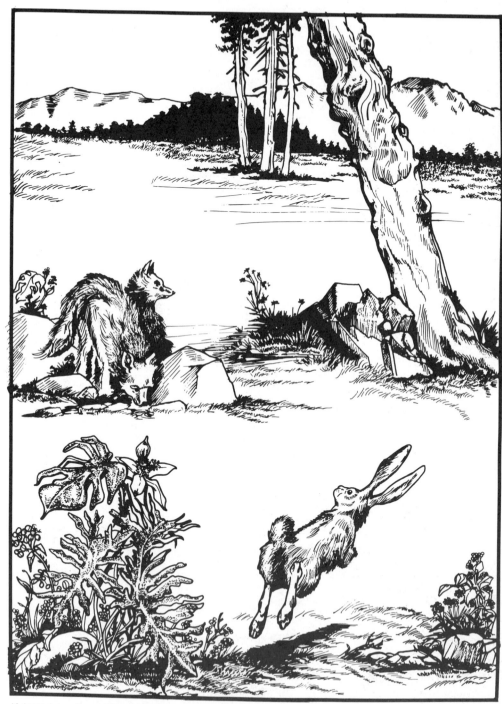

(Adapted courtesy of *Ecology Action Pack*, McDonald's Corporation, 1974.)

FIGURE 35
NEVER OPEN THE DOOR FOR
STRANGERS

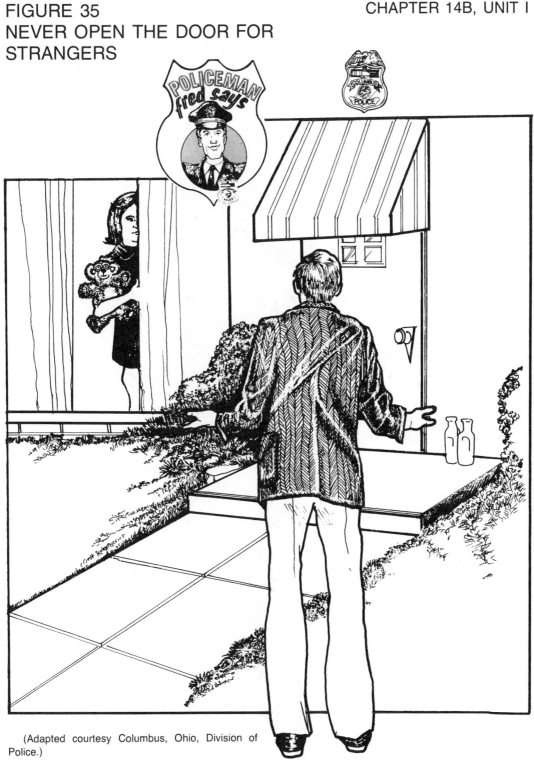

(Adapted courtesy Columbus, Ohio, Division of Police.)

FIGURE 36
OBEY TRAFFIC SIGNALS

CHAPTER 14B, UNIT II

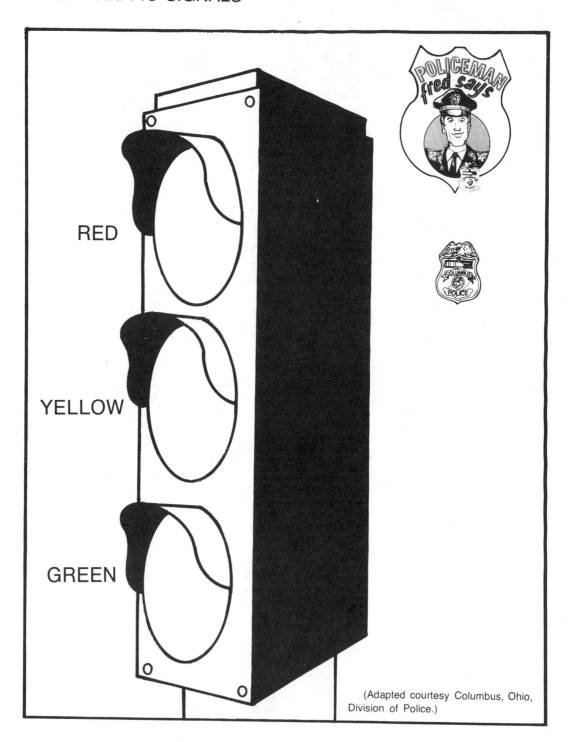

RED

YELLOW

GREEN

(Adapted courtesy Columbus, Ohio, Division of Police.)

FIGURE 37
BE EXTRA CAREFUL ON
RAINY DAYS

CHAPTER 14B, UNIT II

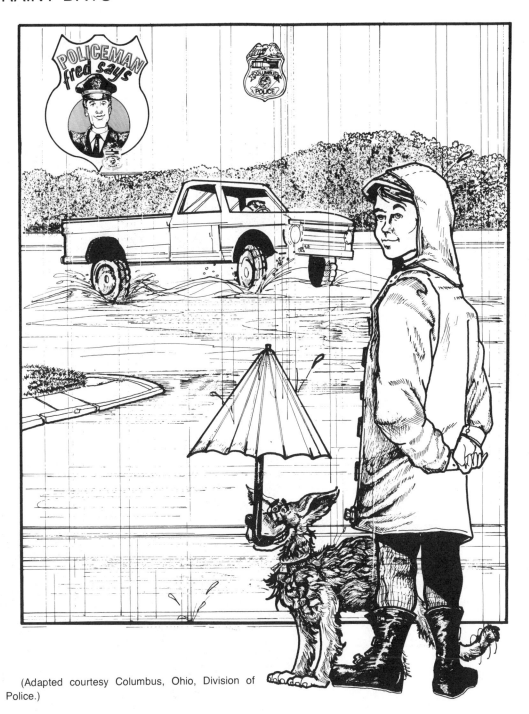

(Adapted courtesy Columbus, Ohio, Division of Police.)

FIGURE 38
RIDING DOUBLE LEADS TO TROUBLE

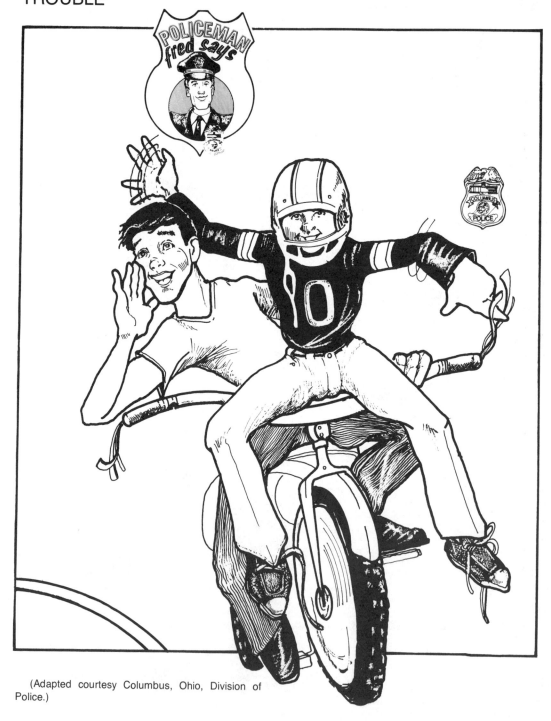

(Adapted courtesy Columbus, Ohio, Division of Police.)

FIGURE 39
ALWAYS USE BIKE HAND SIGNALS—OBEY ALL TRAFFIC SIGNS AND SIGNALS

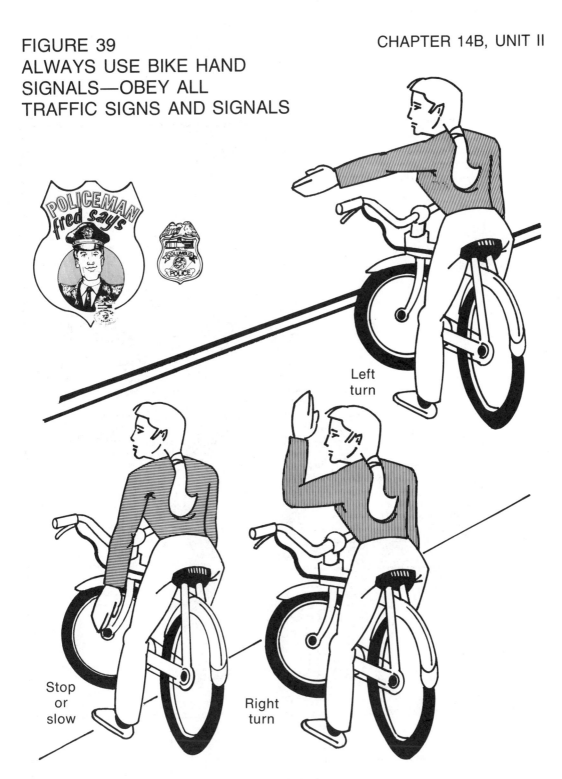

Left turn

Stop or slow

Right turn

(Adapted courtesy Columbus, Ohio, Division of Police.)

FIGURE 40
OBEY YOUR SCHOOL
PATROL

CHAPTER 14B, UNIT I

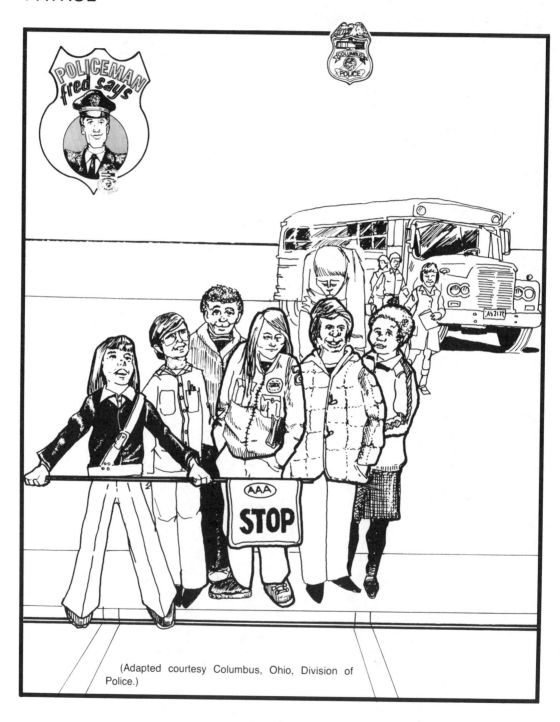

(Adapted courtesy Columbus, Ohio, Division of Police.)

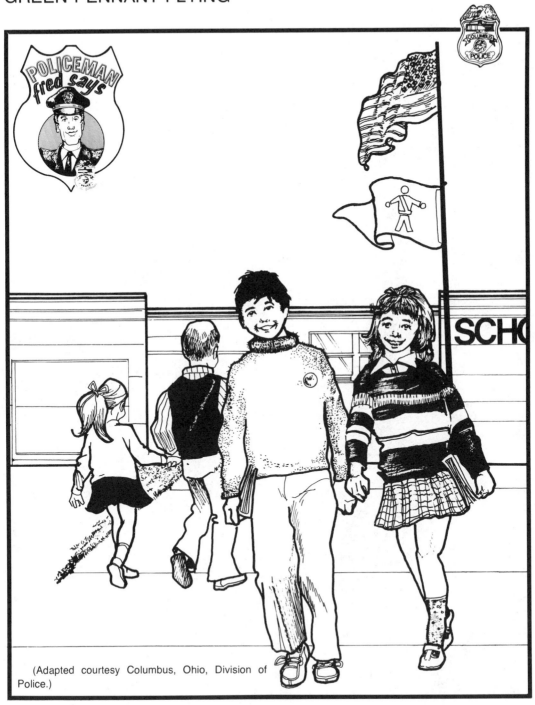

(Adapted courtesy Columbus, Ohio, Division of Police.)

FIGURE 42
IF YOU ARE LOST OR GO
ASTRAY...

CHAPTER 14B, UNIT III

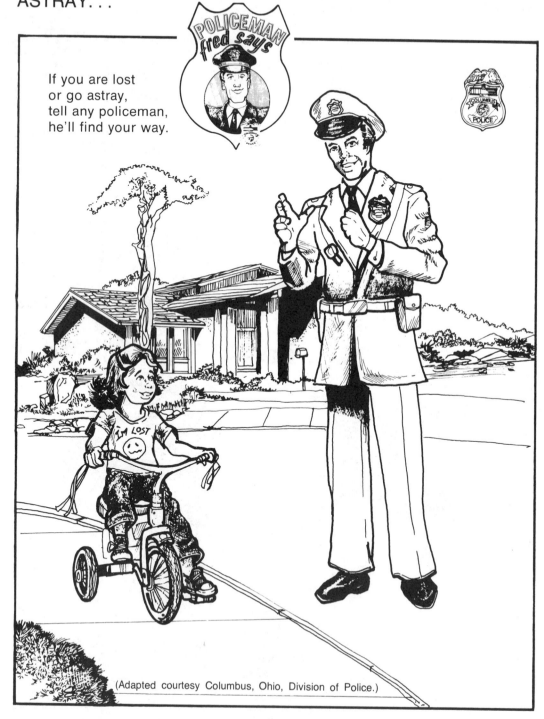

POLICEMAN *fred says*

If you are lost
or go astray,
tell any policeman,
he'll find your way.

COLUMBUS POLICE

I'M LOST

(Adapted courtesy Columbus, Ohio, Division of Police.)

FIGURE 43
TAKING CANDY FROM A STRANGER

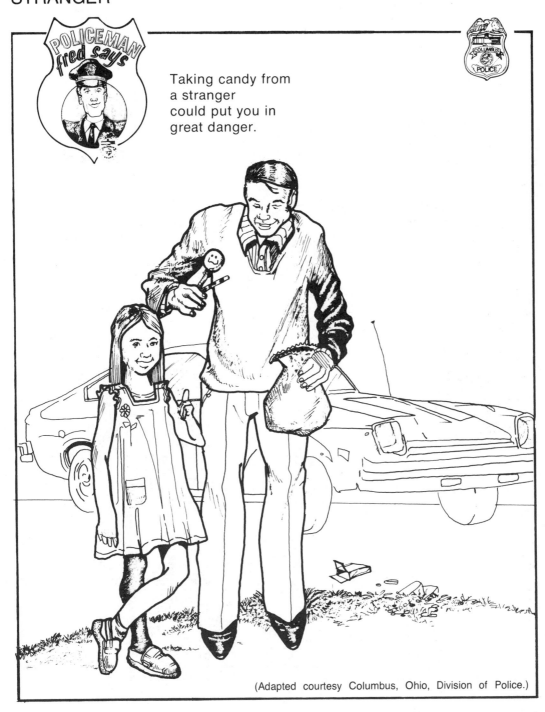

POLICEMAN *fred says*

Taking candy from a stranger could put you in great danger.

(Adapted courtesy Columbus, Ohio, Division of Police.)

FIGURE 44
A TRIP THROUGH
SAFETYLAND

CHAPTER 14B, UNIT III

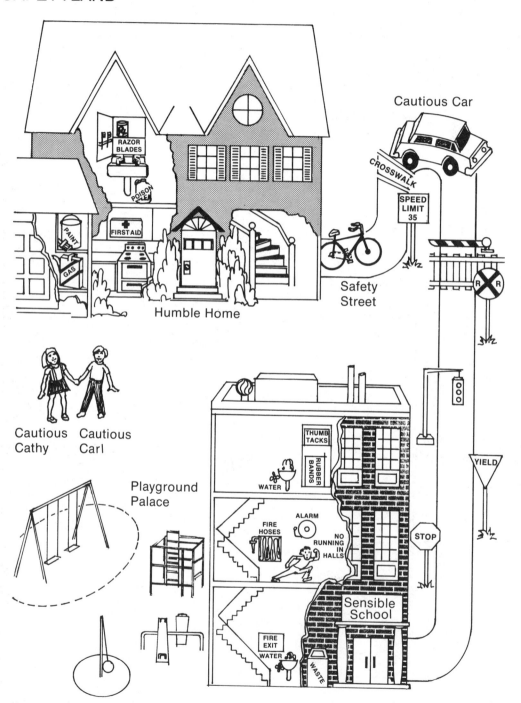

FIGURE 45
SCALES

CHAPTER 15B, UNIT III

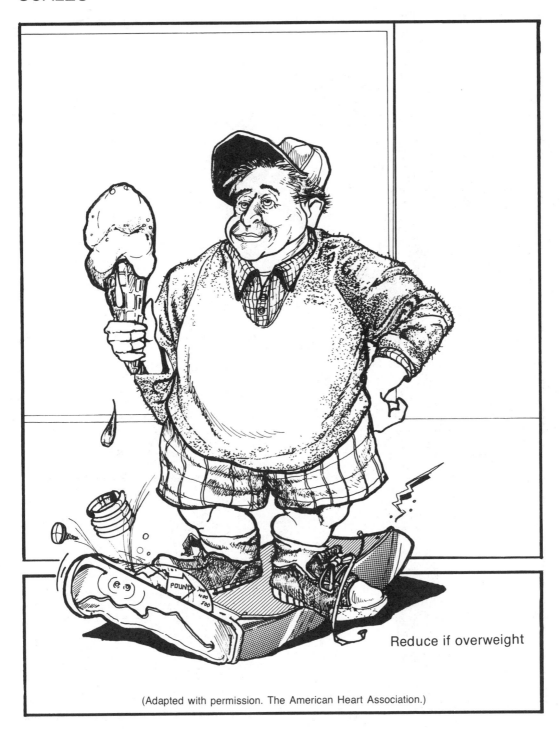

Reduce if overweight

(Adapted with permission. The American Heart Association.)

FIGURE 46
THERMOMETER

CHAPTER 15B, UNIT III

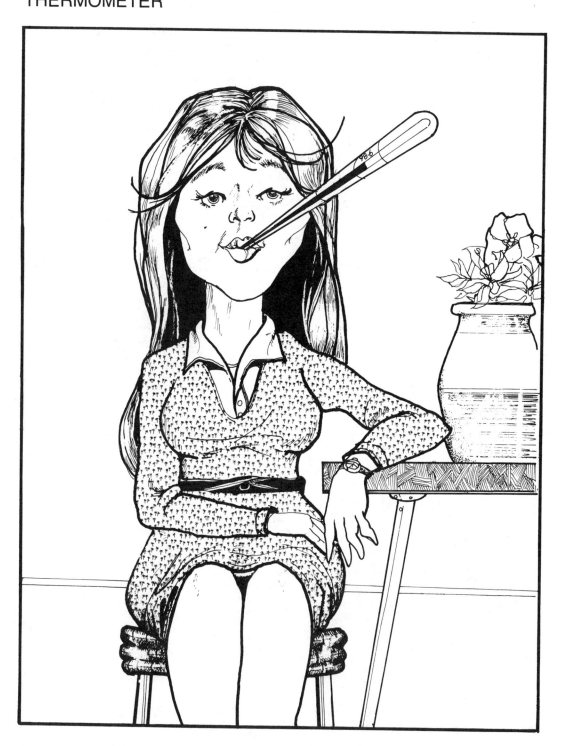

FIGURE 47
SPHYGMOMANOMETER

CHAPTER 15B, UNIT III

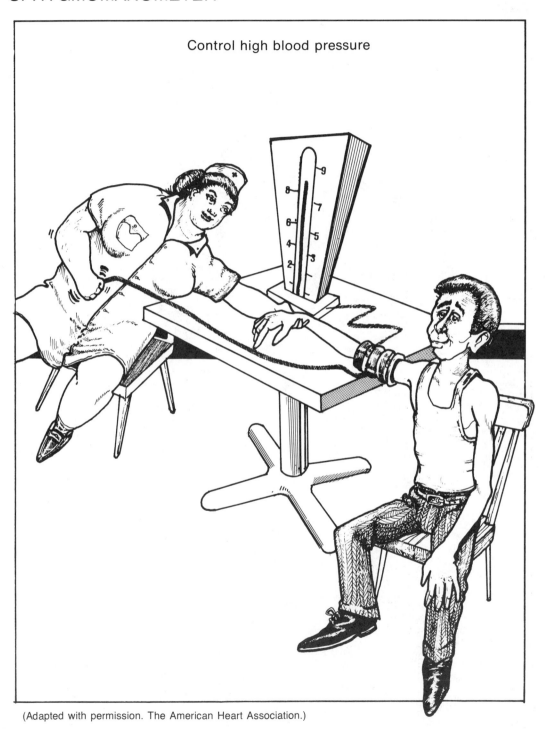

Control high blood pressure

(Adapted with permission. The American Heart Association.)

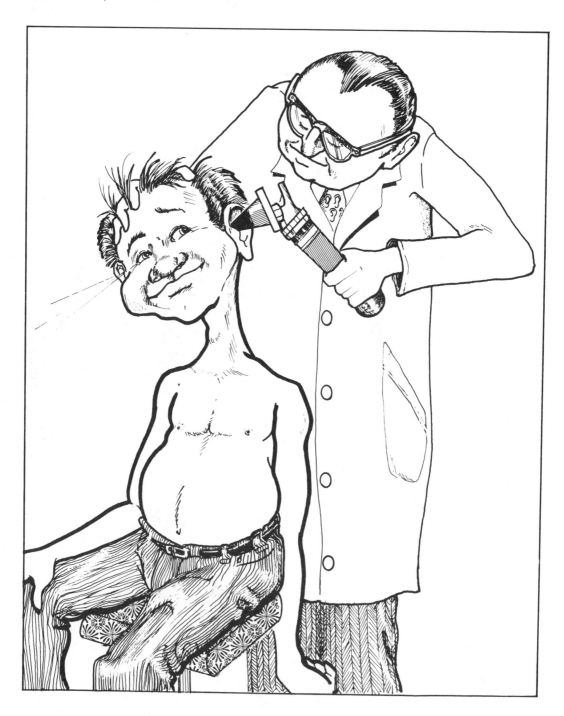

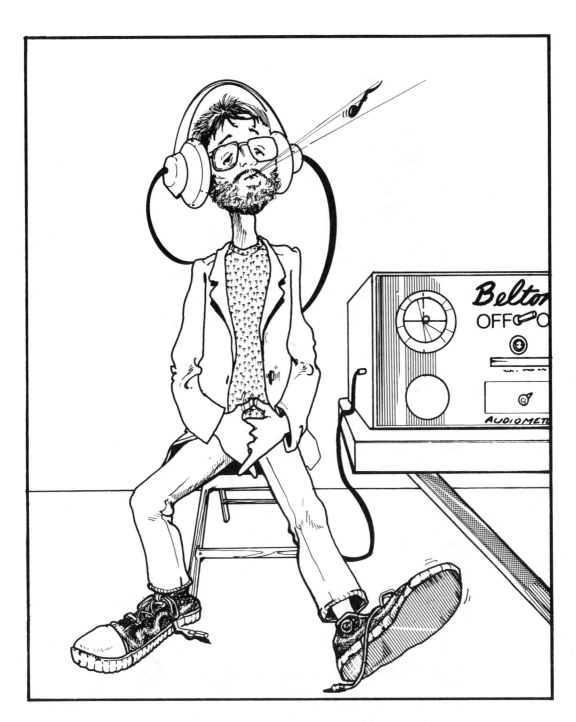

FIGURE 50
TONGUE DEPRESSOR

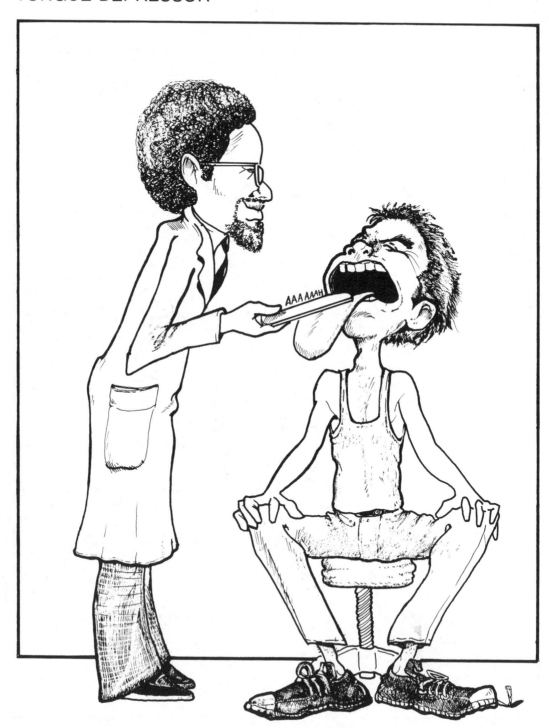

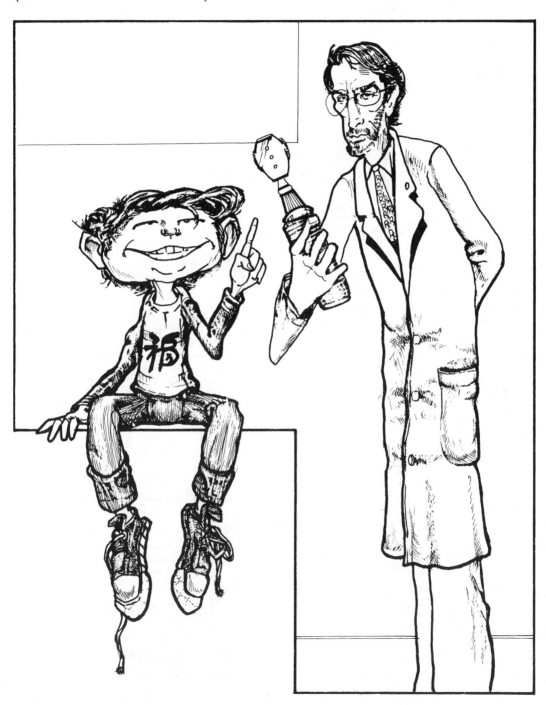

FIGURE 52
EYE CHART

CHAPTER 15B, UNIT III

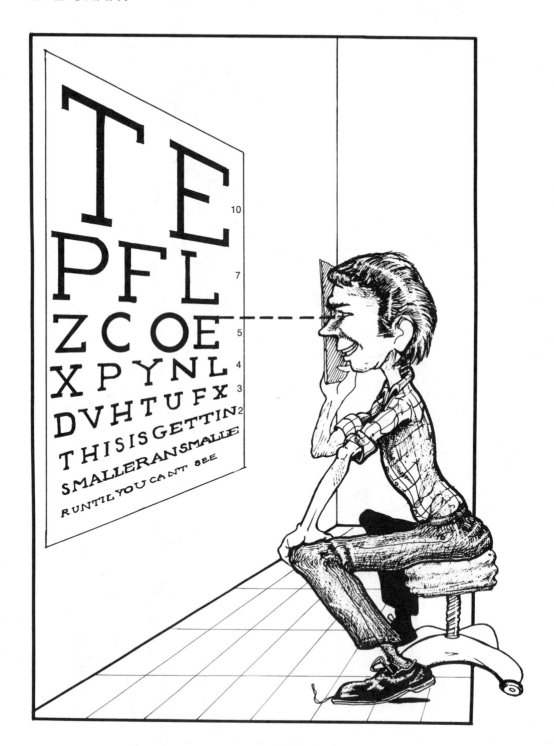

FIGURE 53
REFRACTOR MACHINE USED
FOR PRESCRIBING EYEGLASSES
AND EXAMINING EYES

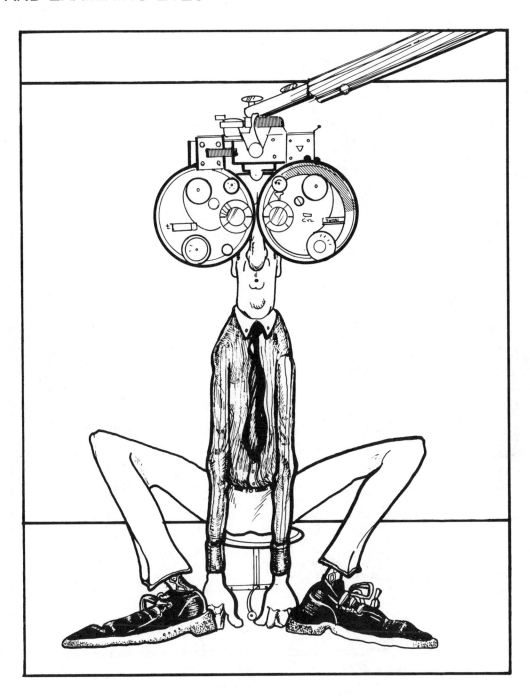

FIGURE 54
STETHOSCOPE

CHAPTER 15B, UNIT III

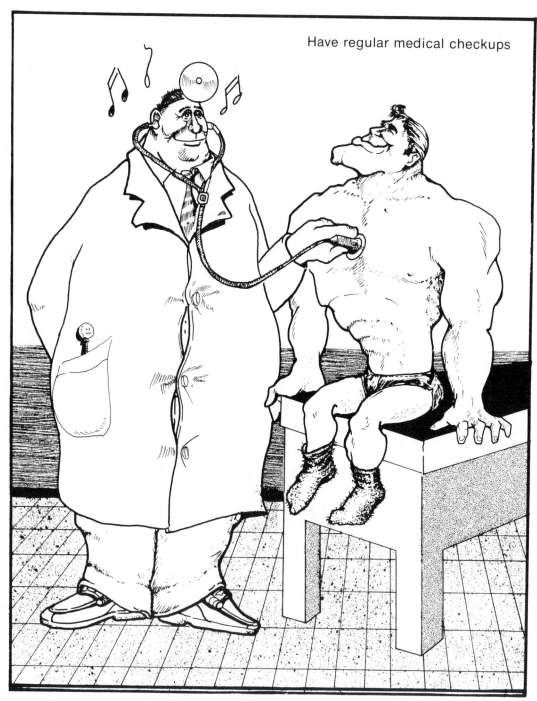

(Adapted with permission. The American Heart Association.)

FIGURE 55
HYPODERMIC SYRINGE

CHAPTER 15B, UNIT III

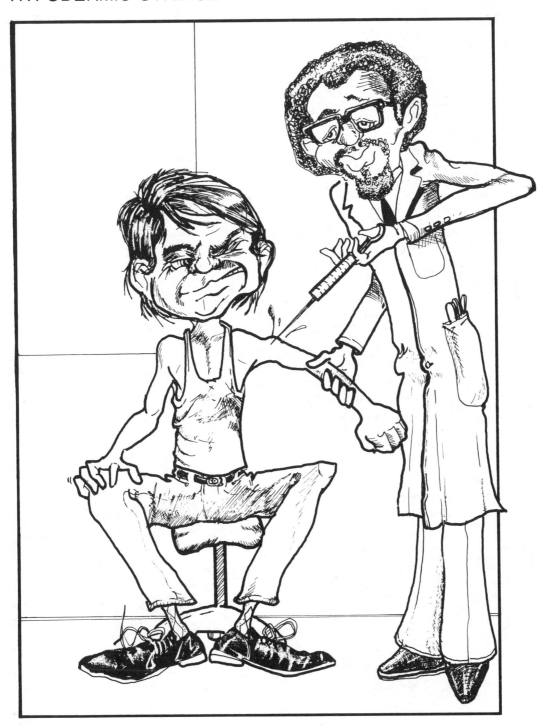

FIGURE 56
X-RAY MACHINE

CHAPTER 15B, UNIT III

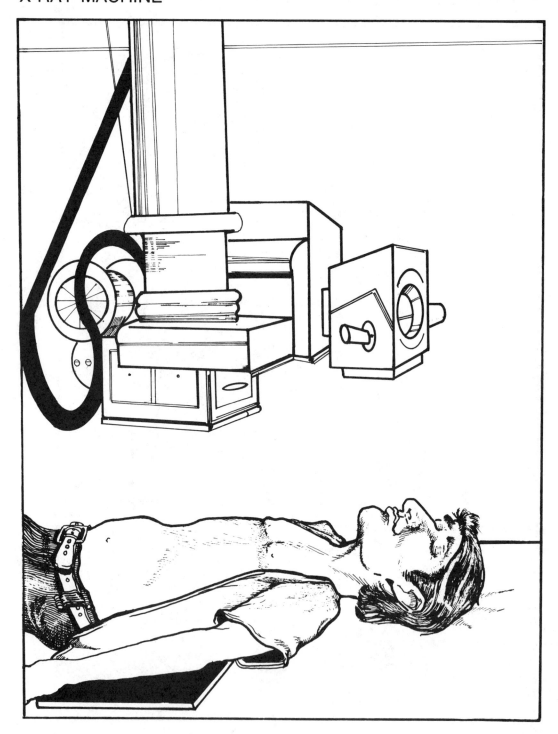

FIGURE 57
STRUCTURE OF THE
HUMAN EAR

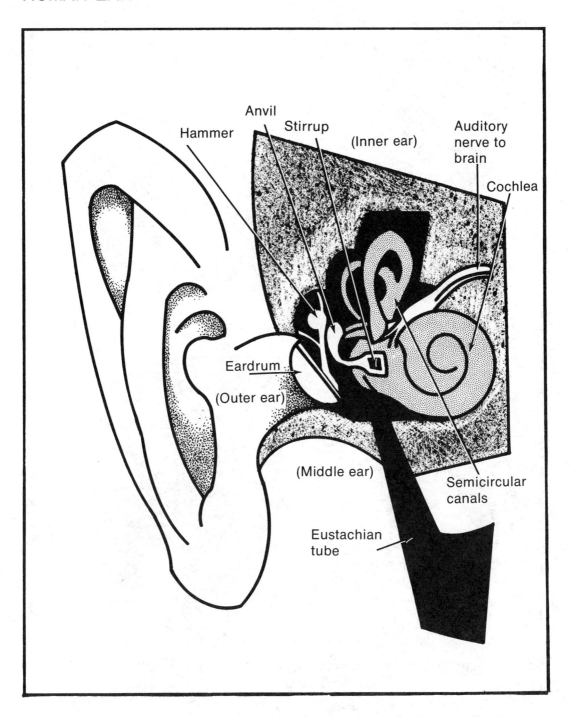

The lens acts like a crazy projector, focusing the light rays upside down on the back of the eye (retina).

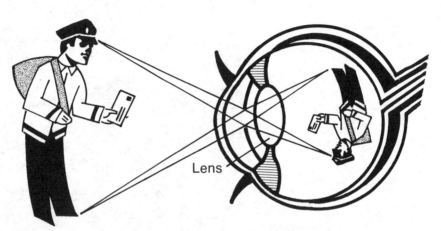

The optic nerve is like a mailman, carrying messages from the eye (retina) to the brain.

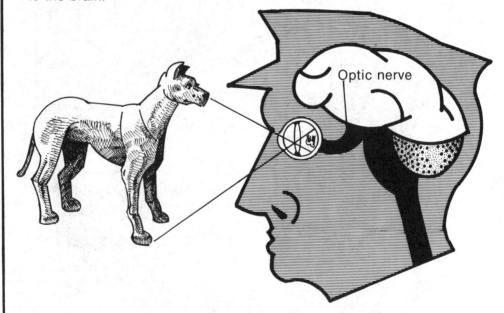

The brain receives the message and turns it right side up!

FIGURE 59
STRUCTURE OF THE EYE

CHAPTER 8B, UNIT VII

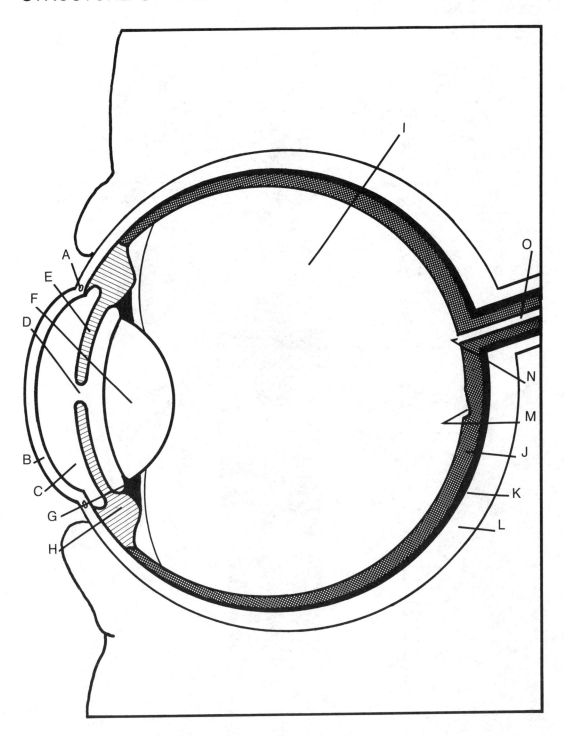

FIGURE 60
SYMBOLS OF VOLUNTARY HEALTH AGENCIES

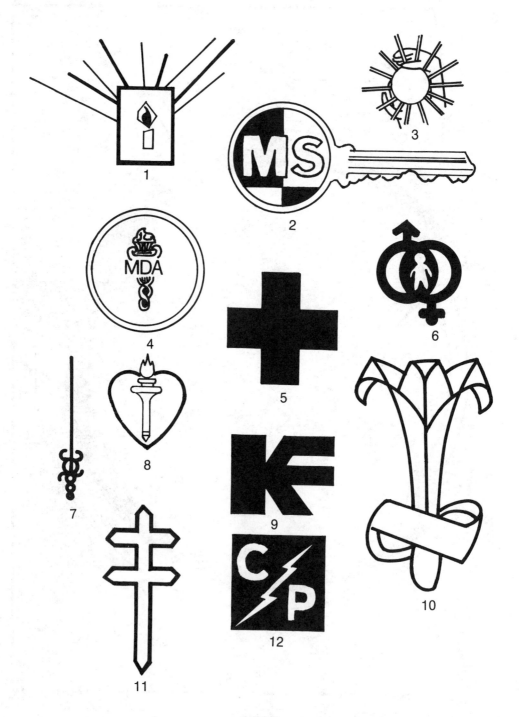

CHAPTER 16B
GAMES AND OTHER ACTIVITIES FOR CLASSROOM USE

The instructional materials in this section may be used in any order, but have been included under Chapter headings to correlate with additional information provided in the textbook.

Chapter 7B Teaching About Drugs, Alcohol and Tobacco

Figure 61, The Hi-Lo Memorial Golf Courses Drug Education Game (gameboard includes four game sheets; one sheet of Feeling High cards; one sheet of Feeling Low cards)

Figure 62, Drug Abuse Crossword Puzzle

Figure 63, Methyl/Ethyl Gameboard and Game Cards

Figure 64, In Touch with Feelings Crossword Puzzle

Figure 65, Study Sheet: Need + Blocking = Anger

Chapter 8B Teaching About the Human Body and Grooming

Figure 66, Human Skeleton Pattern (three pages)

Figure 67, Study Sheet: Comparison of Bone Names

Figure 68, What's Your Muscle Power? Crossword Puzzle and Questions

Figure 69, Worksheet: Inside the Human Heart

Figure 70, Worksheet: Trace the Passage of Air into the Lungs

Figure 71, Digestion Game (two sheets) and Game Cards (two sheets)

Figure 72, Worksheet: Outline of the Digestive System

Figure 73, The Brain Maze

Figure 74, Worksheet: The Nervous System

Figure 75, Sample Cards for Bull's-Eye Game

Figure 76, Sample Cards for Ear-Opener Game

Figure 77, Fertilization: A Game of Chance (gameboard and game cards)

Figure 78, Female Reproductive System (puzzle pieces)

Figure 79, Male Reproductive System (puzzle pieces)

Figure 80, Worksheet: This is Me!

Figure 81, Grooming Rally (gameboard) (Should be enlarged)

Figure 82, Grooming Grand Prix Checklist

Figure 83, Worksheet: Body Tune-up

Chapter 9B Teaching About Exercise, Rest and Relaxation

Figure 84, Normal Artery

Figure 85, Abnormal Artery

Figure 86, Worksheet: Stars for Sleep

Chapter 11B Teaching About Dental Health

Figure 87, Orally Safe and Hazardous Snacks

Figure 88, Worksheet: Mystery Mouth

Chapter 12B Teaching About Disease Control and Prevention

Figure 89, VD Game No. 1

Figure 90, VD Game No. 2 (game board and game cards)

Chapter 13B Teaching About the Environment

Figure 91, Environment Puzzle

Figure 92, Puzzle: What's in the Terrarium?

Figure 93, Terrarium Jigsaw Puzzle

Figure 94, Environment Word Search

Figure 95, Environment Crossword Puzzle

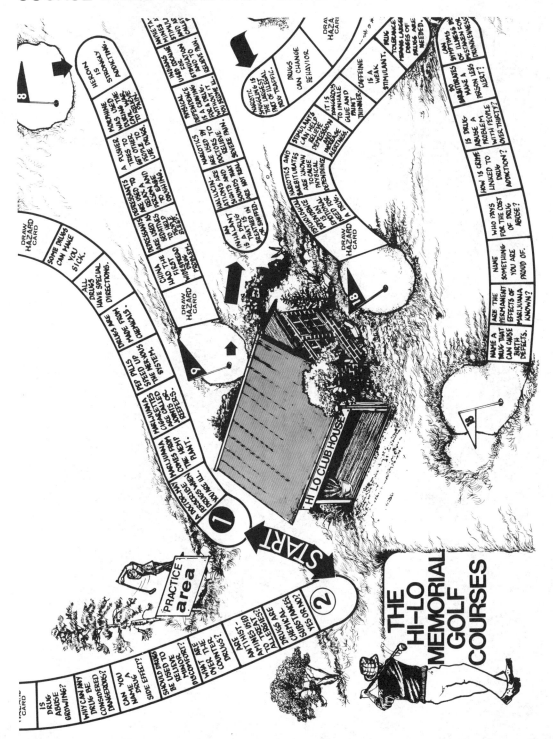

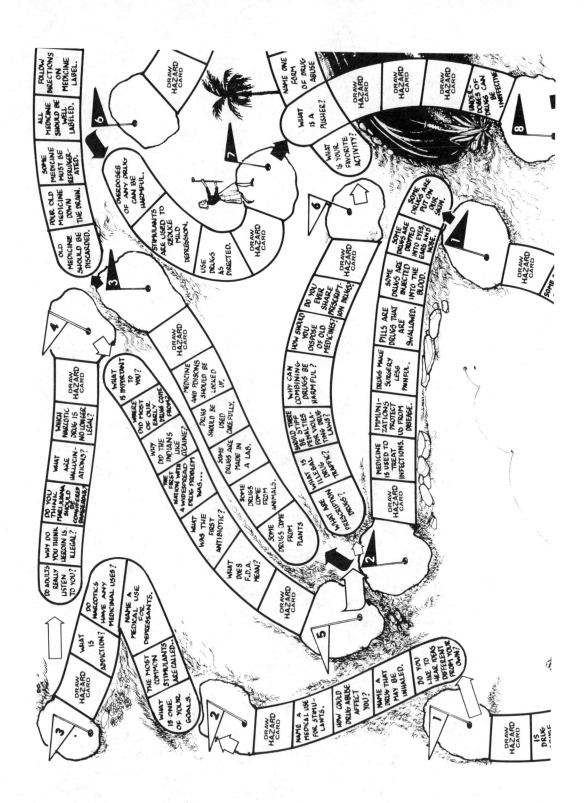

FOLLOW DIRECTIONS ON MEDICINE LABEL.

ALL MEDICINE SHOULD BE WELL LABELED.

SOME MEDICINE MUST BE REFRIGERATED.

POUR OLD MEDICINE DOWN THE DRAIN.

OLD MEDICINE SHOULD BE DISCARDED.

OVERDOSES OF ANY DRUG CAN BE HARMFUL.

STIMULANTS ARE USED TO REDUCE MILD DEPRESSION.

USE DRUGS AS DIRECTED.

DRAW HAZARD CARD

NAME ONE FORM OF DRUG ABUSE

WHAT IS A PUSHER?

WHAT IS YOUR FAVORITE ACTIVITY?

DRAW HAZARD CARD

DRAW HAZARD CARD

DRAW HAZARD CARD

LARGE DOSES OF DRUGS CAN BE INEFFECTIVE?

SOME DRUGS ARE PUT ON OUR SKIN.

SOME DRUGS ARE DROPPED INTO EYES, EARS, AND THE NOSE.

SOME DRUGS ARE INJECTED INTO THE BLOOD.

PILLS ARE DRUGS THAT ARE SWALLOWED.

DRAW HAZARD CARD

DRAW HAZARD CARD

DRAW HAZARD CARD

WHICH NARCOTIC DRUG IS NO LONGER LEGAL?

WHAT ARE HALLUCINATIONS?

DO YOU THINK MARIJUANA SHOULD BE CONSIDERED DANGEROUS?

WHAT IS IMPORTANT TO YOU?

WHERE DID MOST OF OUR EARLY DRUGS COME FROM?

WHY DID THE INDIANS LIKE COCAINE?

MEDICINE AND POISONS SHOULD BE LOCKED UP.

DRUGS SHOULD BE USED CAREFULLY.

SOME DRUGS ARE MADE IN A LAB.

HOW SHOULD YOU DISPOSE OF OLD MEDICINES?

DO YOU EVER SHARE PRESCRIPTION DRUGS?

DRAW HAZARD CARD

WHY DO YOU THINK HEROIN IS ILLEGAL?

THE FIRST NATION WITH A WIDESPREAD DRUG PROBLEM WAS....

WAS THE FIRST ANTIBIOTIC?

SOME DRUGS COME FROM ANIMALS.

SOME DRUGS COME FROM PLANTS

WHY CAN COMBINING DRUGS BE HARMFUL?

SHOULD THERE BE STIFF PENALTIES FOR VIOLATING DRUG LAWS?

DO ADULTS REALLY LISTEN TO YOU?

WHAT DOES F.D.A. MEAN?

WHAT IS ILLEGAL DRUG TRAFFIC?

WHAT ARE PRESCRIPTION DRUGS?

MEDICINE IS USED TO TREAT INFECTIONS.

IMMUNIZATIONS PROTECT US FROM DISEASE.

DRUGS MAKE SURGERY LESS PAINFUL.

DRAW HAZARD CARD

DO NARCOTICS HAVE ANY MEDICINAL USES?

NAME A MEDICAL USE FOR DEPRESSANTS.

WHAT IS ADDICTION?

DRAW HAZARD CARD

THE MOST COMMON STIMULANTS ARE CALLED...

WHAT IS ONE OF YOUR GOALS.

NAME A MEDICAL USE FOR STIMULANTS.

HOW COULD DRUG ABUSE AFFECT YOU?

NAME A DRUG THAT MAY BE INHALED.

DO YOU LIKE TO HEAR IDEAS DIFFERENT FROM YOUR OWN?

DRAW HAZARD CARD

DRAW HAZARD CARD

IS DRUG USE

512

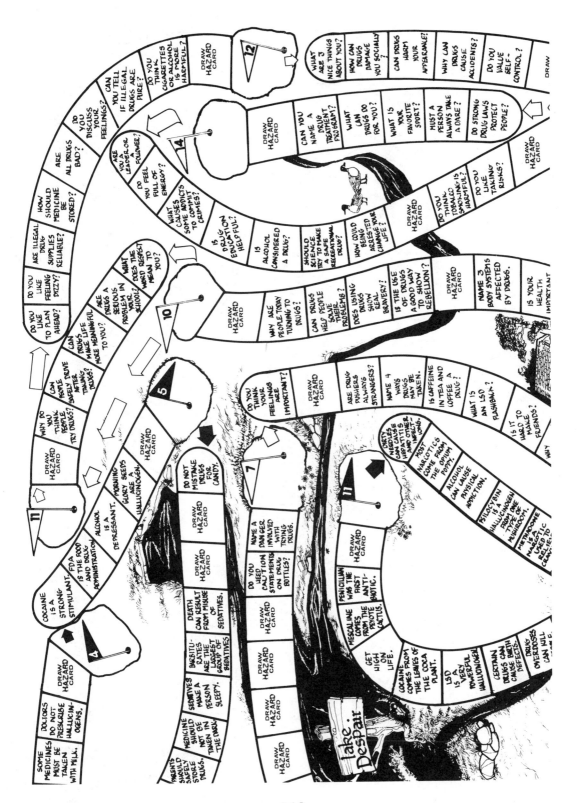

513

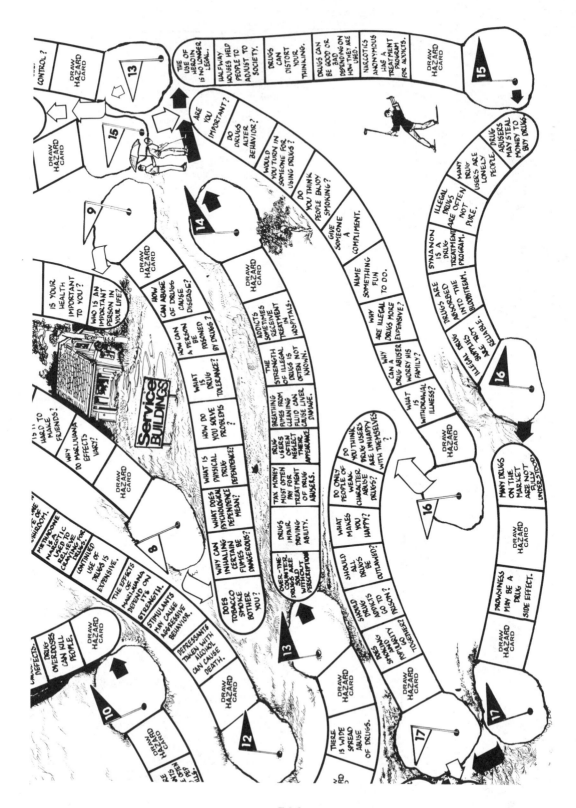

514

FEELING LOW

Glue this sheet to blue construction paper and cut out individual cards: Hazard cards or feeling low.	You are allergic to the drug you just received. Lose your next turn.	You are suffering from a bad drug side effect. Lose your next turn.	You took more medicine than was prescribed for you and are very ill. Lose your next turn.
You did not take the amount of medicine that was prescribed for you and have not gotten well. Lose your next turn.	You took some medicine, thinking it was candy, and now you are ill. Lose your next turn.	You did not turn on your light to read the medicine label and took the wrong medicine by mistake. Lose your next turn.	You were supposed to take a certain medicine with milk but you did not. Lose your next turn.
You took a medicine from the medicine cabinet without your parents' permission or supervision. Lose your next turn.	You took some medicine that had been on the shelf for a long time and was no longer effective. Lose your next turn.	You do not know how to properly dispose of old medicine. Lose your next turn.	You took a medicine without a label on the bottle. Lose your next turn.
You took a pill that your friend gave you. Lose your next turn.	You have become dependent upon sleeping pills. Lose your next turn.	You drank too much alcohol and became drunk. Lose your next turn.	You took some prescription medicine that was prescribed for someone else. Lose your next turn.
You ate some strange berries that made you sick. Lose your next turn.	You ate some poisonous mushrooms and became ill. Lose your next turn.	You accepted a dare to sniff glue. Lose your next turn.	You were curious about sniffing varnish, paint thinner, and kerosene. The strong chemicals made you feel sick. Lose your next turn.
You bought some medicine for your father and tossed it on the table where your little brother could reach it. Lose your next turn.	You rely on amphetamines to help you lose weight. Lose your next turn.	You sample pills to just learn what they are like. Lose your next turn.	You did not store your medicines in a safe place. Lose your next turn.
You accepted candy or pills from a stranger. Lose your next turn.	You think all medicines must be safe if purchased from a pharmacy. Lose your next turn.	You do not know who to call in an emergency. Lose your next turn.	You think it is safe to drive an automobile after consuming several alcoholic drinks. Lose your next turn.
You drank some liquid that had a skull and crossbones on the label. Lose your next turn.	You believe television ads that show drugs as a way to solve personal problems. Lose your next turn.	You tried smoking a cigarette and started coughing and choking. Lose your next turn.	You smoke marijuana daily. Lose your next turn.

FEELING HIGH

Glue this sheet to yellow construction paper and cut out individual cards.	A person just told you how nice you look and you're feeling high! Take another turn!	You have just seen a beautiful sunset and are feeling happy! Take another turn!	You saw an opportunity to help someone less fortunate than yourself and now you're happy that you could help. Take another turn!
You just finished drawing a picture and your mother wants to frame it. Take another turn!	You just finished building a tree shack and you're feeling good! Take another turn!	You just found a really neat colored rock and are feeling happy! Take another turn!	You have just been invited to a picnic and are very excited! Take another turn!
You just made a home-run for your softball team and everybody is congratulating you. Take another turn!	You raised larger tomatoes in your garden last summer than anyone else in your neighborhood. Take another turn!	You have just been invited to go camping with your best friend. Take another turn!	It is your birthday and you and your friends are going to an amusement park and then to an ice cream parlor. Take another turn!
You just hugged your friend's new furry little puppy and are feeling happy. Take another turn!	It is time for your favorite television program. Take another turn!	You just won a roller skating race and are very excited. Take another turn!	The circus is coming to town and you have two free tickets. Take another turn!
You have been invited to spend the weekend at your cousin's farm and see their new colt. Take another turn!	You just got an A on a tough exam. Take another turn!	Your family is going on a neat three-week vacation and you're all packed. Take another turn!	You just caught a huge fish and had your picture taken with it. Take another turn!
You get to help your mother bake cookies and lick the bowl. Take another turn!	You just learned how to dive and are feeling very proud of yourself. Take another turn!	A letter just arrived for you from a good friend that you have not seen in a long time. Take another turn!	Your mother just told you that you could have anything you wanted for dinner tonight. Take another turn!
Your father and you are going to a large field to fly your new airplane. Take another turn!	You just learned how to ride a skateboard. Take another turn!	While walking in the woods you unexpectedly came across a beautiful deer and were able to photograph it. Take another turn!	You just got a part in your school play. Take another turn!
You just earned a President's Physical Fitness Award and are going to try for another one. Take another turn!	You are finally going to be able to receive the music lessons you have wanted. Take another turn!	You just made a present for your grandmother that you know she will like! Take another turn!	Your class is going on a field trip tomorrow and you are very excited! Take another turn!

FIGURE 62
DRUG ABUSE CROSSWORD PUZZLE

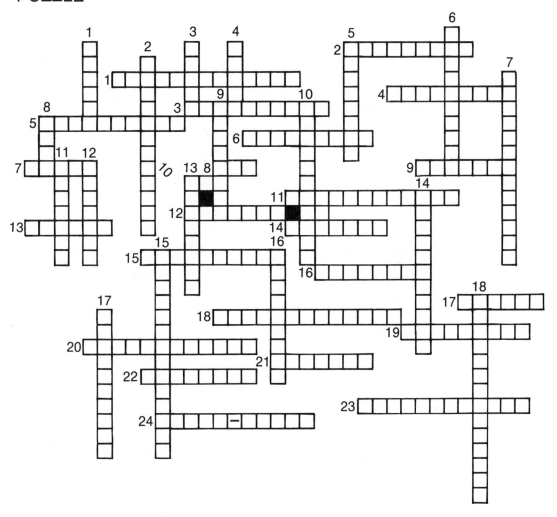

DRUG ABUSE CROSSWORD PUZZLE CLUES

DOWN

1. A person who tries to get other people to use drugs.
2. The most well known and dangerous kind of sedatives.
3. Chemical substances which have an effect on the body or mind.
4. The drug that caused many Chinese workers to lose interest in their work.
5. A narcotic used commonly during the Civil War.
6. A type of painkiller.
7. An emotional need for a drug is called _____ dependence.
8. Amount of anything given or taken at one time.
9. A drug that is breathed in or sniffed.
10. A drug that caused thousands of babies to be born deformed.
11. Unusual sensitivity to certain substances.
12. A drug used as far back as the Stone Age.
13. The feeling that often occurs after taking narcotics.
14. Drugs taken into the body are eventually absorbed into the _____.
15. Effects of LSD where sights, sounds, or feelings are not real.
16. If a person takes repeated doses of a certain drug he may develop a _____.
17. The first antibiotic discovered.
18. Drugs used to treat allergies.

ACROSS

1. Used to change a person's mood and calm a nervous upset.
2. Pot or grass.
3. Uppers.
4. A disease of the liver sometimes spread through the use of dirty syringes (needles).
5. A feeling of sadness and discontent.
6. A narcotic used to treat people dependent upon other narcotics.
7. Breathing in of an aerosol spray has been known to cause _____.
8. The most powerful of the hallucinogens.
9. The chemical substance in liquors that makes them intoxicating.
10. A newborn baby usually receives drops in each _____.
11. Diseases passed from one person to another.
12. The power or strength of drugs.
13. A narcotic drug that is no longer legal or used medically.
14. A kind of drug abuser who does not use medicine properly is called a drug _____.
15. A person licensed to prepare and distribute medicines.
16. The plant from which marijuana comes.
17. An effect of narcotics on the digestive system may be _____.
18. People who try a drug or drugs for nonmedical reasons may be _____.
19. The largest part of the illegal drug traffic is the business of smuggling _____.
20. Drunkenness or excitement beyond self-control.
21. A drug derived from the leaves of the coca plant.
22. A mild stimulant.
23. The kind of drugs that must have medical supervision for safe use.
24. The natural source of most narcotics (two words).

FIGURE 63
METHYL/ETHYL
GAMEBOARD AND GAME
CARDS

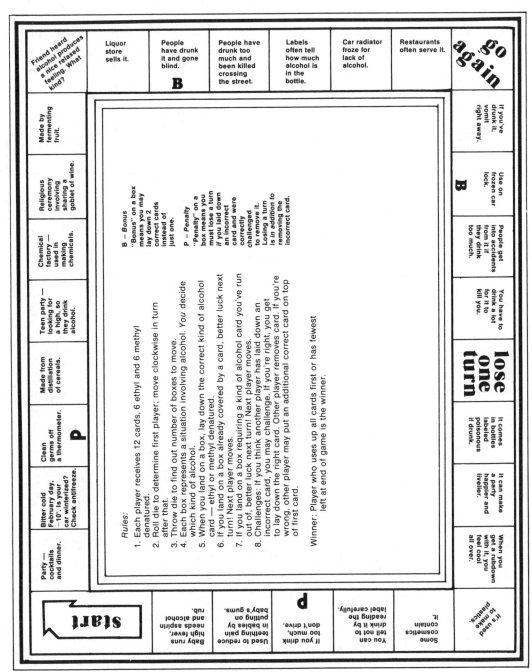

PLAYER 1			PLAYER 2			PLAYER 3			PLAYER 4		
Ethyl alcohol	Ethyl alcohol	Ethyl alcohol	Ethyl alcohol	Ethyl alcohol	Ethyl alcohol	Ethyl alcohol	Ethyl alcohol	Ethyl alcohol	Ethyl alcohol	Ethyl alcohol	Ethyl alcohol
Ethyl alcohol	Ethyl alcohol	Ethyl alcohol	Ethyl alcohol	Ethyl alcohol	Ethyl alcohol	Ethyl alcohol	Ethyl alcohol	Ethyl alcohol	Ethyl alcohol	Ethyl alcohol	Ethyl alcohol
Ethyl alcohol	Ethyl alcohol	Ethyl alcohol	Ethyl alcohol	Ethyl alcohol	Ethyl alcohol	Ethyl alcohol	Ethyl alcohol	Ethyl alcohol	Ethyl alcohol	Ethyl alcohol	Ethyl alcohol
Methyl alcohol or denatured alcohol	Methyl alcohol or denatured alcohol	Methyl alcohol or denatured alcohol	Methyl alcohol or denatured alcohol	Methyl alcohol or denatured alcohol	Methyl alcohol or denatured alcohol	Methyl alcohol or denatured alcohol	Methyl alcohol or denatured alcohol	Methyl alcohol or denatured alcohol	Methyl alcohol or denatured alcohol	Methyl alcohol or denatured alcohol	Methyl alcohol or denatured alcohol
Methyl alcohol or denatured alcohol	Methyl alcohol or denatured alcohol	Methyl alcohol or denatured alcohol	Methyl alcohol or denatured alcohol	Methyl alcohol or denatured alcohol	Methyl alcohol or denatured alcohol	Methyl alcohol or denatured alcohol	Methyl alcohol or denatured alcohol	Methyl alcohol or denatured alcohol	Methyl alcohol or denatured alcohol	Methyl alcohol or denatured alcohol	Methyl alcohol or denatured alcohol
Methyl alcohol or denatured alcohol	Methyl alcohol or denatured alcohol	Methyl alcohol or denatured alcohol	Methyl alcohol or denatured alcohol	Methyl alcohol or denatured alcohol	Methyl alcohol or denatured alcohol	Methyl alcohol or denatured alcohol	Methyl alcohol or denatured alcohol	Methyl alcohol or denatured alcohol	Methyl alcohol or denatured alcohol	Methyl alcohol or denatured alcohol	Methyl alcohol or denatured alcohol

(Courtesy: *Alcohol and Alcohol Safety,* A Curriculum Manual for Elementary Level, Teacher's Activities Guide, Department of Transportation, Highway Traffic Safety Administration Washington DC 20590.)

FIGURE 64
IN TOUCH WITH FEELING
CROSSWORD PUZZLE

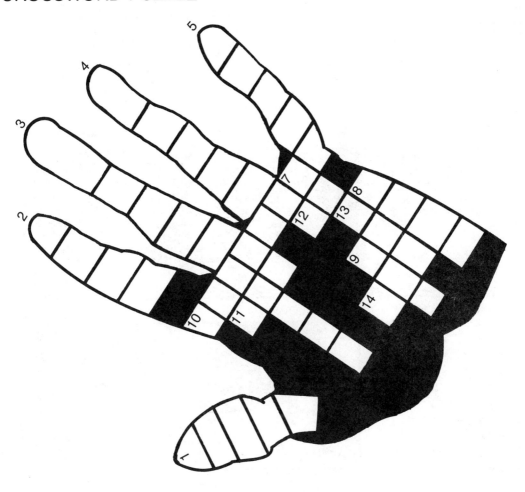

DOWN
1. It would make me _____ to be your friend.
2. Strong affection for another person is called. _____.
3. The little boy _____ jumped off the diving board.
4. Snoopy was _____ as to what was in the box.
5. The clown looked _____ in his ridiculous clothes.
6. We have learned helpful ways to deal with _____ and frustration.
7. When a person is not intoxicated or drunk, we say he or she is _____.
8. You may *know* that thunder cannot hurt you, but sometimes you may _____ afraid of it.
9. Another word for not happy is _____.

ACROSS
9. It makes me happy to _____ you and hear your voice.
10. To envy or resent someone who is successful is called _____.
11. You should not be ashamed of _____ feeling that you have.
12. Feelings always affect your body, _____ it is important to learn about them.
13. An abbreviation for boldface is _____.
14. Would you accept a dangerous _____ to win the approval of other children?

521

STUDY SHEET: NEED + BLOCKING = ANGER

PEOPLE MAY BECOME ANGRY WHEN SOMETHING OR SOMEONE KEEPS THEM FROM WORKING OUT THEIR NEEDS OR FEELINGS.

Sometimes people put a block between us and the feelings we would like to have, such as feeling secure or important. Then we feel angry.

NEED   +   BLOCKING   =   ANGER

Let's see how this works.

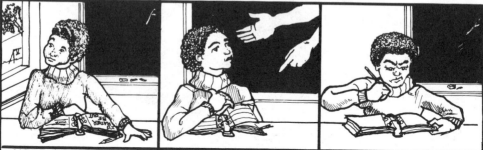

NEED FOR REST   +   BLOCKING   =   ANGER

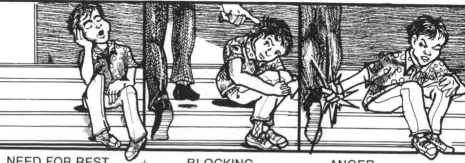

NEED FOR PHYSICAL +   BLOCKING   =   ANGER
ACTIVITY

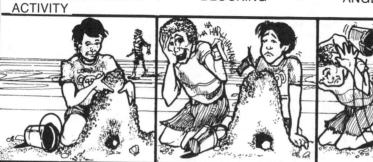

NEED FOR COUNTING +   BLOCKING   =   ANGER
FOR SOMETHING

(Courtesy: *A World to Grow In*, Student Book, Grade Five, The Educational Research Council of America, 1972.)

FIGURE 66
HUMAN SKELETON PATTERN

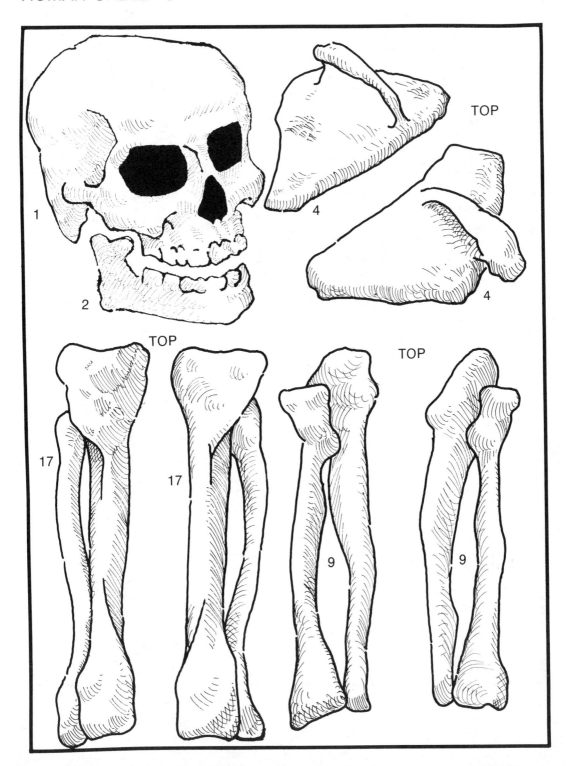

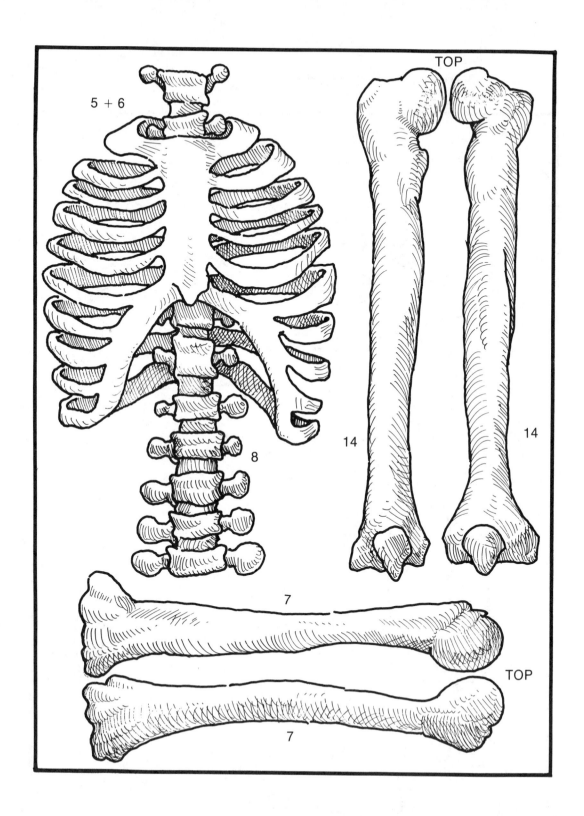

5 + 6

8

14

14

TOP

7

7

TOP

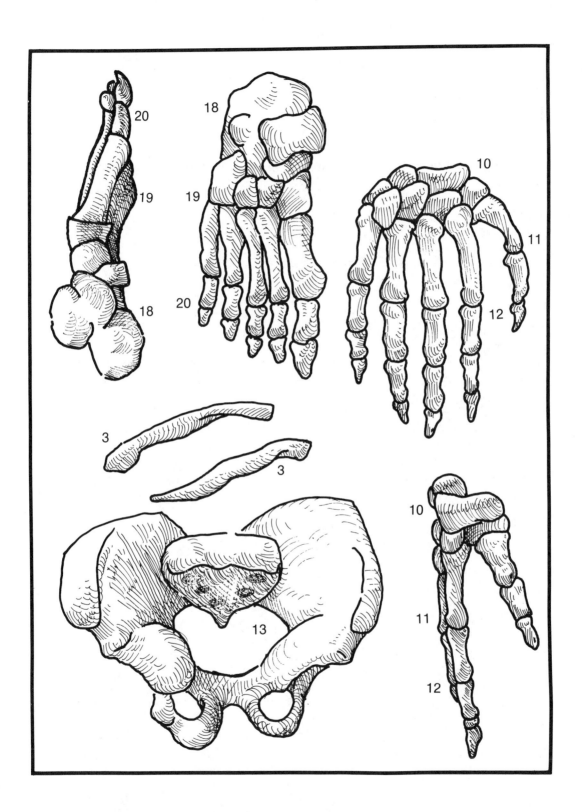

FIGURE 67
STUDY SHEET: COMPARISON OF BONE NAMES

	Scientific names	Common names	Butcher's names
1.	Skull	Head bone	
2.	Mandible	Jawbone	
3.	Clavicle	Collarbone	
4.	Scapula	Shoulder blade	Blade
5.	Sternum	Breastbone	
6.	Rib	Rib	Rib
7.	Humerus	Upper arm bone	Shoulder
8.	Vertebral column	Backbone	Chuck bone (part of backbone)
9.	Radius and ulna	Lower arm bones	Shank bone
10.	Carpal bone	Wrist bone	
11.	Metacarpal bone	Hand bone	
12.	Phalange	Finger bone	
13.	Pelvis	Hipbone	Aitchbone and hipbone
14.	Femur	Thighbone	Thighbone
15.	Patella	Kneecap	
16.	Tibia	Shinbone	Shinbone
17.	Fibula	Calf bone	
18.	Tarsal	Anklebone	
19.	Metatarsal	Foot bone	
20.	Phalange	Toe bone	

(Reprinted from *Bones, Teacher's Guide*, by Elementary Science Study, copyright 1965, with permission of Webster/McGraw-Hill.)

FIGURE 68
CHAPTER 8B, UNIT II

WHAT'S YOUR MUSCLE
POWER? CROSSWORD
PUZZLE AND QUESTIONS

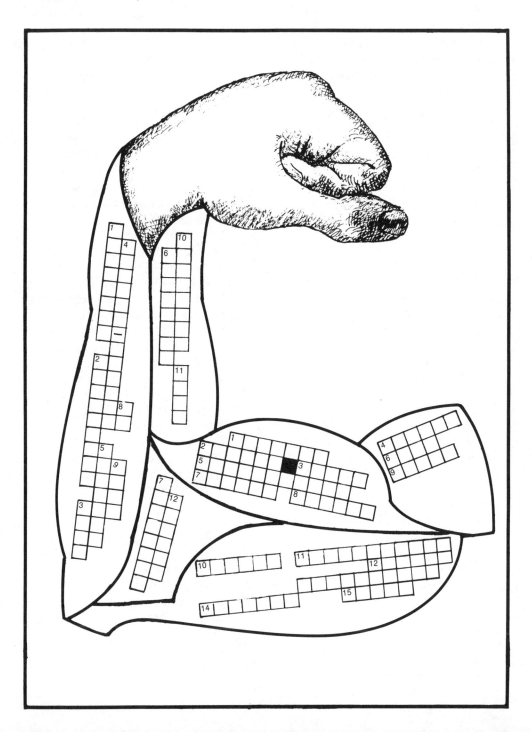

DOWN

1. What type of muscles is fastened to bones? (8 letters)
2. What do we call muscles that are attached to our skeleton and we have some control over? (9 letters)
3. What do we eat to provide our muscles with energy so they can work for us? (4 letters)
4. What is a waste product produced in the muscle? (hyphenated word)
5. What is a safeguard against muscle strain? (It is what we feel after a lot of hard work.) (7 letters)
6. What do the more than 600 skeletal muscles attached to our bones by tendons make possible? (8 letters)
7. What enlarges the fibers that make up our muscles and increases our circulation? (8 letters)
8. Should you participate in strenuous activities when you are out of condition or very tired? (2 letters)
9. If possible, what kind of shower should you take after exercising to help increase circulation of the blood and to relieve sore muscles? (4 letters)
10. What is the name of the tendon that is located just above our heel and helps us to move our heel and foot? (8 letters)
11. How may your muscles feel if the muscle fibers are torn after a lot of strenuous exercise? (4 letters)
12. How is a muscle described when it is without tone and tires easily? (6 letters)

ACROSS

1. What helps hold our bones in place, focus the lenses of our eyes, and draw air into our lungs? (7 letters)
2. What is the cordlike end of a muscle which attaches the muscle to a bone called? (6 letters)
3. What is the name of the muscle that is located on the front of the upper arm? (5 letters)
4. Our muscles can work because food and oxygen are chemically changed to release _____. (6 letters)
5. When a muscle gets shorter and thicker it is _____. (11 letters)
6. What cannot move without a muscle? (4 letters)
7. What occurs when a ligament connecting a bone or supporting a joint is torn? (It is painful; a cold pack may help to relieve the swelling.) (6 letters)
8. What does the circulatory system carry besides food to the muscles so they can work well? (6 letters)
9. The faster your muscles move, the faster your _____ pumps. (5 letters)
10. What may occur by taking a wrong step and stretching the muscle that supports the ankle? (If it happens, rest the injured part and apply heat.) (6 letters)
11. What do we call muscles that we cannot control and are found in the walls of our stomach and intestines? (11 letters)
12. What muscle is located on the back of the upper arm? (6 letters)
13. Which body system supplies food and oxygen to all of our body cells and takes away wastes? (11 letters)
14. When a muscle expands and becomes longer and thinner it is _____. (7 letters)
15. Our muscles, like the bicep and tricep, work in _____. (5 letters)

FIGURE 69
WORKSHEET: INSIDE THE HUMAN HEART

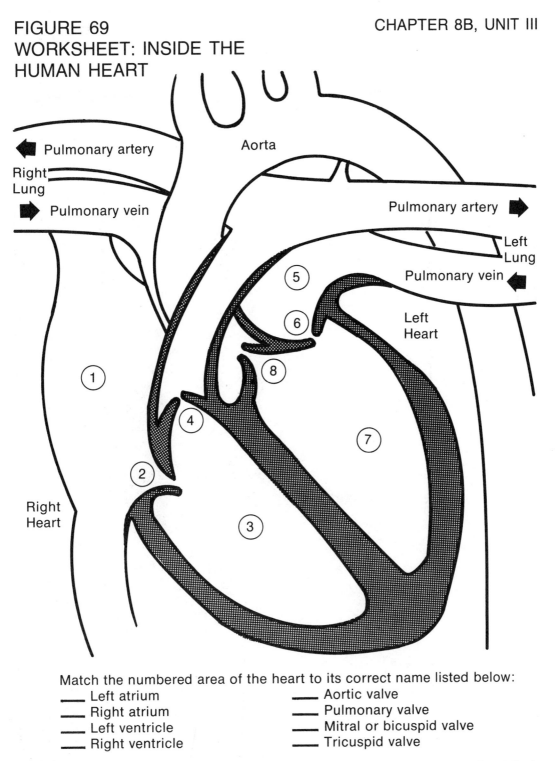

Match the numbered area of the heart to its correct name listed below:

___ Left atrium   ___ Aortic valve
___ Right atrium   ___ Pulmonary valve
___ Left ventricle   ___ Mitral or bicuspid valve
___ Right ventricle   ___ Tricuspid valve

(Illustration adapted with permission from *Your Heart and How It Works,* The American Heart Association.)

FIGURE 70
CHAPTER 8B, UNIT IV
WORKSHEET: TRACE THE PASSAGE
OF AIR INTO THE LUNGS

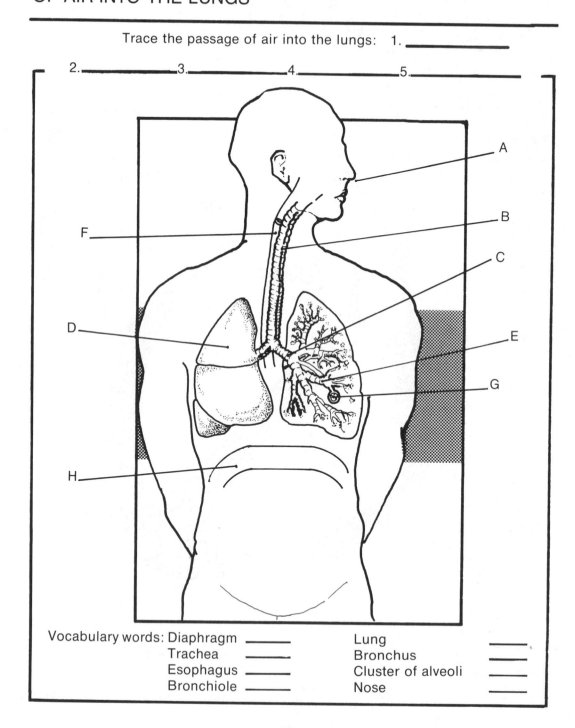

Trace the passage of air into the lungs: 1. _____

2. _____ 3. _____ 4. _____ 5. _____

A

B

C

F

D

E

G

H

Vocabulary words: Diaphragm _____   Lung
Trachea _____   Bronchus   _____
Esophagus _____   Cluster of alveoli   _____
Bronchiole _____   Nose   _____

FIGURE 71

CHAPTER 8B, UNIT V

DIGESTION DRAG TRACK GAME (TWO SHEETS)
AND GAME CARDS (TWO SHEETS)

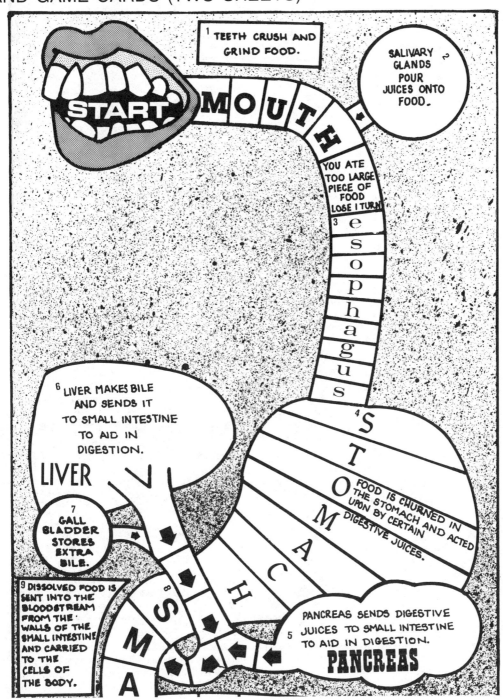

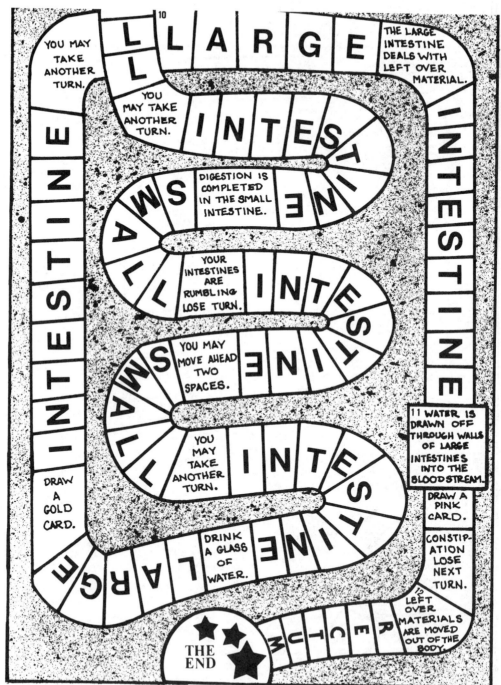

*Adapted from the comic book, *Mulligan Stew*, with permission of Extension, 4H, U.S. Dept of Agriculture in cooperation with State Extension Services of the Land Grant Universities; and from *Health and Growth*, Book 5, Teacher's Edition, by Julius B. Richmond, et al. Copyright © 1971 by Scott, Foresman & Co. Reprinted by permission.

YELLOW CARDS

True or *false*: One serving of milk each day is plenty for a good diet.	What vitamin can you get from orange juice and other citrus fruits? (Vitamin C)	One serving of fruit and vegetables each day is plenty for a balanced diet. (False)	Carbohydrates give us energy for work and play. (True)
We should eat at least four servings of food from the meat group each day. (False)	Potatoes and bread have lots of protein in them. (False, they have lots of carbohydrates)	Protein builds strong muscles and helps to repair our body tissues. (True)	The more you eat the better you feel. (False, it's now how much but what you eat that counts)
What food group has been left out of this breakfast? Bacon and eggs, toast, butter, milk. (Fruit & Veg. group)	Are nutrients carried to our body cells by the blood stream? (Yes)	Food can travel down our trachea and reach our stomach. (NO)	What are two things in our mouth that aid digestion? (Teeth, salivary glands)
What do most foods contain if they smell like burning feathers when they are burned? (Protein)	Protein is found in eggs, milk, meat, cheese, fish, and poultry. (Yes)	Carbohydrates are sweet or starchy foods. (True)	Saliva in our mouth changes some starch to sugar. (Yes)
If a drop of iodine is dropped on food that contains starch the color will change from brown to a purple-black. (Yes)	Any food which contains fat or oil will leave a grease spot on paper. (Yes)	You can enjoy more food (containing calories) when you're active. (Yes)	How does our body use the minerals calcium and phosphorus? (To build strong bones and teeth)

PINK CARDS

From the esophagus food goes into what part of your body? (Stomach)	What is in your mouth besides your tongue and teeth that aids digestion? (Saliva)	You would get all the nutrients you need by eating lots of meat every day. (False)	Move ahead one space.
Which food group is better for giving us fats: Milk or fruits and vegetables? (Milk)	What is the best food for calcium? (Milk)	Iron is especially needed by red blood cells to help carry oxygen. (True)	What is an important use of Vitamin A? (For healthy skin, Good vision at night)
What is an important use of Vitamin C? (Increases resistance to infection; healthy gums and skin.)	What disease can you get if you do not get enough Vitamin D from milk and sunshine? (Rickets)	Water is needed to carry nutrients to cells and to carry away their waste products. (Yes)	Water is especially important to drink when you are fighting an infection. (Yes)

BLUE CARDS

Name one way you can help prevent constipation. (Drink plenty of water; exercise daily.)	What gives us our energy? (The food we eat)	Why is it important to chew your food thoroughly before swallowing it? (Saliva mixed with small pieces of food is easier to digest.)	What muscle in our mouth moves our food around to be chewed? (tongue)
The stomach is a long, muscular tube. (False)	The stomach is a swollen, hollow bag with two openings at opposite ends. (True)	The stomach is a muscle lined with glands which manufacture hydrochloric acid which aids in digestion. (True)	What is an organ that aids in the process of digestion although no food ever passes through it? (liver, pancreas, gallbladder)
Digested food passes through the capillaries in the walls of the small intestine and move into the bloodstream. (True)	All of the foods that we eat are able to be dissolved. (False)	What happens to undigested food in the small intestine? (It passes into the large intestine.)	The large intestine absorbs most of the liquid, leaving a soft, solid, waste material. (True)
The rectum gets rid of waste material that cannot be digested. (True)	The rectum is actually not a part of the digestive system; it belongs to the ___ system. (excretory)	When we are constipated, our food stays in the rectum and water keeps being absorbed by the large intestine. (True)	It is a good idea to set aside a regular time for a bowel movement. (True)
Saliva is a juice that contains water, mucus, and a digestive enzyme. (True)	Digestive enzymes are substances that cause chemical changes to take place in foods. (True)	Strong muscles in the stomach walls churn food into ___ . (a thick paste)	Vitamins and minerals from your food dissolve and pass from the large intestine into the blood. (False, they pass from small intestine.)

PINK CARDS

As the digested food enters your bloodstream, it travels first to the liver. (True)	Your liver is an amazing chemical factory that you need to live. (True)	Much of the fat you eat is stored ___ where it prevents body heat from escaping too quickly. (just under the skin)	Why is it better to be happy and relaxed when eating? (so the stomach will freely produce gastric juice to mix with our food)
When we are worried, unhappy or upset, the gastric juice in our stomach does not flow as well. (True)	Does your stomach work better when you are fairly quiet or exercising after a meal? (fairly quiet)	Alcoholic drinks make the stomach red and sore looking. (True)	Which foods stay in the stomach longer—bread and potatoes or meat and eggs? (meat and eggs)
Go to #2, Salivary Glands (Pour juices onto food.)	Go to #6, Liver (Spend turn making bile.)	Go to #7, gallbladder (Spend turn storing extra bile.)	Go to #5, Pancreas (Spend turn sending digestive juices to the small intestine.)

Label the following organs. On the back of this paper describe a function for each of these organs.

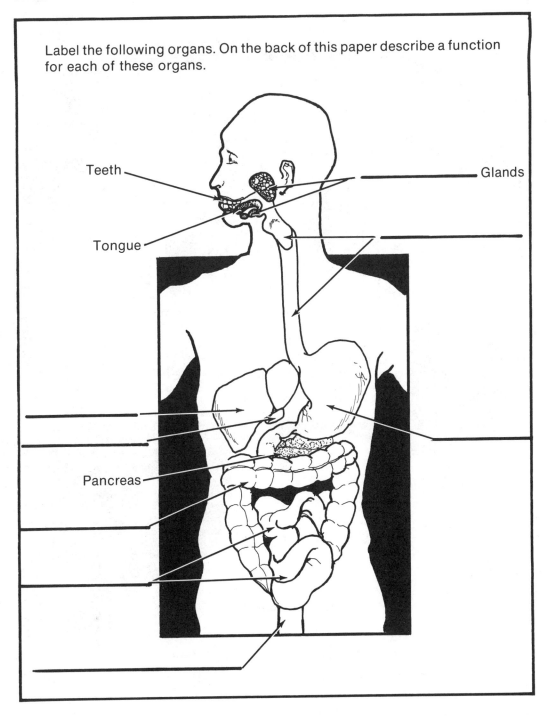

Teeth

Glands

Tongue

Pancreas

FIGURE 73
THE BRAIN MAZE

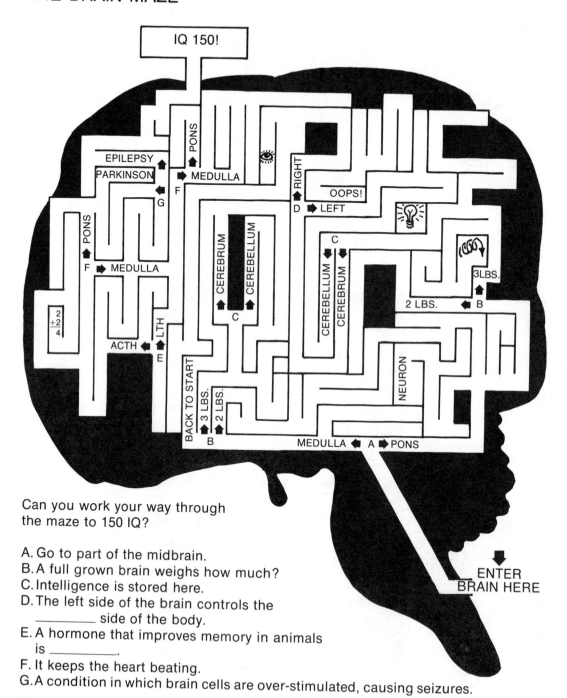

Can you work your way through the maze to 150 IQ?

A. Go to part of the midbrain.
B. A full grown brain weighs how much?
C. Intelligence is stored here.
D. The left side of the brain controls the
   _____ side of the body.
E. A hormone that improves memory in animals
   is _____.
F. It keeps the heart beating.
G. A condition in which brain cells are over-stimulated, causing seizures.

(Adapted from *Current Health: The Continuing Guide to Health Education* 2: 7, March 1976, Curriculum Innovations, Inc.)

FIGURE 74
WORKSHEET: THE
NERVOUS SYSTEM

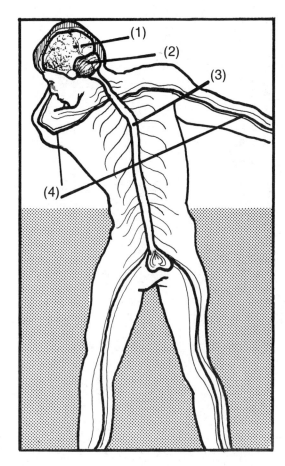

The three main divisions
of the brain are:

I. Forebrain
Including the Cerebrum

II. Midbrain
Including the Pons

III. Hindbrain
Including the Cerebellum
and Medulla Oblongata

Can you name parts numbered
on the drawing?

1._____
2._____
3._____
4._____

Can you match the structure with its
correct function?

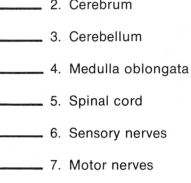

_____ 1. Skull

_____ 2. Cerebrum

_____ 3. Cerebellum

_____ 4. Medulla oblongata

_____ 5. Spinal cord

_____ 6. Sensory nerves

_____ 7. Motor nerves

A. A long cord of connective tissue
that provides a passageway for
nerves.

B. Carries messages from eyes, ears,
skin, etc. to the brain.

C. Carries orders for action from
the brain to the muscles.

D. Bones that help protect the brain.

E. Controls your muscles; Reflex center.

F. Helps regulate your breathing,
digestion of food, and blood
circulation.

G. Controls your voluntary actions;
Enables you to think and remember.

SAMPLE CARDS FOR BULL'S-EYE GAME
(Duplicate this page to make 50 cards—25 pairs)

Use extra care when opening cans of *acid* or other strong liquids. Do not keep your face close to the can!	Avoid *self-diagnosis* and self-medication. Use remedies only if advised by your physician.	Wash your *hands* thoroughly before you examine your eye.	Bandage a *cut eye* lightly with a sterile gauze patch and call a doctor. Do not try to remove an object stuck in the eye.	An *ophthalmologist* is a medical doctor who specializes in the diagnosis and treatment of eye defects and diseases.
Be extra *careful* when working with *tools* (wear safety glasses).	How can ice picks, scissors, and other sharp instruments be *stored* out of children's reach?	*Don't rub* your eyes with dirty hands or if there is a foreign object in your eye.	For a *black eye*, apply cold compresses immediately for about 15 minutes per hour. See a doctor, since there may be serious internal damage to the eyeball.	Excessive blinking, rubbing eyes often, tilting head to one side, and holding a book close to the eyes may indicate *vision problems*.
Have your *eyes* and visual acuity *checked* at least every two years.	Show the class a *safe toy* and an unsafe toy (representing eye safety).	Never look directly at the *sun*, even while wearing sunglasses.	If a speck does not wash out, keep the eye *closed* with a light dressing and seek medical attention.	*Extra care* must be taken if you wear contact lenses. Do not wear them while sleeping; wash your hands before handling the lens; clean lens container daily.
See that you have *good light* (without glare) when you read and study.	Be careful when playing with sticks, stones, arrows, air guns, etc., and *do not throw* these objects at children.	Obtain the approval of a qualified physician before wearing *colored glasses* continuously.	If a speck gets in your eye, lift the upper eyelid over the lower lid and let *tears wash* out the particle.	It is dangerous to wet a *contact lens* with saliva before inserting it.
Wear *Safety Glasses* where there is danger to your eyes.	Search your home for *sharp objects* that stick out at eye level and move them to a safer place.	How can children hurt their eyes by using *fireworks*?	If you need glasses, *wear them* (or your contact lenses).	A *burn* in the eye should be flushed with water immediately for about 15 minutes. See a doctor as soon as possible.

FIGURE 76 CHAPTER 8B, UNIT VII

SAMPLE CARDS FOR EAR-OPENER GAME
(Duplicate this page to make 50 cards—25 pairs)

Tinnitus is a ringing or buzzing sound in the ear. May be caused by many different things.	A fairly loud ticking watch should be audible at a distance of four feet.	If you become *hoarse,* inhaling steam, drinking plenty of liquids, and resting your voice will help.	Besides using an audiometer to test hearing, a *tuning fork* and *word discrimination test* may be used.	Did you know that severe infectious diseases are sometimes complicated by ear trouble?
An *otoscope* is an instrument that lights up the ear so the doctor can see your eardrum and deposits of wax.	An *audiometer* is an instrument that produces electrical tones and is used to test hearing.	You should keep your ear canals free from excess *wax* so it won't obstruct the canal and interfere with hearing.	If an *insect* flies into your friend's ear, you may drop light mineral oil into the canal to suffocate the insect. Have a doctor remove the insect.	Do you think it would be worthwhile for someone to join an organization to *fight noise* or to support antinoise legislation?
An *otorhinolaryngologist* is a doctor who specializes in treating the ear, nose, and throat.	*Cauliflower ear* means an enlarged and disfigured ear commonly seen in boxers and wrestlers.	*Mixed-loss deafness* is a combination of both conductive and nerve deafness.	*Surgery* is often successful in treating conductive deafness.	*Protect your hearing* through regular check-ups; by buying quiet appliances; turning down volume of radio, TV, and stereo; and wearing earplugs where there is a lot of noise.
An *audiologist* is a trained specialist who conducts hearing tests.	*Otosclerosis* is a disease in which the tiny bones in the ear fail to function, resulting in deafness. Corrected with surgery.	*Nerve-loss deafness* involves some destruction of the nerves that carry the sensations of sound from the cochlea to the brain.	Vigorous *nose blowing* is dangerous, because it may force nasal secretions into the middle ear through the eustachian tube and cause an infection.	*Noise pollution* is continuous exposure to excessive noise. It can *increase* tension, industrial accidents, and blood pressure and cause mental disorientation.
An *otologist* is an ear physician who can diagnose the type and extent of a hearing loss and treat defects and diseases.	*Otitis* is an inflammation of the ear.	*Conductive deafness* has to do with the way sound is brought from the eardrum by the three moving bones to the inner ear.	Two *functions* of the *ear* are to detect vibrations, called sound waves, and help us maintain balance.	A *hearing aid* may fit snugly behind the ear, worn on the body, or worn attached to eyeglasses.

The *cochlea* and *semicircular canal* are found in the *inner* ear.	During athletic sports that may cause a sharp blow to the head, wear a *helmet*.	An *optometrist* is not a medical doctor but specializes in correcting vision defects by means of glasses, contact lenses, and eye exercises.	*Deaf* people may learn to *communicate* through sign language or lip-reading.	Most insects hear very poorly, if at all. Many can detect various kinds of vibrations with their antennae. Moths have excellent hearing.
The *hammer, anvil,* and *stirrup* are the three bones that stretch across the *middle* ear.	The normal healthy ear needs *little attention* other than to be washed with a washcloth covering the end of your finger and dried after shower or swimming.	In *astigmatism,* incoming light rays focus at more than one point because of an uneven curvature of the cornea.	We can detect air vibrations through three senses: hearing, seeing, and touching.	The *auditory nerve* connects the ear to the brain.
Symptoms of hearing problems may include asking for words to be repeated; ability to read lips; pain, tenderness, or swelling in or about the ear.	*Picking the ear canal* with a toothpick, hairpin, or similar objects can be dangerous, causing infection or puncturing eardrum.	*Farsightedness* results when the eyeball is too short and light rays focus behind the retina.	Adults over age 35 should have their eyes tested with a *tonometer* to discover *glaucoma* in early stage.	The semicircular canals contain fluid and nerve endings that detect movement and tell the brain. The brain may send return impulses to muscles for restoring balance.
Symptoms of hearing problems may include dizziness, buzzing or ringing in the ears, failure to locate the source of a sound, and poor progress in school.	*Wax* in the middle ear protects it from drying and scaling and from damage while swimming. Excess wax should be removed by a doctor.	*Nearsightedness* results when the eyeball is too long (the lens bends the light rays so that they come to a focus before reaching the retina.	One should not borrow or lend personal towels or eye makeup, because of chance of *infection.*	The eardrum separates the outer ear from the middle ear. The *middle ear* contains three tiny bones and the eustachian tube which leads into the throat.
Symptoms of hearing problems may include turning head toward source of sound, inability to follow directions, and inattention to what others say.	The *outer ear,* because of its prominence and thin, tight skin, is subject to sunburn and frostbite and should be protected.	*Our eyes are protected* by bony ridges, eyelids, tears, and eyebrows.	An *optician* specializes in grinding lenses and fitting glasses.	Sounds (air vibrations) travel through our *outer ear* into the *auditory canal* and then reach the *eardrum.*

FERTILIZATION: A GAME OF
CHANCE (GAMEBOARD AND GAME CARDS)

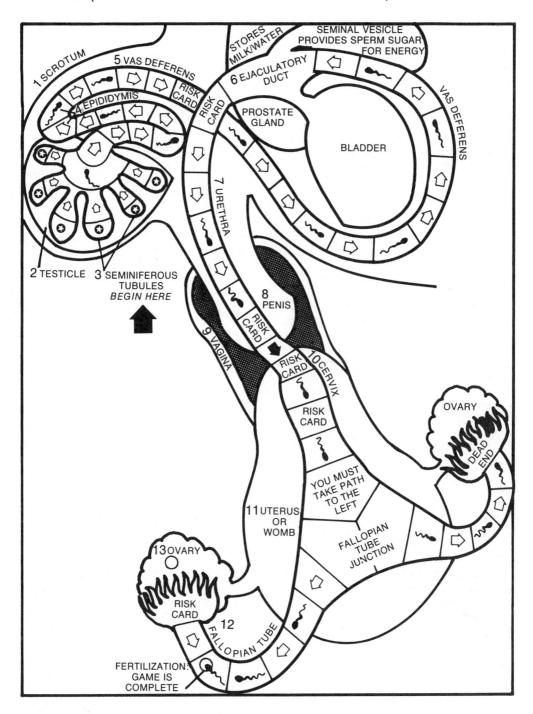

SPERM CARDS

If fertilized, where does the cell normally attach itself to grow into a baby? (Wall of uterus)	What composes the discharge from the vagina during menstruation? (blood—also cells lining the uterus)	What does the scrotum do? (It contains the testes and regulates temperature)	What is one thing that the testes do? (Produce male sex hormone and produce sperm)
Where are sperm produced? (In the testes, specifically the seminiferous tubules)	Of what use is seminal fluid from the seminal vesicle? (Provides sperm with sugar for energy)	What is one thing that the ovaries do? (Produce female sex hormones and produce eggs)	What does FSH do? (It is sent by the pituitary gland to the ovaries and testes to wake them up—or stimulate them to start growing)
Do urine and semen ever travel down the urethra at the same time? (No)	Where is the epididymis located? (On the top of each testes)	How is a sperm like a tadpole? (It has a head and a tail and it can swim)	How old is a boy when he usually starts to make sperms? (11 or 12)
How long does the menstrual flow usually last? (3–5 days, once a month)	What does a girl wear to collect the menstrual blood? (Sanitary napkin or tampon)	If a baby is going to be produced, where do the egg and sperm first meet? (Fallopian tube)	What is a word used to describe a mother with a baby growing inside of her uterus? (Pregnant)
What is the real name for a mark left on a baby showing where it was connected to its mother? (Navel)	When a boy begins making semen, he may overflow at night as he dreams. This is called (seminal emission) "wet dream"	What happens to the penis when semen is going to come out? (It becomes very hard)	What is the name of the short path between the vas deferens and the urethra? (Ejaculatory duct)
What is the name of the long tube inside the penis? (Urethra)	What is it called when the egg and sperm meet and form a partnership? (Fertilization)	Where does the baby grow inside the mother? (Uterus)	What kind of changes that are visible happen to a girl at puberty? (Hips become wider, breasts develop, hair under arms)
How does a baby get food when it is inside the mother? (Through the umbilical cord that is attached to the placenta)	What is the name of the tunnel between the mother's legs that the baby comes through when it is born? (Vagina)	After a girl starts to menstruate regularly, how many nests will her body make each year in preparation for a baby? (Twelve)	How long does the baby grow inside its mother? (9 months)
RISK! Oops! The testes have just been immersed into very hot water resulting in temporary sterility—lose 1 turn.	**RISK!** Oops! Heat from a blast furnace has resulted in a high incidence of defective sperm—Lose one turn.	**RISK!** Oops! Lots of stress has reduced the number of sperm. Lose one turn.	**RISK!** Oops! You have come in contact with too much radiation. Lose one turn.

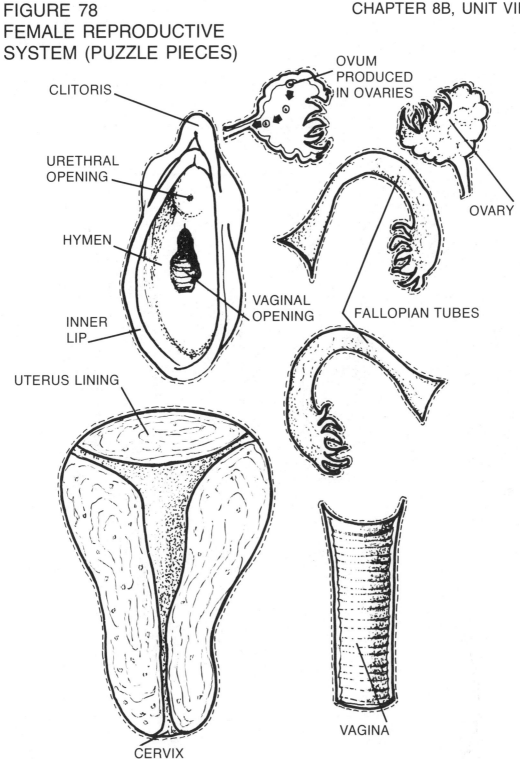

FIGURE 78
FEMALE REPRODUCTIVE
SYSTEM (PUZZLE PIECES)

CLITORIS

OVUM
PRODUCED
IN OVARIES

URETHRAL
OPENING

OVARY

HYMEN

VAGINAL
OPENING

INNER
LIP

FALLOPIAN TUBES

UTERUS LINING

VAGINA

CERVIX

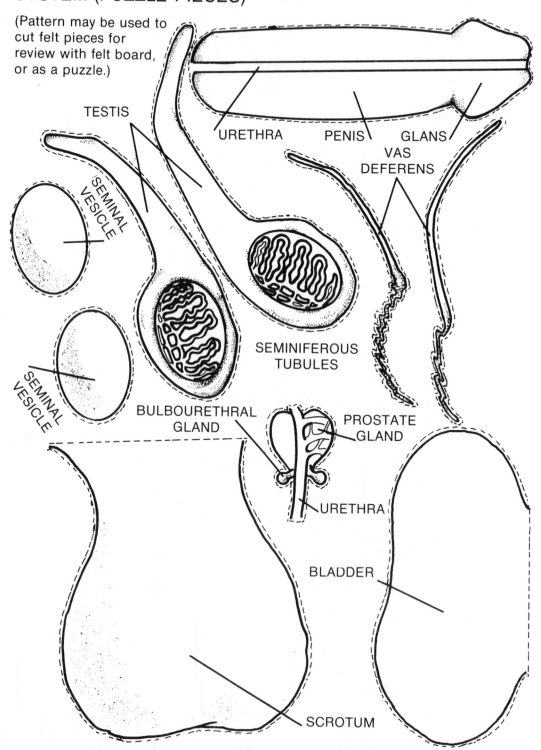

FIGURE 79
MALE REPRODUCTIVE
SYSTEM (PUZZLE PIECES)

(Pattern may be used to
cut felt pieces for
review with felt board,
or as a puzzle.)

TESTIS

URETHRA   PENIS   GLANS

VAS
DEFERENS

SEMINAL
VESICLE

SEMINIFEROUS
TUBULES

SEMINAL
VESICLE

BULBOURETHRAL
GLAND

PROSTATE
GLAND

URETHRA

BLADDER

SCROTUM

FIGURE 80
WORKSHEET: THIS IS ME!

CHAPTER 8B, UNIT VIII

MY NAME IS _____

I like using my EYES _____

I like using my BRAIN _____

I like using my EARS _____

I like using my NOSE _____

I like using my TEETH _____

I like using my TONGUE _____

I like using my HEART _____

I like using my LUNGS _____

I like using my MUSCLES _____

I like using my BONES _____

I like using my STOMACH _____

I like using my LIVER _____

I like to TOUCH _____

I also like to FEEL _____

My LEGS are especially good at _____

I like to EAT _____

I like to SLEEP _____

I like being a boy/girl because _____

Five words that DESCRIBE me are: 1. _____

I think having good health means _____

2. _____
3. _____
4. _____
5. _____

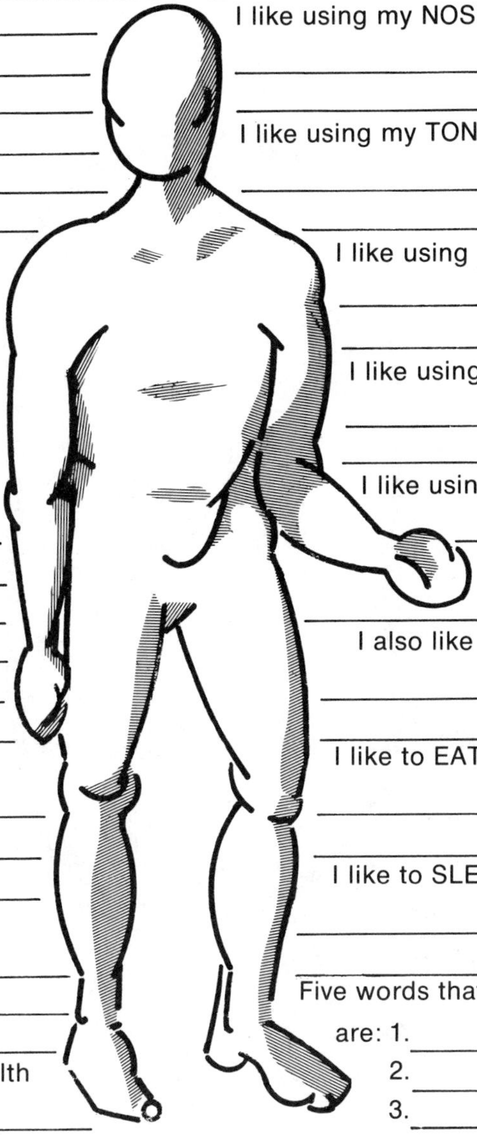

I like my FEET _____

FIGURE 81
GROOMING RALLY (Should
be enlarged)

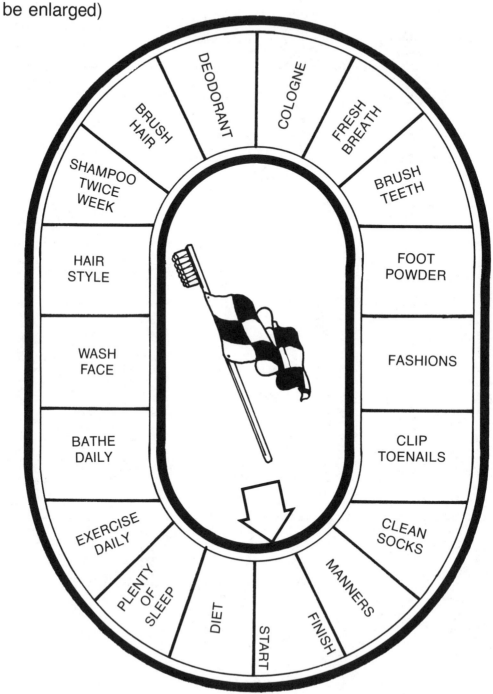

(Adapted with permission from *Avon's Grooming Rally*.)

FIGURE 82
GROOMING GRAND PRIX
CHECKLIST

CHAPTER 8B, UNIT IX

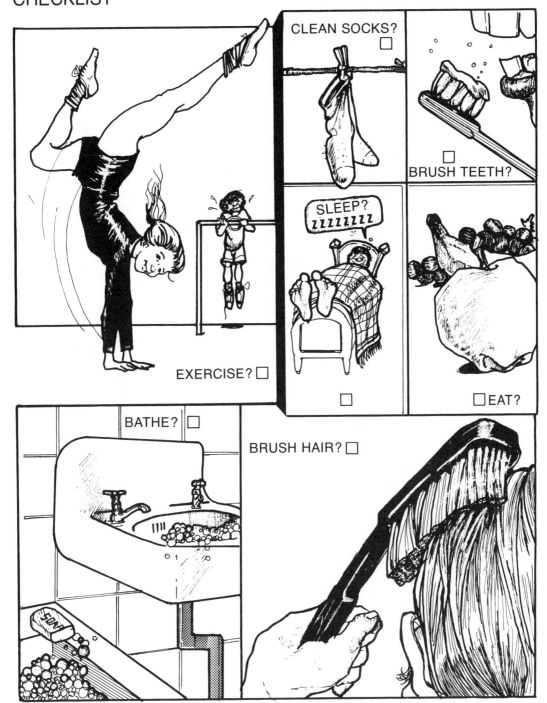

FIGURE 83
WORSHEET: BODY
TUNE-UP

CHAPTER 8B, UNIT IX

My tool is _____.

I think it is important because _____

_____

_____.

I use this tool for _____

_____.

(Show the class how to use your tool.)

I use this tool _____ times a day.

It helps keep my body in running order by _____

_____

_____.

I take care of this tool by _____

_____.

You can buy this tool _____

_____.

FIGURE 84
NORMAL ARTERY

CHAPTER 9B, UNIT I

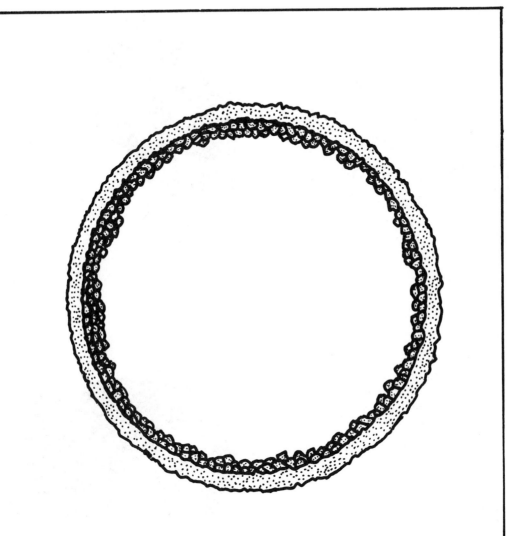

Smooth wide channel carries blood to the heart.

(Adapted from *Heart Project* with permission of The American Heart Association.)

FIGURE 85
ABNORMAL ARTERY

CHAPTER 9B, UNIT I

Cholesterol and other
fatty deposits thicken and
roughen the channel
lining.
These deposits thicken so
that the artery is
completely closed.

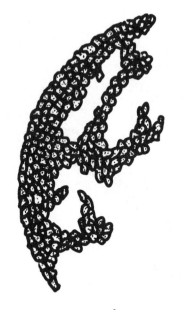

As blood flows through
a narrow channel, the
roughened surface can
cause a clot to form and
plug the artery.

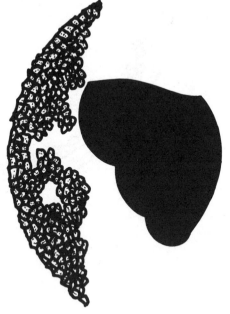

(Cut this page in half and
use as two overlays with
the normal artery
illustration.)

(Adapted from *Heart Project* with permission of The American Heart Association.)

FIGURE 86
WORKSHEET: STARS FOR
SLEEP

CHAPTER 9B, UNIT II

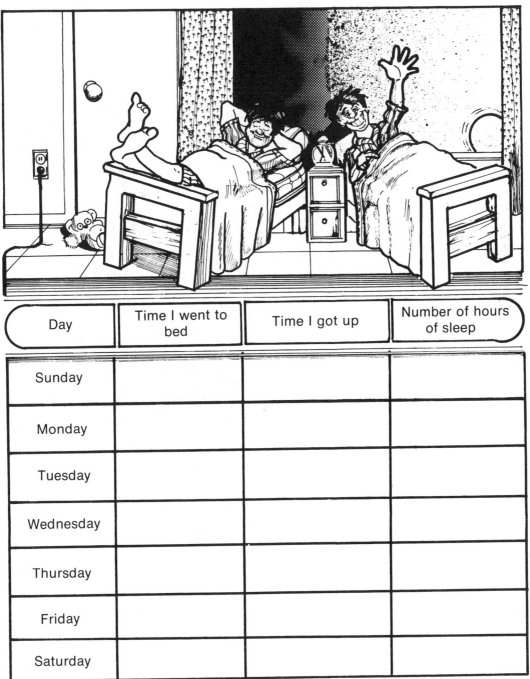

Day	Time I went to bed	Time I got up	Number of hours of sleep
Sunday			
Monday			
Tuesday			
Wednesday			
Thursday			
Friday			
Saturday			

(Adapted from "My Sleep Inventory," National Dairy Council.)

FIGURE 87

CHAPTER 11B, UNIT V

ORALLY SAFE AND HAZARDOUS SNACKS

Poor Snacks will hurt our teeth; Good snacks will keep them stronger. Of these good snacks we'll eat. Our teeth will last much longer! (In the spaces below draw and color snacks that you enjoy.)

Good and Juicy	Something Crunchy	Thirsty?	Really Hungry?	Snacks to Avoid

Raw fruit:
  apples
  blackberries
  grapefruit
  grapes
  oranges
  peaches
  pears
  plums
  raspberries
  strawberries
  tangerines
Tomatoes
Olives
Dill pickles
Yogurt (plain)
	Cabbage wedges
	Carrot strips
	Cauliflower flowerets
	Celery (plain or stuffed
	  with cheese)
	Cucumber strips or
	  slices
	Green onions
	Lettuce wedges
	Popcorn
	Radishes
	Peppers, raw slices
	Corn chips
	Potato chips
		White milk
		Buttermilk
		Tomato juice
		Juices (no sugar
		  added):
		  orange
		  grapefruit
		  pineapple
		  apple
		  Other fruit juices
		Beverages which do not
		  have sugar added
			Meat Cubes:
			  chicken
			  beef
			  ham
			  lamb
			  lunch meat
			  pork
			  turkey
			Vienna sausages
			Sardines
			Shrimp
			Cheese cubes
			Eggs—hard-boiled or
			  deviled
			Peanuts and other nuts
			Whole wheat bread
			Tacos
			Pizza
			Cheeseburgers
				Sweetened fruits and
				  juices
				Chocolate milk/cocoa
				Carbonated drinks
				Other sweetened drinks
				Honey
				Jams and jellies
				Syrups
				Sugar-coated cereals
				Dried fruits
				Cake and pastries
				Candy
				Cookies
				Crackers
				Pie
				Doughnuts
				Gelatin desserts
				Regular and bubble
				  gum
				Breath mints
				Cough drops

Orally safe snacks are not necessarily nutritious snacks. While dill pickles and artificially sweetened soda pop do not promote dental caries, they also are practically devoid of nutrients. On the other hand, raisins are a nutritious snack because of their iron content but orally hazardous because of their sugar content and stickiness. Ideally, a child should choose snacks that are both nutritious and orally safe.

FIGURE 88
WORKSHEET: MYSTERY
MOUTH

By looking at this open mouth, can you determine the approximate age of its owner? _____

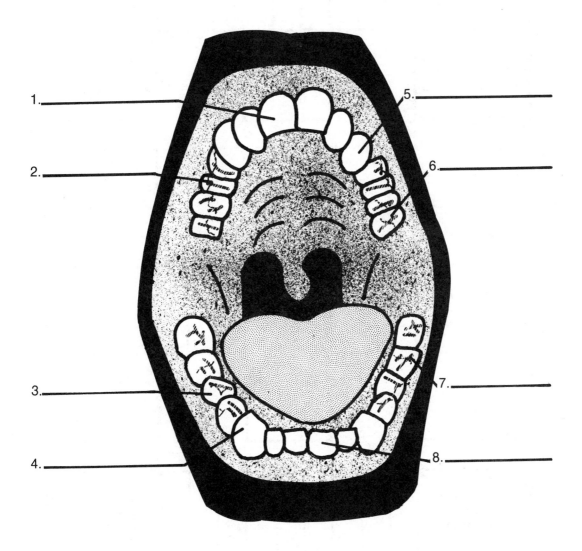

Each tooth has a name. Do you know what these names are?

FIGURE 89
VD GAME #1

CHAPTER 12B, UNIT IV

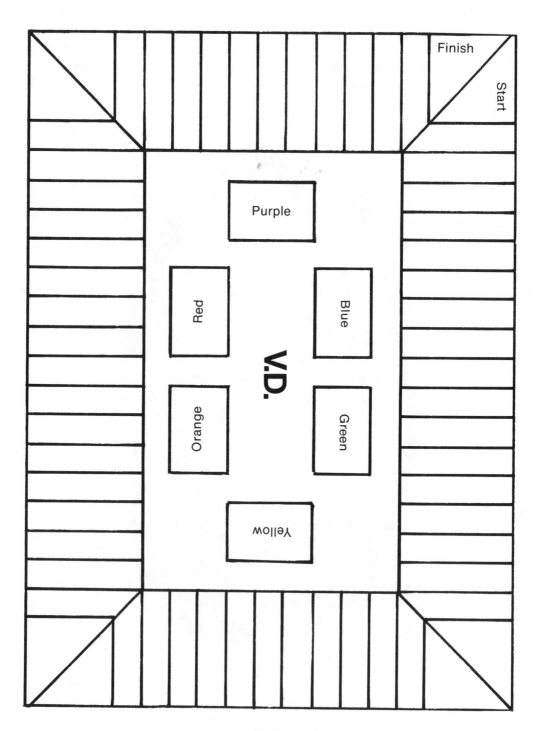

FIGURE 90
VD GAME #2

CHAPTER 12B, UNIT IV

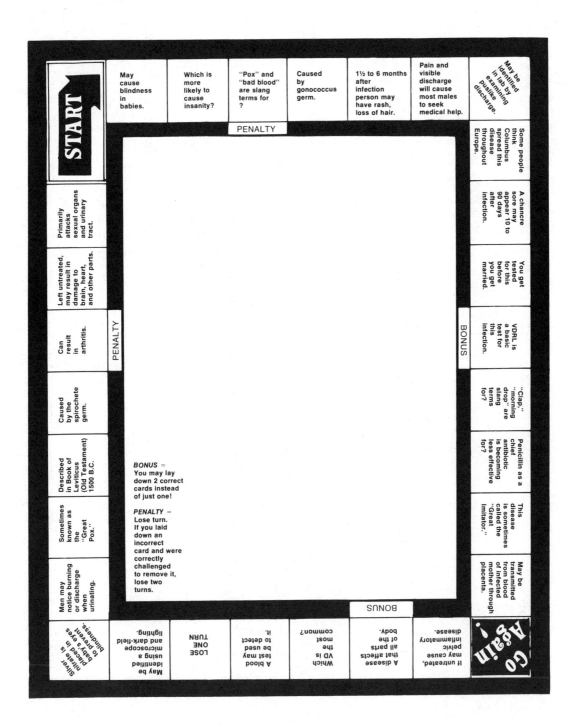

PLAYING CARDS FOR VD GAME #2

PLAYER 1		PLAYER 2		PLAYER 3		PLAYER 4	
Syphilis	Syphilis	Syphilis	Syphilis	Syphilis	Syphilis	Syphilis	Syphilis
Syphilis	Syphilis	Syphilis	Syphilis	Syphilis	Syphilis	Syphilis	Syphilis
Syphilis	Syphilis	Syphilis	Syphilis	Syphilis	Syphilis	Syphilis	Syphilis
Gonorrhea	Gonorrhea	Gonorrhea	Gonorrhea	Gonorrhea	Gonorrhea	Gonorrhea	Gonorrhea
Gonorrhea	Gonorrhea	Gonorrhea	Gonorrhea	Gonorrhea	Gonorrhea	Gonorrhea	Gonorrhea
Gonorrhea	Gonorrhea	Gonorrhea	Gonorrhea	Gonorrhea	Gonorrhea	Gonorrhea	Gonorrhea

(Answers, clockwise from start: G, S, S, G, S, G, G, S, S, S, S, S, G, G, S, G, none, G, S, G, S, none, S, G, none, S, G, S, G, S, G)

FIGURE 91
ENVIRONMENT PUZZLE

CHAPTER 13B, UNIT II

The picture on the other page is not very pretty, but you can fix it up. Cut around the pieces below, on the dotted lines. Each piece fits on a part of the picture, like a puzzle. See what happens to the picture when all of the pieces are on it. Can you think of some real ways that real places could be fixed up? Is there anything *you* could do?

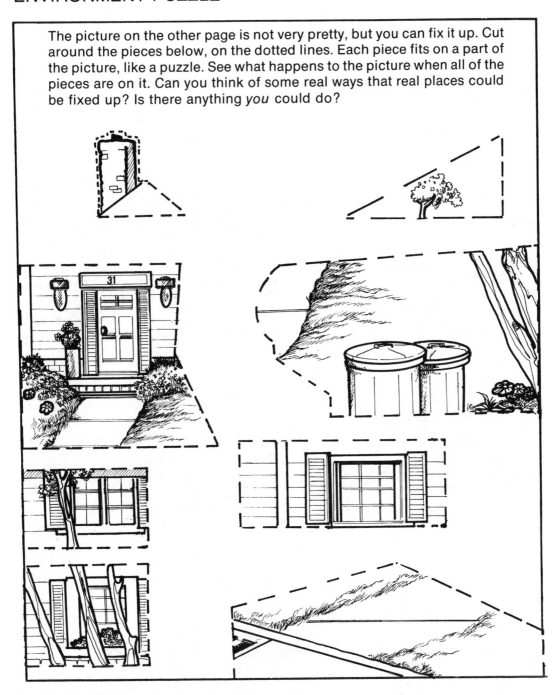

(Adapted with permission from the Environmental Information and Education Division, National Audubon Society, 950 Third Avenue, New York, NY 10022.)

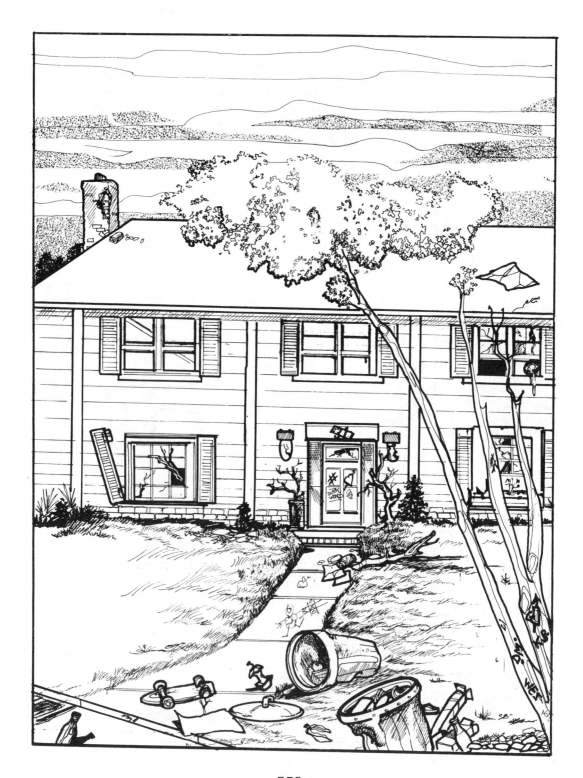

FIGURE 92
PUZZLE: WHAT'S IN THE TERRARIUM?

Have the students fill in the numbered blanks with the corresponding letter. Use the names of plants and animals the class will find in their terrarium.

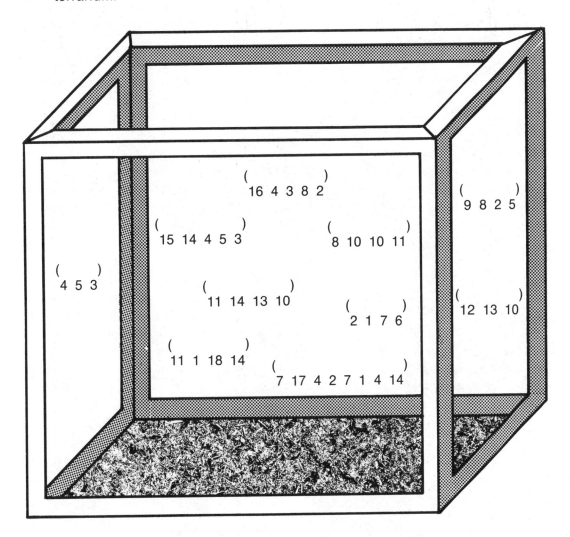

R	A	F	E	N	O	G	U	P	H	C	S	W	B	T	K	L	I
2	4	9	8	5	1	10	13	15	17	7	11	16	12	3	6	14	18

(By Janet Gilchrist, teacher at Glenbrook Elementary School, Euclid, Ohio.)

FIGURE 93
TERRARIUM JIGSAW PUZZLE

CHAPTER 13B, UNIT III

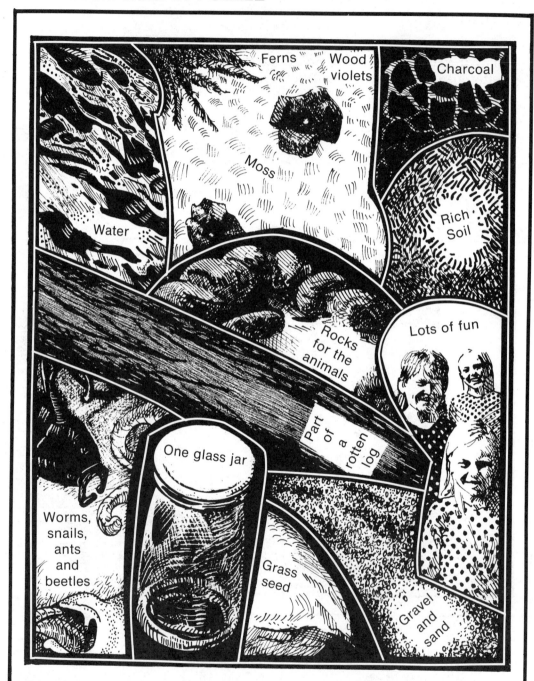

(Adapted with permission from puzzle prepared by Center for the Development of Environmental Curriculum, Willoughby-Eastlake City Schools, Willoughby, Ohio; and Ohio Department of Education, Columbus, Ohio.)

FIGURE 94
ENVIRONMENT WORD SEARCH

B	W	A	I	R	P	U	S	O	C	H	F	E	V	R	E	S	N	O	C
A	E	H	E	A	L	T	H	Y	A	G	A	R	V	P	F	J	U	I	K
R	L	W	E	Q	U	D	N	O	N	C	W	Z	H	I	E	A	E	N	T
E	G	S	A	K	D	I	S	E	A	S	E	B	F	R	A	N	T	P	O
C	V	R	H	T	F	E	Z	Y	T	U	M	O	C	O	V	R	S	S	M
O	N	E	A	O	E	C	K	S	U	R	O	L	A	I	W	T	A	O	Z
S	O	S	R	T	Y	R	O	J	R	Q	L	K	R	S	N	A	W	I	S
Y	S	A	N	I	T	A	R	I	A	N	I	O	M	T	L	O	E	V	R
S	M	L	Q	U	T	P	E	A	L	G	N	S	K	I	U	Y	C	W	P
T	O	L	U	S	E	L	I	N	R	M	E	T	S	G	N	T	O	I	E
E	G	O	B	I	C	R	O	S	E	B	V	N	P	V	G	L	T	A	D
M	C	R	U	Y	O	A	C	N	S	O	G	Y	O	T	S	I	S	J	I
B	G	U	C	M	L	O	T	S	O	F	M	J	I	Y	T	S	R	C	C
N	R	E	T	S	O	W	V	U	U	A	U	Q	N	O	R	A	U	Q	I
O	R	T	M	N	G	P	E	A	R	L	O	S	K	Z	K	E	R	A	T
I	A	S	K	Z	Y	L	I	L	C	H	I	D	R	E	U	N	V	Y	S
S	U	A	Y	L	L	I	T	T	E	R	B	U	G	B	A	U	N	E	E
E	B	P	L	O	Z	T	R	P	S	P	O	L	L	U	T	I	O	N	P

FIGURE 95
ENVIRONMENT CROSSWORD
PUZZLE

CHAPTER 13B, UNIT V

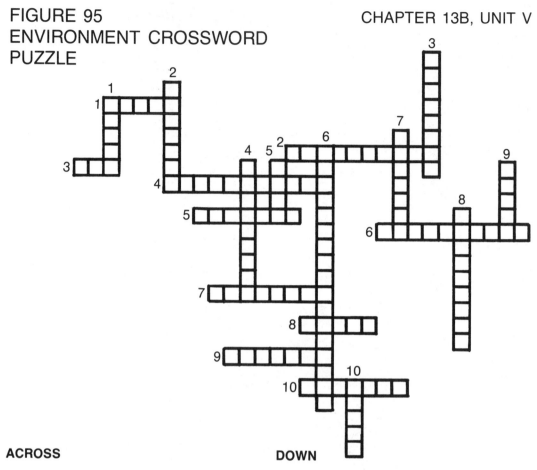

ACROSS

1. Another word for garbage.
2. Inspects our cafeteria and restaurants for cleanliness.
3. The number one polluter of air.
4. All the things around us.
5. The science which studies the relationship between people and their environment and the environment and people.
6. Kills house and garden pests.
7. What we must do for our trees and natural resources.
8. The type of pollution which effects our hearing.
9. Invented the process of purifying milk.
10. A clean environment helps to keep us _____.

DOWN

1. Sewage pollutes our _____.
2. What we should do with our paper, bottles, and cans.
3. Who is responsible for keeping our environment clean and healthy?
4. Everything that makes our air, land, and water dirty.
5. Another name of the haze in Los Angeles.
6. Another word for gas, oil, and water.
7. Improper disposal of garbage can transmit _____.
8. A natural community made up of living and nonliving things.
9. Another name for a person who throws garbage on the ground or out a car window.
10. Air pollution can affect these body organs.

FIGURE 96
POTENTIAL HOME HAZARDS
CHECKLIST

CHAPTER 14B, I

Yes No

____ ____ 1. Are floor surfaces nonskid and floor coverings fastened down?

____ ____ 2. Are all steps (indoors and outdoors) kept uncluttered?

____ ____ 3. Do stairways have sturdy railings?

____ ____ 4. Are electrical extension cords in good condition?

____ ____ 5. Does everyone in the household know how to turn off gas, water, and electricity if the need arises?

____ ____ 6. Do you only use proper size fuses?

____ ____ 7. Are normal walking paths free of electrical extension cords stretched across them.

____ ____ 8. Do you have and use a fireplace screen?

____ ____ 9. Do you have and know how to use an approved fire extinguisher?

____ ____ 10. Are emergency telephone numbers kept close to the telephone?

____ ____ 11. Is lead free paint used on all objects accessible to children?

____ ____ 12. Are window curtains out of reach of candles and the stove?

____ ____ 13. Are stairways, the stove, and sink well lighted?

____ ____ 14. Do you regularly inspect furnaces and flues?

____ ____ 15. Are knives, medicines, and cleaning agents stored out of the reach of small children?

____ ____ 16. Are razor blades properly stored or disposed of?

____ ____ 17. Are children's toys and play apparatus checked for sharp edges and loose parts?

____ ____ 18. Do you keep all electrical appliances away from water?

____ ____ 19. Is an approved and freshly stocked first-aid kit readily available?

____ ____ 20. Are grease, water, and other spilled liquids or foods immediately wiped up?

____ ____ 21. Do all family members refrain from smoking in bed?

____ ____ 22. Do you use a sturdy stepladder for climbing?

____ ____ 23. Is your room properly ventilated when using sprays, solvents, or a room heater?

____ ____ 24. Are entrances to your home well lighted?

FIGURE 97
SPORT AND ACTIVITY
WORD SEARCH

CHAPTER 14B, UNIT IV

How many sports and activities can you find? Words may be written across, backwards, up, down, or diagonally.

Circle the words.
Write a safety rule for each activity.

R	E	B	G	N	I	D	D	E	L	S	O	C	C	E	R
A	F	L	Y	I	N	G	A	R	C	A	M	P	I	N	G
C	L	I	M	B	O	T	R	O	P	I	C	N	I	C	N
I	A	B	A	S	K	E	T	B	A	L	L	U	G	F	I
N	H	O	R	L	W	N	S	A	C	I	D	H	O	I	T
G	U	W	K	I	A	N	H	S	K	N	P	O	L	S	A
N	N	L	O	D	L	I	U	E	R	G	T	Y	F	H	K
I	T	I	M	E	K	S	S	B	B	B	R	E	O	I	S
M	I	N	N	I	J	Q	T	A	A	I	K	C	N	N	B
M	N	G	N	E	U	R	O	L	L	R	K	J	O	G	O
I	G	G	S	S	D	C	L	L	L	E	C	I	U	A	X
W	E	R	H	K	O	R	E	O	Y	T	D	H	N	T	I
S	I	N	G	P	I	L	A	C	R	O	S	S	E	G	N
T	C	A	N	O	E	I	N	G	G	N	I	W	O	R	G
C	A	R	V	E	D	A	N	C	E	L	C	A	R	R	Y
A	T	J	U	M	P	I	N	G	F	E	N	C	I	N	G

FIGURE 98
A MEDICINE CABINET
CHECKLIST

CHAPTER 14B, UNIT V

Directions: Survey your home medicine cabinet with the help of an adult and place a check by the items you find listed below. These items are considered essentials by many different doctors. Did you find anything else in your cabinet? Is it really necessary?

_____ Gauze bandages: one roll of 1-inch wide gauze
one roll of 2-inch gauze
one 2- or 3-inch elastic bandage

_____ Several sterile gauze pads, packaged individually in sealed envelopes, 2x2 inches and 4x4 inches.

_____ Adhesive strip bandages (e.g. Band-Aids or Curads).

_____ Adhesive tape: 1- or 2-inch roll.

_____ Absorbent, sterile cotton.

_____ One package cotton-tipped swabs.

_____ Oral thermometer (rectal thermometer if there is an infant in the house).

_____ Hydrogen peroxide, for use as skin antiseptic.

_____ Vaseline or petroleum jelly.

_____ Aspirin tablets.

_____ Nonprescription medications that have been *specifically recommended* by your physician.

_____ Prescription medicines your physician has prescribed for current or chronic ills, each clearly labeled with name of medicine and person for whom it was prescribed. *Note:* Powerful medications such as strong sleeping tablets and narcotics should be kept apart from the family medicine chest.

_____ Syrup of ipecac: an emetic, or agent to produce vomiting, in cases of accidental poisoning is sometimes recommended if there are preschool-age children in the house.

Other Useful Items

_____ Heating pad

_____ Ice bag or flexible cold packs

_____ Hot water bottle

_____ Flashlight

_____ Steam inhalator (vaporizer)

_____ Scissors

FIGURE 99
BODY ORGANS COLORING ACTIVITY

CHAPTER 15B, UNIT II

Color these organs to match
their correct body system:

Color organs that belong
to the CIRCULATORY
SYSTEM *red.*
Color organs that belong
to the ENDOCRINE
SYSTEM *yellow.*
Color organs that belong
to the REPRODUCTIVE
SYSTEM *dark blue.*
Color organs that belong
to the NERVOUS
SYSTEM *orange.*
Color organs that belong
to the EXCRETORY
SYSTEM *brown.*
Color organs that belong
to the SKELETAL
SYSTEM *white.*
Color organs that belong
to the DIGESTIVE
SYSTEM *pink.*
Color organs that belong
to the MUSCULAR·
SYSTEM *green.*
Color organs that belong
to the RESPIRATORY
SYSTEM *light blue.*

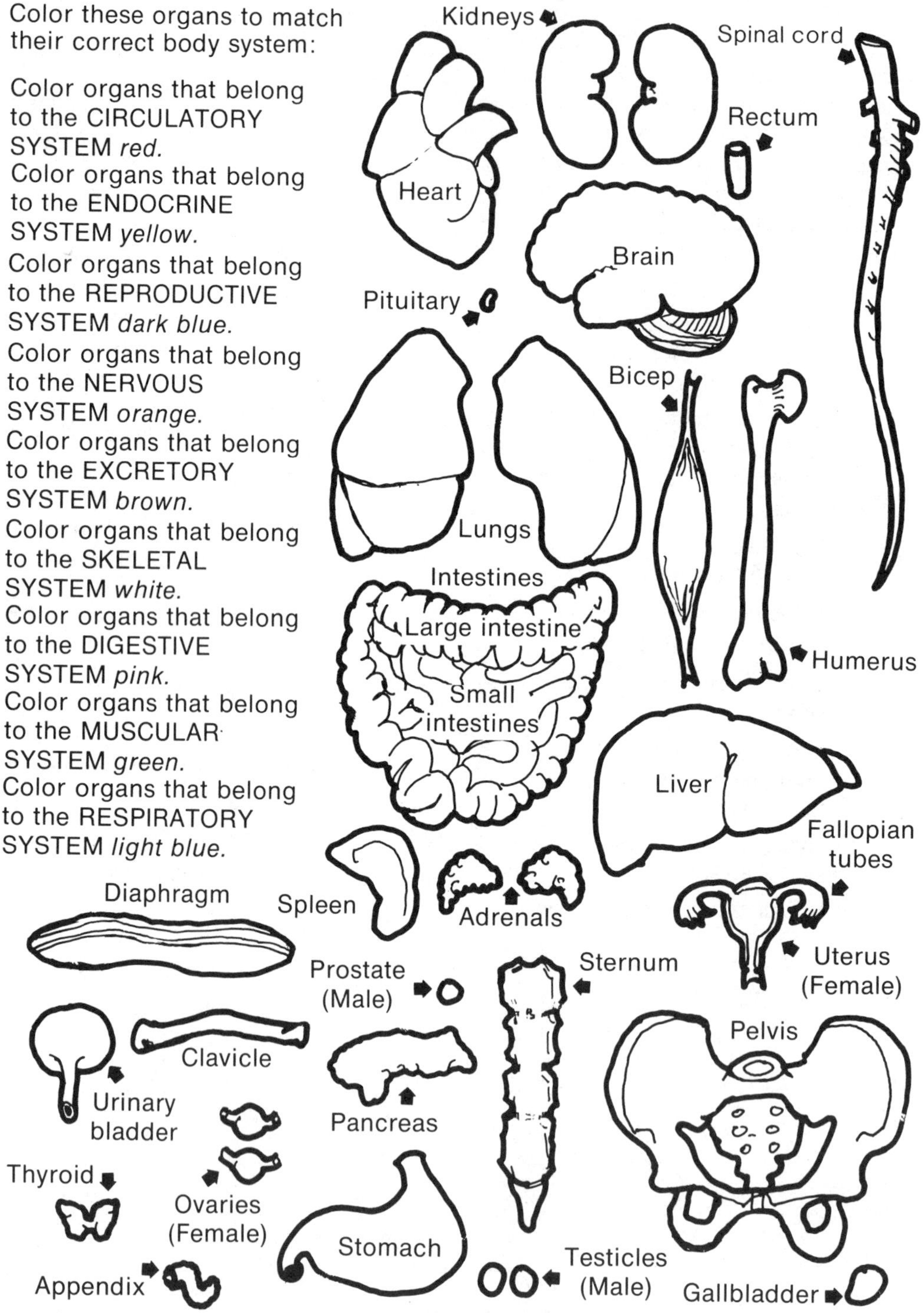

Kidneys

Spinal cord

Rectum

Heart

Brain

Pituitary

Bicep

Lungs

Humerus

Intestines

Large intestine

Small
intestines

Liver

Fallopian
tubes

Diaphragm

Spleen

Adrenals

Sternum

Uterus
(Female)

Prostate
(Male)

Pelvis

Clavicle

Urinary
bladder

Pancreas

Thyroid

Ovaries
(Female)

Stomach

Testicles
(Male)

Gallbladder

Appendix

FIGURE 100
BODY ORGANS PATTERN

CHAPTER 15B, UNIT II

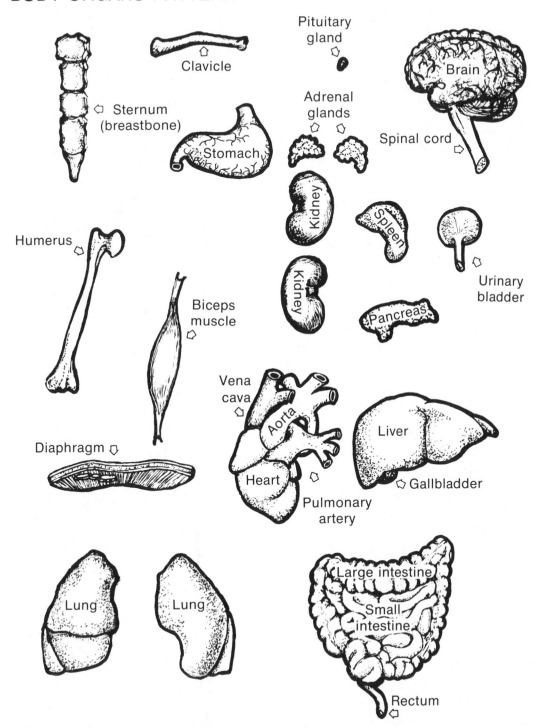

FIGURE 101
HUMAN FORM OUTLINE

CHAPTER 15B, UNIT II

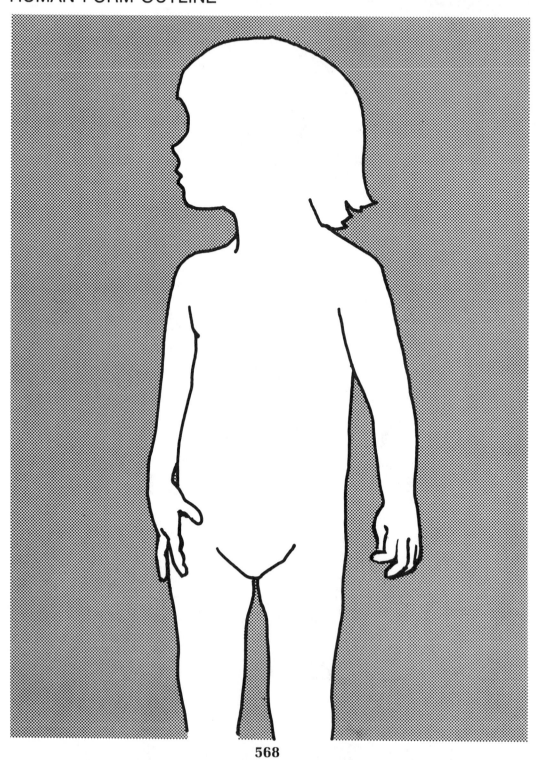

FIGURE 102
FAMILY MEDICAL RECORD

A simple, comprehensive format for keeping vital family health information organized and ready for the times when you need to have it at your fingertips. Faithfully kept, your family medical record not only will help you with school and travel records, insurance forms, and routine medical consultations, but can also prove a valuable diagnostic tool for your physician and an important legacy for your children.

IMPORTANT TELEPHONE NUMBERS

Physicians:
Dr. _____
Dr. _____
Dr. _____
Dr. _____
Dentists:
Dr. _____
Dr. _____
Pharmacist _____

Police Emergency _____
Fire Emergency _____
Ambulance Service _____
Poison Control Center _____
Health Department _____
Health Insurance Agent _____
Medicare Information _____
Medicaid Information _____
Local Medical Society _____

FAMILY HEALTH HISTORY

Information about the health of your immediate family can prove helpful in early diagnosis and treatment of diseases that are known either to be genetic or to occur more commonly in some families. Make a note of *any* serious or chronic diseases in your family, with special attention to those listed at the right. It also helps to note the age when the disease first occurred.

Be sure to include:

- Allergies
- Arthritis
- Cancer
- Diabetes
- Epilepsy
- Hearing defects
- Heart defects
- Hypertension
- Mental illness
- Mental retardation
- Obesity
- Tuberculosis
- Visual defects
- Other recurring family diseases

NAME	BIRTH DATE	BLOOD TYPE & Rh	OCCUPATION	DISEASES, ETC.	IF DECEASED, AGE AND CAUSE
HUSBAND					
his father					
his mother					
brothers and sisters					

NAME	BIRTH DATE	BLOOD TYPE & Rh	OCCUPATION	DISEASES, ETC.	IF DECEASED, AGE AND CAUSE
WIFE					
her father					
her mother					
brothers and sisters					

CHILDREN'S BIRTH RECORD

Be sure to note such details as duration of pregnancy, length of labor, Cesarean delivery, use of forceps, newborn respiratory distress, jaundice, or birth defects. If you are Rh-negative and the child was Rh-positive, were you given the Rh vaccine?

NAME	DATE	SEX	WT.	BLOOD TYPE & Rh	APGAR SCORE	HOSPITAL, CITY	PHYSICIAN	DETAILS

INCOMPLETE PREGNANCIES

A complete reproductive history includes details of spontaneous or induced abortions, miscarriages, and stillbirths. If you are Rh-negative and the fetus was Rh-positive, whether or not you were given the Rh vaccine is relevant here, too.

TERMINATION	DURATION	CIRCUMSTANCES	TERMINATION	DURATION	CIRCUMSTANCES

IMMUNIZATION SCHEDULE AND RECORD

The American Academy of Pediatrics recommends that children be immunized and given tuberculin testing according to the immunization schedule below. Vaccine combinations and schedules are improved frequently, however, so your physician can recommend what is best for you. As each immunization is completed, it should be registered in the immunization record, also below.

IMMUNIZATION SCHEDULE

2 months	Diphtheria/Tetanus/Pertussis (whooping cough) vaccine, first shot; polio vaccine, first dose
3 months	DTP, second shot
4 months	Polio vaccine, second dose; DTP completed
6 months	Polio vaccine completed
12 months	Tuberculin test; rubeola (measles) vaccine
1-12 years	Rubella (German measles) vaccine
15-18 months	Polio booster; DTP booster
4-6 years	Polio booster; DTP booster
12-14 years	Tetanus/diphtheria toxoid (adult form); mumps vaccine
Thereafter	Tetanus/diphtheria toxoid every 10 years

IMMUNIZATION RECORD

Enter month and year of completed series, boosters, single immunizations

IMMUNIZATIONS	CHILD	CHILD	CHILD	CHILD	CHILD	MOTHER	FATHER
DTP completed							
Boosters							
Polio completed							
Boosters							
Tuberculin test							
Rubeola (measles)							
Rubella (German measles)							
Tetanus/diphtheria toxoid							
Mumps							
Other							

PERIODIC PHYSICAL EXAMINATIONS

NAME	DATE	PHYSICIAN/CLINIC	HT.	WT.	BLOOD PRESSURE	FINDINGS, ADVICE, OR INSTRUCTIONS

PERIODIC PHYSICAL EXAMINATIONS

NAME	DATE	PHYSICIAN/CLINIC	HT.	WT.	BLOOD PRESSURE	FINDINGS, ADVICE, OR INSTRUCTIONS

INDIVIDUAL PROBLEMS, MEDICATIONS, ALLERGIES

Note any medications that are taken regularly, any   and any allergies.
substances that must be avoided for medical reasons,

NAME	CONDITIONS	SPECIAL INSTRUCTIONS OR MEDICATIONS

RECORD OF FAMILY ILLNESSES

List accidents, surgery, and illnesses, including chicken pox, mononucleosis, hepatitis, measles, German measles, mumps, strep throat, and whooping cough. If there was surgery, specify what was repaired or removed and note X-rays taken, medications, and diet.

NAME	DATE	NATURE OF ILLNESS, INJURY OR SURGERY	PHYSICIAN	OFFICE, CLINIC, HOSPITAL	TREATMENT

HEALTH AND ACCIDENT INSURANCE INFORMATION

NAME	POLICY NUMBER	DATE ISSUED	COMPANY	TYPE OF COVERAGE	PREMIUM	PAYMENTS REC'D	PAYMENTS REC'D

FIGURE 103
WHAT IS YOUR "EYE-Q"?

CHAPTER 15B, UNIT IV

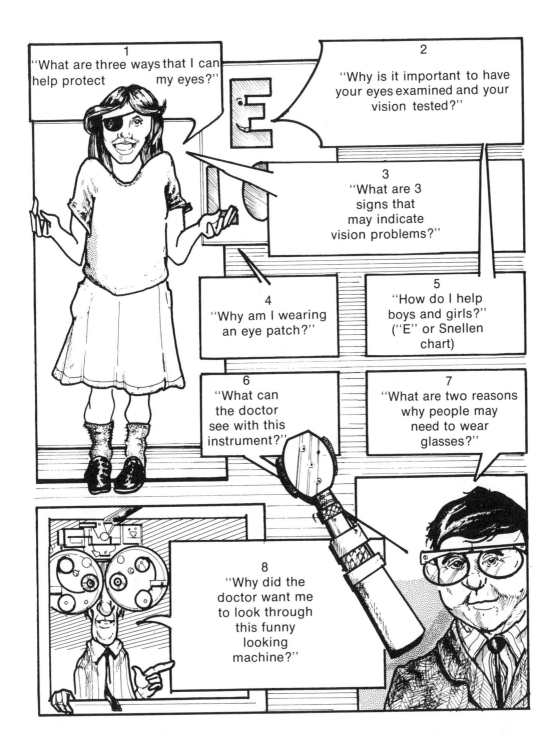

FIGURE 104
CHILDREN'S HOSPITAL

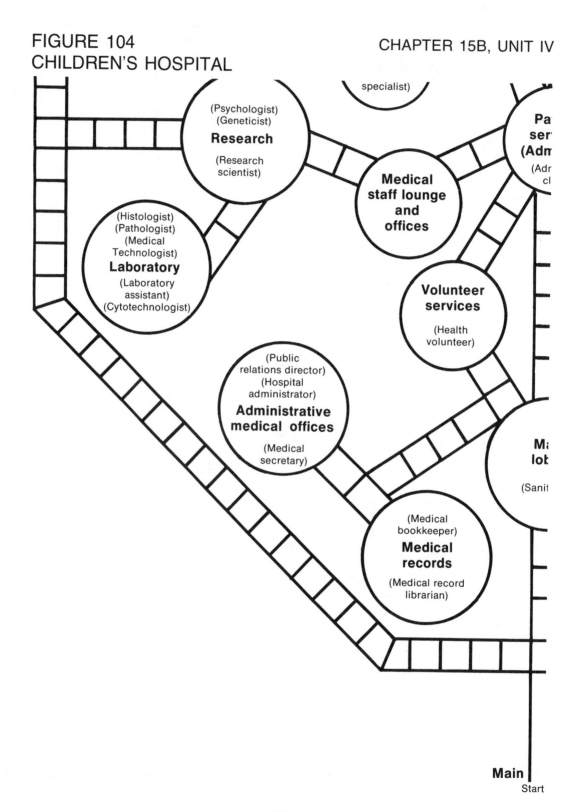

(specialist)

(Psychologist)
(Geneticist)
Research

(Research
scientist)

Pa
ser
(Adm

(Adr
cl

**Medical
staff lounge
and
offices**

(Histologist)
(Pathologist)
(Medical
Technologist)
Laboratory

(Laboratory
assistant)
(Cytotechnologist)

**Volunteer
services**

(Health
volunteer)

(Public
relations director)
(Hospital
administrator)
**Administrative
medical offices**

(Medical
secretary)

Ma
lob

(Sani

(Medical
bookkeeper)
**Medical
records**

(Medical record
librarian)

Main
Start

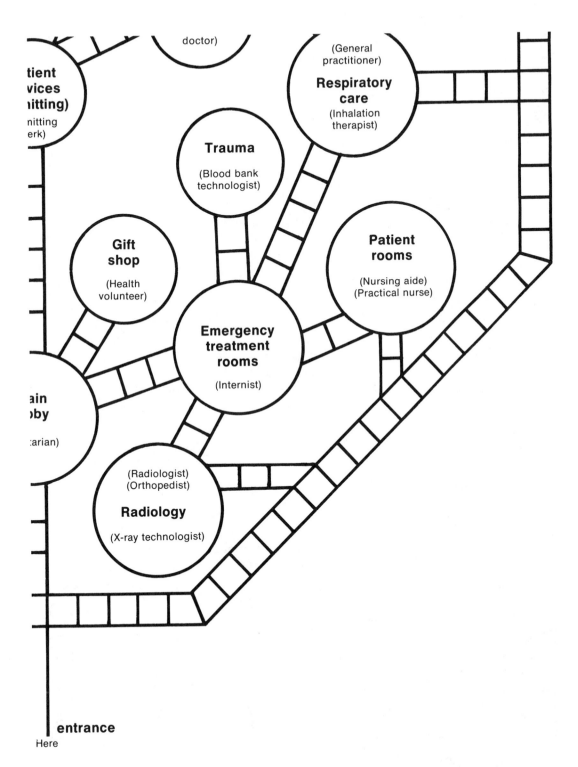

(doctor)

(General practitioner)
Respiratory care
(Inhalation therapist)

tient vices nitting)
(nitting erk)

Trauma
(Blood bank technologist)

Gift shop
(Health volunteer)

Patient rooms
(Nursing aide)
(Practical nurse)

Emergency treatment rooms
(Internist)

ain by
(arian)

(Radiologist)
(Orthopedist)
Radiology
(X-ray technologist)

entrance
Here

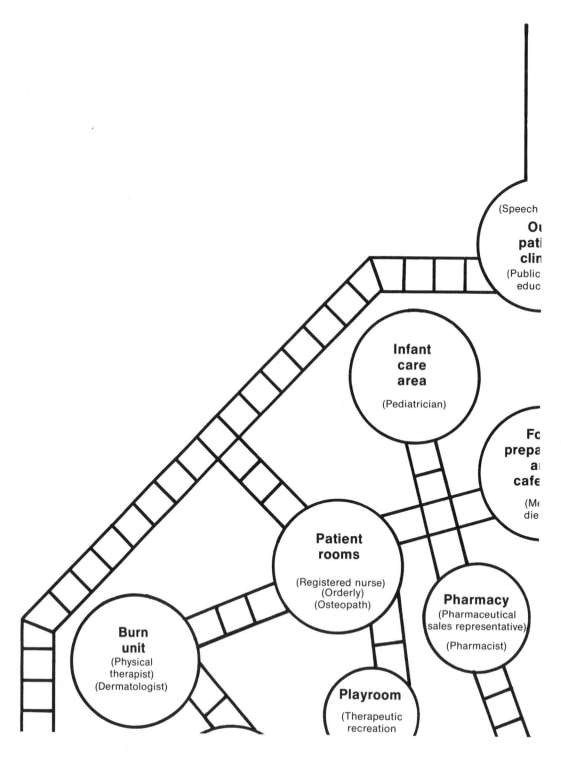

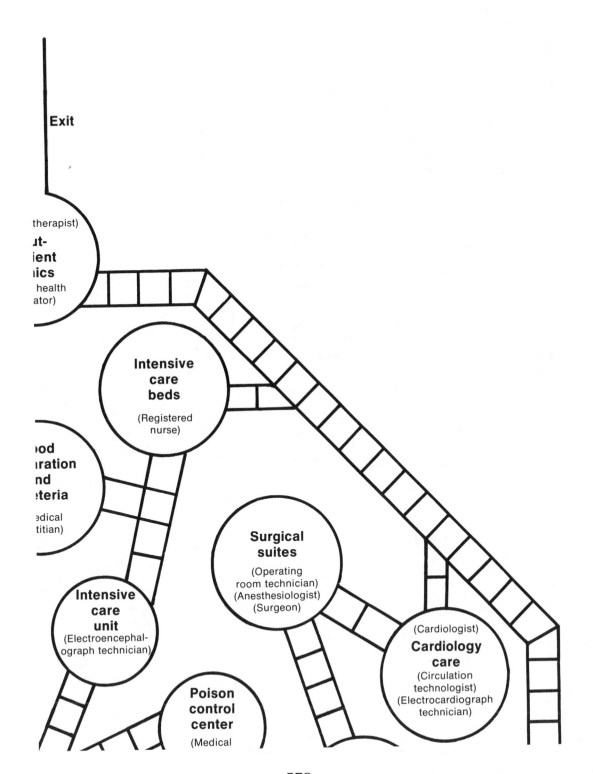

Exit

(therapist)

ut-
ient
ics

(health
ator)

Intensive
care
beds

(Registered
nurse)

od
ration
nd
eteria

(edical
titian)

Intensive
care
unit
(Electroencephal-
ograph technician)

Surgical
suites
(Operating
room technician)
(Anesthesiologist)
(Surgeon)

(Cardiologist)
Cardiology
care
(Circulation
technologist)
(Electrocardiograph
technician)

Poison
control
center
(Medical

FIGURE 105
CHILDREN'S HOSPITAL
FIRST-FLOOR MAZE

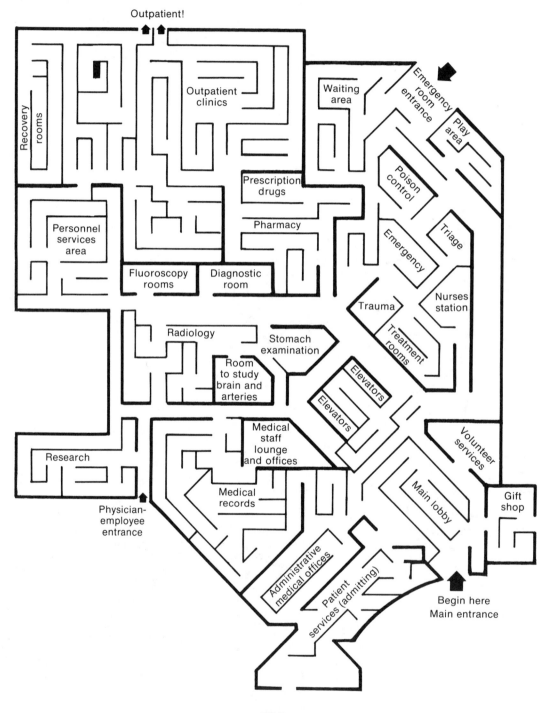

INDEX

*Page numbers in boldface refer to Atlas figures;
page numbers in italics refer to lessons.

INDEX